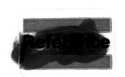

Atlas of
Interventional
Pain Management

Atlas of Interventional Pain Management

Third Edition

Steven D. Waldman, MD, JD

Director
Pain Consortium of Greater Kansas City
Leawood, Kansas

Clinical Professor of Anesthesiology
University of Missouri at Kansas City
School of Medicine
Kansas City, Missouri

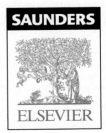

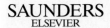

SAUNDERS
ELSEVIER

1600 John F. Kennedy Boulevard
Suite 1800
Philadelphia, PA 19103-2899

ATLAS OF INTERVENTIONAL PAIN MANAGEMENT   ISBN: 978-1-4160-9994-9

Notice

Knowledge and best practice in this field are constantly changing. As new research and experience broaden our knowledge, changes in practice, treatment and drug therapy may become necessary or appropriate. Readers are advised to check the most current information provided (i) on procedures featured or (ii) by the manufacturer of each product to be administered, to verify the recommended dose or formula, the method and duration of administration, and contraindications. It is the responsibility of the practitioner, relying on his or her own experience and knowledge of the patient, to make diagnoses, to determine dosages and the best treatment for each individual patient, and to take all appropriate safety precautions. To the fullest extent of the law, neither the Publisher nor the Editors assume any liability for any injury and/or damage to persons or property arising out of or related to any use of the material contained in this book.

The Publisher

Library of Congress Cataloging-in-Publication Data

Waldman, Steven D.
    Atlas of interventional pain management / Steven D. Waldman.—3rd ed.
        p. ; cm.
    Includes index.
    ISBN 978-1-4160-9994-9
    1. Nerve block—Atlases.   2. Analgesia—Atlases.   I. Title.
    [DNLM: 1. Nerve Block—methods—Atlases.   2. Pain—therapy—Atlases.   WO 517 W164a 2009]
    RD84.W35 2009
    615′.783—dc22   2009004293

Acquisitions Editor: Pamela Hetherington
Developmental Editor: Liliana Kim
Publishing Services Manager: Tina Rebane
Senior Project Manager: Amy Cannon
Senior Book Designer: Lou Forgione
Multimedia Producer: Dan Martinez

Current Procedural Terminology (CPT) is copyright 2009 American Medical Association. All Rights Reserved. No fee schedules, basic units, relative values, or related listings are included in CPT. The AMA assumes no liability for the data contained herein. Applicable FARS/DFARS restrictions apply to government use.

Cover Photo

Photo Researchers Picture Number: SA5159
Credit: David Gifford / Photo Researchers, Inc
Description: Back pain. Artwork of a man holding his lower back in pain. The pain is represented by the cracked orange area. Lower back pain, or lumbago, affects most people at some stage of their lives. It is commonly caused by strain, resulting in temporary injury to soft tissues (such as tendons, muscles and ligaments) around bones of the spine. People who lift heavy objects, or those who spend long periods sitting in one position, are most likely to suffer from back pain. Treatment includes correcting the posture used when resting or lifting objects, and taking painkillers.
Link: http://db2.photoresearchers.com/search/SA5159
    Photo Researchers, Inc.
    60 East 56th Street, 6th Floor
    New York, NY 10022
    Tel: 212-758-3420
    Fax: 212-355-0731
    http://www.photoresearchers.com
    info@photoresearchers.com
Images and Text Copyright © 2008 Photo Researchers, Inc. All Rights Reserved.

Printed in China

Last digit is the print number: 9   8   7   6   5   4   3   2   1

To my wife, Kathy

Preface

In fall 1992, I was asked to organize an educational program sponsored by the Dannemiller Memorial Educational Foundation in conjunction with the International Association for the Study of Pain World Congress. At that time, controversy was raging among the leaders of our nascent specialty of pain management as to what our specialty was really about. On one side were the "pill pushers," who said that the foundation of the specialty of pain management was expertise in the use of pharmacologic agents to treat pain with procedures such as nerve blocks, spinal cord stimulation, and neurosurgical procedures relegated to a purely adjunctive role. On the other side were the "needle wavers," those pain management specialists who believed that the first step in any plan to relieve pain was to perform a nerve block or implant a pump or stimulator. As time and the maturation of our specialty has shown, neither side was completely correct, and both approaches are equally necessary to optimally manage pain.

In 1992 the answer was much less clear (at least in my mind) so I decided to put together a meeting that was solely devoted to nerve blocks, pumps, stimulators, and the like. Although today such meetings are commonplace, at that time it was a radical notion and there was much discussion among the Dannemiller Memorial Educational Foundation board members as to whether anyone would even attend this meeting.

One of our big problems was what to call it. Borrowing from our radiology colleagues who were going through a similar controversy within their specialty, I coined the phrase *interventional pain management*. At first, my dear friend Alon Winnie, MD, hated this term; he noted that whether you gave the patient a pill or a nerve block it was an intervention. But nobody could come up with a better name, so the specialty of interventional pain management was born. In summer 1993, the first educational program devoted solely to interventional pain management (aptly titled "Interventional Pain Management") was held in front of a sold-out crowd of more than 300 in Nice, France.

Following the meeting, Alon and I together edited a textbook entitled *Interventional Pain Management* that was published by WB Saunders. More words than pictures and more *why* than *how*, the book was a reasonable first attempt to provide pain management specialists with a standard reference for the new subspecialty. Although the book was very popular, clinicians clamored for a book that was more *how* than *why* and more pictures than words. This clamoring resulted in the first edition of *Atlas of Interventional Pain Management*, which was published in early 1998. As noted in the Preface of the second edition of this book, which was published in 2004, the first edition of *Atlas of Interventional Pain Management* became the largest selling specialty pain management text in the world and led WB Saunders to expand their offerings in this area.

Fast forwarding to 2009, the subspecialty of interventional pain management has evolved as its parent specialty has evolved. The controversy over whether pills or nerve blocks are better seems almost laughable now that all pain management programs train new doctors in both. Pain management was once a specialty made up overwhelmingly of anesthesiologists. Today, the specialty of pain management and the subspecialty of interventional pain management are made up of doctors from all specialties. Large numbers of physical medicine and rehabilitation physicians and neurologists are joining our ranks as pathways to Board certification in pain management become open. With the new physicians comes a need for this updated third edition of *Atlas of Interventional Pain Management*.

In writing this latest edition, I retained all of the user-friendly features that made the first two editions so popular. This edition contains 20 new chapters and more than 100 new fluoroscopic, MR, and CT images. The reader of the current edition of *Atlas of Interventional Pain Management* will find the familiar how-to-do-it approach and vivid full-color artwork as well as a CPT-2009 procedure code for each technique presented. An expanded "Clinical Pearls" section for each chapter provides the clinician with added tricks of the trade to help improve clinical outcomes and avoid complications.

I trust that you will enjoy reading this latest edition and will use the text in your day-to-day practice of pain management.

Steven D. Waldman, MD, JD

Acknowledgment

A special thanks to my colleagues Milt Landers, DO, Mark Greenfield, MD, Frank Judilla, MD, and Mauricio Garcia, MD, for their generosity in freely sharing their knowledge, expertise, and fluoroscopic images for this edition of *Atlas of Interventional Pain Management.*

Steven D. Waldman, MD, JD

Contents

SECTION 3

Shoulder and Upper Extremity

SECTION 4

Thorax and Chest Wall

SECTION 7

Lower Extremity

SECTION **8**

**Advanced Interventional
Pain Management
Techniques**

DVD Video Contents

Section 1

Head

CHAPTER 1

Atlanto-occipital Block Technique

CPT-2009 CODE

First Joint	64470
Second Joint	64472
Neurolytic First Joint	64626
Neurolytic Second Joint	64627

Relative Value Units

First Joint	12
Second Joint	12
Neurolytic First Joint	20
Neurolytic Second Joint	20

INDICATIONS

Atlanto-occipital block is useful in the diagnosis and treatment of painful conditions involving trauma or inflammation of the atlanto-occipital joint. These problems manifest clinically as neck pain or suboccipital headache pain and occasionally as suboccipital pain that radiates into the temporomandibular joint region.

CLINICALLY RELEVANT ANATOMY

The atlanto-occipital joint is dissimilar from the functional units of the lower cervical spine. The joint is not a true facet joint because it lacks posterior articulations characteristic of a true zygapophyseal joint. The atlanto-occipital joint allows the head to nod forward and backward with an isolated range of motion of about 35 degrees. This joint is located anterior to the posterolateral columns of the spinal cord. Neither the atlas nor axis has intervertebral foramen to accommodate the first or second cervical nerves. These nerves are primarily sensory and, after leaving the spinal canal, travel through muscle and soft tissue laterally and then superiorly to contribute fibers to the greater and lesser occipital nerves.

The atlanto-occipital joint is susceptible to arthritic changes and trauma secondary to acceleration-deceleration injuries. Such damage to the joint results in pain secondary to synovial joint inflammation and adhesions.

TECHNIQUE

Atlanto-occipital block is usually done under fluoroscopic guidance because of the proximity of the joint to the spinal cord and vertebral artery, although some pain specialists have gained sufficient familiarity with the procedure to perform it safely without fluoroscopy. The patient is placed in a prone position. Pillows are placed under the chest to allow moderate flexion of the cervical spine without discomfort to the patient. The forehead is allowed to rest on a folded blanket.

If fluoroscopy is used, the beam is rotated in a sagittal plane from an anterior to a posterior position, which allows identification and visualization of the foramen magnum. Just lateral to the foramen magnum is the atlanto-occipital joint. A total of 5 mL of contrast medium suitable for intrathecal use is drawn up in a sterile 12-mL syringe. Then, 3 mL of preservative-free local anesthetic is drawn up in a separate 5-mL sterile syringe. When treating pain thought to be secondary to an inflammatory process, a total of 40 mg of depot-steroid is added to the local anesthetic with the first block, and 20 mg of depot-steroid is added with subsequent blocks.

After preparation of the skin with antiseptic solution, a skin wheal of local anesthetic is raised at the site of needle insertion. An 18-gauge, 1-inch needle is inserted at the site to serve as an introducer. The fluoroscopy beam is aimed directly through the introducer needle, which appears as a small point on the fluoroscopy screen. The introducer needle is then repositioned under fluoroscopic guidance until this small point is visualized over the posterolateral aspect of the atlanto-occipital joint (Figs. 1-1 and 1-2). This lateral placement avoids trauma to the vertebral artery, which lies medial to the joint at this level.

A 25-gauge, 3½-inch styletted spinal needle is then inserted through the 18-gauge introducer. If bony contact is made, the spinal needle is withdrawn and the introducer needle repositioned over the lateral aspect of the

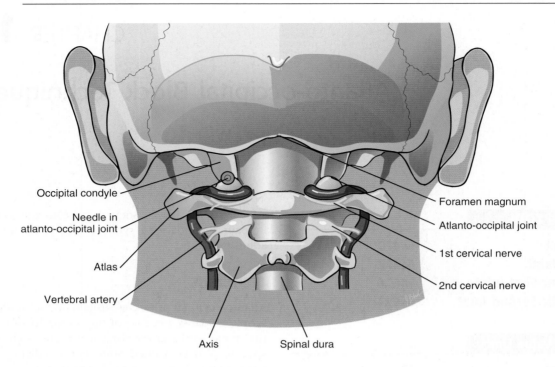

Occipital condyle

Needle in
atlanto-occipital joint

Atlas

Vertebral artery

Foramen magnum

Atlanto-occipital joint

1st cervical nerve

2nd cervical nerve

Axis

Spinal dura

Figure 1-1.

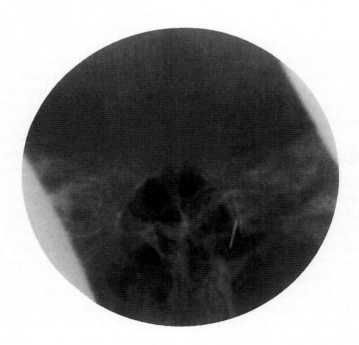

Figure 1-2.
Needle over posterolateral aspect of atlanto-occipital joint.

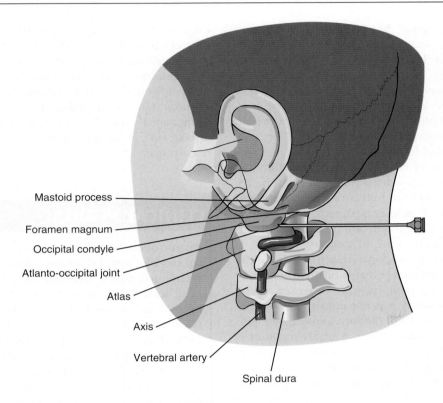

Mastoid process

Foramen magnum

Occipital condyle

Atlanto-occipital joint

Atlas

Axis

Vertebral artery

Spinal dura

Figure 1-3.

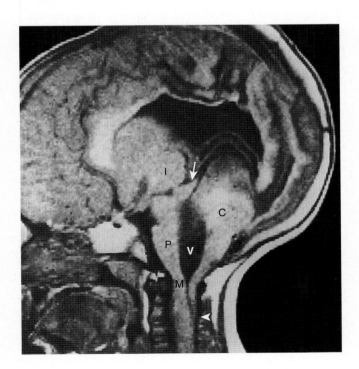

Figure 1-4.
Chiari II malformation: 6-year-old girl. Midline sagittal T1-weighted image demonstrates marked elongation of the cerebellum (C) and fourth ventricle (V). The surface of the inferior vermis is smooth. There is caudal displacement of the medulla (M), vermis, and tonsils into the cervical spinal canal (*arrowhead*) through an enlarged foramen magnum. The superior and inferior colliculi (*arrow*) are fused and form a peak posteriorly. The sylvian aqueduct is not seen. The massa intermedia (I) is large, and the posterior aspect of the corpus callosum is quite thin. P, pons. (From Edelman RR, Hesselink JR, Zlatkin MB, Crues JV: Clinical Magnetic Resonance Imaging, 3rd ed. Philadelphia, WB Saunders, 2006, p 1718.)

joint. The 25-gauge spinal needle is then readvanced until a pop is felt, indicating placement within the atlanto-occipital joint. It is essential to then confirm that the needle is actually in the joint, which is anterior to the posterolateral aspect of the spinal cord (Fig. 1-3). This is accomplished by rotating the C-arm to the horizontal plane and confirming needle placement within the joint. If intra-articular placement cannot be confirmed, the needle should be withdrawn.

After confirmation of needle placement within the atlanto-occipital joint, the stylet is removed from the 25-gauge spinal needle, and the hub is observed for blood or cerebrospinal fluid. If neither is present, gentle aspiration of the needle is carried out, and if no blood or cerebrospinal fluid is seen, 1 mL of contrast medium is slowly injected under fluoroscopy. An arthrogram of the normal atlanto-occipital joint reveals a bilateral concavity representing the intact joint capsule. However, if the joint has been traumatized, it is not unusual to see contrast medium flow freely from the torn joint capsule into the cervical epidural space. If the contrast medium is seen to rapidly enter the venous plexus rather than outline the joint, the needle is almost always not within the joint space. If this occurs, the needle should be repositioned into the joint before injection. If the contrast medium remains within the joint or if it outlines the joint and a small amount leaks into the epidural space, 1 to 1.5 mL of the local anesthetic and steroid is slowly injected through the spinal needle.

SIDE EFFECTS AND COMPLICATIONS

The proximity to the brain stem and spinal cord makes it imperative that this procedure be carried out only by those well versed in the regional anatomy and experienced in performing interventional pain management techniques. Fluoroscopic guidance is recommended for most practitioners because neural trauma is a possibility even in the most experienced hands. The proximity to the vertebral artery, combined with the vascular nature of this anatomic region, makes the potential for intravascular injection high. Even small amounts of local anesthetic injected into the vertebral arteries will result in seizures. Given the proximity of the brain and brain stem, ataxia after atlanto-occipital block due to vascular uptake of local anesthetic is not an uncommon occurrence.

CLINICAL PEARLS

Atlanto-occipital block is often combined with atlantoaxial block when treating pain in the previously mentioned areas. Although neither joint is a true facet joint in the anatomic sense of the word, the block is analogous to the facet joint block technique used commonly by pain practitioners and may be viewed as such. Many pain specialists believe that these techniques are currently underused in the treatment of so-called postwhiplash cervicalgia and cervicogenic headaches. These specialists believe that both techniques should be considered when cervical epidural nerve blocks and occipital nerve blocks fail to provide palliation of these headache and neck pain syndromes.

Any patient being considered for atlanto-occipital nerve block should undergo magnetic resonance imaging (MRI) of the head to rule out unsuspected intracranial and brain stem pathology (Fig. 1-4). Furthermore, MRI of the cervical spine should be considered to rule out congenital abnormalities such as Arnold-Chiari malformations or posterior fossa tumors that may be the hidden cause of the patient's headache symptomatology.

CHAPTER 2

Atlantoaxial Block Technique

CPT-2009 CODE	
First Joint	64470
Second Joint	64472
Neurolytic First Joint	64626
Neurolytic Second Joint	64627

Relative Value Units	
First Joint	12
Second Joint	12
Neurolytic First Joint	20
Neurolytic Second Joint	20

INDICATIONS

Atlantoaxial block is useful in the diagnosis and treatment of painful conditions involving trauma or inflammation of the atlantoaxial joint. These problems may manifest clinically as neck pain or suboccipital headache pain and occasionally as suboccipital pain that radiates into the temporomandibular joint region and is worsened with rotation of the joint.

CLINICALLY RELEVANT ANATOMY

The atlantoaxial joint is dissimilar from the functional units of the lower cervical spine. The joint is not a true facet joint because it lacks posterior articulations characteristic of a true zygapophyseal joint. Furthermore, there is no true disk or intervertebral foramen between atlas and axis. The atlantoaxial joint allows the greatest degree of motion of all the joints of the neck in that it not only allows the head to flex and extend about 10 degrees but also allows more than 60 degrees of rotation in the horizontal plane. The integrity and stability of the atlantoaxial joint are almost entirely ligamentous in nature. Even minor injury of the ligaments due to trauma can result in joint dysfunction and pain. Severe disruption of the ligaments has the same effect as a fracture of the odontoid process and can result in paralysis and death.

This joint is located lateral to the posterolateral columns of the spinal cord. Neither the atlas nor the axis has intervertebral foramen to accommodate the first or second cervical nerves. These nerves are primarily sensory, and after leaving the spinal canal, they travel through muscle and soft tissue laterally and then superiorly to contribute fibers to the greater and lesser occipital nerves. The vertebral artery is lateral to the joint compared with the medial position of the artery relative to the atlanto-occipital joint.

The atlantoaxial joint is susceptible to arthritic changes and trauma secondary to acceleration-deceleration injuries. Such damage to the joint results in pain secondary to synovial joint inflammation and adhesions. Rheumatoid arthritis may result in gradual erosion of the odontoid process that may present initially as occipital headaches. This erosion leads to instability of the atlantoaxial joint and ultimately may result in increased susceptibility to dislocation, paralysis, and death following seemingly minor trauma.

TECHNIQUE

Atlantoaxial block is usually done under fluoroscopic guidance because of the proximity to the spinal cord and vertebral artery, although some pain specialists have gained sufficient familiarity with the procedure to perform it safely without fluoroscopy. The patient is placed in a prone position. Pillows are placed under the chest to allow the cervical spine to be moderately flexed without discomfort to the patient. The forehead is allowed to rest on a folded blanket.

If fluoroscopy is used, the beam is rotated in a sagittal plane from an anterior to a posterior position, which allows identification and visualization of the foramen magnum and atlas. Just lateral and inferior to the atlas and to the foramen magnum is the atlantoaxial joint (Fig. 2-1). A total of 5 mL of contrast medium suitable for intrathecal use is drawn up in a sterile 12-mL syringe. Then, 3 mL of preservative-free local anesthetic is drawn

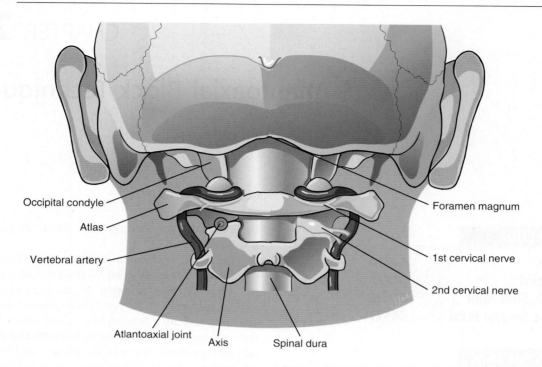

Occipital condyle

Atlas

Vertebral artery

Atlantoaxial joint   Axis   Spinal dura

Foramen magnum

1st cervical nerve

2nd cervical nerve

Figure 2-1.

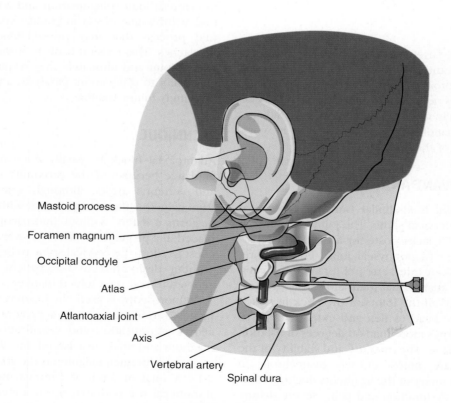

Mastoid process

Foramen magnum

Occipital condyle

Atlas

Atlantoaxial joint

Axis

Vertebral artery

Spinal dura

Figure 2-2.

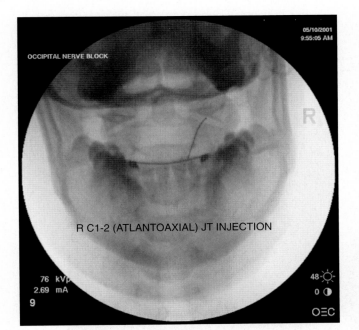

Figure 2-3.

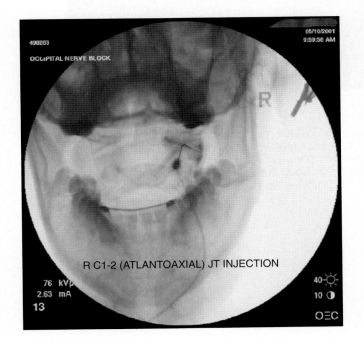

Figure 2-4.

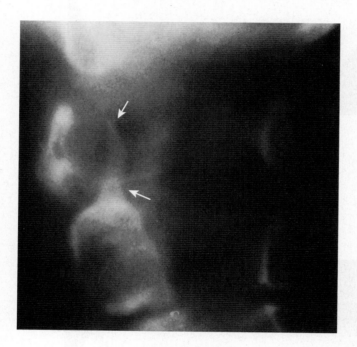

Figure 2-5.
Abnormalities of the cervical spine: odontoid process erosions. Lateral conventional tomogram reveals severe destruction of the odontoid process (*arrows*), which has been reduced to an irregular, pointed protuberance. (From Resnick D, Kransdorf MJ: Bone and Joint Imaging, 3rd ed. Philadelphia, WB Saunders, 2004, p 244.)

up in a separate 5-mL sterile syringe. When treating pain thought to be secondary to an inflammatory process, a total of 40 mg of depot-steroid is added to the local anesthetic with the first block, and 20 mg of depot-steroid is added with subsequent blocks.

After preparation of the skin with antiseptic solution, a skin wheal of local anesthetic is raised at the site of needle insertion. An 18-gauge, 1-inch needle is placed at the insertion site to serve as an introducer. The fluoroscopy beam is aimed directly through the introducer needle, which appears as a small point on the fluoroscopy screen. The introducer needle is then repositioned under fluoroscopic guidance until this small point is visualized over the posterolateral aspect of the atlantoaxial joint (see Fig. 2-1). This lateral placement avoids trauma to the spinal cord, which lies medial to the joint at this level. It should be remembered that the vertebral artery is lateral to the atlantoaxial joint, and care must be taken to avoid arterial trauma or inadvertent intra-arterial injection.

A 25-gauge, 3½-inch styletted spinal needle is then inserted through the 18-gauge introducer. If bony contact is made, the spinal needle is withdrawn, and the introducer needle is repositioned over the lateral aspect of the joint. The 25-gauge spinal needle is then readvanced until a pop is felt, indicating placement within the atlantoaxial joint. It is essential to then confirm that the needle is actually in the joint, which is anterior to the posterolateral aspect of the spinal cord. This is accomplished by rotating the C-arm to the horizontal plane and confirming needle placement within the joint (Figs. 2-2 and 2-3). If intra-articular placement cannot be confirmed, the needle should be withdrawn.

After confirmation of needle placement within the atlantoaxial joint, the stylet is removed from the 25-gauge spinal needle, and the hub is observed for blood or cerebrospinal fluid. If neither is present, gentle aspiration of the needle is carried out, and if no blood or cerebrospinal fluid is seen, 1 mL of contrast medium is slowly injected under fluoroscopy. An arthrogram of the normal atlantoaxial joint reveals a bilateral concavity representing the intact joint capsule (Fig. 2-4). However, if the joint has been traumatized, it is not unusual to see contrast medium flow freely from the torn joint capsule into the cervical epidural space. If the contrast medium is seen to rapidly enter the venous plexus rather than outline the joint, the needle is almost always not within the joint space. If this occurs, the needle should be repositioned into the joint before injection. If the contrast medium remains within the joint or if it outlines the joint and a small amount leaks into the epidural space,

1 to 1.5 mL of the local anesthetic and steroid is slowly injected through the spinal needle.

SIDE EFFECTS AND COMPLICATIONS

The proximity to the brain stem and spinal cord makes it imperative that this procedure be carried out only by those well versed in the regional anatomy and experienced in performing interventional pain management techniques. Fluoroscopic guidance is recommended for most practitioners because neural trauma is a possibility even in the most experienced hands. The proximity to the vertebral artery, combined with the vascular nature of this anatomic region, makes the potential for intravascular injection high. Even small amounts of local anesthetic injected into the vertebral arteries will result in seizures. Given the proximity of the brain and brain stem, ataxia after atlantoaxial block due to vascular uptake of local anesthetic is not an uncommon occurrence. Many patients also complain of a transient increase in headache and cervicalgia after injection of the joint.

CLINICAL PEARLS

Atlantoaxial block is often combined with atlanto-occipital block when treating pain in the previously mentioned areas. Although neither joint is a true facet joint in the anatomic sense of the word, the block is analogous to the facet joint block technique used commonly by pain practitioners and may be viewed as such. Many pain specialists believe that these techniques are currently underused in the treatment of so-called postwhiplash cervicalgia and cervicogenic headaches. These specialists believe that both techniques should be considered when cervical epidural nerve blocks and occipital nerve blocks fail to provide palliation of these headache and neck pain syndromes.

Any patient being considered for atlantoaxial nerve block should undergo magnetic resonance imaging (MRI) of the head to rule out unsuspected intracranial and brain stem pathology. Furthermore, cervical spine x-rays should be considered to rule out congenital abnormalities such as Arnold-Chiari malformations that may be the hidden cause of the patient's headache symptomatology as well as to identify erosion of the odontoid process in patients suffering from rheumatoid arthritis (Fig. 2-5).

CHAPTER 3

Sphenopalatine Ganglion Block: Transnasal Approach

CPT-2009 CODE	
Local Anesthetic	64505
Neurolytic	64640

Relative Value Units	
Local Anesthetic	8
Neurolytic	20

INDICATIONS

Sphenopalatine ganglion block may be used in the treatment of acute migraine headache, acute cluster headache, and a variety of facial neuralgias including Sluder's, Vail's, and Gardner's syndromes. This technique is also useful in the treatment of status migrainosus and chronic cluster headache.

Neurodestructive procedures of the sphenopalatine ganglion with neurolytic agents, radiofrequency lesions, and freezing may be indicated for the palliation of cancer pain and rarely for headache and facial pain syndromes that fail to respond to conservative management.

CLINICALLY RELEVANT ANATOMY

The sphenopalatine ganglion (pterygopalatine, nasal, or Meckel's ganglion) is located in the pterygopalatine fossa, posterior to the middle nasal turbinate. It is covered by a 1- to 1.5-mm layer of connective tissue and mucous membrane. This 5-mm triangular structure sends major branches to the gasserian ganglion, trigeminal nerves, carotid plexus, facial nerve, and superior cervical ganglion. The sphenopalatine ganglion can be blocked by topical application of local anesthetic or by injection.

TECHNIQUE

Sphenopalatine ganglion block through the transnasal approach is accomplished by the application of suitable local anesthetic to the mucous membrane overlying the ganglion. The patient is placed in the supine position, and the anterior nares are inspected for polyps, tumors, and foreign bodies. Three milliliters of either 2% viscous lidocaine or 10% cocaine is drawn up in a 5-mL sterile syringe. The tip of the nose is then drawn upward as if to place a nasogastric tube, and 0.5 mL of local anesthetic is injected into each nostril. The patient is asked to sniff vigorously to draw the local anesthetic posteriorly, which serves the double function of lubricating the nasal mucosa as well as providing topical anesthesia.

Two $3\frac{1}{2}$-inch cotton-tipped applicators are soaked in the local anesthetic chosen, and one applicator is advanced along the superior border of the middle turbinate of each nostril until the tip comes into contact with the mucosa overlying the sphenopalatine ganglion (Fig. 3-1). Then 1 mL of local anesthetic is instilled over each cotton-tipped applicator. The applicator acts as a tampon that allows the local anesthetic to remain in contact with the mucosa overlying the ganglion. The applicators are removed after 20 minutes. The patient's blood pressure, pulse, and respirations are monitored for untoward side effects.

SIDE EFFECTS AND COMPLICATIONS

Because of the highly vascular nature of the nasal mucosa, epistaxis is the major complication of this technique. This vascularity can lead to significant systemic absorption of local anesthetic with resultant local anesthetic toxicity, especially when cocaine is used.

Patients occasionally may experience significant orthostatic hypotension after sphenopalatine ganglion block. This can be a problem because postblock monitoring may be lax because of the benign appearance of the technique. For this reason, patients who undergo sphenopalatine ganglion block should be monitored closely for orthostatic hypotension and allowed to initially ambulate only with assistance.

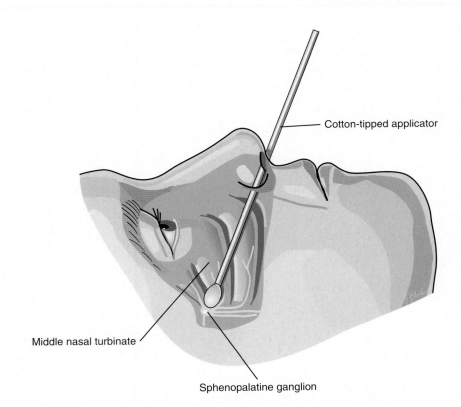

Cotton-tipped applicator

Middle nasal turbinate

Sphenopalatine ganglion

Figure 3-1.

CLINICAL PEARLS

Clinical experience has shown that sphenopalatine ganglion block with local anesthetic is useful in aborting the acute attack of migraine or cluster headache. The simplicity of the transnasal approach lends itself to use at the bedside, in the emergency room, or in the pain clinic. Although cocaine is probably a superior topical anesthetic for use with this technique, the various political issues surrounding the use of controlled substances make the use of other local anesthetics such as viscous lidocaine a more logical choice.

For the acute headache sufferer, this technique can be combined with the inhalation of 100% oxygen via mask through the mouth while the cotton-tipped applicators are in place. Experience has shown that this technique aborts about 80% of cluster headaches. Sphenopalatine ganglion block should be carried out on a daily basis with the endpoint of complete pain relief. This usually occurs within five blocks.

CHAPTER 4

Sphenopalatine Ganglion Block: Greater Palatine Foramen Approach

CPT-2009 CODE	
Local Anesthetic	64505
Neurolytic	64640

Relative Value Units	
Local Anesthetic	8
Neurolytic	20

INDICATIONS

Sphenopalatine ganglion block may be used in the treatment of acute migraine headache, acute cluster headache, and a variety of facial neuralgias including Sluder's, Vail's, and Gardner's syndromes. The technique is also useful in the treatment of status migrainosus and chronic cluster headache. The greater palatine foramen approach to sphenopalatine ganglion block is useful in patients who have an alteration of the nasal anatomy secondary to trauma or malignancy that would preclude use of the transnasal approach.

Neurodestructive procedures of the sphenopalatine ganglion with neurolytic agents, radiofrequency lesions, and freezing may be indicated for the palliation of cancer pain and rarely for headache and facial pain syndromes that fail to respond to conservative management. The transnasal or lateral approach to the sphenopalatine ganglion block may be more suitable for these neurodestructive techniques.

CLINICALLY RELEVANT ANATOMY

The sphenopalatine ganglion (pterygopalatine, nasal, or Meckel's ganglion) is located in the pterygopalatine fossa, posterior to the middle nasal turbinate. It is covered by a 1- to 1.5-mm layer of connective tissue and mucous membrane. This 5-mm triangular structure sends major branches to the gasserian ganglion, trigeminal nerves, carotid plexus, facial nerve, and superior cervical ganglion. The sphenopalatine ganglion can be blocked by topical application of local anesthetic via the transnasal approach or by injection via the lateral approach or through the greater palatine foramen.

TECHNIQUE

Sphenopalatine ganglion block via the greater palatine foramen approach is accomplished by the injection of local anesthetic onto the ganglion. The patient is placed in the supine position with the cervical spine extended over a foam wedge. The greater palatine foramen is identified just medial to the gum line of the third molar on the posterior portion of the hard palate. A dental needle with a 120-degree angle is advanced about 2.5 cm through the foramen in a superior and slightly posterior trajectory (Figs. 4-1 and 4-2). The maxillary nerve is just superior to the ganglion, and if the needle is advanced too deep, a paresthesia may be elicited. After careful, gentle aspiration, 2 mL of local anesthetic is slowly injected.

SIDE EFFECTS AND COMPLICATIONS

Because of the highly vascular nature of this anatomic region, significant systemic absorption of local anesthetic with resultant local anesthetic toxicity is a distinct possibility.

Patients occasionally may experience significant orthostatic hypotension after sphenopalatine ganglion block. Therefore, patients who undergo sphenopalatine ganglion block should be monitored closely for orthostatic hypotension and allowed to initially ambulate only with assistance.

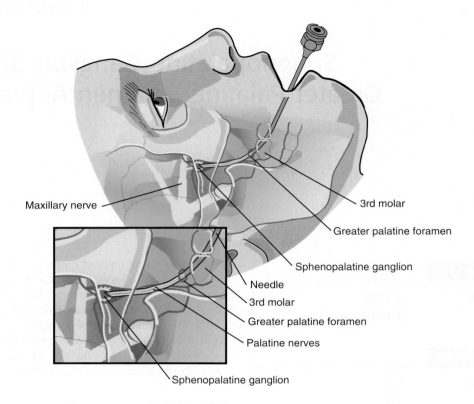

Maxillary nerve

3rd molar

Greater palatine foramen

Sphenopalatine ganglion

Needle

3rd molar

Greater palatine foramen

Palatine nerves

Sphenopalatine ganglion

Figure 4-1.

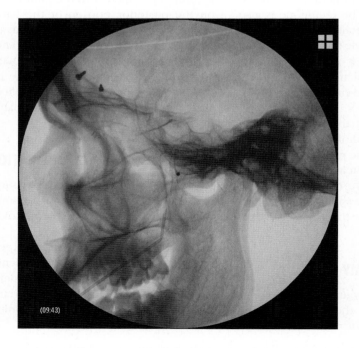

Figure 4-2.
Tip of needle placed through greater palatine foramen.

CLINICAL PEARLS

Clinical experience has shown that sphenopalatine ganglion block with local anesthetic is useful in aborting the acute attack of migraine or cluster headache. The simplicity of the transnasal approach lends itself to use at the bedside, in the emergency room, or in the pain clinic. Although cocaine is probably a superior topical anesthetic for use with this technique, the various political issues surrounding the use of controlled substances make the use of other local anesthetics such as viscous lidocaine a more logical choice.

If previous trauma or tumor precludes the use of the transnasal approach to sphenopalatine ganglion block, injection via the greater palatine foramen represents a good alternative. Because of the proximity of the sphenopalatine ganglion to the maxillary nerve,

care must be taken to avoid inadvertent neurolysis of the maxillary nerve when performing neurodestructive procedures on the sphenopalatine ganglion. Because of the ability to more accurately localize the sphenopalatine ganglion by stimulation, radiofrequency lesioning via the lateral approach probably represents the safest option if destruction of the sphenopalatine ganglion is desired.

For the acute headache sufferer, this technique can be combined with the inhalation of 100% oxygen via mask after the injection of local anesthetic. Experience has shown that this technique aborts about 80% of cluster headaches. Sphenopalatine ganglion block should be carried out on a daily basis with the endpoint of complete pain relief. This usually occurs within five blocks.

CHAPTER 5

Sphenopalatine Ganglion Block: Lateral Approach

INDICATIONS

Sphenopalatine ganglion block may be used in the treatment of acute migraine headache, acute cluster headache, and a variety of facial neuralgias including Sluder's, Vail's, and Gardner's syndromes. The technique is also useful in the treatment of status migrainosus and chronic cluster headache. The lateral approach to sphenopalatine ganglion block is useful in patients who have an alteration of the nasal anatomy secondary to trauma or malignancy that would preclude use of the transnasal approach. It is also the preferred route for neurodestructive procedures of the sphenopalatine ganglion. These neurodestructive procedures of the sphenopalatine ganglion may be performed with neurolytic agents, radiofrequency lesions, and freezing and are indicated for the palliation of cancer pain and rarely for headache and facial pain syndromes that fail to respond to conservative management.

CLINICALLY RELEVANT ANATOMY

The sphenopalatine ganglion (pterygopalatine, nasal, or Meckel's ganglion) is located in the pterygopalatine fossa, posterior to the middle nasal turbinate. It is covered by a 1- to 1.5-mm layer of connective tissue and mucous membrane. This 5-mm triangular structure sends major branches to the gasserian ganglion, trigeminal nerves, carotid plexus, facial nerve, and superior cervical ganglion. The sphenopalatine ganglion can be blocked by topical application of local anesthetic via the transnasal approach, by injection via the pterygopalatine fossa or through the greater palatine foramen, or by lateral placement of a needle via the coronoid notch.

TECHNIQUE

Sphenopalatine ganglion block via the lateral approach is accomplished by the injection of local anesthetic onto the ganglion via a needle placed through the coronoid notch. The patient is placed in the supine position with the cervical spine in the neutral position. The coronoid notch is identified by asking the patient to open and close the mouth several times and palpating the area just anterior and slightly inferior to the acoustic auditory meatus. After the notch is identified, the patient is asked to hold the mouth open in the neutral position.

A total of 2 mL of local anesthetic is drawn up in a 3-mL sterile syringe. Some pain management specialists empirically add a small amount of depot-steroid preparation to the local anesthetic. After the skin overlying the coronoid notch is prepared with antiseptic solution, a 22-gauge, $3\frac{1}{2}$-inch styletted needle is inserted just below the zygomatic arch directly in the middle of the coronoid notch. The needle is advanced about 1.5 to 2 inches in a plane perpendicular to the skull until the lateral pterygoid plate is encountered. At this point, the needle is withdrawn slightly and redirected slightly superior and anterior, with the goal of placing the needle just above the lower aspect of the lateral pterygoid plate so that it can enter the pterygopalatine fossa below the maxillary nerve and in close proximity to the sphenopalatine ganglion (Fig. 5-1). If this procedure is performed under fluoroscopy, the needle tip is visualized just under the lateral nasal mucosa, and its position can be confirmed by injecting 0.5 mL of contrast medium (Fig. 5-2). Additional confirmation of needle position can be obtained by needle stimulation at 50 Hz. If the needle is in the correct position, the patient experiences a buzzing sensation just behind the nose with no stimulation into the distribution of other areas innervated by the maxillary nerve.

After correct needle placement is confirmed, careful aspiration is carried out, and 2 mL of solution is injected in incremental doses. During the injection procedure,

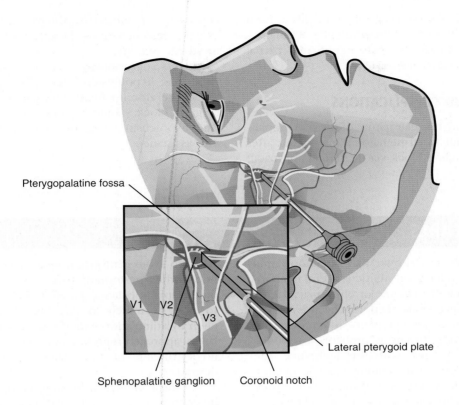

Figure 5-1.

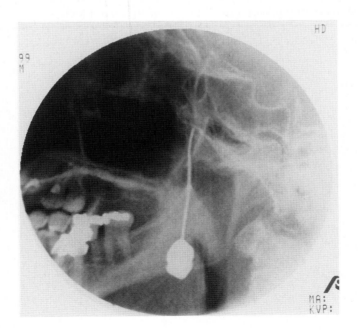

Figure 5-2.
Needle tip in pterygopalatine fossa. (From Waldman SD: Interventional Pain Management, 2nd ed. Philadelphia, WB Saunders, 2001, p 309.)

the patient must be observed carefully for signs of local anesthetic toxicity. Because of the proximity of the maxillary nerve, the patient also may experience partial blockade of the maxillary nerve.

SIDE EFFECTS AND COMPLICATIONS

Because of the highly vascular nature of the pterygopalatine fossa, significant facial hematoma may occur after sphenopalatine ganglion block via the lateral approach.

This vascularity means that the pain specialist should use small, incremental doses of local anesthetic to avoid local anesthetic toxicity.

Patients occasionally may experience significant orthostatic hypotension after sphenopalatine ganglion block. Therefore, patients who undergo sphenopalatine ganglion block should be monitored closely for orthostatic hypotension and allowed to initially ambulate only with assistance.

CLINICAL PEARLS

Clinical experience has shown that sphenopalatine ganglion block with local anesthetic is useful in aborting the acute attack of migraine or cluster headache. The simplicity of the transnasal approach lends itself to use at the bedside, in the emergency room, or in the pain clinic. Although cocaine is probably a superior topical anesthetic for use with this technique, the various political issues surrounding the use of controlled substances make the use of other local anesthetics such as viscous lidocaine a more logical choice.

If previous trauma or tumor precludes the use of the transnasal approach to sphenopalatine ganglion block, injection of local anesthetic via the greater palatine foramen or the lateral approach represents a good alternative. Because of the proximity of the sphenopalatine ganglion to the maxillary nerve, care must be taken to avoid inadvertent neurolysis of the maxillary nerve when performing neurodestructive procedures on the sphenopalatine ganglion. Because of the ability to more accurately localize the sphenopalatine ganglion by stimulation, radiofrequency lesioning via the lateral approach represents probably the safest option if destruction of the sphenopalatine ganglion is desired.

For the acute headache sufferer, this technique can be combined with the inhalation of 100% oxygen via mask after the injection of local anesthetic. Experience has shown that this technique aborts about 80% of cluster headaches. Sphenopalatine ganglion block should be carried out on a daily basis with the endpoint of complete pain relief. This usually occurs within five blocks.

CHAPTER 6

Sphenopalatine Ganglion Block: Radiofrequency Lesioning

INDICATIONS

Radiofrequency lesioning of the sphenopalatine ganglion block may be used in the treatment of chronic cluster headache, cancer pain, and a variety of facial neuralgias including Sluder's, Vail's, and Gardner's syndromes that have failed to respond to more conservative treatments. The lateral approach to sphenopalatine ganglion block is used to place the radiofrequency needle, although the transnasal and greater palatine foramen approach can be used in patients who have an alteration of the nasal anatomy secondary to trauma or malignancy that would preclude use of the lateral approach. Neurodestructive procedures of the sphenopalatine ganglion using the lateral approach may be performed with neurolytic agents, freezing, and radiofrequency lesioning. Radiofrequency lesioning has the added advantage of allowing the use of a stimulating needle, which enhances correct needle placement.

CLINICALLY RELEVANT ANATOMY

The sphenopalatine ganglion (pterygopalatine, nasal, or Meckel's ganglion) is located in the pterygopalatine fossa, posterior to the middle nasal turbinate. It is covered by a 1- to 1.5-mm layer of connective tissue and mucous membrane. This 5-mm triangular structure sends major branches to the gasserian ganglion, trigeminal nerves, carotid plexus, facial nerve, and superior cervical ganglion. The sphenopalatine ganglion can be blocked by topical application of local anesthetic via the transnasal approach, by injection via the pterygopalatine fossa or through the greater palatine foramen, or by lateral placement of a needle via the coronoid notch.

TECHNIQUE

Radiofrequency lesioning of the sphenopalatine ganglion block is accomplished by placing a radiofrequency needle in proximity to the sphenopalatine ganglion using the lateral approach via an introducer needle. The patient is placed in the supine position with the cervical spine in the neutral position. A $3\frac{1}{2}$-inch cotton-tipped applicator is soaked in contrast media and placed between the middle and inferior turbinates to serve as a radiopaque marker (Figs. 6-1 and 6-2).

A total of 2 mL of local anesthetic is drawn up in a 3-mL sterile syringe. After the skin lateral to the angle of the mouth is prepared with antiseptic solution, a 22-gauge, 10-cm insulated blunt curved needle with a 5- to 10-mm active tip is inserted through an introducer needle placed through the previously anesthetized area. The needle is advanced toward the tip of the cotton-tipped applicator, which rests on the mucosa just over the sphenopalatine ganglion at the level of the middle turbinate. The trajectory of the needle should be toward the posterior clinoid. The needle is slowly advanced under fluoroscopic guidance into the pterygopalatine fossa below the maxillary nerve and in close proximity to the sphenopalatine ganglion (Fig. 6-3). The needle tip ultimately is visualized just under the lateral nasal mucosa, and its position can be confirmed by injecting 0.5 mL of contrast medium.

Sensory stimulation is then applied to the needle at 0.5 V at a frequency of 50 Hz. If the needle is in correct position, the patient experiences a buzzing sensation just behind the nose with no stimulation into the distribution of other areas innervated by the maxillary nerve, which is often perceived by the patient as a buzzing sensation in the upper teeth (see "Side Effects and Complications" for pitfalls in needle placement). After correct needle placement is confirmed, pulsed radiofrequency lesioning is performed for 90 seconds at 44°C. Often a second lesion and sometimes a third lesion are necessary to provide long-lasting relief.

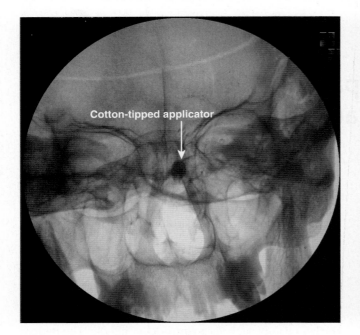

Figure 6-1.

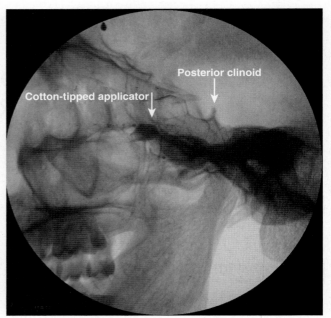

Figure 6-2.

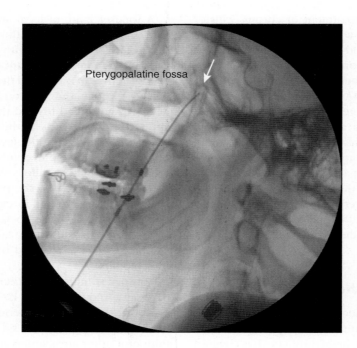

Figure 6-3.

SIDE EFFECTS AND COMPLICATIONS

Because of the highly vascular nature of the pterygopalatine fossa, significant facial hematoma may occur after radiofrequency lesioning of the sphenopalatine ganglion. Owing to the proximity of other nerves, misplacement of the radiofrequency needle can result in damage to the affected nerve with permanent neurologic deficit. Stimulation before lesioning can help detect needle misplacement by identification of specific stimulation patterns (Table 6-1). The stimulation pattern associated with proper placement of the needle is felt at the root of the nose. If the needle is malpositioned in proximity to the maxillary division of nerve, the stimulation pattern is experienced in the upper teeth. Should this occur, the patient should be positioned more caudad. If the needle is malpositioned near the greater and lesser palatine nerves, the stimulation pattern is experienced in the hard palate. Should this occur, the needle should be redirected more medial and posterior.

Patients occasionally may experience significant orthostatic hypotension or bradycardia during stimulation of the sphenopalatine ganglion. This phenomenon is thought to be analogous to the oculocardiac reflex and can be prevented with atropine. Patients who undergo stimulation of the sphenopalatine ganglion should be monitored closely for orthostatic hypotension and bradycardia and allowed to initially ambulate only with assistance.

Table 6-1 ■ IDENTIFICATION OF SPECIFIC STIMULATION PATTERNS

Needle Position	Stimulation Pattern	Corrective Maneuver
Needle in proper position	Stimulation at base of nose	None
Needle in proximity to maxillary nerve	Stimulation in upper teeth	Redirect needle more caudad
Needle in proximity to greater and lesser palatine nerves	Stimulation in hard palate	Redirect needle more posterior

CLINICAL PEARLS

Clinical experience has shown that sphenopalatine ganglion block with local anesthetic is useful in aborting the acute attack of migraine or cluster headache. The simplicity of the transnasal approach lends itself to use at the bedside, in the emergency room, or in the pain clinic. Although cocaine is probably a superior topical anesthetic for use with this technique, the various political issues surrounding the use of controlled substances make the use of other local anesthetics such as viscous lidocaine a more logical choice.

If previous trauma or tumor precludes the use of the transnasal approach to sphenopalatine ganglion block, injection of local anesthetic via the greater palatine foramen or the lateral approach represents a good alternative. Because of the proximity of the sphenopalatine ganglion to the maxillary nerve, care must be taken to avoid inadvertent neurolysis of the maxillary nerve when performing neurodestructive procedures on the sphenopalatine ganglion. Because of the ability to more accurately localize the sphenopalatine ganglion by stimulation, radiofrequency lesioning via the lateral approach represents probably the safest option if destruction of the sphenopalatine ganglion is desired.

CHAPTER 7

Greater and Lesser Occipital Nerve Block

CPT-2009 CODE	
Unilateral	64405
Bilateral	64405-50
Neurolytic	64640

Relative Value Units	
Unilateral	8
Bilateral	12
Neurolytic	20

INDICATIONS

Occipital nerve block is useful in the diagnosis and treatment of occipital neuralgia. This technique is also useful in providing surgical anesthesia in the distribution of the greater and lesser occipital nerves for lesion removal and laceration repair.

CLINICALLY RELEVANT ANATOMY

The greater occipital nerve arises from fibers of the dorsal primary ramus of the second cervical nerve and to a lesser extent from fibers of the third cervical nerve. The greater occipital nerve pierces the fascia just below the superior nuchal ridge along with the occipital artery. It supplies the medial portion of the posterior scalp as far anterior as the vertex (Fig. 7-1).

The lesser occipital nerve arises from the ventral primary rami of the second and third cervical nerves. The lesser occipital nerve passes superiorly along the posterior border of the sternocleidomastoid muscle, dividing into cutaneous branches that innervate the lateral portion of the posterior scalp and the cranial surface of the pinna of the ear (see Fig. 7-1).

TECHNIQUE

The patient is placed in a sitting position with the cervical spine flexed and the forehead on a padded bedside table (Fig. 7-2). A total of 8 mL of local anesthetic is drawn up in a 12-mL sterile syringe. When treating occipital neuralgia or other painful conditions involving the greater and lesser occipital nerves, a total of 80 mg of depot-steroid is added to the local anesthetic with the first block, and 40 mg of depot-steroid is added with subsequent blocks.

The occipital artery is then palpated at the level of the superior nuchal ridge. After preparation of the skin with antiseptic solution, a 22-gauge, $1\frac{1}{2}$-inch needle is inserted just medial to the artery and is advanced perpendicularly until the needle approaches the periosteum of the underlying occipital bone (Fig. 7-3). A paresthesia may be elicited, and the patient should be warned of such. The needle is then redirected superiorly, and after gentle aspiration, 5 mL of solution is injected in a fanlike distribution, with care taken to avoid the foramen magnum, which is located medially (Fig. 7-4; see Fig. 7-3).

The lesser occipital nerve and a number of superficial branches of the greater occipital nerve are then blocked by directing the needle laterally and slightly inferiorly. After gentle aspiration, an additional 3 to 4 mL of solution is injected (Fig. 7-5; see Fig. 7-3).

SIDE EFFECTS AND COMPLICATIONS

The scalp is highly vascular, and this, coupled with the fact that both nerves are in close proximity to arteries, means that the pain specialist should carefully calculate the total milligram dosage of local anesthetic that may be given safely, especially if bilateral nerve blocks are being performed. This vascularity and the proximity to the arterial supply give rise to an increased incidence of postblock ecchymosis and hematoma formation. These complications can be decreased if manual pressure is applied to the area of the block immediately after injection. Despite the vascularity of this anatomic region, this technique can be performed safely in the presence of anticoagulation by using a 25- or 27-gauge needle, albeit at increased risk for hematoma, if the clinical situation dictates a favorable risk-to-benefit ratio. Application of cold packs for 20-minute periods after the block also

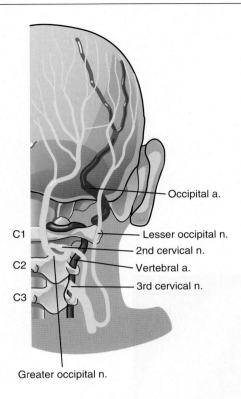

Occipital a.

C1 — Lesser occipital n.

2nd cervical n.

C2 — Vertebral a.

3rd cervical n.

C3

Greater occipital n.

Figure 7-1.

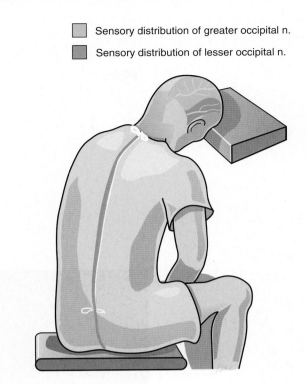

Sensory distribution of greater occipital n.

Sensory distribution of lesser occipital n.

Figure 7-2.

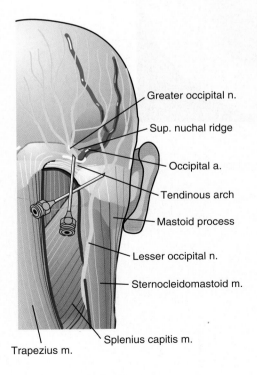

Greater occipital n.

Sup. nuchal ridge

Occipital a.

Tendinous arch

Mastoid process

Lesser occipital n.

Sternocleidomastoid m.

Splenius capitis m.

Trapezius m.

Figure 7-3.

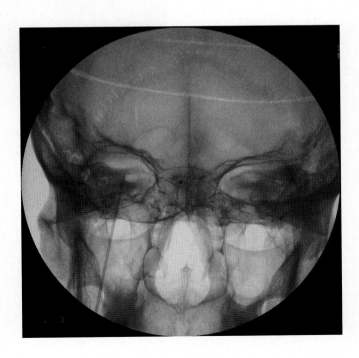

Figure 7-4.
Needle tip in proximity to occipital nerve.

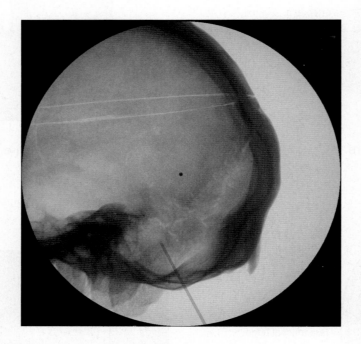

Figure 7-5.
Needle tip in proximity to lesser occipital nerve.

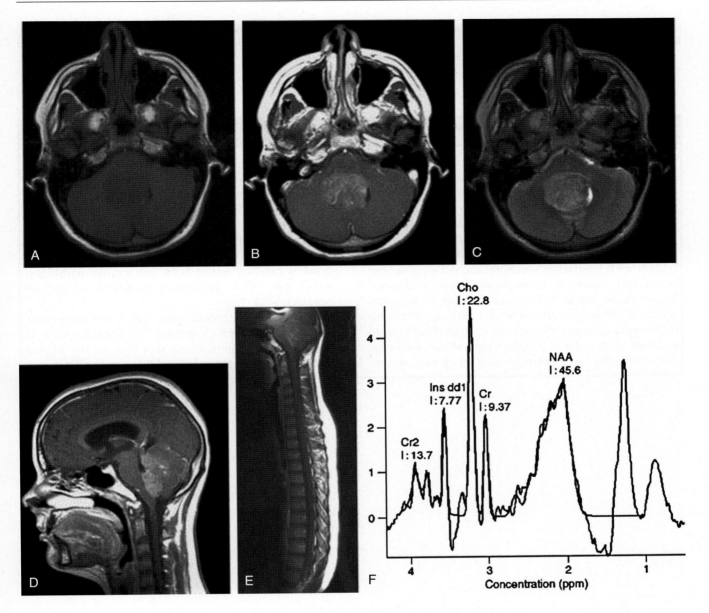

Figure 7-6.

MR scans of a 12-year-old girl who presented with a 4-week history of headaches, drowsiness and vomiting and was found to have medulloblastoma. **A,** Brain axial T1-weighted image without contrast. **B,** Brain axial T1-weighted image with contrast. **C,** Brain axial T2-weighted image. **D,** Brain sagittal T1-weighted image with contrast. **E,** Spinal sagittal T1-weighted image with contrast. **F,** Brain MRS spectrum. There is a midline tumor in the posterior fossa, arising from the cerebellar vermis and projecting into the fourth ventricle cavity, which it fills almost entriely (**A-D**). The tumor is enhanced with gadolinium contrast IV injection in (**B**) and (**D**). It is well circumscribed and is not causing significance edema in the surrounding brain (**B, C**). The third ventricle is dilated due to obstructive hydrocephalus caused by the tumor (**D**). In the spinal views, there is a faint film of enhancement on the pial surface of the spinal cord (**E**), which denotes the presence of metastatic disease. In the spectroscopy analysis (**F**), there is a high Cho peak and comparatively lower NAA peak, giving a low NAA:Cho ratio. Cho, choline; Cr, creatine; Cr2, creatine ethyl ester; I, integral; Ins dd1, inositol; MRS, magnetic resonance spectroscopy; NAA, N-acetyl aspartate. (From Kombogiorgas D, Sgouros S: Medulloblastoma. Encyclopedia of Neuroscience. Philadelphia, Elsevier, 2009, pp 703-711.)

decreases the amount of postprocedure pain and bleeding the patient may experience.

As mentioned earlier, care must be taken to avoid inadvertent needle placement into the foramen magnum because the subarachnoid administration of local anesthetic in this region results in an immediate total spinal anesthetic.

CLINICAL PEARLS

The most common reason that greater and lesser occipital nerve block fails to relieve headache pain is that the headache syndrome being treated has been misdiagnosed as occipital neuralgia. In my experience, occipital neuralgia is an infrequent cause of headaches and rarely occurs in the absence of trauma to the greater and lesser occipital nerves. More often, the patient with headaches involving the occipital region is, in fact, suffering from tension-type headaches. Tension-type headaches do not respond to occipital nerve blocks but are amenable to treatment with antidepressant compounds such as amitriptyline in conjunction with cervical steroid epidural nerve blocks. Therefore, the pain management specialist should reconsider the diagnosis of occipital neuralgia in patients whose symptoms are consistent with occipital neuralgia but who fail to respond to greater and lesser occipital nerve blocks.

Any patient with headaches severe enough to require neural blockade as part of the treatment plan should undergo magnetic resonance imaging of the head to rule out unsuspected intracranial pathology, which may mimic the clinical symptoms of occipital neuralgia (Fig. 7-6).

Furthermore, cervical spine x-rays should be considered to rule out congenital abnormalities such as Arnold-Chiari malformations that may be the hidden cause of the patient's occipital headaches.

CHAPTER 8

Greater and Lesser Occipital Nerve Block: Radiofrequency Lesioning

CPT-2009 CODE	
Neurolytic	64640
Neurolytic-Bilateral	64640-50

Relative Value Units	
Neurolytic	20

INDICATIONS

Radiofrequency lesioning of the occipital nerve block is useful in select patients who have experienced short-term relief with occipital nerve blocks performed with local anesthetic or steroid and have failed to respond to other conservative therapies.

CLINICALLY RELEVANT ANATOMY

The greater occipital nerve arises from fibers of the dorsal primary ramus of the second cervical nerve and to a lesser extent from fibers of the third cervical nerve. The greater occipital nerve pierces the fascia just below the superior nuchal ridge along with the occipital artery. It supplies the medial portion of the posterior scalp as far anterior as the vertex (Fig. 8-1).

The lesser occipital nerve arises from the ventral primary rami of the second and third cervical nerves. The lesser occipital nerve passes superiorly along the posterior border of the sternocleidomastoid muscle, dividing into cutaneous branches that innervate the lateral portion of the posterior scalp and the cranial surface of the pinna of the ear (see Fig. 8-1).

TECHNIQUE

The patient is placed in a sitting position with the cervical spine flexed and the forehead on a padded bedside table. A total of 4 mL of local anesthetic is drawn up in a 12-mL sterile syringe. The occipital artery is then palpated at the level of the superior nuchal ridge. After preparation of the skin with antiseptic solution, a 22-gauge, 10-cm insulated blunt curved needle with a 5- to 10-mm active tip is inserted through an introducer needle just medial to the artery and is advanced perpendicularly until the needle approaches the periosteum of the underlying occipital bone (Fig. 8-2). A paresthesia may be elicited, and the patient should be warned of such. After the needle is in satisfactory position, sensory stimulation to confirm correct needle position is carried out with a frequency of 50 Hz. Amplitude of no greater than 0.5 V should be required. The patient should experience stimulation in the distribution of the greater occipital nerve. Then, 2 mL of 1% lidocaine is injected to provide analgesia. After adequate analgesia has been obtained, two to three 120-second cycles of pulsed radiofrequency at 42°C is carried out.

The lesser occipital nerve and a number of superficial branches of the greater occipital nerve are then lesioned by redirecting the needle laterally and slightly inferiorly (Fig. 8-3). Sensory stimulation to confirm correct needle position is again carried out with a frequency of 50 Hz. Amplitude of no greater than 0.5 V should be required. The patient should experience stimulation in the distribution of the lesser occipital nerve. Then, 2 mL of 1% lidocaine is injected to provide analgesia. After adequate analgesia has been obtained, two to three 120-second cycles of pulsed radiofrequency at 42 degrees is carried out.

SIDE EFFECTS AND COMPLICATIONS

The vascularity and the proximity to the arterial supply in this region give rise to an increased incidence of post-block ecchymosis and hematoma formation. These complications can be decreased if manual pressure is applied to the area of the block immediately after injection. Application of cold packs for 20-minute periods after the block also decreases the amount of postprocedure pain and bleeding the patient may experience.

As mentioned earlier, care must be taken to avoid inadvertent needle placement into the foramen magnum because the subarachnoid administration of local anesthetic in this region results in an immediate total spinal anesthetic.

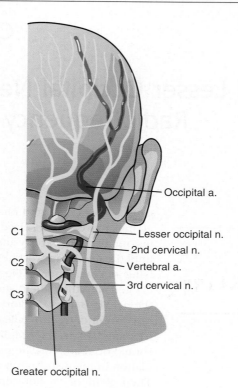

Occipital a.

C1

Lesser occipital n.

2nd cervical n.

C2

Vertebral a.

3rd cervical n.

C3

Greater occipital n.

Figure 8-1.

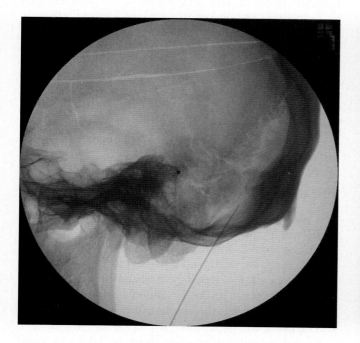

Figure 8-2.
Needle tip in proximity to the greater occipital nerve.

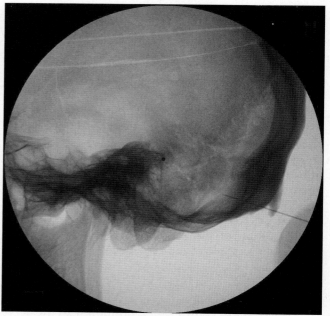

Figure 8-3.
Needle tip in proximity to the lesser occipital nerve.

CLINICAL PEARLS

The most common reason that greater and lesser occipital nerve block fails to relieve headache pain is that the headache syndrome being treated has been misdiagnosed as occipital neuralgia. In my experience, occipital neuralgia is an infrequent cause of headaches and rarely occurs in the absence of trauma to the greater and lesser occipital nerves. More often, the patient with headaches involving the occipital region is in fact suffering from tension-type headaches. Tension-type headaches do not respond to occipital nerve blocks but are amenable to treatment with antidepressant compounds such as amitriptyline in conjunction with cervical steroid epidural nerve blocks. Therefore, the pain management specialist should reconsider the diagnosis of occipital neuralgia in patients whose symptoms are consistent with occipital neuralgia but who fail to respond to greater and lesser occipital nerve blocks.

As with all neurodestructive procedures, the pain management specialist should be sure that the patient fully understands that the numbness experienced after the block may be permanent and that there is no guarantee that the procedure will relieve the patient's pain. Any patient with headaches severe enough to require neural blockade as part of the treatment plan should undergo magnetic resonance imaging of the head to rule out unsuspected intracranial pathology, which may mimic the clinical symptoms of occipital neuralgia.

CHAPTER 9

Gasserian Ganglion Block

CPT-2009 CODE

Unilateral	64400
Neurolytic	64605
	61790 (with radiographic guidance)

Relative Value Units

Unilateral	15
Neurolytic	25

INDICATIONS

Gasserian ganglion block may be used as a part of the diagnostic evaluation of facial pain when the pain management specialist is trying to determine whether a patient's pain is somatic or sympathetic in origin. In addition to its use in anatomic differential neural blockade, gasserian ganglion block may be used in a prognostic manner before neurodestruction of the gasserian ganglion. Gasserian ganglion block also may be used in the acute setting to provide palliation of acute pain emergencies, including trigeminal neuralgia and cancer pain, while waiting for pharmacologic and antiblastic agents to become effective.

Neurodestructive procedures of the gasserian ganglion with neurolytic agents, radiofrequency lesions, balloon compression, and freezing may be indicated for palliation of cancer pain, including that of invasive tumors of the orbit, maxillary sinus, and mandible. Destructive techniques also may be useful in the management of trigeminal neuralgia in patients for whom pharmacologic treatment, as well as nerve blocks with local anesthetic and steroid, has been ineffective and who are not considered candidates for more definitive neurosurgical procedures, including microvascular decompression (Jannetta's procedure). Destruction of the gasserian ganglion has also been used in the management of intractable cluster headache and ocular pain secondary to persistent glaucoma.

CLINICALLY RELEVANT ANATOMY

The gasserian ganglion is formed from two roots that exit the ventral surface of the brain stem at the mid-pontine level. These roots pass in a forward and lateral direction in the posterior cranial fossa across the border of the petrous bone. They then enter a recess called *Meckel's cave*, which is formed by an invagination of the surrounding dura mater into the middle cranial fossa. The dural pouch that lies just behind the ganglion is called the *trigeminal cistern* and contains cerebrospinal fluid (CSF).

The gasserian ganglion is canoe shaped, with the three sensory divisions—the ophthalmic (V1), the maxillary (V2), and the mandibular (V3)—exiting the anterior convex aspect of the ganglion (Fig. 9-1). A small motor root joins the mandibular division as it exits the cranial cavity through the foramen ovale.

TECHNIQUE

The patient is placed in the supine position with the cervical spine extended over a rolled towel. About 2.5 cm lateral to the corner of the mouth, the skin is prepared with antiseptic solution, and sterile drapes are placed (Fig. 9-2). The skin and subcutaneous tissues are then anesthetized with 1% lidocaine with epinephrine.

A 20-gauge, 13-cm styletted needle is advanced through the anesthetized area, traveling perpendicular to the pupil of the eye (when the eye is looking straight ahead). The trajectory of the needle is cephalad toward the acoustic auditory meatus. The needle is advanced until contact is made with the base of the skull (Fig. 9-3). The needle is withdrawn slightly and is "walked" posteriorly into the foramen ovale (Fig. 9-4). Paresthesia of the mandibular nerve will probably be elicited as the needle enters the foramen ovale, and the patient should be warned of such.

When performing gasserian ganglion block under fluoroscopic guidance, the foramen ovale is identified on submental and oblique views (Fig. 9-5). The needle is then advanced under fluoroscopic guidance as described previously toward the foramen ovale. If the base of the

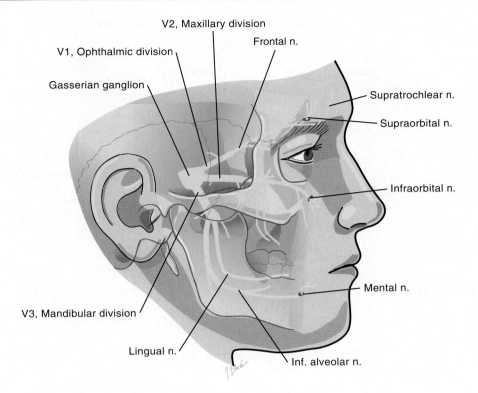

Figure 9-1.

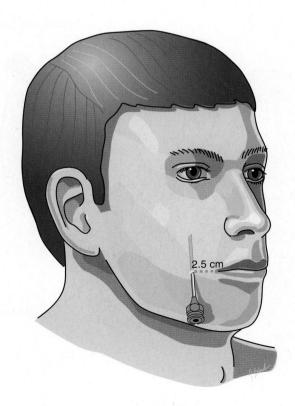

Figure 9-2.

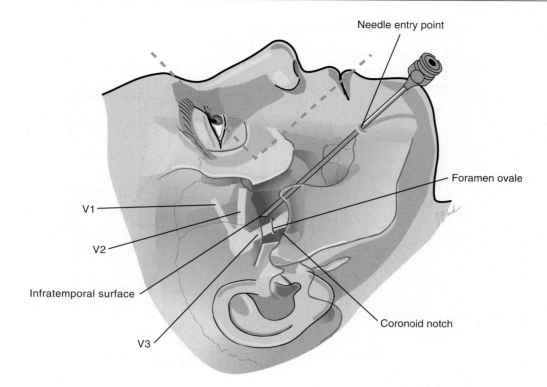

Figure 9-3.

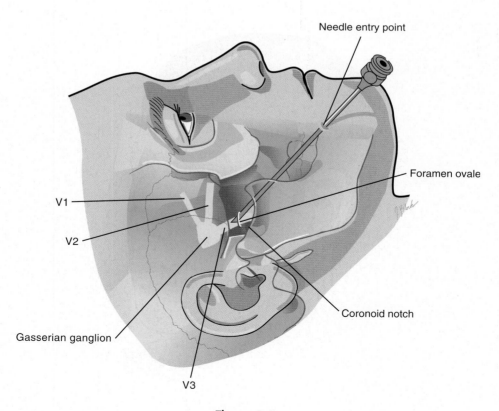

Figure 9-4.

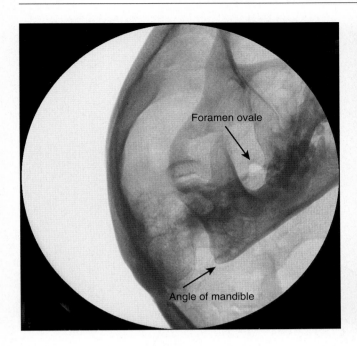

Figure 9-5.
The foramen ovale.

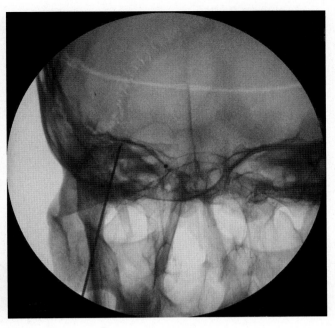

Figure 9-6.
AP view of needle through the foramen ovale.

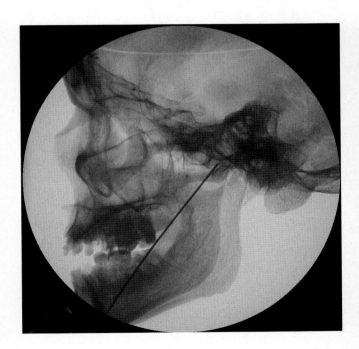

Figure 9-7.
Lateral view of needle through the foramen ovale.

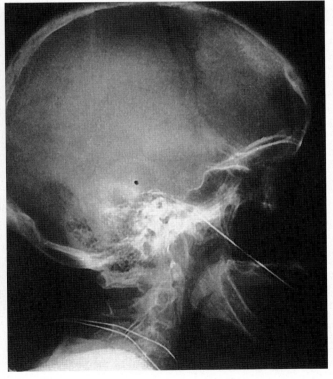

Figure 9-8.
Contrast medium outlining Meckel's cave. (From Waldman SD: Interventional Pain Management, 2nd ed. Philadelphia, WB Saunders, 2001, p 320.)

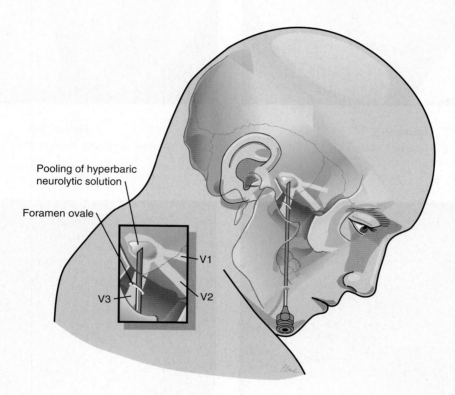

Pooling of hyperbaric
neurolytic solution

Foramen ovale

V1

V3

V2

Figure 9-9.

skull is encountered, the needle is redirected into the foramen ovale (Figs. 9-6 and 9-7).

After the needle enters the foramen ovale, the needle stylet is removed. A free flow of CSF is usually observed. If no CSF is observed, the needle tip is probably anterior to the trigeminal cistern but still may be within Meckel's cave. Needle position can be confirmed by injection of 0.1-mL increments of preservative-free 1% lidocaine and observing the clinical response. Alternatively, 0.1 to 0.4 mL of contrast medium suitable for central nervous system use may be administered under fluoroscopic guidance before injection of the neurolytic substance (Fig. 9-8). Sterile glycerol, 6.5% phenol in glycerin, and absolute alcohol all have been successfully used for neurolysis of the gasserian ganglion. The neurolytic agent should be administered in 0.1-mL increments, with time allotted between additional increments to allow for observation of the clinical response. If hyperbaric neurolytic solutions such as glycerol or phenol in glycerin are used, the patient should be moved to the sitting position with the chin on the chest before injection (Fig. 9-9). This ensures that the solution is placed primarily around the maxillary and mandibular divisions and avoids the ophthalmic division. The patient should be left in the supine position if absolute alcohol is used.

This same approach to the gasserian ganglion may be used to place radiofrequency needles, cryoprobes, compression balloons, and stimulating electrodes.

SIDE EFFECTS AND COMPLICATIONS

Because of the highly vascular nature of the pterygopalatine space, as well as its proximity to the middle meningeal artery, significant hematoma of the face and subscleral hematoma of the eye are common sequelae to gasserian ganglion block. The ganglion lies within the central nervous system, and small amounts of local anesthetic injected into the CSF may lead to total spinal anesthesia. For this reason, it is imperative that small, incremental doses of local anesthetic be injected, with time allowed after each dose to observe the effect of prior doses.

Because of the potential for anesthesia of the ophthalmic division with its attendant corneal anesthesia, corneal sensation should be tested with a cotton wisp after gasserian ganglion block with either local anesthetic or neurolytic solution. If corneal anesthesia is present, sterile ophthalmic ointment should be used and the affected eye patched to avoid damage to the anesthetic cornea. This precaution must be continued for the duration of corneal anesthesia. Ophthalmologic consultation is advisable should persistent corneal anesthesia occur.

Postprocedure dysesthesia, including anesthesia dolorosa, occurs in about 6% of patients who undergo neurodestructive procedures of the gasserian ganglion. These dysesthesias can range from mild pulling or burning sensations to severe postprocedure pain called *anesthesia dolorosa*. These postprocedure symptoms are thought to be due to incomplete destruction of the ganglion. Sloughing of skin in the area of anesthesia also may occur.

In addition to disturbances of sensation, blockade or destruction of the gasserian ganglion may result in abnormal motor function, including weakness of the muscles of mastication and facial asymmetry. Horner's syndrome also may occur as a result of block of the parasympathetic trigeminal fibers. The patient should be warned that all these complications may occur.

CLINICAL PEARLS

Gasserian ganglion block with local anesthetic represents an excellent stopgap measure for patients suffering the uncontrolled pain of trigeminal neuralgia and cancer pain while waiting for pharmacologic and antiblastic treatments to take effect. This block has more side effects and complications than the usual nerve block modalities used by the pain management specialist and thus should be reserved for those special situations in which the pain is truly out of control.

An interesting side effect of gasserian ganglion block is the activation of herpes labialis and, occasionally, of herpes zoster after the procedure. This occurs in about 10% of patients who undergo procedures on the gasserian ganglion, and patients should be forewarned of this possibility.

As mentioned previously, bleeding complications are not uncommon, and given the dramatic and highly visible nature of a facial and subscleral hematoma, all patients undergoing gasserian ganglion block should be warned to expect this side effect to avoid undue anxiety should bleeding complications occur. Infection, although rare, remains an ever-present possibility, especially in the immunocompromised patient. Early detection of infection is crucial to avoid potential life-threatening sequelae.

The pain management specialist should be particularly careful to identify and treat postprocedure corneal anesthesia. Failure to do so can often result in loss of vision. If persistent corneal anesthesia occurs, obtain immediate ophthalmologic consultation to manage any eye-related problems.

CHAPTER 10

Gasserian Ganglion Block: Radiofrequency Lesioning

CPT-2009 CODE

Neurolytic	64605
	61710 (with radiographic guidance)

Relative Value Units

Neurolytic	25

INDICATIONS

Neurodestructive procedures of the gasserian ganglion with neurolytic agents, radiofrequency lesions, balloon compression, and freezing may be indicated for palliation of cancer pain, including that of invasive tumors of the orbit, maxillary sinus, and mandible. Destructive techniques also may be useful in the management of trigeminal neuralgia in patients for whom pharmacologic treatment, as well as nerve blocks with local anesthetic and steroid, has been ineffective and who are not considered candidates for more definitive neurosurgical procedures, including microvascular decompression (Jannetta's procedure). Destruction of the gasserian ganglion has also been used in the management of intractable cluster headache and ocular pain secondary to persistent glaucoma. In recent years, radiofrequency lesioning has supplanted the use of neurolytic agents as the preferred method of destruction of the gasserian ganglion if the patient is not a suitable candidate for more definitive neurosurgical treatment.

CLINICALLY RELEVANT ANATOMY

The gasserian ganglion is formed from two roots that exit the ventral surface of the brain stem at the mid-pontine level. These roots pass in a forward and lateral direction in the posterior cranial fossa across the border of the petrous bone. They then enter a recess called *Meckel's cave*, which is formed by an invagination of the surrounding dura mater into the middle cranial fossa. The dural pouch that lies just behind the ganglion is called

the *trigeminal cistern* and contains cerebrospinal fluid (CSF).

The gasserian ganglion is canoe-shaped, with the three sensory divisions—the ophthalmic (V1), the maxillary (V2), and the mandibular (V3)—exiting the anterior convex aspect of the ganglion (Fig.10-1). A small motor root joins the mandibular division as it exits the cranial cavity via the foramen ovale.

TECHNIQUE

The patient is placed in the supine position with the cervical spine extended over a rolled towel. About 2.5 cm lateral to the corner of the mouth, the skin is prepared with antiseptic solution and sterile drapes are placed. The skin and subcutaneous tissues are then anesthetized with 1% lidocaine with epinephrine.

A 22-gauge, 15-cm insulated blunt curved needle with a 5- to 10-mm active tip is inserted through an introducer needle placed through the previously anesthetized area traveling perpendicular to the pupil of the eye (when the eye is looking straight ahead). The trajectory of the needle is cephalad toward the acoustic auditory meatus. The foramen ovale is then identified on submental and oblique views (Fig. 10-2). The needle is then advanced under fluoroscopic guidance as described previously toward the foramen ovale (Figs. 10-3 and 10-4). If the base of the skull is encountered, the needle is redirected into the foramen ovale (Figs. 10-5 and 10-6). If difficulty is encountered in placing the needle through the foramen ovale into Meckel's cave, submental and oblique views may be beneficial (Figs. 10-7 and 10-8). Paresthesia of the mandibular nerve probably will be elicited as the needle enters the foramen ovale, and the patient should be warned of such.

To confirm that the needle is properly placed, stimulation at 2 Hz with 0.5 to 1.5 V should produce motor stimulation of the ipsilateral muscles of the lower mandible. If no motor response is observed, the needle should be repositioned more medially. If in proximity to the first or second divisions of the gasserian ganglion, no motor response should be observed. A mild paresthesia

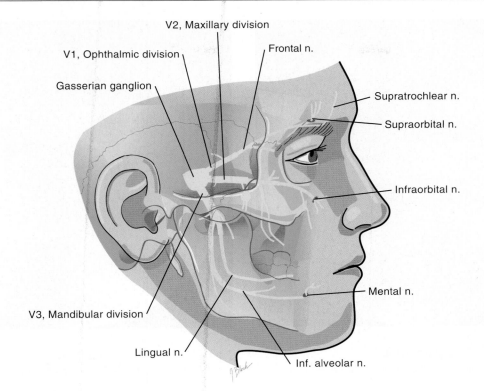

Figure 10-1.

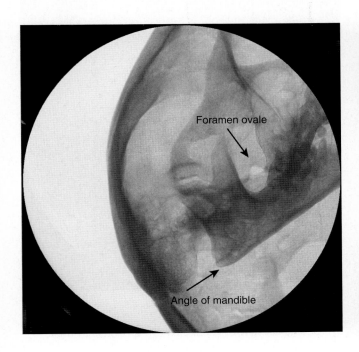

Figure 10-2.
The foramen ovale.

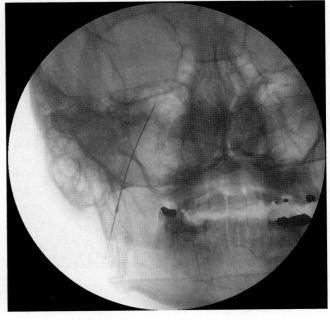

Figure 10-3.
AP view of needle tip approaching the foramen ovale.

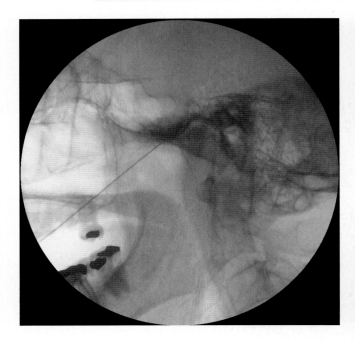

Figure 10-4.
Lateral view of needle approaching the foramen ovale.

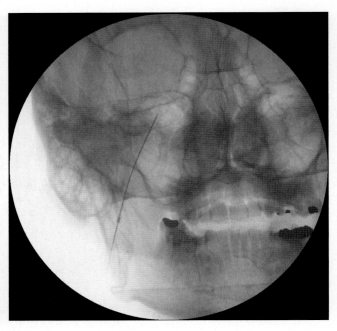

Figure 10-5.
AP view of needle through the foramen ovale.

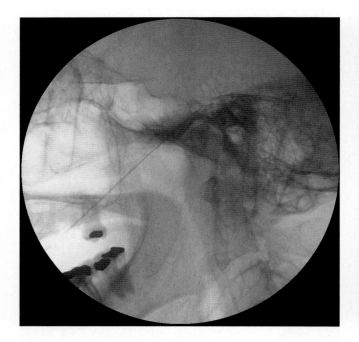

Figure 10-6.
Lateral view of needle through the foramen ovale.

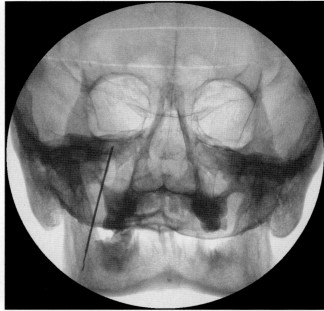

Figure 10-7.
Submental view of needle through the foramen ovale.

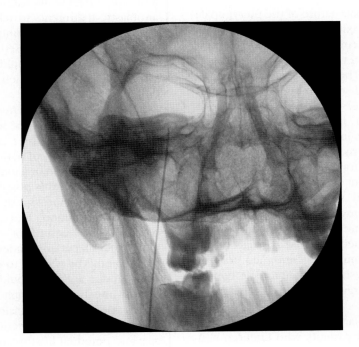

Figure 10-8.
Needle properly placed in the foramen ovale.

in the division that is to be lesioned should then be elicited by stimulating at 50 to 100 Hz with 0.1 to 0.5 V. If higher voltages are required to stimulate a paresthesia, the needle should be repositioned. Careful aspiration for blood and CSF should then be carried out and the needle repositioned until blood is not present. If no CSF or blood is present, 0.25 to 0.5 mL of 0.2% ropivacaine is then injected, and the patient is monitored closely for inadvertent intravascular or subarachnoid injection. After 60 seconds, radiofrequency lesioning is carried out at 60°C for 90 seconds. Care should be taken to verify that the lesion has not produced corneal anesthesia.

SIDE EFFECTS AND COMPLICATIONS

Because of the highly vascular nature of the pterygopalatine space as well as its proximity to the middle meningeal artery, significant hematoma of the face and subscleral hematoma of the eye are common sequelae to gasserian ganglion block. The ganglion lies within the central nervous system, and small amounts of local anesthetic injected into the CSF may lead to total spinal anesthesia. For this reason, it is imperative that small doses of local anesthetic be injected, with time allowed after each dose to observe the effect of prior doses.

Because of the potential for anesthesia of the ophthalmic division with its attendant corneal anesthesia, corneal sensation should be tested with a cotton wisp after lesioning of the gasserian ganglion. If corneal anesthesia is present, sterile ophthalmic ointment should be used and the affected eye patched to avoid damage to the cornea. This precaution must be continued for the duration of corneal anesthesia. Ophthalmologic consultation is advisable should persistent corneal anesthesia occur.

Postprocedure dysesthesia, including anesthesia dolorosa, occurs in about 6% of patients who undergo neurodestructive procedures of the gasserian ganglion. These dysesthesias can range from mild pulling or burning sensations to severe postprocedure pain called *anesthesia dolorosa*. These postprocedure symptoms are thought to be due to incomplete destruction of the ganglion. Sloughing of skin in the area of anesthesia also may occur.

In addition to disturbances of sensation, blockade or destruction of the gasserian ganglion may result in abnormal motor function, including weakness of the muscles of mastication and facial asymmetry. Horner's syndrome also may occur as a result of block of the parasympathetic trigeminal fibers. The patient should be warned that all these complications may occur.

CLINICAL PEARLS

Gasserian ganglion block with local anesthetic represents an excellent stopgap measure for patients suffering the uncontrolled pain of trigeminal neuralgia and cancer pain while waiting for pharmacologic and antiblastic treatments to take effect. This block has more side effects and complications than the usual nerve block modalities used by the pain management specialist and thus should be reserved for those special situations in which the pain is truly out of control.

An interesting side effect of gasserian ganglion block is the activation of herpes labialis and, occasionally, of herpes zoster after the procedure. This occurs in about 10% of patients who undergo procedures on the gasserian ganglion, and patients should be forewarned of this possibility.

As mentioned previously, bleeding complications are not uncommon, and given the dramatic and highly visible nature of a facial and subscleral hematoma, all patients undergoing gasserian ganglion block should be warned to expect this side effect to avoid undue anxiety should bleeding complications occur. Infection, although rare, remains an ever-present possibility, especially in the immunocompromised patient. Early detection of infection is crucial to avoid potential life-threatening sequelae.

The pain management specialist should be particularly careful to identify and treat postprocedure corneal anesthesia. Failure to do so can often result in loss of vision. If persistent corneal anesthesia occurs, obtain immediate ophthalmologic consultation to manage any eye-related problems.

CHAPTER 11

Gasserian Ganglion Block: Balloon Compression Technique

INDICATIONS

Neurodestructive procedures of the gasserian ganglion with neurolytic agents, radiofrequency lesions, balloon compression, and freezing may be indicated for palliation of cancer pain, including that of invasive tumors of the orbit, maxillary sinus, and mandible. Destructive techniques also may be useful in the management of trigeminal neuralgia in patients for whom pharmacologic treatment, as well as nerve blocks with local anesthetic and steroid, has been ineffective and who are not considered candidates for more definitive neurosurgical procedures, including microvascular decompression (Jannetta's procedure). Destruction of the gasserian ganglion has also been used in the management of intractable cluster headache and ocular pain secondary to persistent glaucoma. Balloon compression of the gasserian ganglion is a reasonable choice if the patient is not a suitable candidate for more definitive neurosurgical treatment. This technique has the added advantage of being performed completely under general anesthesia, which makes this ideal for the patient who is unwilling or unable to cooperate with the other percutaneous neurodestructive procedures on the gasserian ganglion that require patient participation.

CLINICALLY RELEVANT ANATOMY

The gasserian ganglion is formed from two roots that exit the ventral surface of the brain stem at the mid-pontine level. These roots pass in a forward and lateral direction in the posterior cranial fossa across the border of the petrous bone. They then enter a recess called *Meckel's cave*, which is formed by an invagination of the surrounding dura mater into the middle cranial fossa. The dural pouch that lies just behind the ganglion is called the *trigeminal cistern* and contains cerebrospinal fluid (CSF).

The gasserian ganglion is canoe shaped, with the three sensory divisions—the ophthalmic (V1), the maxillary (V2), and the mandibular (V3)—exiting the anterior convex aspect of the ganglion (Fig.11-1). A small motor root joins the mandibular division as it exits the cranial cavity through the foramen ovale.

TECHNIQUE

The patient is placed in the supine position with the cervical spine extended over a rolled towel. About 2.5 cm lateral to the corner of the mouth, the skin is prepared with antiseptic solution, and sterile drapes are placed. The skin and subcutaneous tissues are then anesthetized with 1% lidocaine with epinephrine.

An 18-gauge styletted spinal needle is used as an introducer needle and is placed through the previously anesthetized area traveling perpendicular to the pupil of the eye (when the eye is looking straight ahead). The trajectory of the needle is cephalad toward the acoustic auditory meatus. The foramen ovale is then identified on submental and oblique views (Fig. 11-2). A 22-gauge sterile K-wire is then placed through the spinal needle and advanced carefully to the foramen ovale. Proper placement of the K-wire is confirmed on fluoroscopy as being just inside the foramen ovale. An outer cannula is then passed over the K-wire into Meckel's cave. After satisfactory placement of the outer cannula is confirmed with fluoroscopy, a 4-mm Fogarty catheter is placed through the cannula carefully into Meckel's cave. After satisfactory placement of the Fogarty catheter is confirmed with fluoroscopy, the balloon is inflated with 0.7 mL of contrast media for a period of 2 minutes. A pear-shaped image should be observed conforming to the internal bony constraints of Meckel's cave. A failure to observe this pear shape means that the patient has a

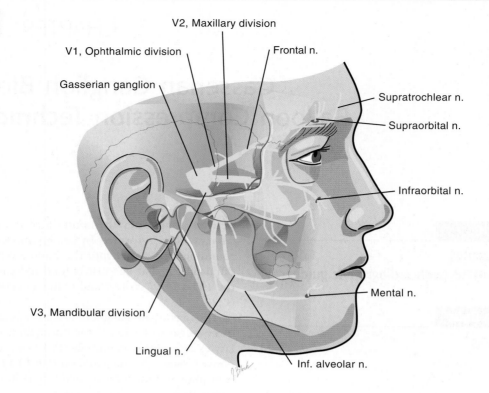

V1, Ophthalmic division
V2, Maxillary division
Gasserian ganglion
Frontal n.
Supratrochlear n.
Supraorbital n.
Infraorbital n.
V3, Mandibular division
Mental n.
Lingual n.
Inf. alveolar n.

Figure 11-1.

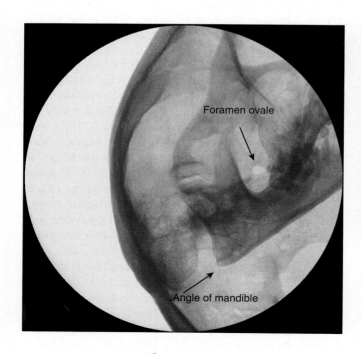

Foramen ovale

Angle of mandible

Figure 11-2.
The foramen ovale.

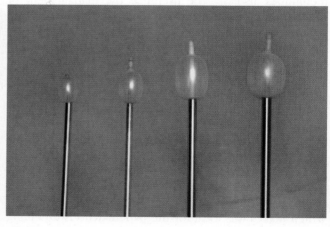

Figure 11-3.
Left to right: Different-sized outer cannulas with Nos. 3, 4, 5, and 6 inflated Fogarty balloons. (From Goerss SJ, Atkinson JLD, Kallmes DF: Variable size percutaneous balloon compression of the gasserian ganglion for trigeminal neuralgia. Surg Neurol 2008 Feb 19 [Epub ahead of print].)

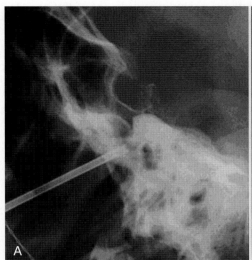
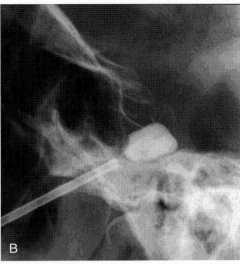

Figure 11-4.
A, Patient with a No. 4 Fogarty balloon maximally inflated for 2 minutes failed to produce any facial hypesthesia, with early recurrence of pain 9 months later. **B,** Repeat balloon compression using a No. 5 Fogarty balloon for 1 minute with resultant perioral hypesthesia and no pain recurrence in 5 years. (From Goerss SJ, Atkinson JLD, Kallmes DF: Variable size percutaneous balloon compression of the gasserian ganglion for trigeminal neuralgia. Surg Neurol 2008 Feb 19 [Epub ahead of print].)

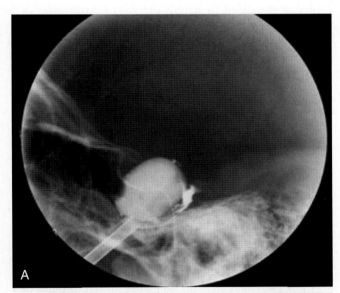

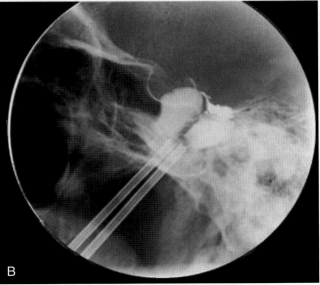

Figure 11-5.
A and **B,** Patient with multiple sclerosis who had failed previous radiofrequency and glycerol tests (note tantalum powder behind balloon) and failed all our balloon compression procedures over a few months. The balloon depicted is a No. 6 Fogarty balloon held in place for 4 minutes. Note the lack of a pear-shaped configuration owing primarily to the large dimensions of Meckel's cave. There was no facial hypesthesia, and her pain continued unabated. **B,** Two No. 4 Fogarty balloons were passed through separate cannulas. Both were inflated and held in place for 2 minutes with resultant perioral hypesthesia and excellent pain relief without medications. (From Goerss SJ, Atkinson JLD, Kallmes DF: Variable size percutaneous balloon compression of the gasserian ganglion for trigeminal neuralgia. Surg Neurol 2008 Feb 19 [Epub ahead of print].)

capacious Meckel's cave and will require a larger Fogarty catheter (Figs. 11-3 through 11-5) A failure to completely compress the gasserian ganglion with a Fogarty catheter with inadequate size results in little or no pain relief. Occasionally, two balloons are required to completely fill Meckel's cave and fully compress the gasserian ganglion. After a 2-minute compression period, the Fogarty balloon catheter is deflated and, along with the introducer cannula, is removed. The patient is then observed for postoperative bleeding.

SIDE EFFECTS AND COMPLICATIONS

Because of the highly vascular nature of the pterygopalatine space, as well as its proximity to the middle meningeal artery, significant hematoma of the face and subscleral hematoma of the eye are common sequelae to gasserian ganglion block. The ganglion lies within the central nervous system, and small amounts of local anesthetic injected into the CSF may lead to total spinal anesthesia. For this reason, it is imperative that small doses of local anesthetic be injected, with time allowed after each dose to observe the effect of prior doses.

Because of the potential for anesthesia of the ophthalmic division with its attendant corneal anesthesia, corneal sensation should be tested with a cotton wisp after lesioning of the gasserian ganglion. If corneal anesthesia is present, sterile ophthalmic ointment should be used and the affected eye patched to avoid damage to the cornea. This precaution must be continued for the duration of corneal anesthesia. Ophthalmologic consultation is advisable should persistent corneal anesthesia occur.

Postprocedure dysesthesia, including anesthesia dolorosa, occurs in about 6% of patients who undergo neurodestructive procedures of the gasserian ganglion. These dysesthesias can range from mild pulling or burning sensations to severe postprocedure pain called *anesthesia dolorosa*. These postprocedure symptoms are thought to be due to incomplete destruction of the ganglion. Sloughing of skin in the area of anesthesia also may occur.

In addition to disturbances of sensation, blockade or destruction of the gasserian ganglion may result in abnormal motor function, including weakness of the muscles of mastication and facial asymmetry. Horner's syndrome also may occur as a result of block of the parasympathetic trigeminal fibers. The patient should be warned that all of these complications may occur.

CLINICAL PEARLS

Gasserian ganglion block with local anesthetic represents an excellent stopgap measure for patients suffering the uncontrolled pain of trigeminal neuralgia and cancer pain while waiting for pharmacologic and antiblastic treatments to take effect. This block has more side effects and complications than the usual nerve block modalities used by the pain management specialist and thus should be reserved for those special situations in which the pain is truly "out of control."

An interesting side effect of gasserian ganglion block is the activation of herpes labialis and, occasionally, of herpes zoster after the procedure. This occurs in about 10% of patients who undergo procedures on the gasserian ganglion, and patients should be forewarned of this possibility.

As mentioned previously, bleeding complications are not uncommon, and given the dramatic and highly visible nature of a facial and subscleral hematoma, all patients undergoing gasserian ganglion block should be warned to expect this side effect to avoid undue anxiety should bleeding complications occur. Infection, although rare, remains an ever-present possibility, especially in the immunocompromised patient. Early detection of infection is crucial to avoid potential life-threatening sequelae.

The pain management specialist should be particularly careful to identify and treat postprocedure corneal anesthesia. Failure to do so can often result in loss of vision. If persistent corneal anesthesia occurs, obtain immediate ophthalmologic consultation to manage any eye-related problems.

CHAPTER 12

Trigeminal Nerve Block: Coronoid Approach

CPT-2009 CODE	
Unilateral	64400
Neurolytic	64605
	64610 (with radiographic guidance)

Relative Value Units	
Unilateral	10
Neurolytic	20

INDICATIONS

Trigeminal nerve block through the coronoid approach is a simple and safe way to block the maxillary and mandibular divisions of the trigeminal nerve. This technique may be used as a part of the diagnostic evaluation of facial pain when the pain management specialist is trying to determine whether a patient's pain is somatic or sympathetic in origin. In addition to its use in anatomic differential neural blockade, trigeminal nerve block through the coronoid approach allows for selective blockade of the maxillary and mandibular divisions to allow the technique to be used in a prognostic manner before neurodestruction of these nerves.

Trigeminal nerve block through the coronoid approach also may be used in the acute setting to provide palliation of acute pain emergencies, including trigeminal neuralgia, facial trauma, and cancer pain, while waiting for pharmacologic and antiblastic agents to become effective. Trigeminal nerve block with local anesthetic may be used as a treatment for trismus and as an aid to awake intubation. Trigeminal nerve block with local anesthetic and steroid through the coronoid approach is also useful as a first-line treatment for the breakthrough pain of trigeminal neuralgia that has previously been controlled with medications. This technique can be used in the treatment of pain associated with acute herpes zoster and postherpetic neuralgia in the distribution of the trigeminal nerve. Atypical facial pain syndromes, including temporomandibular joint dysfunction, also may be amenable to treatment using this technique.

Neurodestructive procedures of the maxillary and mandibular nerves using neurolytic agents, radiofrequency lesions, or freezing may be carried out using the coronoid approach to the trigeminal nerve. These neurodestructive techniques are useful in the palliation of cancer pain, including pain secondary to invasive tumors of the maxillary sinus and mandible.

CLINICALLY RELEVANT ANATOMY

The maxillary division (V2) of the trigeminal nerve is a pure sensory nerve (Fig. 12-1). It exits the middle cranial fossa via the foramen rotundum and crosses the pterygopalatine fossa (Fig. 12-2). Passing through the inferior orbital fissure, it enters the orbit, emerging on the face via the infraorbital foramen. The maxillary nerve can be selectively blocked by placing a needle just above the anterior margin of the lateral pterygoid plate.

The maxillary nerve provides sensory innervation for the dura of the middle cranial fossa, the temporal and lateral zygomatic region, and the mucosa of the maxillary sinus. The nerve also provides sensory innervation for the upper molars, premolars, incisors, canines, and associated oral gingiva as well as the mucous membranes of the cheek. The nasal cavity, lower eyelid, skin of the side of the nose, and upper lip are also subserved by the maxillary nerve.

The mandibular division (V3) is composed of a large sensory root and smaller motor root. Both leave the middle cranial fossa together via the foramen ovale and join to form the mandibular nerve. Branches of the mandibular nerve provide sensory innervation to portions of the dura mater and the mucosal lining of the mastoid sinus. Sensory innervation to the skin overlying the muscles of mastication, the tragus and helix of the ear, the posterior temporomandibular joint, the chin, and the dorsal aspect of the anterior two thirds of the tongue and associated mucosa of the oral cavity is also provided by the mandibular nerve (see Fig. 12-1). The smaller

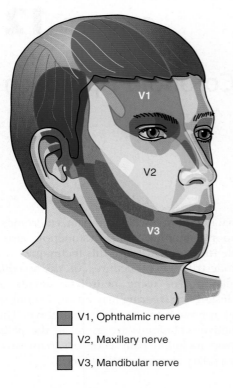

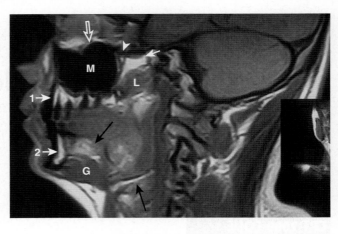

Figure 12-2.

T1-weighted image through the left face medial to the mandible, demonstrating the maxillary sinus (M), orbital surface of the maxilla (*open white arrow*), medial aspect of the pterygopalatine fossa (*white arrowhead*), retroantral fat pad (*solid white arrow*), lateral pterygoid muscle fibers coursing to the proximal mandible (L), marrow in the maxilla (*solid white arrow 1*) and mandible (*solid white arrow 2*), sublingual space (*top black arrow*), geniohyoid muscle (G), and hyoid bone (*bottom black arrow*). (From Stark DD, Bradley WG: Magnetic Resonance Imaging, 3rd ed. St. Louis, Mosby, 1999, p 1747.)

■ V1, Ophthalmic nerve

□ V2, Maxillary nerve

■ V3, Mandibular nerve

Figure 12-1.

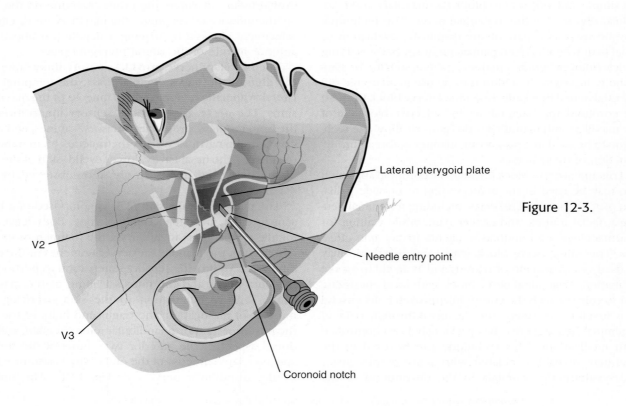

Lateral pterygoid plate

Needle entry point

Coronoid notch

V2

V3

Figure 12-3.

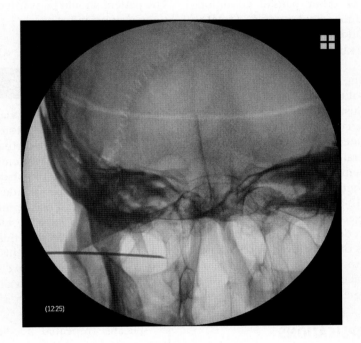

Figure 12-4.
Proper needle placement for trigeminal nerve block using the coronoid approach.

motor branch provides innervation to the masseter, external pterygoid, and temporalis muscles.

TECHNIQUE

The patient is placed in the supine position with the cervical spine in the neutral position. The coronoid notch is identified by asking the patient to open and close the mouth several times and palpating the area just anterior and slightly inferior to the acoustic auditory meatus. After the notch is identified, the patient is asked to hold his or her mouth in neutral position.

A total of 7 mL of local anesthetic is drawn up in a 12-mL sterile syringe. When treating trigeminal neuralgia, atypical facial pain, or other painful conditions involving the maxillary and mandibular nerve, a total of 80 mg of depot-steroid is added to the local anesthetic with the first block, and 40 mg of depot-steroid is added with subsequent blocks.

After the skin overlying the coronoid notch is prepared with antiseptic solution, a 22-gauge, 3½-inch styletted needle is inserted just below the zygomatic arch directly in the middle of the coronoid notch. The needle is advanced about 1½ to 2 inches in a plane perpendicular to the skull until the lateral pterygoid plate is encountered (Fig. 12-3). At this point, if blockade of both the maxillary and mandibular nerves is desired, the needle is withdrawn slightly (Fig. 12-4). After careful aspiration, 7 to 8 mL of solution is injected in incremental doses. During the injection procedure, the patient must be observed carefully for signs of local anesthetic toxicity.

The coronoid approach to blockade of the trigeminal nerve may be used to place radiofrequency needles, cryoprobes, and stimulating electrodes.

SIDE EFFECTS AND COMPLICATIONS

Because of the highly vascular nature of the pterygopalatine fossa, significant facial hematoma may occur after trigeminal nerve block via the coronoid approach. This vascularity means that the pain specialist should use small, incremental doses of local anesthetic to avoid local anesthetic toxicity.

Postprocedure dysesthesia, including anesthesia dolorosa, may occur in a small number of patients who undergo neurodestructive procedures of the branches of the trigeminal nerve. These dysesthesias can range from mild pulling or burning sensations to severe postprocedure pain called *anesthesia dolorosa*. These postprocedure symptoms are thought to be due to incomplete destruction of the neural structures. Sloughing of skin in the area of anesthesia also may occur.

In addition to disturbances of sensation, blockade or destruction of the branches of the trigeminal nerve may result in abnormal motor function, including weakness of the muscles of mastication and secondary facial asymmetry due to muscle weakness or loss of proprioception. The patient should be warned that all of these complications may occur.

CLINICAL PEARLS

Trigeminal nerve block via the coronoid approach with local anesthetic and steroid represents an excellent stopgap measure for patients suffering from the uncontrolled pain of trigeminal neuralgia and cancer pain while waiting for pharmacologic treatments to take effect. The major side effects of this block are related to the vascular nature of the pterygopalatine fossa, and care must be taken to avoid local anesthetic toxicity. Despite this vascularity, by using a 25- or 27-gauge needle, this technique can safely be performed in the presence of anticoagulation, albeit at increased risk for facial hematoma, should the clinical situation dictate a favorable risk-to-benefit ratio.

Because repeated needle punctures of daily or every-other-day blocks may result in small punctate facial scars, patients should be warned of this possibility. Infection, although rare, remains an ever-present possibility, especially in the immunocompromised patient. Early detection of infection is crucial to avoid potential life-threatening sequelae.

CHAPTER 13

Selective Maxillary Nerve Block: Coronoid Approach

CPT-2009 CODE	
Unilateral	64400
Neurolytic	64605
	64610 (with radiographic guidance)

Relative Value Units	
Unilateral	10
Neurolytic	20

INDICATIONS

Trigeminal nerve block via the coronoid approach is a simple and safe way to block the maxillary and mandibular divisions of the trigeminal nerve. This technique may be used as a part of the diagnostic evaluation of facial pain when the pain management specialist is trying to determine whether a patient's pain is somatic or sympathetic in origin. In addition to its use in anatomic differential neural blockade, trigeminal nerve block via the coronoid approach allows for selective blockade of the maxillary and mandibular divisions to allow the technique to be used in a prognostic manner before neurodestruction of these nerves.

Neurodestructive procedures of the maxillary and mandibular nerves using neurolytic agents, radiofrequency lesions, or freezing may be carried out using selective maxillary and mandibular nerve block techniques. These neurodestructive techniques are useful in the palliation of cancer pain, including pain secondary to invasive tumors of the maxillary sinus and mandible.

CLINICALLY RELEVANT ANATOMY

The maxillary division (V2) of the trigeminal nerve is a pure sensory nerve. It exits the middle cranial fossa via the foramen rotundum and crosses the pterygopalatine fossa (Fig. 13-1). Passing through the inferior orbital fissure, it enters the orbit, emerging on the face via the infraorbital foramen. The maxillary nerve can be selectively blocked by placing a needle just above the anterior margin of the lateral pterygoid plate.

The maxillary nerve provides sensory innervation for the dura of the middle cranial fossa, the temporal and lateral zygomatic region, and the mucosa of the maxillary sinus. The nerve also provides sensory innervation for the upper molars, premolars, incisors, canines, and associated oral gingiva as well as the mucous membranes of the cheek (Fig. 13-2). The nasal cavity, lower eyelid, skin of the side of the nose, and upper lip are also subserved by the maxillary nerve.

The mandibular division (V3) is composed of a large sensory root and smaller motor root. Both leave the middle cranial fossa together via the foramen ovale and join to form the mandibular nerve. Branches of the mandibular nerve provide sensory innervation to portions of the dura mater and the mucosal lining of the mastoid sinus. Sensory innervation to the skin overlying the muscles of mastication, the tragus and helix of the ear, the posterior temporomandibular joint, the chin, and the dorsal aspect of the anterior two thirds of the tongue and associated mucosa of the oral cavity is also provided by the mandibular nerve (see Fig. 13-2). The smaller motor branch provides innervation to the masseter, external pterygoid, and temporalis muscles.

TECHNIQUE

The patient is placed in the supine position with the cervical spine in the neutral position. The coronoid notch is identified by asking the patient to open and close the mouth several times and palpating the area just anterior and slightly inferior to the acoustic auditory meatus. After the notch is identified, the patient is asked to hold his or her mouth in neutral position.

A total of 7 mL of local anesthetic is drawn up in a 12-mL sterile syringe. When treating trigeminal neuralgia, atypical facial pain, or other painful conditions involving the maxillary and mandibular nerve, a total of 80 mg of depot-steroid is added to the local anesthetic

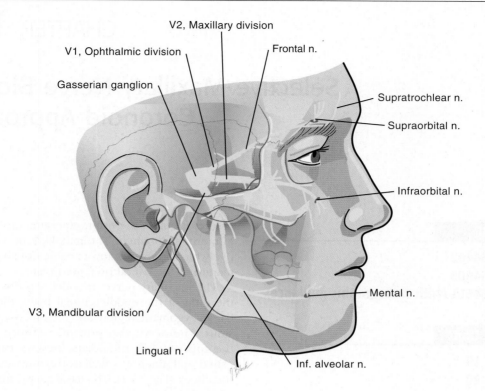

V2, Maxillary division

V1, Ophthalmic division

Frontal n.

Gasserian ganglion

Supratrochlear n.

Supraorbital n.

Infraorbital n.

Mental n.

V3, Mandibular division

Lingual n.

Inf. alveolar n.

Figure 13-1.

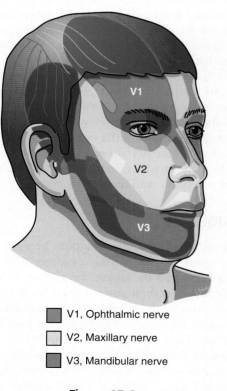

V1

V2

V3

■ V1, Ophthalmic nerve

□ V2, Maxillary nerve

■ V3, Mandibular nerve

Figure 13-2.

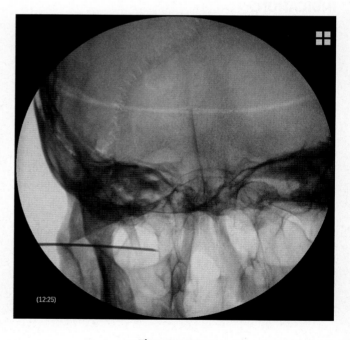

(12:25)

Figure 13-3.
Needle placed through the coronoid notch with tip resting against lateral pterygoid plate.

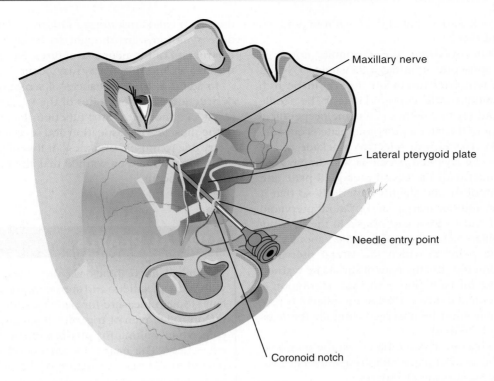

Figure 13-4.

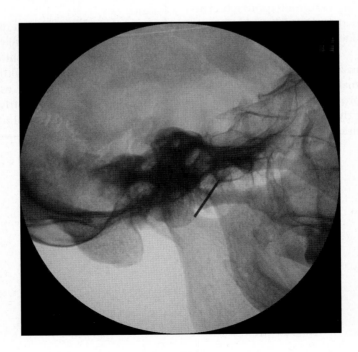

Figure 13-5.
Needle in position in front of anterior margin of the lateral pterygoid plate.

with the first block, and 40 mg of depot-steroid is added with subsequent blocks.

After the skin overlying the coronoid notch is prepared with antiseptic solution, a 22-gauge, 3½-inch styletted needle is inserted just below the zygomatic arch directly in the middle of the coronoid notch. The needle is advanced about 1½ to 2 inches in a plane perpendicular to the skull until the lateral pterygoid plate is encountered (Fig. 13-3). To perform selective blockade of the maxillary nerve, the styletted needle is withdrawn after it comes in contact with the lateral pterygoid plate and is redirected anteriorly and slightly superiorly so that it will slip past the anterior margin of the lateral pterygoid plate (Figs. 13-4 and 13-5). A paresthesia in the distribution of the maxillary nerve is usually elicited about 1 cm deeper than the point at which the lateral pterygoid plate was encountered, and the patient should be warned of such. After careful aspiration, 3 to 5 mL of solution is injected in incremental doses. During the injection procedure, the patient must be observed carefully for signs of local anesthetic toxicity.

The selective maxillary nerve block via the coronoid approach may be used to place radiofrequency needles, cryoprobes, and stimulating electrodes.

SIDE EFFECTS AND COMPLICATIONS

Because of the highly vascular nature of the pterygopalatine fossa, significant facial hematoma may occur after trigeminal nerve block via the coronoid approach. This vascularity means that the pain specialist should use small, incremental doses of local anesthetic to avoid local anesthetic toxicity.

Postprocedure dysesthesia, including anesthesia dolorosa, may occur in a small number of patients who undergo neurodestructive procedures of the branches of the trigeminal nerve. These dysesthesias can range from mild pulling or burning sensations to severe postprocedure pain called *anesthesia dolorosa*. These postprocedure symptoms are thought to be due to incomplete destruction of the neural structures. Sloughing of skin in the area of anesthesia also may occur.

In addition to disturbances of sensation, blockade or destruction of the branches of the trigeminal nerve may result in abnormal motor function, including weakness of the muscles of mastication and secondary facial asymmetry due to muscle weakness or loss of proprioception. The patient should be warned that all of these complications may occur.

CLINICAL PEARLS

Trigeminal nerve block via the coronoid approach with local anesthetic and steroid represents an excellent stopgap measure for patients suffering from the uncontrolled pain of trigeminal neuralgia and cancer pain while waiting for pharmacologic treatments to take effect. The major side effects of this block are related to the vascular nature of the pterygopalatine fossa, and care must be taken to avoid local anesthetic toxicity. Despite this vascularity, by using a 25- or 27-gauge needle, this technique can safely be performed in the presence of anticoagulation, albeit at increased risk for facial hematoma, should the clinical situation dictate a favorable risk-to-benefit ratio.

Because repeated needle punctures of daily or every-other-day blocks may result in small punctate facial scars, patients should be warned of this possibility. Infection, although rare, remains an ever-present possibility, especially in the immunocompromised patient. Early detection of infection is crucial to avoid potential life-threatening sequelae.

CHAPTER 14

Selective Mandibular Nerve Block: Coronoid Approach

CPT-2009 CODE	
Unilateral	64400
Neurolytic	64605
	64610 (with radiographic guidance)

Relative Value Units	
Unilateral	10
Neurolytic	20

INDICATIONS

Trigeminal nerve block via the coronoid approach is a simple and safe way to block the maxillary and mandibular divisions of the trigeminal nerve. This technique may be used as a part of the diagnostic evaluation of facial pain when the pain management specialist is trying to determine whether a patient's pain is somatic or sympathetic in origin. In addition to its use in anatomic differential neural blockade, trigeminal nerve block via the coronoid approach allows for selective blockade of the maxillary and mandibular divisions to allow the technique to be used in a prognostic manner before neurodestruction of these nerves.

Neurodestructive procedures of the maxillary and mandibular nerves using neurolytic agents, radiofrequency lesions, or freezing may be carried out using selective maxillary and mandibular nerve block techniques. These neurodestructive techniques are useful in the palliation of cancer pain, including pain secondary to invasive tumors of the maxillary sinus and mandible.

CLINICALLY RELEVANT ANATOMY

The maxillary division (V2) of the trigeminal nerve is a pure sensory nerve. It exits the middle cranial fossa via the foramen rotundum and crosses the pterygopalatine fossa (Fig. 14-1). Passing through the inferior orbital fissure, it enters the orbit, emerging on the face via the infraorbital foramen. The maxillary nerve can be selectively blocked by placing a needle just above the anterior margin of the lateral pterygoid plate.

The maxillary nerve provides sensory innervation for the dura of the middle cranial fossa, the temporal and lateral zygomatic region, and the mucosa of the maxillary sinus. The nerve also provides sensory innervation for the upper molars, premolars, incisors, canines, and associated oral gingiva as well as the mucous membranes of the cheek (Fig. 14-2). The nasal cavity, lower eyelid, skin of the side of the nose, and upper lip are also subserved by the maxillary nerve.

The mandibular division (V3) is composed of a large sensory root and smaller motor root. Both leave the middle cranial fossa together via the foramen ovale and join to form the mandibular nerve. Branches of the mandibular nerve provide sensory innervation to portions of the dura mater and the mucosal lining of the mastoid sinus. Sensory innervation to the skin overlying the muscles of mastication, the tragus and helix of the ear, the posterior temporomandibular joint, the chin, and the dorsal aspect of the anterior two thirds of the tongue and associated mucosa of the oral cavity is also provided by the mandibular nerve (see Fig. 14-2). The smaller motor branch provides innervation to the masseter, external pterygoid, and temporalis muscles.

TECHNIQUE

The patient is placed in the supine position with the cervical spine in the neutral position. The coronoid notch is identified by asking the patient to open and close the mouth several times and palpating the area just anterior and slightly inferior to the acoustic auditory meatus. After the notch is identified, the patient is asked to hold his or her mouth in neutral position.

After the skin overlying the coronoid notch is prepared with antiseptic solution, a 22-gauge, 3½-inch styletted needle is inserted just below the zygomatic arch directly in the middle of the coronoid notch. The needle is advanced about 1½ to 2 inches in a plane perpendicular to the skull until the lateral pterygoid

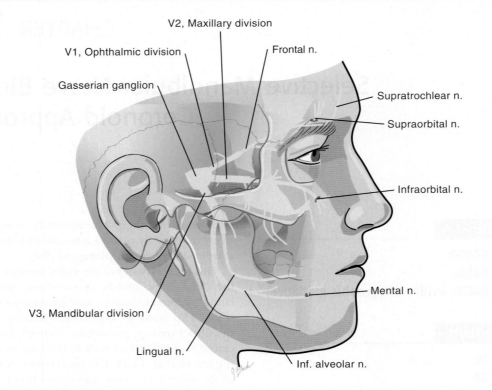

V2, Maxillary division

V1, Ophthalmic division

Frontal n.

Gasserian ganglion

Supratrochlear n.

Supraorbital n.

Infraorbital n.

Mental n.

V3, Mandibular division

Lingual n.

Inf. alveolar n.

Figure 14-1.

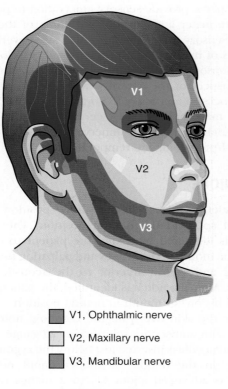

V1

V2

V3

■ V1, Ophthalmic nerve

□ V2, Maxillary nerve

■ V3, Mandibular nerve

Figure 14-2.

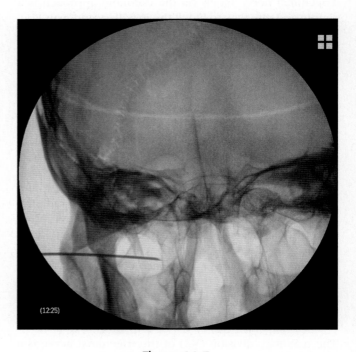

Figure 14-3.
Needle placed through the coronoid notch with tip resting against lateral pterygoid plate.

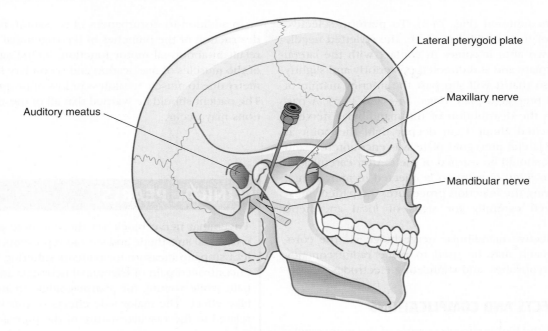

Lateral pterygoid plate

Maxillary nerve

Auditory meatus

Mandibular nerve

Figure 14-4.

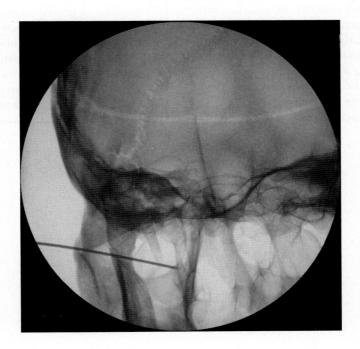

Figure 14-5.
Needle tip placed beyond the inferior margin of lateral pterygoid plate.

plate is encountered (Fig. 14-3). To perform selective blockade of the mandibular nerve, the styletted needle is withdrawn after it comes in contact with the lateral pterygoid plate and is redirected posteriorly and slightly inferiorly so that it will slip past the inferior margin of the lateral pterygoid plate (Figs. 14-4 and 14-5). A paresthesia in the distribution of the mandibular nerve is usually elicited about 1 cm deeper than the point at which the lateral pterygoid plate was encountered, and the patient should be warned of such. After careful aspiration, 3 to 5 mL of solution is injected in incremental doses. During the injection procedure, the patient must be observed carefully for signs of local anesthetic toxicity.

The selective mandibular nerve block via the coronoid approach may be used to place radiofrequency needles, cryoprobes, and stimulating electrodes.

SIDE EFFECTS AND COMPLICATIONS

Because of the highly vascular nature of the pterygopalatine fossa, significant facial hematoma may occur after trigeminal nerve block via the coronoid approach. This vascularity means that the pain specialist should use small, incremental doses of local anesthetic to avoid local anesthetic toxicity.

Postprocedure dysesthesia, including anesthesia dolorosa, may occur in a small number of patients who undergo neurodestructive procedures of the branches of the trigeminal nerve. These dysesthesias can range from mild pulling or burning sensations to severe postprocedure pain called *anesthesia dolorosa*. These postprocedure symptoms are thought to be due to incomplete destruction of the neural structures. Sloughing of skin in the area of anesthesia also may occur.

In addition to disturbances of sensation, blockade or destruction of the branches of the trigeminal nerve may result in abnormal motor function, including weakness of the muscles of mastication and secondary facial asymmetry due to muscle weakness or loss of proprioception. The patient should be warned that all of these complications may occur.

CLINICAL PEARLS

Trigeminal nerve block via the coronoid approach with local anesthetic and steroid represents an excellent stopgap measure for patients suffering from the uncontrolled pain of trigeminal neuralgia and cancer pain while waiting for pharmacologic treatments to take effect. The major side effects of this block are related to the vascular nature of the pterygopalatine fossa, and care must be taken to avoid local anesthetic toxicity. Despite this vascularity, by using a 25- or 27-gauge needle, this technique can safely be performed in the presence of anticoagulation, albeit at increased risk for facial hematoma, should the clinical situation dictate a favorable risk-to-benefit ratio.

Because repeated needle punctures of daily or every-other-day blocks may result in small punctate facial scars, patients should be warned of this possibility. Infection, although rare, remains an ever-present possibility, especially in the immunocompromised patient. Early detection of infection is crucial to avoid potential life-threatening sequelae.

CHAPTER 15

Supraorbital Nerve Block

CPT-2009 CODE	
Unilateral	64400
Bilateral	64400-50
Neurolytic	64600

Relative Value Units	
Unilateral	5
Bilateral	10
Neurolytic	20

INDICATIONS

Supraorbital nerve block is useful in the diagnosis and treatment of painful conditions in areas subserved by the supraorbital nerve, including supraorbital neuralgia and pain secondary to herpes zoster. This technique is also useful in providing surgical anesthesia in the distribution of the supraorbital nerve for lesion removal and laceration repair.

CLINICALLY RELEVANT ANATOMY

The supraorbital nerve arises from fibers of the frontal nerve, which is the largest branch of the ophthalmic nerve. The frontal nerve enters the orbit via the superior orbital fissure and passes anteriorly beneath the periosteum of the roof of the orbit. The frontal nerve gives off a larger lateral branch, the supraorbital nerve, and a smaller medial branch, the supratrochlear nerve. Both exit the orbit anteriorly. The supraorbital nerve sends fibers all the way to the vertex of the scalp and provides sensory innervation to the forehead, upper eyelid, and anterior scalp (Fig. 15-1).

TECHNIQUE

The patient is placed in a supine position. A total of 3 mL of local anesthetic is drawn up in a 10-mL sterile syringe.

When treating supraorbital neuralgia, acute herpes zoster, postherpetic neuralgia, or other painful conditions involving the supraorbital nerve, a total of 80 mg of depot-steroid is added to the local anesthetic with the first block, and 40 mg of depot-steroid is added with subsequent blocks.

The supraorbital notch on the affected side is then identified by palpation. The skin overlying the notch is prepared with antiseptic solution, with care being taken to avoid spillage into the eye. A 25-gauge, 1½-inch needle is inserted at the level of the supraorbital notch and is advanced medially about 15 degrees off the perpendicular to avoid entering the foramen. The needle is advanced until it approaches the periosteum of the underlying bone (Figs. 15-2 and 15-3). A paresthesia may be elicited, and the patient should be warned of such. The needle should not enter the supraorbital foramen, and should this occur, the needle should be withdrawn and redirected slightly more medially.

Because of the loose alveolar tissue of the eyelid, a gauze sponge should be used to apply gentle pressure on the upper eyelid and supraorbital tissues before injection of solution to prevent the injectate from dissecting inferiorly into these tissues. This pressure should be maintained after the procedure to avoid periorbital hematoma and ecchymosis.

After gentle aspiration, 3 mL of solution is injected in a fanlike distribution. If blockade of the supratrochlear nerve is also desired, the needle is then redirected medially, and after careful aspiration, an additional 3 mL of solution is injected in a fanlike manner.

SIDE EFFECTS AND COMPLICATIONS

The forehead and scalp are highly vascular, and the pain specialist should carefully calculate the total milligram dosage of local anesthetic that may be given safely, especially if bilateral nerve blocks are being performed. This vascularity gives rise to an increased incidence of postblock ecchymosis and hematoma formation. Despite the vascularity of this anatomic region, this technique can safely be performed in the presence of anticoagulation

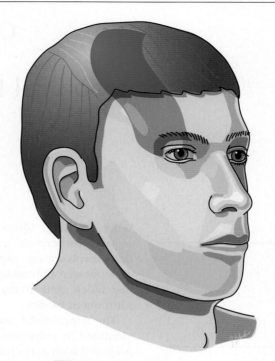

Sensory distribution of supraorbital nerve

Figure 15-1.

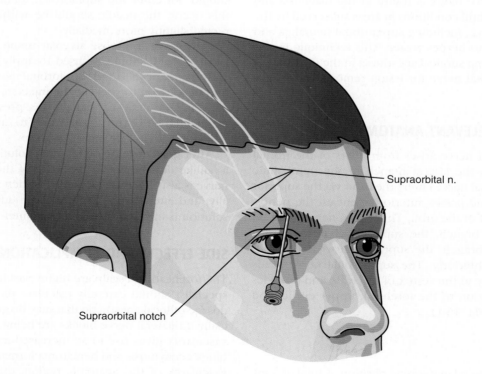

Supraorbital n.

Supraorbital notch

Figure 15-2.

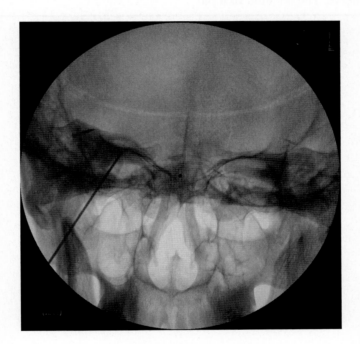

Figure 15-3.
Needle tip in proximity of the supraorbital nerve.

by using a 25- or 27-gauge needle, albeit at increased risk for hematoma, if the clinical situation dictates a favorable risk-to-benefit ratio. These complications can be decreased if manual pressure is applied to the area of the block immediately after injection. Application of cold packs for 20-minute periods after the block also decreases the amount of postprocedure pain and bleeding the patient may experience.

CLINICAL PEARLS

Supraorbital nerve block is especially useful in the palliation of pain secondary to acute herpes zoster involving the ophthalmic division and its branches. In this setting, the pain management specialist also has to block the supratrochlear nerve. The addition of tepid aluminum acetate soaks helps dry weeping lesions and makes the patient more comfortable. Care should be taken to avoid spillage of the aluminum acetate solution into the eye.

CHAPTER 16

Supratrochlear Nerve Block

CPT-2009 CODE	
Unilateral	64400
Bilateral	64400-50
Neurolytic	64600

Relative Value Units	
Unilateral	5
Bilateral	10
Neurolytic	20

INDICATIONS

Supratrochlear nerve block is useful in the diagnosis and treatment of painful conditions in areas subserved by the supratrochlear nerve, including supratrochlear neuralgia and pain secondary to herpes zoster. This technique is also useful in providing surgical anesthesia in the distribution of the supratrochlear nerve for lesion removal and laceration repair.

CLINICALLY RELEVANT ANATOMY

The supratrochlear nerve arises from fibers of the frontal nerve, which is the largest branch of the ophthalmic nerve. The frontal nerve enters the orbit via the superior orbital fissure and passes anteriorly beneath the periosteum of the roof of the orbit. The frontal nerve gives off a larger lateral branch, the supraorbital nerve, and a smaller medial branch, the supratrochlear nerve. Both exit the orbit anteriorly. The supratrochlear nerve sends fibers to provide sensory innervation to the inferomedial section of the forehead, the bridge of the nose, and the medial portion of the upper eyelid (Fig. 16-1).

TECHNIQUE

The patient is placed in a supine position. A total of 3 mL of local anesthetic is drawn up in a 10-mL sterile syringe.

When treating supratrochlear neuralgia, acute herpes zoster, postherpetic neuralgia, or other painful conditions involving the supratrochlear nerve, a total of 80 mg of depot-steroid is added to the local anesthetic with the first block, and 40 mg of depot-steroid is added with subsequent blocks.

The supraorbital ridge on the affected side is then identified by palpation. The skin at the point where the bridge of the nose abuts the supraorbital ridge is prepared with antiseptic solution, with care being taken to avoid spillage into the eye. A 25-gauge, 16½-inch needle is inserted just lateral to the junction of the bridge of the nose and the supraorbital ridge and is advanced medially into the subcutaneous tissue (Fig. 16-2). A paresthesia may be elicited, and the patient should be warned of such. Because of the loose alveolar tissue of the eyelid, a gauze sponge should be used to apply gentle pressure on the upper eyelid and supratrochlear tissues before injection of solution to prevent the injectate from dissecting inferiorly into these tissues. This pressure should be maintained after the procedure to avoid periorbital hematoma and ecchymosis. After gentle aspiration, 3 mL of solution is injected in a fanlike distribution.

SIDE EFFECTS AND COMPLICATIONS

The forehead and scalp are highly vascular, and the pain specialist should carefully calculate the total milligram dosage of local anesthetic that may be given safely, especially if bilateral nerve blocks are being performed. This vascularity gives rise to an increased incidence of post-block ecchymosis and hematoma formation. Despite the vascularity of this anatomic region, this technique can safely be performed in the presence of anticoagulation by using a 25- or 27-gauge needle, albeit at increased risk for hematoma, if the clinical situation dictates a favorable risk-to-benefit ratio. These complications can be decreased if manual pressure is applied to the area of the block immediately after injection. Application of cold packs for 20-minute periods after the block also decreases the amount of postprocedure pain and bleeding the patient may experience.

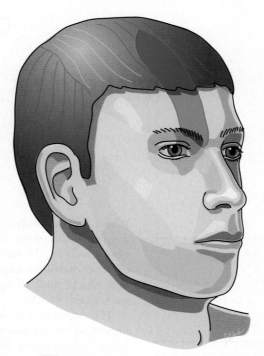

Sensory distribution of supratrochlear nerve

Figure 16-1.

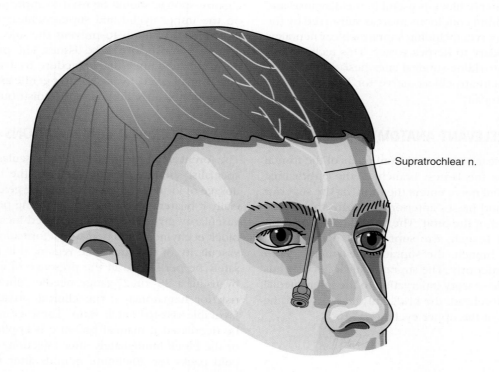

Supratrochlear n.

Figure 16-2.

CLINICAL PEARLS

Supratrochlear nerve block is especially useful in the palliation of pain secondary to acute herpes zoster involving the ophthalmic division and its branches. In this setting, the pain management specialist also has to block the supraorbital nerve. The addition of tepid aluminum acetate soaks helps dry weeping lesions and makes the patient more comfortable. Care should be taken to avoid spillage of the aluminum acetate solution into the eye.

CHAPTER 17

Infraorbital Nerve Block: Extraoral Approach

CPT-2009 CODE

Unilateral	64400
Bilateral	64400-50
Neurolytic	64600

Relative Value Units

Unilateral	5
Bilateral	10
Neurolytic	20

INDICATIONS

Infraorbital nerve block is useful in the diagnosis and treatment of painful conditions in areas subserved by the infraorbital nerve, including infraorbital neuralgia and pain secondary to herpes zoster. This technique is also useful in providing surgical anesthesia in the distribution of the infraorbital nerve for lesion removal and laceration repair.

CLINICALLY RELEVANT ANATOMY

The infraorbital nerve arises from fibers of the maxillary nerve. The infraorbital nerve enters the orbit via the inferior orbital fissure and passes along the floor of the orbit in the infraorbital groove. The nerve exits the orbit via the infraorbital foramen and provides cutaneous branches that innervate the lower eyelid, lateral naris, and upper lip (Fig. 17-1). The superior alveolar branch of the infraorbital nerves provides sensory innervation to the upper incisor, canine, and associated gingiva.

TECHNIQUE

The patient is placed in a supine position. A total of 3 mL of local anesthetic is drawn up in a 10-mL sterile syringe. When treating infraorbital neuralgia, facial trauma, or other painful conditions involving the infraorbital nerve, a total of 80 mg of depot-steroid is added to the local anesthetic with the first block, and 40 mg of depot-steroid is added with subsequent blocks.

The infraorbital notch on the affected side is then identified by palpation. The skin overlying the notch is prepared with antiseptic solution, with care taken to avoid spillage into the eye. A 25-gauge, 1$\frac{1}{2}$-inch needle is inserted at the level of the infraorbital notch and is advanced medially about 15 degrees off the perpendicular to avoid entering the foramen. The needle is advanced until it approaches the periosteum of the underlying bone (Figs. 17-2 and 17-3). A paresthesia may be elicited, and the patient should be warned of such. The needle should not enter the infraorbital foramen, and should this occur, the needle should be withdrawn and redirected slightly more medially. Because of the loose alveolar tissue of the eyelid, a gauze sponge should be used to apply gentle pressure on the lower eyelid and infraorbital tissues before injection of solution to prevent the injectate from dissecting upward into these tissues. This pressure should be maintained after the procedure to avoid periorbital hematoma and ecchymosis. After gentle aspiration, 3 mL of solution is injected in a fanlike distribution.

SIDE EFFECTS AND COMPLICATIONS

The face is highly vascular, and the pain specialist should carefully calculate the total milligram dosage of local anesthetic that may be given safely, especially if bilateral nerve blocks are being performed. This vascularity gives rise to an increased incidence of postblock ecchymosis and hematoma formation. Despite the vascularity of this anatomic region, this technique can safely be performed in the presence of anticoagulation by using a 25- or 27-gauge needle, albeit at increased risk for hematoma, if the clinical situation dictates a favorable risk-to-benefit ratio. These complications can be decreased if manual pressure is applied to the area of the block immediately after injection. Application of cold packs for 20-minute periods after the block also decreases the amount of

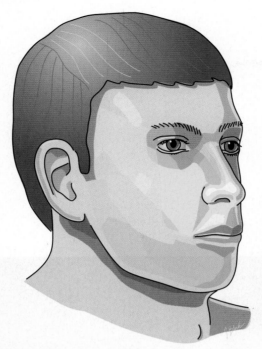

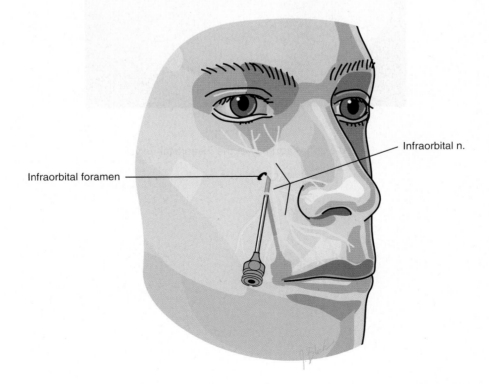

Sensory distribution of infraorbital nerve

Figure 17-1.

Infraorbital n.

Infraorbital foramen

Figure 17-2.

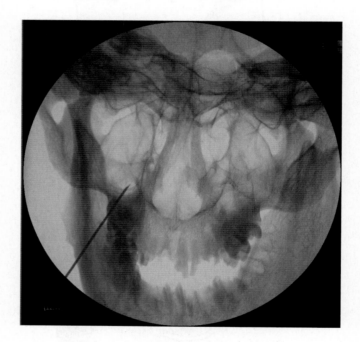

Figure 17-3.
Needle tip in proximity of the infraorbital nerve.

postprocedure pain and bleeding the patient may experience.

The pain management specialist should avoid inserting the needle directly into the infraorbital foramen because the nerve may be damaged as solution is injected into the bony canal, resulting in a compression neuropathy.

CLINICAL PEARLS

Infraorbital nerve block is useful in the palliation of pain secondary to facial trauma and neuropathic pain involving the infraorbital nerve. For use in the pediatric population or for repair of facial lacerations, the intraoral approach to blockade of the infraorbital nerve should be considered.

Because repeated needle punctures of daily or every-other-day blocks may result in small punctate facial scars, patients should be warned of this possibility. Infection, although rare, remains an ever-present possibility, especially in the immunocompromised patient. Early detection of infection is crucial to avoid potential life-threatening sequelae.

CHAPTER 18

Infraorbital Nerve Block: Intraoral Approach

CPT-2009 CODE	
Unilateral	64400
Bilateral	64400-5
Neurolytic	64600

Relative Value Units	
Unilateral	5
Bilateral	10
Neurolytic	20

INDICATIONS

Infraorbital nerve block is useful in the diagnosis and treatment of painful conditions in areas subserved by the infraorbital nerve, including infraorbital neuralgia and pain secondary to herpes zoster. The intraoral approach to infraorbital nerve block is especially useful in providing surgical anesthesia in the distribution of the infraorbital nerve for lesion removal and laceration repair when a cosmetic result is desired because this approach avoids distortion of the facial anatomy from local anesthetic infiltration at the surgical site. The intraoral approach is also useful in the pediatric population.

CLINICALLY RELEVANT ANATOMY

The infraorbital nerve arises from fibers of the maxillary nerve. The infraorbital nerve enters the orbit via the inferior orbital fissure and passes along the floor of the orbit in the infraorbital groove. The nerve exits the orbit via the infraorbital foramen and provides cutaneous branches that innervate the lower eyelid, lateral naris, and upper lip. The superior alveolar branch of the infraorbital nerves provides sensory innervation to the upper incisor, canine, and associated gingiva.

TECHNIQUE

The patient is placed in a supine position. A total of 3 mL of local anesthetic is drawn up in a 10-mL sterile syringe. When treating infraorbital neuralgia, facial trauma, or other painful conditions involving the infraorbital nerve, a total of 80 mg of depot-steroid is added to the local anesthetic with the first block, and 40 mg of depot-steroid is added with subsequent blocks.

The infraorbital notch on the affected side is then identified by palpation. The upper lip is then pulled backward, and a cotton ball soaked in 10% cocaine solution or 2% viscous lidocaine is placed in the alveolar sulcus, just inferior to the infraorbital foramen. After adequate topical anesthesia of the mucosa is obtained, a 25-gauge, 1½-inch needle is advanced through the anesthetized mucosa toward the infraorbital foramen (Fig. 18-1). A paresthesia may be elicited, and the patient should be warned of such. Because of the loose alveolar tissue of the eyelid, a gauze sponge should be used to apply gentle pressure on the lower eyelid and infraorbital tissues before injection of solution to prevent the injectate from dissecting upward into these tissues. This pressure should be maintained after the procedure to avoid periorbital hematoma and ecchymosis. After gentle aspiration, 3 mL of solution is injected in a fanlike distribution.

SIDE EFFECTS AND COMPLICATIONS

The face is highly vascular, and the pain specialist should carefully calculate the total milligram dosage of local anesthetic that may be given safely, especially if bilateral nerve blocks are being performed. This vascularity gives rise to an increased incidence of postblock ecchymosis and hematoma formation. Despite the vascularity of this anatomic region, this technique can safely be performed in the presence of anticoagulation by using a 25- or 27-gauge needle, albeit at increased risk for hematoma, if the clinical situation dictates a favorable risk-to-benefit

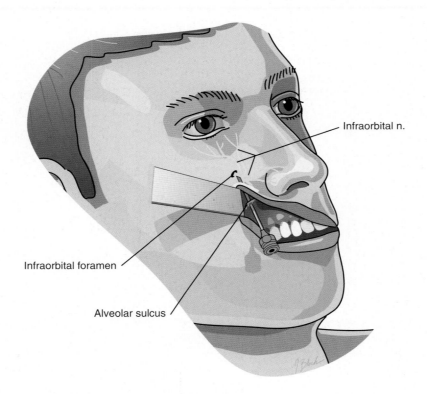

Infraorbital n.

Infraorbital foramen

Alveolar sulcus

Figure 18-1.

ratio. These complications can be decreased if manual pressure is applied to the area of the block immediately after injection. Application of cold packs for 20-minute periods after the block also decreases the amount of postprocedure pain and bleeding the patient may experience.

CLINICAL PEARLS

Infraorbital nerve block is useful in the palliation of pain secondary to facial trauma and neuropathic pain involving the infraorbital nerve. For use in the pediatric population or for repair of facial lacerations, the intraoral approach to blockade of the infraorbital nerve should be considered. When using the intraoral approach with children, the child's mother or father can actually place the anesthetic-soaked cotton ball in the alveolar sulcus under the pain management specialist's direction.

CHAPTER 19

Mental Nerve Block: Extraoral Approach

CPT-2009 CODE	
Unilateral	**64400**
Bilateral	**64400-50**
Neurolytic	**64600**

Relative Value Units	
Unilateral	**5**
Bilateral	**10**
Neurolytic	**20**

INDICATIONS

Mental nerve block is useful in the diagnosis and treatment of painful conditions in areas subserved by the mental nerve, including mental neuralgia, facial trauma, and pain secondary to herpes zoster. This technique is also useful in providing surgical anesthesia in the distribution of the mental nerve for lesion removal and laceration repair.

CLINICALLY RELEVANT ANATOMY

The mental nerve arises from fibers of the mandibular nerve. The mental nerve exits the mandible via the mental foramen at the level of the second premolar, where it makes a sharp turn superiorly. The nerve provides cutaneous branches that innervate the lower lip, chin, and corresponding oral mucosa (Fig. 19-1).

TECHNIQUE

The patient is placed in a supine position. A total of 3 mL of local anesthetic is drawn up in a 10-mL sterile syringe.

When treating mental neuralgia, facial trauma, or other painful conditions involving the mental nerve, a total of 80 mg of depot-steroid is added to the local anesthetic with the first block, and 40 mg of depot-steroid is added with subsequent blocks.

The mental notch on the affected side is then identified by palpation. The skin overlying the notch is prepared with antiseptic solution. A 25-gauge, 1½-inch needle is inserted at the level of the mental notch and is advanced medially about 15 degrees off the perpendicular to avoid entering the foramen. The needle is advanced until it approaches the periosteum of the underlying bone (Figs. 19-2 and 19-3). A paresthesia may be elicited, and the patient should be warned of such. The needle should not enter the mental foramen, and should this occur, the needle should be withdrawn and redirected slightly more medially. After gentle aspiration, 3 mL of solution is injected in a fanlike distribution.

The face is highly vascular, and the pain specialist should carefully calculate the total milligram dosage of local anesthetic that may be given safely, especially if bilateral nerve blocks are being performed. This vascularity gives rise to an increased incidence of postblock ecchymosis and hematoma formation. Despite the vascularity of this anatomic region, this technique can safely be performed in the presence of anticoagulation by using a 25- or 27-gauge needle, albeit at increased risk for hematoma, if the clinical situation dictates a favorable risk-to-benefit ratio. These complications can be decreased if manual pressure is applied to the area of the block immediately after injection. Application of cold packs for 20-minute periods after the block also decreases the amount of postprocedure pain and bleeding the patient may experience.

The pain management specialist should avoid inserting the needle directly into the mental foramen because the nerve may be damaged as solution is injected into the bony canal, resulting in a compression neuropathy.

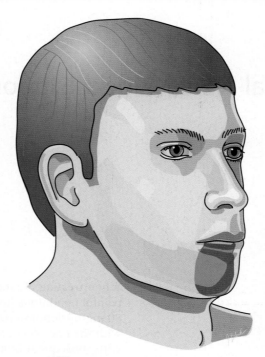

Sensory distribution of mental nerve

Figure 19-1.

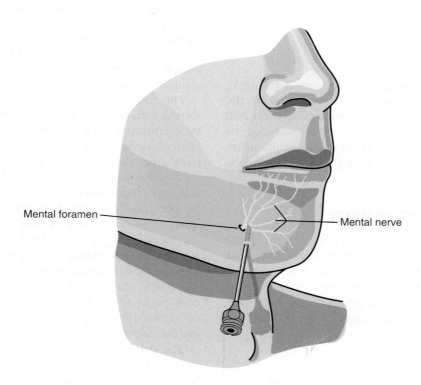

Mental foramen ————————————— ——— Mental nerve

Figure 19-2.

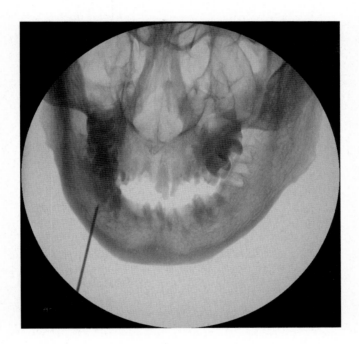

Figure 19-3.
Needle tip in proximity to the mental nerve.

CLINICAL PEARLS

Mental nerve block is useful in the palliation of pain secondary to facial trauma and neuropathic pain involving the mental nerve. For use in the pediatric population or for repair of facial lacerations, the intraoral approach to blockade of the mental nerve should be considered.

Because repeated needle punctures of daily or every-other-day blocks may result in small punctate facial scars, patients should be warned of this possibility. Infection, although rare, remains an ever-present possibility, especially in the immunocompromised patient. Early detection of infection is crucial to avoid potential life-threatening sequelae.

The pain specialist should carefully examine the patient before performing mental nerve block to identify preexisting neural compromise because the mental nerve is especially vulnerable to blunt trauma owing to the acute angle at which the mental nerve exits the mental foramen. This preblock assessment helps identify subtle neurologic changes that might subsequently be erroneously attributed to the block.

CHAPTER 20

Mental Nerve Block: Intraoral Approach

CPT-2009 CODE	
Unilateral	64400
Bilateral	64400-50
Neurolytic	64600

Relative Value Units	
Unilateral	5
Bilateral	10
Neurolytic	20

INDICATIONS

Mental nerve block is useful in the diagnosis and treatment of painful conditions in areas subserved by the mental nerve, including mental neuralgia, facial trauma, and pain secondary to herpes zoster.

The intraoral approach to mental nerve block is especially useful in providing surgical anesthesia in the distribution of the mental nerve for lesion removal and laceration repair when a cosmetic result is desired because this approach avoids distortion of the facial anatomy from local anesthetic infiltration at the surgical site.

CLINICALLY RELEVANT ANATOMY

The mental nerve arises from fibers of the mandibular nerve. The mental nerve exits the mandible via the mental foramen at the level of the second premolar, where it makes a sharp turn superiorly. The nerve provides cutaneous branches that innervate the lower lip, chin, and corresponding oral mucosa.

TECHNIQUE

The patient is placed in a supine position. A total of 3 mL of local anesthetic is drawn up in a 10-mL sterile syringe. When treating mental neuralgia, facial trauma, or other painful conditions involving the mental nerve, a total of 80 mg of depot-steroid is added to the local anesthetic with the first block, and 40 mg of depot-steroid is added with subsequent blocks.

The mental notch on the affected side is then identified by palpation. The lower lip is then pulled downward, and a cotton ball soaked in 10% cocaine solution or 2% viscous lidocaine is placed in the alveolar sulcus, just above the mental foramen. After adequate topical anesthesia of the mucosa is obtained, a 25-gauge, $1\frac{1}{2}$-inch needle is advanced through the anesthetized mucosa toward the mental foramen (Fig. 20-1). A paresthesia may be elicited, and the patient should be warned of such. After gentle aspiration, 3 mL of solution is injected in a fanlike distribution.

SIDE EFFECTS AND COMPLICATIONS

The face is highly vascular, and the pain specialist should carefully calculate the total milligram dosage of local anesthetic that may be given safely, especially if bilateral nerve blocks are being performed. This vascularity gives rise to an increased incidence of postblock ecchymosis and hematoma formation. Despite the vascularity of this anatomic region, this technique can safely be performed in the presence of anticoagulation by using a 25- or 27-gauge needle, albeit at increased risk for hematoma, if the clinical situation dictates a favorable risk-to-benefit ratio. These complications can be decreased if manual pressure is applied to the area of the block immediately after injection. Application of cold packs for 20-minute periods after the block also decreases the amount of postprocedure pain and bleeding the patient may experience.

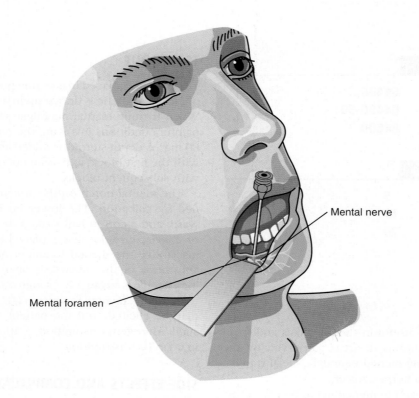

Mental nerve

Mental foramen

Figure 20-1.

CLINICAL PEARLS

Mental nerve block is useful in the palliation of pain secondary to facial trauma and neuropathic pain involving the mental nerve. For use in the pediatric population or for repair of facial lacerations, the intraoral approach to blockade of the mental nerve should be considered. When using the intraoral approach in the pediatric population, the child's mother or father can actually place the anesthetic-soaked cotton ball in the alveolar sulcus under the pain management specialist's direction.

The pain specialist should carefully examine the patient before performing mental nerve block to identify preexisting neural compromise because the mental nerve is especially vulnerable to blunt trauma owing to the acute angle at which the mental nerve exits the mental foramen. This preblock assessment helps identify subtle neurologic changes that might subsequently be erroneously attributed to the block.

CHAPTER 21

Inferior Alveolar Nerve Block

CPT-2009 CODE	
Unilateral	64400
Bilateral	64400-50
Neurolytic	64600

Relative Value Units	
Unilateral	5
Bilateral	10
Neurolytic	20

INDICATIONS

Inferior alveolar nerve block is useful in the diagnosis and treatment of painful conditions in areas subserved by the inferior alveolar nerve, including post-traumatic neuralgias and pain secondary to intraoral malignancies. Inferior alveolar nerve block is especially useful in providing surgical anesthesia in the distribution of the inferior alveolar nerve for lesion removal, dental surgery, and laceration repair.

CLINICALLY RELEVANT ANATOMY

The inferior alveolar nerve arises from fibers of the mandibular nerve. The inferior alveolar nerve passes inferiorly to enter the mandibular canal. The nerve travels forward through the body of the mandible, providing sensory innervation to the molars and premolars as well as their associated gingiva. As the inferior alveolar nerve approaches the mental foramen, it divides into two branches. The incisor branch provides sensory innervation to the canines and incisors. The mental branch passes through the mental foramen to provide sensory innervation to the lower lip and corresponding gingival surface.

TECHNIQUE

The patient is placed in a supine position with the mouth wide open. A total of 5 mL of local anesthetic is drawn up in a 10-mL sterile syringe. When treating neuralgias involving the inferior alveolar nerve, facial trauma, or other painful or inflammatory conditions involving the inferior alveolar nerve, a total of 80 mg of depot-steroid is added to the local anesthetic with the first block, and 40 mg of depot-steroid is added with subsequent blocks. Neurolytic blocks with small amounts of 6.5% aqueous phenol can be performed for intractable pain secondary to malignancy.

The anterior margin of the mandible just above the last molar on the affected side is then identified by palpation. Topical anesthesia of the gingiva overlying this area is then obtained with either 10% cocaine solution or 2% viscous lidocaine applied via a $3\frac{1}{2}$-inch cotton-tipped applicator. After adequate topical anesthesia of the mucosa is obtained, a 25-gauge, 2-inch needle is advanced submucosally through the anesthetized area along the inner surface of the mandible (Figs. 21-1 and 21-2). A paresthesia may be elicited, and the patient should be warned of such. Three to 5 mL of solution is injected as the needle is slowly advanced.

SIDE EFFECTS AND COMPLICATIONS

The face is highly vascular, and the pain specialist should carefully calculate the total milligram dosage of local anesthetic that may be given safely, especially if bilateral nerve blocks are being performed. This vascularity gives rise to an increased incidence of postblock ecchymosis and hematoma formation. Despite the vascularity of this anatomic region, this technique can safely be performed in the presence of anticoagulation by using a 25- or 27-gauge needle, albeit at increased risk for hematoma, if the clinical situation dictates a favorable risk-to-benefit ratio. These complications can be decreased if manual pressure is applied to the area of the block immediately after injection.

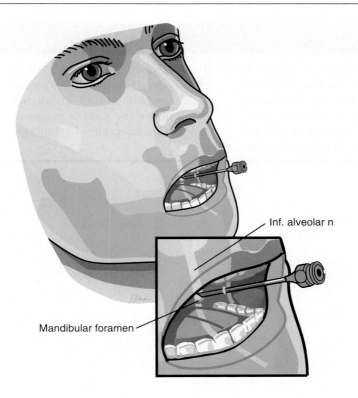

Figure 21-1.

Inf. alveolar n.

Mandibular foramen

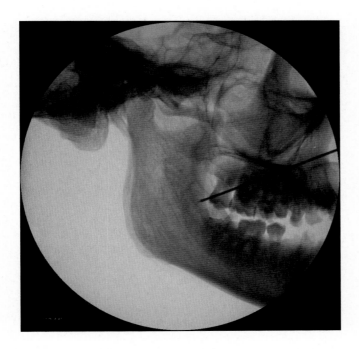

Figure 21-2.
Needle tip in proximity to inferior alveolar nerve.

CLINICAL PEARLS

Inferior alveolar nerve block is useful in the palliation of pain secondary to facial trauma and neuropathic pain involving the inferior alveolar nerve. For use in the pediatric population or for repair of intraoral lacerations, topical anesthesia of the mucosa should be considered before proceeding with injection of the local anesthetic. When using the technique in the pediatric population, the child's mother or father can hold the anesthetic-soaked cotton-tipped applicators in place under the pain management specialist's direction before injection of solution.

CHAPTER 22

Auriculotemporal Nerve Block

CPT-2009 CODE

Unilateral	64450
Bilateral	64450-50
Neurolytic	64640

Relative Value Units

Unilateral	10
Bilateral	20
Neurolytic	20

INDICATIONS

Auriculotemporal nerve block is useful in the diagnosis and treatment of painful conditions in areas subserved by the auriculotemporal nerve, including post-traumatic neuralgia, atypical facial pain involving the temporomandibular joint, acute herpes zoster involving the external auditory meatus, and pain secondary to malignancy. This technique is also useful in providing surgical anesthesia in the distribution of the auriculotemporal nerve for lesion removal and laceration repair.

CLINICALLY RELEVANT ANATOMY

The auriculotemporal nerve arises from fibers of the mandibular nerve. The auriculotemporal nerve courses upward through the parotid gland, passing between the temporomandibular joint and the external auditory meatus, where it gives off branches that provide sensory innervation to the temporomandibular joint and portions of the pinna of the ear and the external auditory meatus. Ascending over the origin of the zygomatic arch, the auriculotemporal nerve continues upward along with the temporal artery, providing sensory innervation to the temporal region and lateral scalp.

TECHNIQUE

The patient is placed in the supine position with the head turned away from the side to be blocked. A total of 5 mL of local anesthetic is drawn up in a 12-mL sterile syringe. When treating painful conditions involving the auriculotemporal nerve that may have an inflammatory component, a total of 80 mg of depot-steroid is added to the local anesthetic with the first block, and 40 mg of depot-steroid is added with subsequent blocks.

The temporal artery is identified at a point just above the origin of the zygoma on the affected side. After preparation of the skin with antiseptic solution, a 25-gauge, 1½-inch needle is inserted at this point and is advanced perpendicularly until the needle approaches the periosteum of the underlying bone (Fig. 22-1). A paresthesia may be elicited, and the patient should be warned of such. After gentle aspiration, 3 mL of solution is injected. The needle is then redirected in a cephalad trajectory, and after careful aspiration, the remaining 2 mL of solution is injected in a fanlike manner.

SIDE EFFECTS AND COMPLICATIONS

The scalp is highly vascular, and the auriculotemporal nerve is in close proximity to the temporal artery at the point at which the nerve is blocked. Therefore, the pain specialist should carefully calculate the total milligram dosage of local anesthetic that may be given safely, especially if bilateral nerve blocks are being performed. This vascularity gives rise to an increased incidence of post-block ecchymosis and hematoma formation. Despite the vascularity of this anatomic region, this technique can safely be performed in the presence of anticoagulation by using a 25- or 27-gauge needle, albeit at increased risk for hematoma, if the clinical situation dictates a favorable risk-to-benefit ratio. These complications can be decreased if manual pressure is applied to the area of the block immediately after injection. Application of cold packs for 20-minute periods after the block also decreases the amount of postprocedure pain and bleeding the patient may experience.

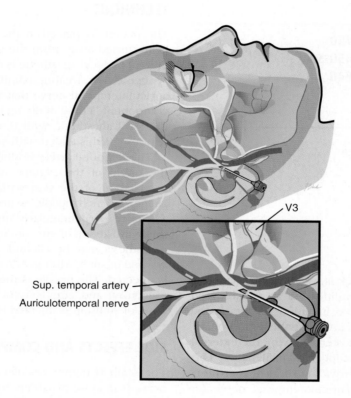

V3

Sup. temporal artery

Auriculotemporal nerve

Figure 22-1.

CLINICAL PEARLS

Auriculotemporal nerve block is especially useful in the palliation of pain secondary to acute herpes zoster involving the geniculate ganglion, such as Ramsay Hunt syndrome, when combined with facial nerve block. Aluminum acetate used as tepid soaks helps dry weeping lesions of the external auditory meatus and helps make the patient more comfortable.

Auriculotemporal nerve block is also useful in the management of atypical facial pain syndromes involving the temporomandibular joint. Blockade of the auriculotemporal nerve allows the physical therapist to more aggressively treat temporomandibular joint dysfunction.

CHAPTER 23

Greater Auricular Nerve Block

CPT-2009 CODE

Unilateral	64450
Bilateral	64450-50
Neurolytic	64640

Relative Value Units

Unilateral	8
Bilateral	12
Neurolytic	20

INDICATIONS

Greater auricular nerve block is useful in the diagnosis and treatment of painful conditions in areas subserved by the greater auricular nerve, including greater auricular neuralgia and pain secondary to herpes zoster. This technique is also useful in providing surgical anesthesia in the distribution of the greater auricular nerve for lesion removal and laceration repair.

CLINICALLY RELEVANT ANATOMY

The greater auricular nerve arises from fibers of the primary ventral ramus of the second and third cervical nerves. The greater auricular nerve pierces the fascia inferior and lateral to the lesser occipital nerve. It passes superiorly and forward and then curves around the sternocleidomastoid muscle, moving more superficially to provide cutaneous sensory innervation to the ear, external auditory canal, angle of the jaw, and the skin overlying a portion of the parotid gland (Fig. 23-1).

TECHNIQUE

The patient is placed in a sitting position with the cervical spine flexed and the forehead on a padded bedside table. A total of 5 mL of local anesthetic is drawn up in a 12-mL sterile syringe. When treating greater auricular neuralgia or other painful conditions involving the greater auricular nerve, a total of 80 mg of depot-steroid is added to the local anesthetic with the first block, and 40 mg of depot-steroid is added with subsequent blocks.

The mastoid process on the affected side is then identified by palpation. After preparation of the skin with antiseptic solution, a 22-gauge, $1\frac{1}{2}$-inch needle is inserted at the level of the mastoid process and is advanced perpendicularly until the needle approaches the periosteum of the underlying bone (Figs. 23-2 and 23-3). A paresthesia may be elicited, and the patient should be warned of such. The needle is then redirected toward the lobe of the ear. After gentle aspiration, 3 mL of solution is injected in a fanlike distribution. The needle is then redirected medially, and after careful aspiration, the remaining 2 mL of solution is injected in a fanlike manner (Fig. 23-4).

SIDE EFFECTS AND COMPLICATIONS

The scalp is highly vascular, and the pain specialist should carefully calculate the total milligram dosage of local anesthetic that may be given safely, especially if bilateral nerve blocks are being performed. This vascularity gives rise to an increased incidence of postblock ecchymosis and hematoma formation. Despite the vascularity of this anatomic region, this technique can safely be performed in the presence of anticoagulation by using a 25- or 27-gauge needle, albeit at increased risk for hematoma, if the clinical situation dictates a favorable risk-to-benefit ratio. These complications can be decreased if manual pressure is applied to the area of the block immediately after injection. Application of cold packs for 20-minute periods after the block also decreases the amount of postprocedure pain and bleeding the patient may experience.

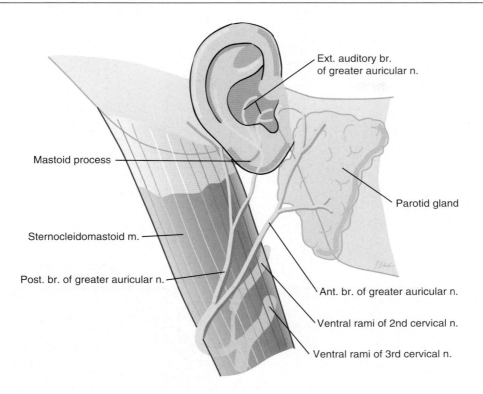

Ext. auditory br.
of greater auricular n.

Mastoid process

Parotid gland

Sternocleidomastoid m.

Post. br. of greater auricular n.

Ant. br. of greater auricular n.

Ventral rami of 2nd cervical n.

Ventral rami of 3rd cervical n.

Figure 23-1.

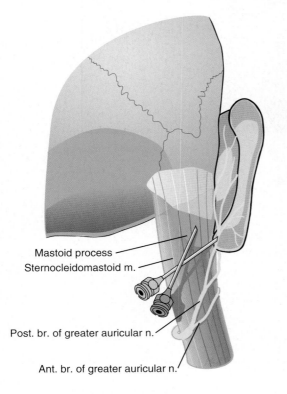

Mastoid process
Sternocleidomastoid m.

Post. br. of greater auricular n.

Ant. br. of greater auricular n.

Figure 23-2.

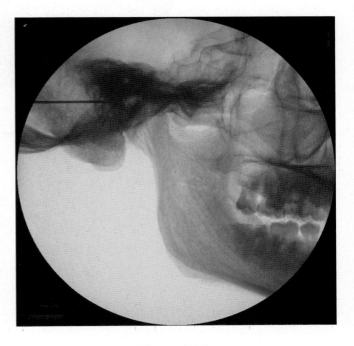

Figure 23-3.
Needle tip in proximity to the auriculotemporal nerve.

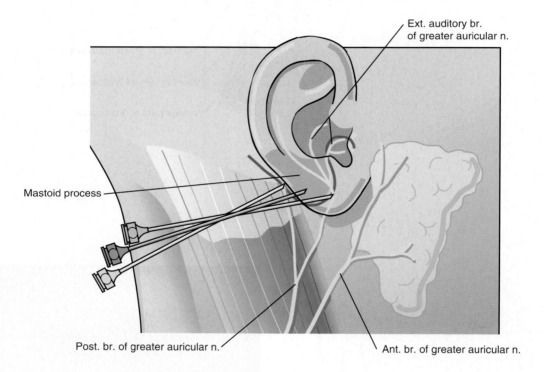

Ext. auditory br.
of greater auricular n.

Mastoid process

Post. br. of greater auricular n.

Ant. br. of greater auricular n.

Figure 23-4.

CLINICAL PEARLS

Greater auricular nerve block is especially useful in the palliation of pain secondary to acute herpes zoster involving the geniculate ganglion, such as Ramsay Hunt syndrome, when combined with facial nerve block. Aluminum acetate used as tepid soaks helps dry weeping lesions in the external auditory meatus and helps make the patient more comfortable.

Section 2

Neck

CHAPTER 24

Glossopharyngeal Nerve Block: Extraoral Approach

CPT-2009 CODE	
Unilateral	64999
Neurolytic	64640

Relative Value Units	
Unilateral	12
Neurolytic	20

INDICATIONS

In addition to applications for surgical anesthesia, glossopharyngeal nerve block with local anesthetic can be used as a diagnostic tool when performing differential neural blockade on an anatomic basis in the evaluation of head and facial pain. If destruction of the glossopharyngeal nerve is being considered, this technique is useful as a prognostic indicator of the degree of motor and sensory impairment that the patient may experience. Glossopharyngeal nerve block with local anesthetic may be used to palliate acute pain emergencies, including glossopharyngeal neuralgia and cancer pain, while waiting for pharmacologic, surgical, and antiblastic methods to become effective. Glossopharyngeal nerve block is also useful as an adjunct to awake endotracheal intubation.

Destruction of the glossopharyngeal nerve is indicated for the palliation of cancer pain, including invasive tumors of the posterior tongue, hypopharynx, and tonsils. This technique is especially useful in the management of the pain of glossopharyngeal neuralgia for those patients for whom medical management has not been effective or for patients who are not candidates for surgical microvascular decompression of the glossopharyngeal nerve.

Because of the desperate nature of many patients suffering from aggressively invasive head and face malignancies, blockade of the glossopharyngeal nerve using a 25-gauge needle may be carried out in the presence of coagulopathy or anticoagulation, albeit with an increased risk for ecchymosis and hematoma formation.

CLINICALLY RELEVANT ANATOMY

The glossopharyngeal nerve contains both motor and sensory fibers. The motor fibers innervate the stylopharyngeus muscle. The sensory portion of the nerve innervates the posterior third of the tongue, palatine tonsil, and mucous membranes of the mouth and pharynx. Special visceral afferent sensory fibers transmit information from the taste buds of the posterior third of the tongue. Information from the carotid sinus and body that helps control blood pressure, pulse, and respiration is carried via the carotid sinus nerve, which is a branch of the glossopharyngeal nerve. Parasympathetic fibers pass via the glossopharyngeal nerve to the otic ganglion. Post-ganglionic fibers from the ganglion carry secretory information to the parotid gland.

The glossopharyngeal nerve exits from the jugular foramen in proximity to the vagus and accessory nerves and the internal jugular vein (Figs. 24-1 and 24-2). All three nerves lie in the groove between the internal jugular vein and internal carotid artery.

The key landmark for extraoral glossopharyngeal nerve block is the styloid process of the temporal bone. This osseous process represents the calcification of the cephalad end of the stylohyoid ligament. Although usually easy to identify, the styloid process may be difficult to locate with the exploring needle if ossification is limited.

TECHNIQUE

The patient is placed in the supine position. An imaginary line is visualized running from the mastoid process to the angle of the mandible (Fig. 24-3). The styloid process should lie just below the midpoint of this line. The skin is prepped with antiseptic solution. A 22-gauge, 1½-inch needle attached to a 10-mL syringe is advanced at this midpoint location in a plane perpendicular to the

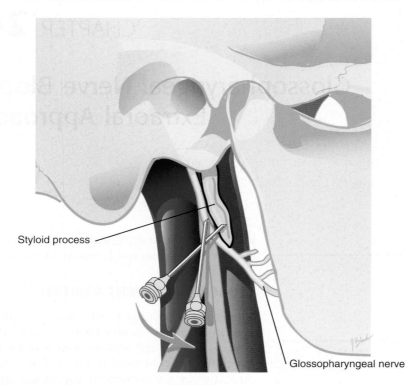

Figure 24-1.

Styloid process

Glossopharyngeal nerve

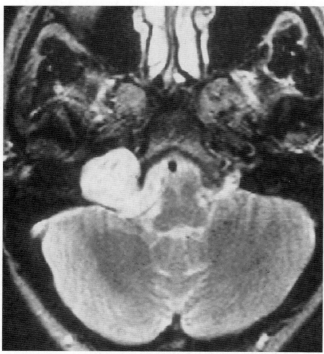

Figure 24-2.
Jugular fossa schwannoma in a 32-year-old woman. Axial T2-weighted magnetic resonance image. The sharply defined tumor centered in the right jugular foramen is well seen. The tumor represents a benign schwannoma with smooth expansion of the skull base but no involvement of the right internal auditory canal. (From Stark DD, Bradley WG: Magnetic Resonance Imaging, 3rd ed. St. Louis, Mosby, 1999, p 1217.)

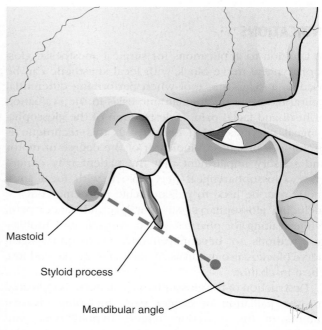

Mastoid

Styloid process

Mandibular angle

Figure 24-3.

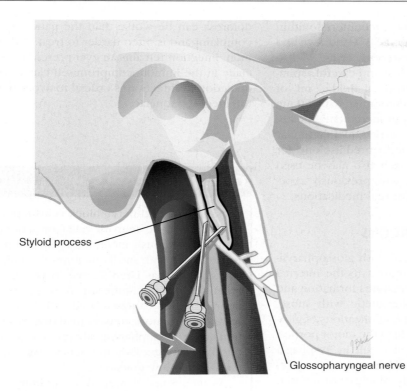

Figure 24-4.

Styloid process

Glossopharyngeal nerve

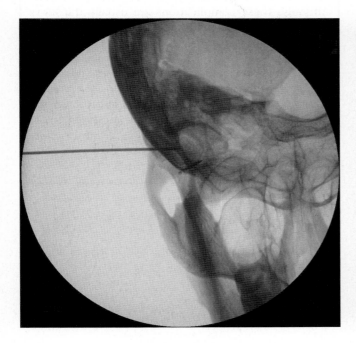

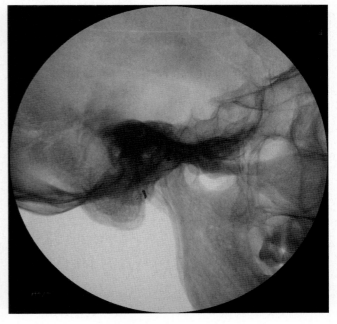

Figure 24-5.
AP view of the needle tip just behind the posterior aspect of the styloid process.

Figure 24-6.
Lateral view of the needle tip just behind the posterior aspect of the styloid process.

skin. The styloid process should be encountered within 3 cm. After contact is made, the needle is withdrawn and walked off the styloid process posteriorly (Figs. 24-4 to 24-6). As soon as bony contact is lost and careful aspiration reveals no blood or cerebrospinal fluid, 7 mL of 0.5% preservative-free lidocaine combined with 80 mg of methylprednisolone is injected in incremental doses. Subsequent daily nerve blocks are carried out in a similar manner, substituting 40 mg of methylprednisolone for the initial 80-mg dose. This approach also may be used for breakthrough pain in patients who previously experienced adequate pain control with oral medications.

SIDE EFFECTS AND COMPLICATIONS

The major complications associated with glossopharyngeal nerve block are related to trauma to the internal jugular vein and carotid artery. Hematoma formation and intravascular injection of local anesthetic with subsequent toxicity are not uncommon complications of glossopharyngeal nerve block. Blockade of the motor portion of the glossopharyngeal nerve can result in dysphagia secondary to weakness of the stylopharyngeus muscle. If the vagus nerve is inadvertently blocked, as is often the case during glossopharyngeal nerve block, dysphonia secondary to paralysis of the ipsilateral vocal cord may occur. A reflex tachycardia secondary to vagal nerve block is also observed in some patients. Inadvertent block of the hypoglossal and spinal accessory nerves during glossopharyngeal nerve block results in weakness of the tongue and trapezius muscle.

A small percentage of patients who undergo chemical neurolysis or neurodestructive procedures of the glossopharyngeal nerve experience postprocedure dysesthesias in the area of anesthesia. These symptoms range from a mildly uncomfortable burning or pulling sensation to severe pain. When this severe postprocedure pain occurs, it is called *anesthesia dolorosa*. Anesthesia dolorosa can be worse than the patient's original pain complaint and is often harder to treat. Although uncommon, infection remains an ever-present possibility, especially in the immunocompromised cancer patient. Early detection of infection is crucial to avoid potentially life-threatening sequelae.

CLINICAL PEARLS

Glossopharyngeal nerve block is a simple technique that can produce dramatic relief for patients suffering from the previously mentioned pain complaints. Neurolytic block with small quantities of alcohol, phenol, and glycerol has been shown to provide long-term relief for patients suffering from glossopharyngeal neuralgia and cancer-related pain who have not responded to more conservative treatments. Destruction of the glossopharyngeal nerve can also be carried out by creating a radiofrequency lesion under biplanar fluoroscopic guidance.

As mentioned earlier, the proximity of the glossopharyngeal nerve to major vasculature makes postblock hematoma and ecchymosis a distinct possibility. Although these complications are usually transitory in nature, their dramatic appearance can be quite upsetting to the patient, and therefore the patient should be warned of such before the procedure. The vascularity of this region also increases the incidence of inadvertent intravascular injection. Even small amounts of local anesthetic injected into the carotid artery at this level will result in local anesthetic toxicity and seizures. Incremental dosing while carefully monitoring the patient for signs of local anesthetic toxicity helps avoid this complication.

CHAPTER 25

Glossopharyngeal Nerve Block: Intraoral Approach

CPT-2009 CODE	
Unilateral	64999
Neurolytic	64640

Relative Value Units	
Unilateral	12
Neurolytic	20

INDICATIONS

Glossopharyngeal nerve block via the intraoral approach is used when anatomic distortion secondary to tumor or prior surgery makes the extraoral approach impossible. Its indications are the same as for the extraoral approach and include applications for surgical anesthesia and use as a diagnostic tool when performing differential neural blockade on an anatomic basis in the evaluation of head and facial pain. If destruction of the glossopharyngeal nerve is being considered, this technique is useful as a prognostic indicator of the degree of motor and sensory impairment that the patient may experience. Glossopharyngeal nerve block with local anesthetic may be used to palliate acute pain emergencies, including glossopharyngeal neuralgia and cancer pain, while waiting for pharmacologic, surgical, and antiblastic methods to become effective. Glossopharyngeal nerve block is also useful as an adjunct to awake endotracheal intubation.

Destruction of the glossopharyngeal nerve is indicated for the palliation of cancer pain, including invasive tumors of the posterior tongue, hypopharynx, and tonsils. In this setting, the extraoral approach may be preferred to avoid injection through tumor mass or distorted anatomy. This technique is especially useful in the management of the pain of glossopharyngeal neuralgia for those patients for whom medical management has not been effective or for patients who are not candidates for surgical microvascular decompression of the glossopharyngeal nerve.

Because of the desperate nature of many patients suffering from aggressively invasive head and face malignancies, blockade of the glossopharyngeal nerve using a 25-gauge needle may be carried out in the presence of coagulopathy or anticoagulation, albeit with an increased risk for ecchymosis and hematoma formation.

CLINICALLY RELEVANT ANATOMY

The key landmark for intraoral glossopharyngeal nerve block is the palatine tonsil. The glossopharyngeal nerve lies submucosally just medial to the palatine tonsil. The internal carotid artery lies just posterior and lateral to the nerve, making inadvertent intra-arterial needle placement a distinct possibility.

The glossopharyngeal nerve contains both motor and sensory fibers. The motor fibers innervate the stylopharyngeus muscle. The sensory portion of the nerve innervates the posterior third of the tongue, palatine tonsil, and mucous membranes of the mouth and pharynx. Special visceral afferent sensory fibers transmit information from the taste buds of the posterior third of the tongue. Information from the carotid sinus and body that helps control blood pressure, pulse, and respiration is carried via the carotid sinus nerve, which is a branch of the glossopharyngeal nerve. Parasympathetic fibers pass via the glossopharyngeal nerve to the otic ganglion. Postganglionic fibers from the ganglion carry secretory information to the parotid gland.

The glossopharyngeal nerve exits from the jugular foramen in proximity to the vagus and accessory nerves and the internal jugular vein (Fig. 25-1). All three nerves lie in the groove between the internal jugular vein and internal carotid artery. The nerve proceeds inferiorly and courses medially, where it lies submucosally behind the palatine tonsil, allowing easy access via the intraoral approach.

TECHNIQUE

The patient is placed in the supine position. The tongue is anesthetized with 2% viscous lidocaine. The patient

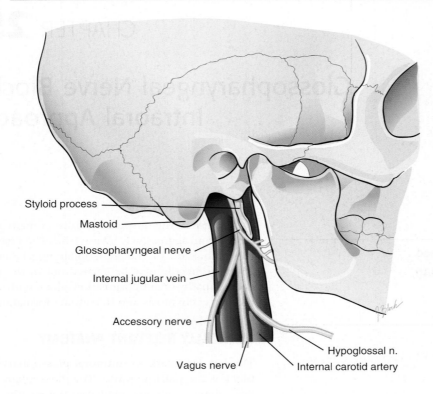

Styloid process

Mastoid

Glossopharyngeal nerve

Internal jugular vein

Accessory nerve

Vagus nerve

Hypoglossal n.

Internal carotid artery

Figure 25-1.

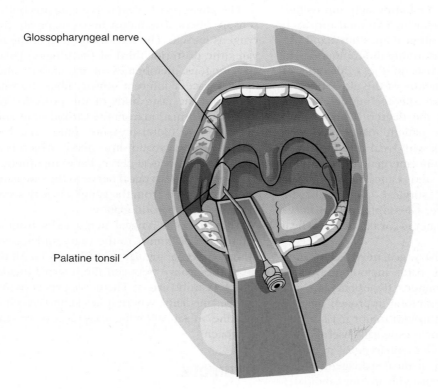

Glossopharyngeal nerve

Palatine tonsil

Figure 25-2.

opens the mouth wide, and the tongue is then retracted inferiorly with a tongue depressor or laryngoscope blade. A 22-gauge, $3\frac{1}{2}$-inch spinal needle that has been bent about 25 degrees is inserted through the mucosa at the lower lateral portion of the posterior tonsillar pillar (Fig. 25-2). The needle is advanced approximately 0.5 cm. After careful aspiration for blood and cerebrospinal fluid, 7 mL of 0.5% preservative-free lidocaine combined with 80 mg of methylprednisolone is injected in incremental doses. Subsequent daily nerve blocks are carried out in a similar manner, substituting 40 mg of methylprednisolone for the initial 80-mg dose.

SIDE EFFECTS AND COMPLICATIONS

The major complications associated with glossopharyngeal nerve block are related to trauma to the internal jugular vein and carotid artery. Hematoma formation and intravascular injection of local anesthetic with subsequent toxicity are not uncommon after glossopharyngeal nerve block. Blockade of the motor portion of the glossopharyngeal nerve can result in dysphagia secondary to weakness of the stylopharyngeus muscle.

A small percentage of patients who undergo chemical neurolysis or neurodestructive procedures of the glossopharyngeal nerve experience postprocedure dysesthesias in the area of anesthesia. These symptoms range from a mildly uncomfortable burning or pulling sensation to severe pain. When this severe postprocedure pain occurs, it is called *anesthesia dolorosa*. Anesthesia dolorosa can be worse than the patient's original pain complaint and is often harder to treat.

Although uncommon, infection remains an ever-present possibility, especially in the immunocompromised cancer patient. Early detection of infection is crucial to avoid potentially life-threatening sequelae.

CLINICAL PEARLS

The intraoral approach to glossopharyngeal nerve block is used when anatomic distortion secondary to tumor or prior surgery makes the extraoral approach impossible. Glossopharyngeal nerve block is a simple technique that can produce dramatic relief for patients suffering from the previously mentioned pain complaints. Neurolytic block with small quantities of alcohol, phenol, and glycerol has been shown to provide long-term relief for patients suffering from glossopharyngeal neuralgia and cancer-related pain who have not responded to more conservative treatments. Destruction of the glossopharyngeal nerve can also be carried out by creating a radiofrequency lesion under biplanar fluoroscopic guidance.

As mentioned earlier, the proximity of the glossopharyngeal nerve to major vasculature makes post-block hematoma and ecchymosis a distinct possibility. Although these complications are usually transitory in nature, their dramatic appearance can be quite upsetting to the patient, and therefore the patient should be warned of such before the procedure. The vascularity of this region also increases the incidence of inadvertent intravascular injection. Even small amounts of local anesthetic injected into the carotid artery at this level will result in local anesthetic toxicity and seizures. Incremental dosing while carefully monitoring the patient for signs of local anesthetic toxicity helps avoid this complication.

CHAPTER 26

Glossopharyngeal Nerve Block: Radiofrequency Lesioning

CPT-2009 CODE	
Unilateral	64999
Neurolytic	64640

Relative Value Units	
Unilateral	12
Neurolytic	20

INDICATIONS

Destruction of the glossopharyngeal nerve is indicated for the palliation of cancer pain, including invasive tumors of the posterior tongue, hypopharynx, and tonsils. This technique is especially useful in the management of the pain of glossopharyngeal neuralgia for those patients for whom medical management has not been effective or for patients who are not candidates for surgical microvascular decompression of the glossopharyngeal nerve. In recent years, radiofrequency lesioning has gained in popularity as the technique of choice when destruction of the glossopharyngeal nerve is indicated.

CLINICALLY RELEVANT ANATOMY

The glossopharyngeal nerve contains both motor and sensory fibers. The motor fibers innervate the stylopharyngeus muscle. The sensory portion of the nerve innervates the posterior third of the tongue, palatine tonsil, and mucous membranes of the mouth and pharynx. Special visceral afferent sensory fibers transmit information from the taste buds of the posterior third of the tongue. Information from the carotid sinus and body that helps control blood pressure, pulse, and respiration is carried via the carotid sinus nerve, which is a branch of the glossopharyngeal nerve. Parasympathetic fibers pass via the glossopharyngeal nerve to the otic ganglion. Postganglionic fibers from the ganglion carry secretory information to the parotid gland.

The glossopharyngeal nerve exits from the jugular foramen in proximity to the vagus and accessory nerves and the internal jugular vein (Fig. 26-1). All three nerves lie in the groove between the internal jugular vein and internal carotid artery.

The key landmark for extraoral glossopharyngeal nerve block is the styloid process of the temporal bone. This osseous process represents the calcification of the cephalad end of the stylohyoid ligament. Although usually easy to identify, the styloid process may be difficult to locate with the exploring needle if ossification is limited.

TECHNIQUE

The patient is placed in the supine position. An imaginary line is visualized running from the mastoid process to the angle of the mandible (Fig. 26-2). The styloid process should lie just below the midpoint of this line. The skin is prepped with antiseptic solution, and local anesthetic is injected into the skin and subcutaneous tissues at the intended site of needle entry. A 20-gauge, 10-cm blunt curved radiofrequency needle with a 10-mm active tip is placed via a 16-gauge introducer needle through the previously anesthetized area until the tip rests against the styloid process (Figs. 26-3 and 26-4). The styloid process should be encountered within 3 cm. After contact is made, the needle is withdrawn and walked off the styloid process posteriorly (Fig. 26-5). As soon as bony contact is lost and careful aspiration reveals no blood or cerebrospinal fluid, a small amount of nonionic contrast media can be injected to demonstrate proper needle position and confirm the absence of vascular runoff. Sensory stimulation up to 1 V at 50 Hz should produce stimulation at the base of the tongue, pharynx, and ipsilateral tonsillar fossa. The patient should be carefully observed for stimulation-induced bradycardia or hypotension. Motor stimulation at 2 to 2.5 V at 2 Hz is then carried out to demonstrate the lack of stimulation of the muscles innervated by the phrenic and spinal accessory nerves. Then, 2 mL of 1% lidocaine is injected, and after allowing for the drug to produce

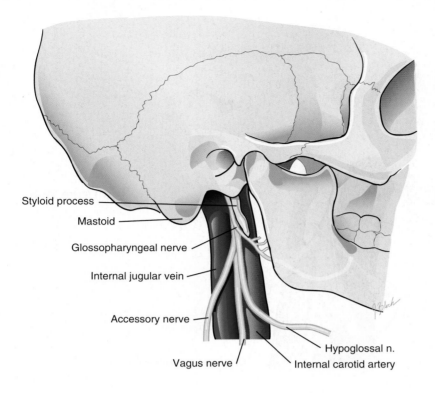

Figure 26-1.

Styloid process

Mastoid

Glossopharyngeal nerve

Internal jugular vein

Accessory nerve

Vagus nerve

Hypoglossal n.

Internal carotid artery

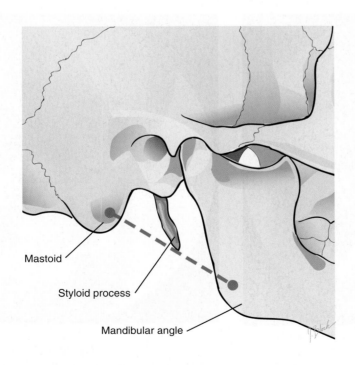

Figure 26-2.

Mastoid

Styloid process

Mandibular angle

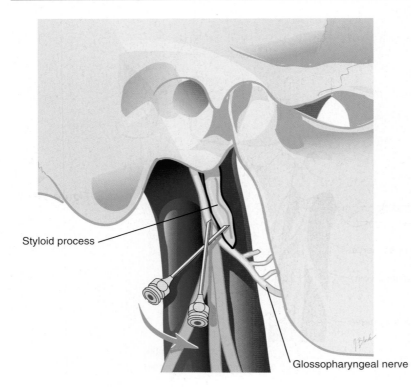

Figure 26-3.

Styloid process

Glossopharyngeal nerve

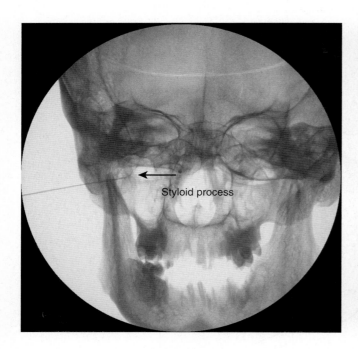

Figure 26-4.
Needle tip resting against the styloid process.

Styloid process

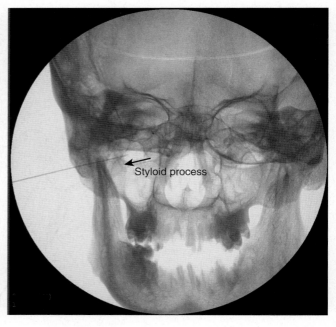

Figure 26-5.
Needle tip just behind the posterior aspect of the styloid process in proximity to the glossopharyngeal nerve.

Styloid process

anesthesia, pulsed radiofrequency lesioning is carried out at a rate of 2 Hz with a pulse width of 20 milliseconds at a temperature of 42°C for a duration of 120 seconds. This sequence is repeated 2 or 3 times.

SIDE EFFECTS AND COMPLICATIONS

The major complications associated with radiofrequency lesioning of the glossopharyngeal nerve are related to trauma to the internal jugular vein and carotid artery. Hematoma formation and intravascular injection of local anesthetic with subsequent toxicity are not uncommon complications of glossopharyngeal nerve block. The patient should be informed that blockade of the motor portion of the glossopharyngeal nerve can result in dysphagia secondary to weakness of the stylopharyngeus muscle. If the vagus nerve is inadvertently blocked, as is often the case during glossopharyngeal nerve block, dysphonia secondary to paralysis of the ipsilateral vocal cord may occur. A reflex tachycardia secondary to vagal nerve block also is observed in some patients. Inadvertent block of the hypoglossal and spinal accessory nerves during glossopharyngeal nerve block results in weakness of the tongue and trapezius muscle.

A small percentage of patients who undergo chemical neurolysis or neurodestructive procedures of the glossopharyngeal nerve experience postprocedure dysesthesias in the area of anesthesia. These symptoms range from a mildly uncomfortable burning or pulling sensation to severe pain. When this severe postprocedure pain occurs, it is called *anesthesia dolorosa*. Anesthesia dolorosa can be worse than the patient's original pain complaint and is often harder to treat. Although uncommon, infection remains an ever-present possibility, especially in the immunocompromised cancer patient. Early detection of infection is crucial to avoid potentially life-threatening sequelae.

CLINICAL PEARLS

Glossopharyngeal nerve block is a simple technique that can produce dramatic relief for patients suffering from the previously mentioned pain complaints. Neurolytic block with small quantities of alcohol, phenol, and glycerol has been shown to provide long-term relief for patients suffering from glossopharyngeal neuralgia and cancer-related pain who have not responded to more conservative treatments. Destruction of the glossopharyngeal nerve can also be carried out by creating a radiofrequency lesion under biplanar fluoroscopic guidance. Stimulation during radiofrequency lesioning of the glossopharyngeal nerve can induce bradycardia and hypotension in some patients.

As mentioned earlier, the proximity of the glossopharyngeal nerve to major vasculature makes post-block hematoma and ecchymosis a distinct possibility. Although these complications are usually transitory in nature, their dramatic appearance can be quite upsetting to the patient, and therefore the patient should be warned of such before the procedure. The vascularity of this region also increases the incidence of inadvertent intravascular injection. Even small amounts of local anesthetic injected into the carotid artery at this level will result in local anesthetic toxicity and seizures. Incremental dosing while carefully monitoring the patient for signs of local anesthetic toxicity helps avoid this complication.

CHAPTER **27**

Vagus Nerve Block

CPT-2009 CODE	
Unilateral	64408
Neurolytic	64640

Relative Value Units	
Unilateral	12
Neurolytic	20

INDICATIONS

Vagus nerve block with local anesthetic can be used as a diagnostic tool when performing differential neural blockade on an anatomic basis in the evaluation of head and facial pain. If destruction of the vagus nerve is being considered, this technique is useful as a prognostic indicator of the degree of motor and sensory impairment that the patient may experience. Vagus nerve block with local anesthetic may be used to palliate acute pain emergencies, including vagal neuralgia and cancer pain, while waiting for pharmacologic, surgical, and antiblastic methods to become effective. Vagus nerve block is used as a diagnostic and therapeutic maneuver in those patients suspected of suffering from vagal neuralgia. Destruction of the vagus nerve is indicated for the palliation of cancer pain, including invasive tumors of the larynx, hypopharynx, and pyriform sinus and occasionally intrathoracic malignancies.

Because of the desperate nature of many patients suffering from aggressively invasive head and neck malignancies, blockade of the vagus nerve using a 25-gauge needle may be carried out in the presence of coagulopathy or anticoagulation, albeit with an increased risk for ecchymosis and hematoma formation.

CLINICALLY RELEVANT ANATOMY

The vagus nerve contains both motor and sensory fibers. The motor fibers innervate the pharyngeal muscle and provide fibers for the superior and recurrent laryngeal nerves. The sensory portion of the nerve innervates the dura mater of the posterior fossa, the posterior aspect of the external auditory meatus, the inferior aspect of the tympanic membrane, and the mucosa of the larynx below the vocal cords. The vagus nerve also provides fibers to the intrathoracic contents, including the heart, lungs, and major vasculature.

The vagus nerve exits from the jugular foramen in close proximity to the spinal accessory nerve (Fig. 27-1). The vagus nerve lies just caudad to the glossopharyngeal nerve and is superficial to the internal jugular vein. The vagus nerve courses downward from the jugular foramen within the carotid sheath along with the internal jugular vein and internal carotid artery.

Blockade of the vagus nerve is carried out in a manner analogous to glossopharyngeal nerve block. The key landmark for vagus nerve block is the styloid process of the temporal bone. This osseous process represents the calcification of the cephalad end of the stylohyoid ligament. Although usually easy to identify, the styloid process may be difficult to locate with the exploring needle if ossification is limited.

TECHNIQUE

The patient is placed in the supine position. An imaginary line is visualized running from the mastoid process to the angle of the mandible. The styloid process should lie just below the midpoint of this line. The skin is prepared with antiseptic solution. A 22-gauge, 1½-inch needle attached to a 10-mL syringe is advanced at this midpoint location in a plane perpendicular to the skin. The styloid process should be encountered within 3 cm (Figs. 27-2 and 27-3). After contact is made, the needle is withdrawn and walked off the styloid process posteriorly and in a slightly inferior trajectory. The needle is advanced about 0.5 cm past the depth at which the styloid process was identified. If careful aspiration reveals no blood or cerebrospinal fluid, 5 mL of 0.5% preservative-free lidocaine combined with 80 mg of methylprednisolone is injected in incremental doses. Subsequent daily nerve blocks are carried out in a similar manner,

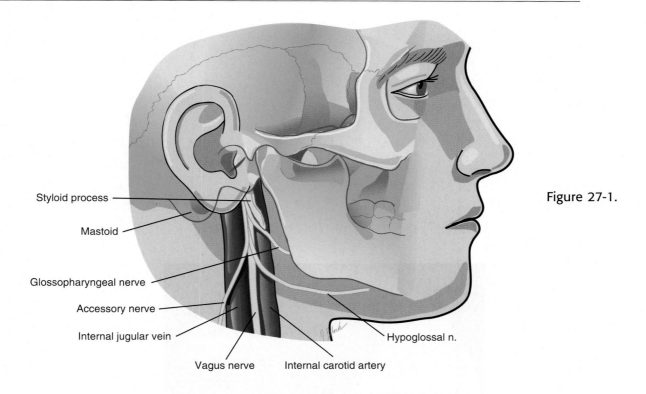

Styloid process

Mastoid

Glossopharyngeal nerve

Accessory nerve

Internal jugular vein

Vagus nerve   Internal carotid artery

Hypoglossal n.

Figure 27-1.

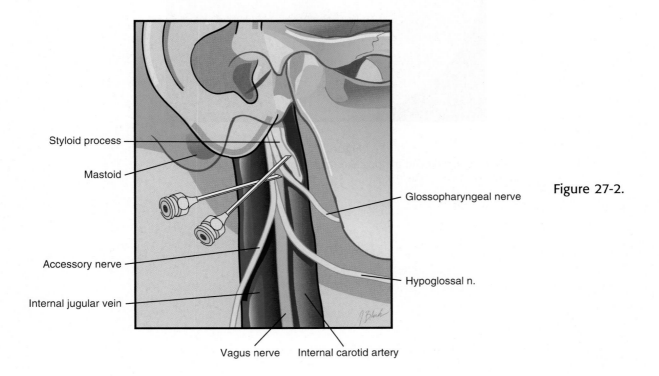

Styloid process

Mastoid

Glossopharyngeal nerve

Accessory nerve

Hypoglossal n.

Internal jugular vein

Vagus nerve   Internal carotid artery

Figure 27-2.

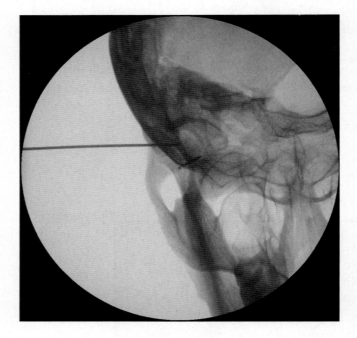

Figure 27-3.
Needle tip just behind the posterior aspect of the styloid process in proximity to the vagus nerve.

substituting 40 mg of methylprednisolone for the initial 80-mg dose. This approach also may be used for breakthrough pain in patients who previously experienced adequate pain control with oral medications.

SIDE EFFECTS AND COMPLICATIONS

The major complications associated with vagus nerve block are related to trauma to the internal jugular vein and carotid artery. Hematoma formation and intravascular injection of local anesthetic with subsequent toxicity are not uncommon after vagus nerve block. Blockade of the motor portion of the vagus nerve can result in dys-

phonia and difficulty coughing due to blockade of the superior and recurrent laryngeal nerves. A reflex tachycardia secondary to vagal nerve block is also observed in some patients. Inadvertent block of the glossopharyngeal, hypoglossal, and spinal accessory nerves during vagus nerve block will result in weakness of the tongue and trapezius muscle and numbness in the distribution of the glossopharyngeal nerve.

Although uncommon, infection remains an ever-present possibility, especially in the immunocompromised cancer patient. Early detection of infection is crucial to avoid potentially life-threatening sequelae.

CLINICAL PEARLS

Vagus nerve block should be considered in two clinical situations: (1) in patients with vagal neuralgia and (2) in patients with cancer in the previously mentioned areas who suffer persistent ill-defined pain that fails to respond to conservative measures. Vagal neuralgia is clinically analogous to trigeminal and glossopharyngeal neuralgia. It is characterized by paroxysms of shocklike pain into the thyroid and laryngeal areas. Pain may occasionally radiate into the jaw and upper thoracic region. Attacks of vagal neuralgia may be precipitated by coughing, yawning, and swallowing. Excessive salivation also may be present. This is a rare pain syndrome and should be considered a diagnosis of exclusion.

Neurolytic block with small quantities of alcohol, phenol, and glycerol has been shown to provide long-term relief for patients suffering from vagus neuralgia and cancer-related pain who have not responded to

more conservative treatments. Destruction of the vagus nerve can be also carried out by creating a radiofrequency lesion under biplanar fluoroscopic guidance.

As mentioned earlier, the proximity of the vagus nerve to major vasculature makes postblock hematoma and ecchymosis a distinct possibility. Although these complications are usually transitory in nature, their dramatic appearance can be quite upsetting to the patient, and therefore the patient should be warned of such before the procedure. The vascularity of this region also increases the incidence of inadvertent intravascular injection. Even small amounts of local anesthetic injected into the carotid artery at this level will result in local anesthetic toxicity and seizures. Incremental dosing while carefully monitoring the patient for signs of local anesthetic toxicity helps avoid this complication.

CHAPTER 28

Spinal Accessory Nerve Block

INDICATIONS

Spinal accessory nerve block is useful in the diagnosis and treatment of spasm of the sternocleidomastoid or trapezius muscle. It is also occasionally useful as a diagnostic maneuver to determine whether spasm of these muscles is being mediated via the spinal accessory nerve. Spinal accessory nerve block with local anesthetic is also used in a prognostic manner before destruction of the spinal accessory nerve for the palliation of spastic conditions of the sternocleidomastoid or trapezius muscle. Neurodestruction of the spinal accessory nerve may be carried out by chemoneurolysis, cryoneurolysis, radiofrequency lesioning, surgical crushing, or resection of the nerve.

CLINICALLY RELEVANT ANATOMY

The spinal accessory nerve arises from the nucleus ambiguus. The nerve has two roots, which leave the cranium together along with the vagus nerve via the jugular foramen. The fibers of the spinal root pass inferiorly and posteriorly to provide motor innervation to the superior portion of the sternocleidomastoid muscle. The spinal accessory exits the posterior border of the sternocleidomastoid muscle in the upper third of the muscle. The nerve, in combination with the cervical plexus, provides innervation to the trapezius muscle.

TECHNIQUE

The patient is placed in a supine position with the head turned away from the side to be blocked. A total of 10 mL of local anesthetic is drawn up in a 20-mL sterile syringe. When treating conditions that are mediated via the spinal accessory nerve that are thought to have an inflammatory component, a total of 80 mg of depot-steroid is added to the local anesthetic with the first block, and 40 mg of depot-steroid is added with subsequent blocks.

The patient is then asked to raise his or her head against the resistance of the pain specialist's hand to aid in identification of the posterior border of the sternocleidomastoid muscle. The posterior border of the upper third of the muscle is then identified. At a point just behind the posterior border of the upper third of the sternocleidomastoid muscle, after preparation of the skin with antiseptic solution, a 1½-inch needle is inserted with a slightly anterior trajectory (Fig. 28-1). After inserting the needle to a depth of about ¾ inch, gentle aspiration is carried out to identify blood or cerebrospinal fluid. If the aspiration test is negative and no paresthesia into the brachial plexus is elicited, 10 mL of solution is slowly injected in a fanlike manner, with close monitoring of the patient for signs of local anesthetic toxicity or inadvertent subarachnoid injection.

SIDE EFFECTS AND COMPLICATIONS

The proximity to the external jugular vein and other large vessels suggests the potential for inadvertent intravascular injection or local anesthetic toxicity from intravascular absorption. The pain specialist should carefully calculate the total milligram dosage of local anesthetic that may be given safely. This vascularity also gives rise to an increased incidence of postblock ecchymosis and hematoma formation. Despite the vascularity of this anatomic region, this technique can safely be performed in the presence of anticoagulation by using a 25- or 27-gauge needle, albeit at increased risk for hematoma, if the clinical situation dictates a favorable risk-to-benefit

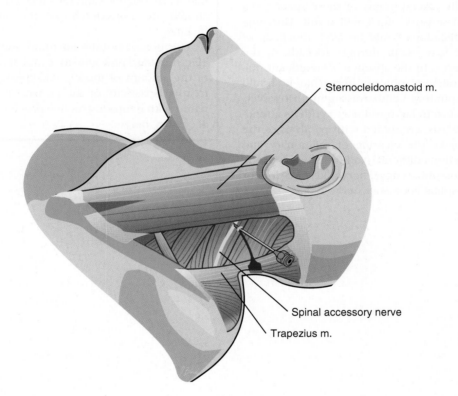

Sternocleidomastoid m.

Spinal accessory nerve

Trapezius m.

Figure 28-1.

ratio. These complications can be decreased if manual pressure is applied to the area of the block immediately after injection. Application of cold packs for 20 minutes on, 20 minutes off, after the block also decreases the amount of postprocedure pain and bleeding the patient may experience.

In addition to the potential for complications involving the vasculature, the proximity of the spinal accessory nerve to the central neuraxial structures and the phrenic nerve can result in side effects and complications. If the needle is placed too deep, the potential for inadvertent epidural, subdural, or subarachnoid injection is a possibility. If the volume of local anesthetic used for this block is accidentally placed in any of these spaces, significant motor and sensory block will result. Unrecognized, these complications could be fatal. Blockade of the phrenic nerve may occur during blockade of the spinal accessory nerve. In the absence of significant pulmonary disease, unilateral phrenic nerve block should rarely create respiratory embarrassment. However, blockade of the recurrent laryngeal nerve with its attendant vocal cord paralysis, combined with paralysis of the diaphragm, may make the clearing of pulmonary and upper airway secretions difficult. Additionally, blockade of the vagus and glossopharyngeal nerves also may occur when performing spinal accessory nerve block.

CLINICAL PEARLS

A clear diagnosis of the cause of spastic conditions of the cervical musculature should be ascertained before spinal accessory nerve block. Demyelinating disease, the cervical dystonias (including spasmodic torticollis), and posterior fossa and brain-stem tumors must be ruled out. The workup should include magnetic resonance imaging of the head, with special attention to the posterior fossa and brain stem, as well as electromyograms and, if indicated, trimodal evoked potentials. Laboratory testing for the inflammatory myopathies and the collagen vascular diseases should be considered as the clinical situation dictates.

The use of botulinum toxin administered under electromyographic guidance may allow better control of the amount of muscle weakness produced when treating spasticity of the cervical musculature compared with neurodestructive procedures of the spinal accessory nerve.

CHAPTER 29

Phrenic Nerve Block

CPT-2009 CODE	
Unilateral	64410
Neurolytic	64640

Relative Value Units	
Unilateral	12
Neurolytic	20

INDICATIONS

Phrenic nerve block is useful in the diagnosis and treatment of intractable hiccups. It is also occasionally useful as both a diagnostic and therapeutic maneuver to determine whether pain from subdiaphragmatic processes, including abscess and malignancy, is being mediated via the phrenic nerve. Phrenic nerve block with local anesthetic is also used in a prognostic manner before destruction of the phrenic nerve for palliation of intractable hiccups. Neurodestruction of the phrenic nerve may be carried out by chemoneurolysis, cryoneurolysis, radiofrequency lesioning, surgical crushing, or resection of the nerve.

CLINICALLY RELEVANT ANATOMY

The phrenic nerve arises from fibers of the primary ventral ramus of the fourth cervical nerve, with contributions from the third and fifth cervical nerves. The phrenic nerve passes inferiorly between the omohyoid and sternocleidomastoid muscles and exits the root of the neck between the subclavian artery and vein to enter the mediastinum. The right phrenic nerve follows the course of the vena cava to provide motor innervation to the right hemidiaphragm. The left phrenic nerve descends to provide motor innervation to the left hemidiaphragm in a course parallel to that of the vagus nerve.

TECHNIQUE

The patient is placed in a supine position with the head turned away from the side to be blocked. A total of 10 mL of local anesthetic is drawn up in a 20-mL sterile syringe. When treating painful conditions associated with inflammation that are mediated via the phrenic nerve, a total of 80 mg of depot-steroid is added to the local anesthetic with the first block, and 40 mg of depot-steroid is added with subsequent blocks.

The patient is then asked to raise his or her head against the resistance of the pain specialist's hand to aid in identification of the posterior border of the sternocleidomastoid muscle. In most patients, a groove between the posterior border of the sternocleidomastoid muscle and the anterior scalene muscle can be palpated. At a point 1 inch above the clavicle, at this groove or just slightly behind the posterior border of the sternocleidomastoid muscle, after preparation of the skin with antiseptic solution, a 1½-inch needle is inserted with a slightly anterior trajectory (Fig. 29-1). After inserting the needle to a depth of about 1 inch, gentle aspiration is carried out to identify blood or cerebrospinal fluid. If the aspiration test is negative and no paresthesia into the brachial plexus is elicited, 10 mL of solution is slowly injected in a fanlike manner, with close monitoring of the patient for signs of local anesthetic toxicity or inadvertent subarachnoid injection.

SIDE EFFECTS AND COMPLICATIONS

The proximity to the external jugular vein and other large vessels suggests the potential for inadvertent intravascular injection or local anesthetic toxicity from intravascular absorption. The pain specialist should carefully calculate the total milligram dosage of local anesthetic that may be given safely. This vascularity also gives rise to an increased incidence of postblock ecchymosis and hematoma formation. Despite the vascularity of this anatomic region, this technique can safely be performed in the presence of anticoagulation by using a 25- or 27-

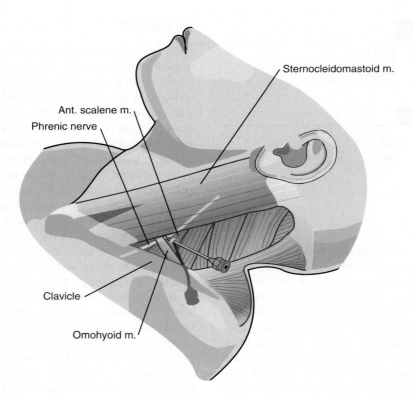

Sternocleidomastoid m.

Ant. scalene m.

Phrenic nerve

Clavicle

Omohyoid m.

Figure 29-1.

gauge needle, albeit at increased risk for hematoma, if the clinical situation dictates a favorable risk-to-benefit ratio. These complications can be decreased if manual pressure is applied to the area of the block immediately after injection. Application of cold packs for 20 minutes on, 20 minutes off, after the block also decreases the amount of postprocedure pain and bleeding the patient may experience.

In addition to the potential for complications involving the vasculature, the proximity of the phrenic nerve to the central neuraxial structures and the spinal accessory nerve can result in side effects and complications. If the needle is placed too deep, the potential for inadvertent epidural, subdural, or subarachnoid injection is a possibility. If the volume of local anesthetic used for this block is accidentally placed in any of these spaces, significant motor and sensory block will result. Unrecognized, these complications could be fatal. In the absence of significant pulmonary disease, unilateral phrenic nerve block should rarely create respiratory embarrassment. However, blockade of the recurrent laryngeal nerve with its attendant vocal cord paralysis, combined with paralysis of the diaphragm, may make the clearing of pulmonary and upper airway secretions difficult.

CLINICAL PEARLS

Phrenic nerve block is useful in both the diagnosis and palliation of pain secondary to malignancies of the subdiaphragmatic region that produce ill-defined referred pain in the supraclavicular region. This referred pain is known as Kerr's sign and generally does not respond to treatments focused on the primary subdiaphragmatic tumor. The use of phrenic nerve block for intractable hiccups can be of great value to patients with this distressing problem for whom pharmacologic management has failed. A cause should be determined for the intractable hiccups before destruction of the phrenic nerve. The workup should include magnetic resonance imaging of the head, with special attention to the posterior fossa and brain stem as well as a careful evaluation of the subdiaphragmatic region. Additionally, the pain specialist should be aware that there is a high incidence of intractable hiccups associated with the macroglobulinemias, and such a possibility should be evaluated.

CHAPTER **30**

Facial Nerve Block

INDICATIONS

Facial nerve block is useful in the diagnosis and treatment of painful conditions and facial spasms subserved by the facial nerve, including geniculate neuralgia, atypical facial neuralgias, the pain associated with Bell's palsy, herpes zoster involving the geniculate ganglion (Ramsay Hunt syndrome), and spastic conditions including hemifacial spasm.

CLINICALLY RELEVANT ANATOMY

The facial nerve provides both motor and sensory fibers to the head. The facial nerve arises from the brain stem at the inferior margin of the pons. The sensory portion of the facial nerve is called the *nervus intermedius*. As it leaves the pons, the nervus intermedius is susceptible to compression, producing a "trigeminal neuralgia–like" syndrome called geniculate neuralgia (Fig. 30-1). After leaving the pons, the fibers of the facial nerve travel across the subarachnoid space and enter the internal auditory meatus to pass through the petrous temporal bone. The nerve then exits the base of the skull via the stylomastoid foramen. It passes downward and then turns forward to pass through the parotid gland, where it divides into fibers that provide innervation to the muscles of facial expression (Fig. 30-2).

TECHNIQUE

The patient is placed in a supine position with the head turned away from the side to be blocked to allow easy access to the mastoid process on the affected side. A total of 3 mL of local anesthetic is drawn up in a 12-mL sterile syringe. When treating geniculate neuralgia, herpes zoster, or other painful conditions involving the facial nerve, a total of 80 mg of depot-steroid is added to the local anesthetic with the first block, and 40 mg of depot-steroid is added with subsequent blocks.

The mastoid process on the affected side is then identified by palpation. After preparation of the skin with antiseptic solution, a 22-gauge, $1\frac{1}{2}$-inch needle is inserted at the anterior border of the mastoid process immediately below the external auditory meatus and at the level of the middle of the ramus of the mandible. The needle is then advanced perpendicularly until the needle approaches the periosteum of the underlying mastoid bone (Figs. 30-3 and 30-4). The needle is then redirected slightly more anteriorly until it slides past the anterior border of the mastoid. The needle is slowly advanced about $\frac{1}{2}$ inch beyond the edge of the mastoid (Fig. 30-5). This places the needle in proximity to the point at which the facial nerve exits the stylomastoid foramen. After gentle aspiration for blood and cerebrospinal fluid, 3 to 4 mL of solution is injected in incremental doses.

SIDE EFFECTS AND COMPLICATIONS

This anatomic region is highly vascular, and because of the proximity to major vessels, the pain specialist should carefully observe the patient for signs of local anesthetic toxicity during injection. This vascularity and proximity to major blood vessels also give rise to an increased incidence of postblock ecchymosis and hematoma formation, and the patient should be warned of such. Despite the vascularity of this anatomic region, this technique can safely be performed in the presence of anticoagulation by using a 25- or 27-gauge needle, albeit at increased risk for hematoma, if the clinical situation dictates a favorable risk-to-benefit ratio. These complications can be decreased if manual pressure is applied to the area of the block immediately after injection. Application of cold packs for 20 minutes on, 20 minutes off, after the block also decreases the amount of postprocedure pain and bleeding the patient may experience.

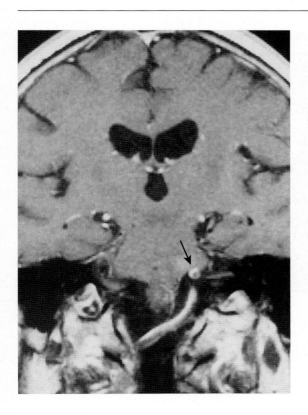

Figure 30-1.
Vascular compression of the left seventh nerve in an elderly patient with hemifacial spasm. Coronal view showing the vascular compression of the left seventh nerve with a "loop" of the basilar artery adjacent to the root exit zone. (From Stark DD, Bradley WG: Magnetic Resonance Imaging, 3rd ed. St. Louis, Mosby, 1999, p 1215.)

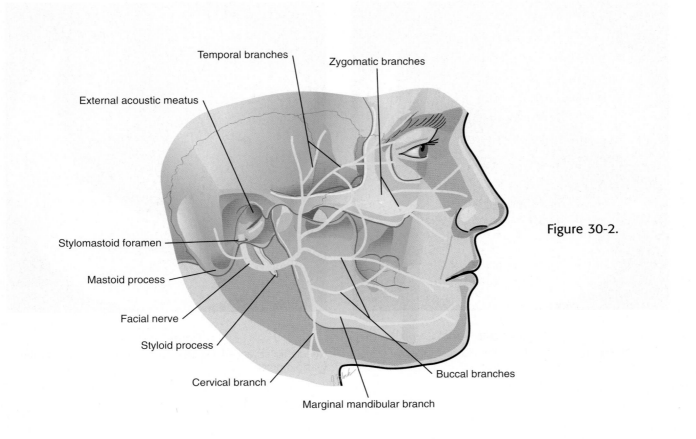

Figure 30-2.

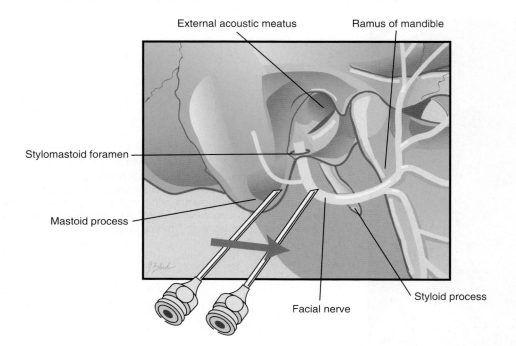

External acoustic meatus

Ramus of mandible

Stylomastoid foramen

Mastoid process

Facial nerve

Styloid process

Figure 30-3.

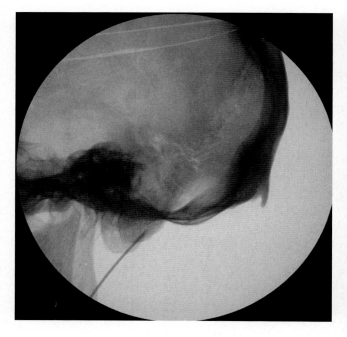

Figure 30-4.
Needle tip resting against the mastoid process.

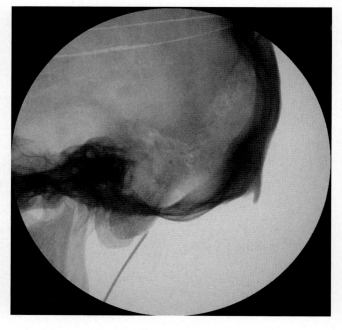

Figure 30-5.
Needle tip advanced just beyond the posterior aspect of the mastoid process.

Because of the proximity to the spinal column, it is also possible to inadvertently inject the local anesthetic into the epidural, subdural, or subarachnoid space. At this level, even small amounts of local anesthetic placed into the subarachnoid space may result in a total spinal anesthetic.

CLINICAL PEARLS

Facial nerve block is especially useful in the palliation of pain secondary to acute herpes zoster involving the geniculate ganglion (Ramsay Hunt syndrome). The addition of tepid aluminum acetate soaks helps dry weeping lesions and makes the patient more comfortable. Facial nerve block is also useful in the management of geniculate neuralgia that has failed to respond to pharmacologic management. Geniculate neuralgia is a rare unilateral facial pain syndrome analogous to trigeminal and glossopharyngeal neuralgia. It is characterized by paroxysms of shocklike pain deep in the ear that are triggered by talking and swallowing. Brainstem tumors involving the facial nerve may mimic this syndrome, and magnetic resonance imaging, with special attention to the posterior fossa and brain stem, and brain-stem evoked response testing are indicated when the diagnosis of geniculate neuralgia is suspected.

CHAPTER 31

Superficial Cervical Plexus Block

CPT-2009 CODE	
Unilateral	64413
Neurolytic	64613

Relative Value Units	
Unilateral	10
Neurolytic	20

INDICATIONS

Superficial cervical plexus block is useful in the diagnosis and treatment of painful conditions subserved by the nerves of the superficial cervical plexus, including post-trauma pain and pain of malignant origin. This technique also is used to provide surgical anesthesia in the distribution of the superficial cervical plexus for lesion removal, laceration repair, and carotid endarterectomy. Neurodestructive procedures of the superficial cervical plexus may be indicated for pain of malignant origin that fails to respond to conservative measures.

CLINICALLY RELEVANT ANATOMY

The superficial cervical plexus arises from fibers of the primary ventral rami of the first, second, third, and fourth cervical nerves. Each nerve divides into an ascending and a descending branch providing fibers to the nerves above and below, respectively. This collection of nerve branches makes up the cervical plexus, which provides both sensory and motor innervation. The most important motor branch is the phrenic nerve, with the plexus also providing motor fibers to the spinal accessory nerve and to the paravertebral and deep muscles of the neck. Each nerve, with the exception of the first cervical nerve, provides significant cutaneous sensory innervation. These nerves converge at the midpoint of the sternocleidomastoid muscle at its posterior margin to provide sensory innervation to the skin of the lower mandible, neck, and supraclavicular fossa. Terminal sensory fibers

of the superficial cervical plexus contribute to nerves including the greater auricular and lesser occipital nerves.

TECHNIQUE

The patient is placed in a supine position with the head turned away from the side to be blocked. A total of 15 mL of local anesthetic is drawn up in a 20-mL sterile syringe. When treating painful conditions involving the superficial cervical plexus, a total of 80 mg of depot-steroid is added to the local anesthetic with the first block, and 40 mg of depot-steroid is added with subsequent blocks.

The midpoint of the posterior border of the sternocleidomastoid muscle is identified by careful palpation. After preparation of the skin with antiseptic solution, a 22-gauge, $1\frac{1}{2}$-inch needle is inserted at this point and is advanced just past the sternocleidomastoid muscle (Fig. 31-1). After gentle aspiration, 5 mL of solution is slowly injected. The needle is then redirected in a line that would pass just behind the lobe of the ear. After gentle aspiration, an additional 5 mL of solution is injected in a fanlike distribution. The needle is then redirected inferiorly toward the ipsilateral nipple, and after careful aspiration, the remaining 5 to 6 mL of solution is injected in a fanlike manner.

SIDE EFFECTS AND COMPLICATIONS

The proximity to the external jugular vein and other large vessels suggests the potential for inadvertent intravascular injection or local anesthetic toxicity from intravascular absorption. The pain specialist should carefully calculate the total milligram dosage of local anesthetic that may be given safely, especially if bilateral nerve blocks are being performed. This vascularity also gives rise to an increased incidence of postblock ecchymosis and hematoma formation. Despite the vascularity of this anatomic region, this technique can be performed safely in the presence of anticoagulation by using a 25- or 27-gauge needle, albeit at increased risk for hematoma, if

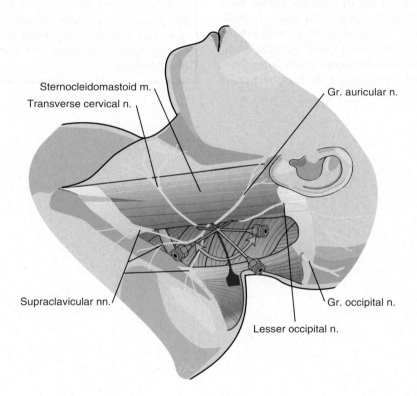

Figure 31-1.

the clinical situation dictates a favorable risk-to-benefit ratio. These complications can be decreased if manual pressure is applied to the area of the block immediately after injection. Application of cold packs for 20 minutes on, 20 minutes off, after the block also decreases the amount of postprocedure pain and bleeding the patient may experience.

In addition to the potential for complications involving the vasculature, the proximity of the superficial cervical plexus to the central neuraxial structures and the phrenic nerve can result in side effects and complications. If the needle is placed too deep, the potential for inadvertent epidural, subdural, or subarachnoid injection is a possibility. If the volume of local anesthetic used for this block is accidentally placed in any of these spaces, significant motor and sensory block will result. Unrecognized, these complications could be fatal. Additionally, blockade of the phrenic nerve occurs commonly after superficial cervical plexus block. In the absence of significant pulmonary disease, unilateral phrenic nerve block should rarely create respiratory embarrassment. However, if bilateral block is used for surgical indications, respiratory complications can occur.

CLINICAL PEARLS

Superficial cervical plexus block is useful in the palliation of pain secondary to malignancies of the neck, including malignant melanoma, that may result in superficial tissue damage but may not invade the deep structures of the neck. Careful monitoring of the patient's respiratory status should be undertaken any time bilateral superficial cervical plexus blocks are performed because the phrenic nerve is often also blocked.

CHAPTER 32

Deep Cervical Plexus Block

CPT-2009 CODE	
Unilateral	64413
Neurolytic	64613

Relative Value Units	
Unilateral	12
Neurolytic	20

INDICATIONS

Deep cervical plexus block is useful in the diagnosis and treatment of painful conditions subserved by the deep cervical plexus, including post-trauma pain and pain of malignant origin. This technique is also used to provide surgical anesthesia in the distribution of the nerves of the deep cervical plexus for lesion removal, laceration repair, carotid endarterectomy, and other surgeries of the neck that require muscle relaxation. Blockade of the plexus with botulinum toxin has been shown to be useful in the palliation of cervical dystonias. Neurodestructive procedures of the deep cervical plexus may be indicated for pain of malignant origin that fails to respond to other conservative measures.

CLINICALLY RELEVANT ANATOMY

The deep cervical plexus arises from fibers of the primary ventral rami of the first, second, third, and fourth cervical nerves. Each nerve divides into an ascending and a descending branch providing fibers to the nerves above and below, respectively. This collection of nerve branches makes up the cervical plexus, which provides both sensory and motor innervation. The most important motor branch of the cervical plexus is the phrenic nerve. The plexus also provides motor fibers to the spinal accessory nerve and to the paravertebral and deep muscles of the neck. Each nerve, with the exception of the first cervical nerve, provides significant cutaneous sensory innervation. Terminal sensory fibers of the deep cervical plexus contribute fibers to the greater auricular and lesser occipital nerves.

TECHNIQUE

The patient is placed in a supine position with the head turned away from the side to be blocked. A total of 15 mL of local anesthetic is drawn up in a 20-mL sterile syringe. When treating painful conditions involving the deep cervical plexus, a total of 80 mg of depot-steroid is added to the local anesthetic with the first block, and 40 mg of depot-steroid is added with subsequent blocks.

A line is drawn between the mastoid process and the posterior aspect of the insertion of the sternocleidomastoid muscle at the clavicle. A point about 2 inches below the mastoid process is then identified (Fig. 32-1). After preparation of the skin with antiseptic solution, a 22-gauge, 1½-inch needle is inserted about ½ inch in front of the previously identified point on the line. This places the needle at the C3 or C4 level and allows a single needle to be used to block the deep cervical plexus. The needle is advanced to a depth of about 1 inch in a slightly anterior and caudad direction to avoid entering a neural foramen or slipping between the transverse process and entering the vertebral artery. A paresthesia will usually be elicited, and the patient should be warned of such. If a paresthesia is not elicited, the needle should be withdrawn and redirected in a slightly anterior trajectory. Once a paresthesia is obtained and gentle aspiration reveals no evidence of blood or cerebrospinal fluid, 15 mL of solution is slowly injected in incremental doses, with monitoring of the patient for signs of local anesthetic toxicity or inadvertent subarachnoid injection.

SIDE EFFECTS AND COMPLICATIONS

The proximity to the external jugular vein and other large vessels suggests the potential for inadvertent intravascular injection or local anesthetic toxicity from intravascular absorption. The pain specialist should carefully calculate the total milligram dosage of local anesthetic

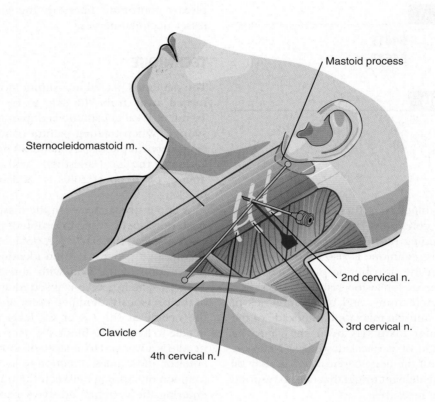

Figure 32-1.

that may be given safely, especially if bilateral nerve blocks are being performed. This vascularity also gives rise to an increased incidence of postblock ecchymosis and hematoma formation. Despite the vascularity of this anatomic region, this technique can be performed safely in the presence of anticoagulation by using a 25- or 27-gauge needle, albeit at increased risk for hematoma, if the clinical situation dictates a favorable risk-to-benefit ratio. These complications can be decreased if manual pressure is applied to the area of the block immediately after injection. Application of cold packs for 20 minutes on, 20 minutes off, after the block also decreases the amount of postprocedure pain and bleeding the patient may experience.

In addition to the potential for complications involving the vasculature, the proximity of the deep cervical plexus to the central neuraxial structures and the phrenic nerve can result in side effects and complications. If the needle is placed too deep, the potential for inadvertent epidural, subdural, or subarachnoid injection is a possibility. If the volume of local anesthetic used for this block is accidentally placed in any of these spaces, significant motor and sensory block will result. Unrecog-

nized, these complications could be fatal. Additionally, blockade of the phrenic nerve occurs commonly after deep cervical plexus block. In the absence of significant pulmonary disease, unilateral phrenic nerve block should rarely create respiratory embarrassment. However, if bilateral block is used for surgical indications, respiratory complications can occur.

CLINICAL PEARLS

Deep cervical plexus block is useful in the palliation of pain secondary to malignancies of the neck that have invaded the deep structures of the neck. The use of botulinum toxin to block the deep cervical plexus has represented a great advance in the treatment of cervical dystonias, including spasmodic torticollis, a syndrome that has been notoriously hard to treat. Careful monitoring of the patient's respiratory status should be undertaken any time bilateral deep cervical plexus blocks are performed because the phrenic nerve is often blocked.

CHAPTER 33

Superior Laryngeal Nerve Block

CPT-2009 CODE	
Unilateral	64408
Bilateral	64408-50
Neurolytic	64640

Relative Value Units	
Unilateral	10
Bilateral	20
Neurolytic	20

INDICATIONS

Superior laryngeal nerve block is useful in the diagnosis and treatment of painful conditions of the larynx and pharynx above the glottis, including pain of malignant origin. Bilateral superior laryngeal nerve block is also useful as an adjunct to topical anesthesia when performing awake intubation, laryngoscopy, bronchoscopy, and transesophageal echocardiography.

CLINICALLY RELEVANT ANATOMY

The superior laryngeal nerve arises from the vagus nerve with a small contribution from the superior cervical ganglion. The nerve passes inferiorly and anteriorly behind the carotid arteries to pass the lateral extent of the hyoid bone. The internal branch of this nerve provides sensory innervation to the mucous membranes of the lower portion of the epiglottis inferiorly to the area just above the vocal cords. An external branch provides innervation to the cricothyroid muscle.

TECHNIQUE

The patient is placed in a supine position with the head turned slightly away from the side to be blocked. A total of 4 mL of local anesthetic is drawn up in a 10 mL sterile syringe. When treating conditions that are mediated via the superior laryngeal nerve that are thought to have an inflammatory component, including pain of malignant origin, a total of 80 mg of depot-steroid is added to the local anesthetic with the first block, and 40 mg of depot-steroid is added with subsequent blocks. Neurolytic blocks may be performed with small, incremental doses of 6.5% aqueous phenol or absolute alcohol.

The lateral border of the hyoid bone and the upper outer margin of the thyroid cartilage are identified. At a point between these two, after preparation of the skin with antiseptic solution, a 25-gauge, $\frac{5}{8}$-inch needle is inserted perpendicular to the skin (Fig. 33-1). After inserting the needle to a depth of about $\frac{1}{2}$ inch, gentle aspiration is carried out to identify blood or air that would indicate intratracheal placement. If the aspiration test is negative, 2 mL of solution is slowly injected, with close monitoring of the patient for signs of local anesthetic toxicity.

SIDE EFFECTS AND COMPLICATIONS

The proximity to the carotid artery, external jugular vein, and other vessels suggests the potential for inadvertent intravascular injection or local anesthetic toxicity from intravascular absorption. The pain specialist should carefully calculate the total milligram dosage of local anesthetic that may be given safely. This vascularity also gives rise to an increased incidence of postblock ecchymosis and hematoma formation. Despite the vascularity of this anatomic region, this technique can be performed safely in the presence of anticoagulation by using a 25- or 27-gauge needle, albeit at increased risk for hematoma, if the clinical situation dictates a favorable risk-to-benefit ratio. These complications can be decreased if manual pressure is applied to the area of the block immediately after injection. Application of cold packs for 20 minutes on, 20 minutes off, after the block also decreases the amount of postprocedure pain and bleeding the patient may experience.

In addition to the potential for complications involving the vasculature, the proximity of the superior laryn-

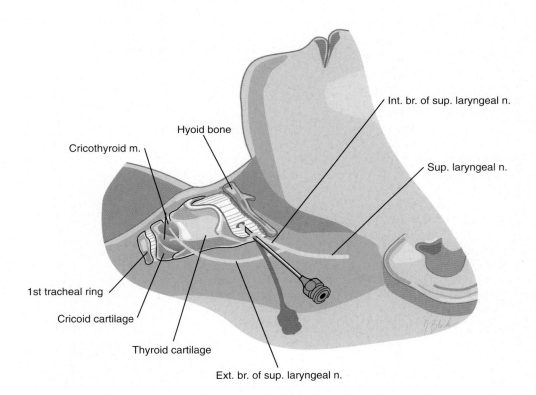

Int. br. of sup. laryngeal n.

Hyoid bone

Cricothyroid m.

Sup. laryngeal n.

1st tracheal ring

Cricoid cartilage

Thyroid cartilage

Ext. br. of sup. laryngeal n.

Figure 33-1.

geal nerve to the trachea makes intratracheal injection a possibility. Blockade of the superior laryngeal nerve puts the patient at risk for occult aspiration, especially if bilat- eral block is performed for diagnostic or therapeutic purposes.

CLINICAL PEARLS

Superior laryngeal nerve block is a useful technique in the palliation of pain secondary to upper airway malig- nancies. Although bilateral block is often required, it is recommended that only one side be blocked at a time to minimize untoward effects of the block.

CHAPTER 34

Recurrent Laryngeal Nerve Block

CPT-2009 CODE

Unilateral	64408
Bilateral	64408-50
Neurolytic	64640

Relative Value Units

Unilateral	10
Bilateral	20
Neurolytic	20

INDICATIONS

Recurrent laryngeal nerve block is useful in the diagnosis and treatment of painful conditions of the larynx arising below the vocal cords and the tracheal mucosa, including pain of malignant origin.

CLINICALLY RELEVANT ANATOMY

The recurrent laryngeal nerves arise from the vagus nerve. The right and left nerves follow different paths to reach the larynx and trachea. The right recurrent laryngeal nerve loops underneath the innominate artery and then ascends in the lateral groove between the trachea and esophagus to enter the inferior portion of the larynx. The left recurrent laryngeal nerve loops below the arch of the aorta and then ascends in the lateral groove between the trachea and esophagus to enter the inferior portion of the larynx (Fig. 34-1). These nerves provide the innervation to all the intrinsic muscles of the larynx except the cricothyroid muscle as well as providing the sensory innervation for the mucosa below the vocal cords.

TECHNIQUE

The patient is placed in a supine position with the head turned slightly away from the side to be blocked. A total of 4 mL of local anesthetic is drawn up in a 10-mL sterile syringe. When treating conditions that are mediated via the recurrent laryngeal nerve that are thought to have an inflammatory component, including pain of malignant origin, a total of 80 mg of depot-steroid is added to the local anesthetic with the first block, and 40 mg of depot-steroid is added with subsequent blocks. Neurolytic blocks may be performed with small, incremental doses of 6.5% aqueous phenol or absolute alcohol.

The medial border of the sternocleidomastoid muscle is identified at the level of the first tracheal ring (Fig. 34-2). At this point, after preparation of the skin with antiseptic solution, a 25-gauge, $\frac{5}{8}$-inch needle is inserted perpendicular to the skin. After inserting the needle to a depth of about $\frac{1}{2}$ inch, gentle aspiration is carried out to identify blood or air that would indicate intratracheal placement. If the aspiration test is negative, 2 mL of solution is slowly injected, with close monitoring of the patient for signs of local anesthetic toxicity.

SIDE EFFECTS AND COMPLICATIONS

The proximity to the carotid artery, external jugular vein, and other vessels suggests the potential for inadvertent intravascular injection or local anesthetic toxicity from intravascular absorption. The pain specialist should carefully calculate the total milligram dosage of local anesthetic that may be given safely. This vascularity also gives rise to an increased incidence of postblock ecchymosis and hematoma formation. Despite the vascularity of this anatomic region, this technique can be performed safely in the presence of anticoagulation by using a 25- or 27-gauge needle, albeit at increased risk for hematoma, if the clinical situation dictates a favorable risk-to-benefit ratio. These complications can be decreased if manual pressure is applied to the area of the block immediately after injection. Application of cold packs for 20 minutes on, 20 minutes off, after the block also decreases the amount of postprocedure pain and bleeding the patient may experience.

Because the recurrent laryngeal nerves provide the innervation to all the intrinsic muscles of the larynx except the cricothyroid muscle, bilateral recurrent laryn-

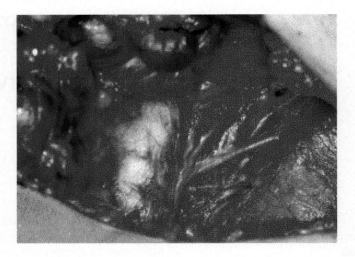

Figure 34-1.

Left recurrent laryngeal nerve with its trifurcations. (From Guglielmo A, Revelli L, D'Alatri L, et al: Revisited anatomy of the recurrent laryngeal nerves. Am J Surg 187:249-253, 2004.)

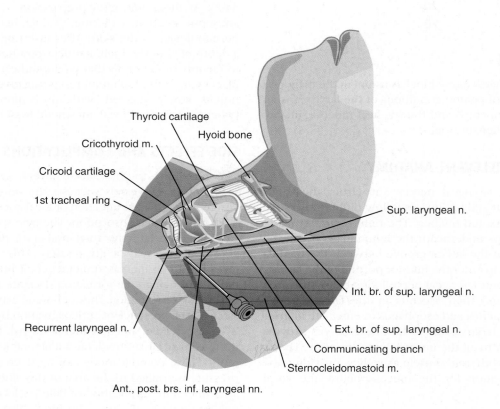

Figure 34-2.

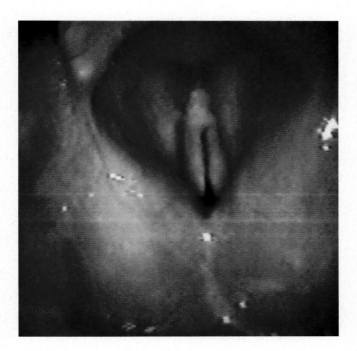

Figure 34-3.
Both vocal cords are immobile in the paramedian position with a slightly glottic gap. (From Endo K, Okabe Y, Maruyama Y, et al: Bilateral vocal cord paralysis caused by laryngeal mask airway. Am J Otolaryngol 28:126-129, 2007.)

geal nerve block is reserved for those patients who have undergone laryngectomy or tracheostomy because the resulting bilateral vocal cord paralysis could result in airway obstruction.

CLINICAL PEARLS

Recurrent laryngeal nerve block is a useful technique in the palliation of pain secondary to upper airway malignancies. Bilateral block should be reserved for those patients who have undergone previous laryngectomy to avoid airway obstruction from bilateral vocal cord paralysis (Fig. 34-3). When treating cancer pain of the larynx and upper trachea, recurrent laryngeal nerve block often has to be combined with superior laryngeal nerve block to obtain adequate pain control.

CHAPTER 35

Stellate Ganglion Block: Anterior Approach

CPT-2009 CODE	
Unilateral	64510
Neurolytic	64680

Relative Value Units	
Unilateral	12
Neurolytic	20

INDICATIONS

Stellate ganglion block is indicated in the treatment of acute herpes zoster in the distribution of the trigeminal nerve and cervical and upper thoracic dermatomes as well as frostbite and acute vascular insufficiency of the face and upper extremities. Stellate ganglion block is also indicated in the treatment of reflex sympathetic dystrophy of the face, neck, upper extremity, and upper thorax, Raynaud's syndrome of the upper extremities, and sympathetically mediated pain of malignant origin. There are clinical reports to suggest that stellate ganglion blocks also may be useful in the acute palliation of some atypical vascular headaches.

CLINICALLY RELEVANT ANATOMY

The stellate ganglion is located on the anterior surface of the longus colli muscle. This muscle lies just anterior to the transverse processes of the seventh cervical and first thoracic vertebrae. The stellate ganglion is made up of the fused portion of the seventh cervical and first thoracic sympathetic ganglia. The stellate ganglion lies anteromedial to the vertebral artery and is medial to the common carotid artery and jugular vein. The stellate ganglion is lateral to the trachea and esophagus.

TECHNIQUE

The patient is placed in the supine position with the cervical spine in neutral position. From 7 to 10 mL of local anesthetic without preservative is drawn into a 12-mL sterile syringe. For disease processes that have a component of inflammation, such as acute herpes zoster, or disease processes with associated edema, such as reflex sympathetic dystrophy, 80 mg of methylprednisolone is added for the first block, and 40 mg of methylprednisolone is added for subsequent blocks.

The medial edge of the sternocleidomastoid muscle is identified at the level of the cricothyroid notch (C6). The sternocleidomastoid muscle is then displaced laterally with two fingers, and the tissues overlying the transverse process of C6 (Chassaignac's tubercle) are compressed. The pulsations of the carotid artery are then identified under the palpating fingers (Fig. 35-1). The skin medial to the carotid pulsation is prepared with antiseptic solution, and a 22-gauge, 1½-inch needle is advanced until contact is made with the transverse process of C6 (Fig. 35-2). If bony contact is not made with needle insertion to a depth of 1 inch, the needle is probably between the transverse processes of C6 and C7. If this occurs, the needle should be withdrawn and reinserted with a more cephalad trajectory. After bony contact is made, the needle is then withdrawn about 2 mm to bring the needle tip out of the body of the longus colli muscle. Careful aspiration is carried out, and 7 to 10 mL of solution is then injected (Fig. 35-3). Figure 35-4 demonstrates the extensive spread of contrast medium above and below the site of injection.

SIDE EFFECTS AND COMPLICATIONS

This anatomic region is highly vascular, and because of the proximity of major vessels, the pain specialist should carefully observe the patient for signs of local anesthetic toxicity during injection. This vascularity and proximity to major blood vessels also give rise to an increased incidence of postblock ecchymosis and hematoma formation, and the patient should be warned of such. Despite the vascularity of this anatomic region, this technique can be performed safely in the presence of anticoagulation by using a 25- or 27-gauge needle, albeit at increased risk for hematoma, if the clinical situation

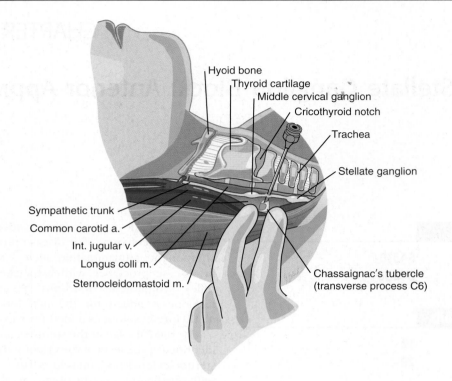

Figure 35-1.

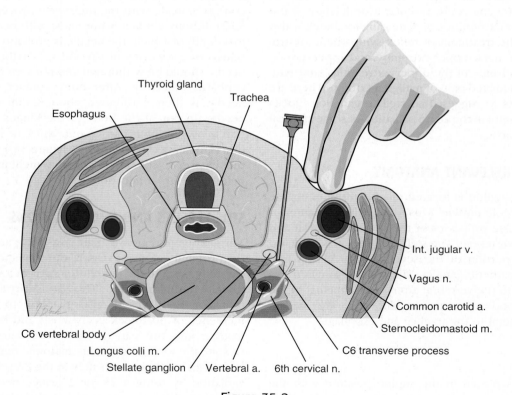

Figure 35-2.

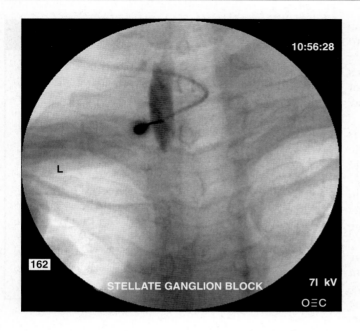

Figure 35-3.
Contrast medium surrounding the stellate ganglion.

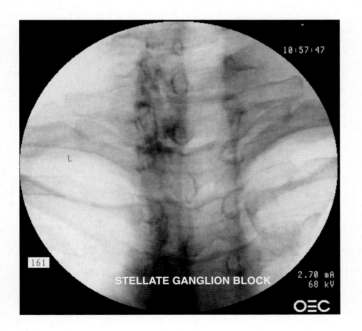

Figure 35-4.
Extensive spread of contrast medium after injection for stellate ganglion block.

dictates a favorable risk-to-benefit ratio. These complications can be decreased if manual pressure is applied to the area of the block immediately after injection. The application of cold packs for 20 minutes on, 20 minutes off, after the block also decreases the amount of postprocedure pain and bleeding the patient may experience.

Because of the proximity to the spinal column, it is also possible to inadvertently inject the local anesthetic solution into the epidural, subdural, or subarachnoid space. At this level, even small amounts of local anesthetic placed into the subarachnoid space may result in total spinal anesthesia. If needle placement is too inferior, pneumothorax is possible because the dome of the lung lies at the level of the C7-T1 interspace.

Additional side effects associated with stellate ganglion block include inadvertent block of the recurrent laryngeal nerve with associated hoarseness and dysphagia and the sensation that there is a lump in the throat when swallowing. Horner's syndrome occurs when the superior cervical sympathetic ganglion is also blocked during stellate ganglion block. The patient should be forewarned of the possibility of these complications before stellate ganglion block.

CLINICAL PEARLS

Properly performed stellate ganglion block is a safe and effective technique for treatment of the previously mentioned pain syndromes. Improperly performed, it can be one of the most dangerous regional anesthetic techniques used in pain management. Almost all the complications associated with stellate ganglion block can be avoided if two simple rules are always followed: (1) the C6 level must always be accurately identified and double-checked by identifying the cricothyroid notch; and (2) the needle tip must always make bony contact with the transverse process of C6 before the injection of any drugs. Always forewarn the patient of the potential side effects associated with this technique because these side effects invariably occur.

CHAPTER 36

Stellate Ganglion Block: Posterior Approach

CPT-2009 CODE	
Unilateral	64510
Neurolytic	64680

Relative Value Units	
Unilateral	12
Neurolytic	20

INDICATIONS

The posterior approach to the stellate ganglion is used in two clinical situations: (1) when infection, trauma, or tumor precludes use of the traditional anterior approach to stellate ganglion block, and (2) when neurolysis of the sympathetic innervation of the upper extremity is desired. The posterior approach to stellate ganglion block is preferred when neurolytic solutions are being used because this approach allows the needle to be placed at the more inferior T1 or T2 level, thus avoiding the possibility of superior spread of neurolytic solution with resultant permanent Horner's syndrome. Neurolysis of the sympathetic chain also can be accomplished via the anterior vertebral approach using radiofrequency lesioning.

The anterior approach to stellate ganglion block is preferred in the routine treatment of acute herpes zoster in the distribution of the trigeminal nerve and cervical and upper thoracic dermatomes as well as frostbite and acute vascular insufficiency of the face and upper extremities. The anterior approach to the stellate ganglion is also indicated in the treatment of reflex sympathetic dystrophy of the face, neck, upper extremity, and upper thorax; Raynaud's syndrome of the upper extremities; and sympathetically mediated pain of malignant origin. There are clinical reports to suggest that stellate ganglion blocks also may be useful in the acute palliation of some atypical vascular headaches.

CLINICALLY RELEVANT ANATOMY

The stellate ganglion is located on the anterior surface of the longus colli muscle. This muscle lies just anterior to the transverse processes of the seventh cervical and first thoracic vertebrae. The stellate ganglion is made up of the fused portion of the seventh cervical and first thoracic sympathetic ganglia. The stellate ganglion lies anteromedial to the vertebral artery and is medial to the common carotid artery and jugular vein. The stellate ganglion is lateral to the trachea and esophagus. At the T1 and T2 levels, the sympathetic chain lies just anterior to the neck of the rib, lateral to the longus colli muscle. The apex of the lung lies just lateral to the sympathetic chain at this level, making pneumothorax a distinct possibility. For this reason, it is recommended that this block be performed under computed tomography (CT) or fluoroscopic guidance.

TECHNIQUE

The patient is placed in the prone position with the cervical spine in neutral position. From 5 to 7 mL of local anesthetic without preservative is drawn into a 12-mL sterile syringe. For disease processes that have a component of inflammation, such as acute herpes zoster, or disease processes with associated edema, such as reflex sympathetic dystrophy, 80 mg of methylprednisolone is added for the first block, and 40 mg of methylprednisolone is added for subsequent blocks.

A point 4 cm lateral to the spinous process of T1-T2 is identified. The skin at this area is then prepared with antiseptic solution, and the skin and subcutaneous tissues are anesthetized with local anesthetic. A 22-gauge, 10-cm needle is advanced until contact is made with the lamina of the target vertebra (Fig. 36-1). If bony contact is not made with needle insertion to a depth of $1\frac{1}{2}$ inches, the needle is probably either between the transverse processes of adjacent vertebrae or too lateral. If this occurs, the needle should be withdrawn and reinserted with a more caudad and medial trajectory. After bony contact is made, the needle is then withdrawn and redirected

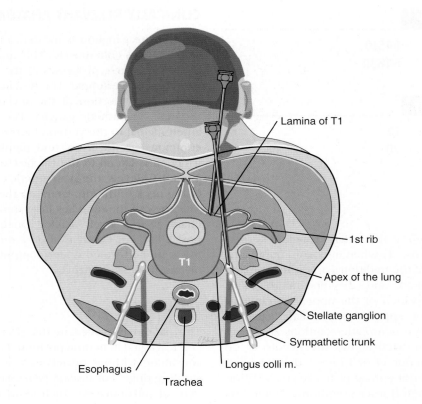

Lamina of T1

1st rib

Apex of the lung

Stellate ganglion

Sympathetic trunk

Longus colli m.

T1

Esophagus

Trachea

Figure 36-1.

slightly laterally and inferiorly. This allows the needle to slide beneath the transverse process and rib. Ultimately the needle tip should rest just adjacent to the antero-lateral border of the vertebral body in a manner analogous to the final needle position when performing lumbar sympathetic block. Careful aspiration is carried out, and 5 to 7 mL of solution is then injected. If neurolytic block is performed, small incremental doses of 6.5% aqueous phenol or absolute alcohol should be injected while observing the patient's clinical response.

SIDE EFFECTS AND COMPLICATIONS

The main complication of the posterior approach to stellate ganglion block is pneumothorax. The use of CT guidance should help decrease this complication. Proximity to the aorta also represents a potential risk that can be decreased with careful attention to technique and the use of CT guidance.

Because of the proximity to the spinal column, it is also possible to inadvertently inject the local anesthetic solution into the epidural, subdural, or subarachnoid space. At this level, even small amounts of local anesthetic placed into the subarachnoid space may result in a total spinal anesthetic. Trauma to exiting spinal roots is also a distinct possibility, especially if bony contact with the lamina of the target vertebra does not occur and the needle continues to be advanced.

Inadvertent block of the recurrent laryngeal nerve with associated hoarseness and dysphagia can occur if the injectate comes in contact with this nerve. Should neurolytic solution be inadvertently injected onto this nerve, these side effects could be permanent, with devastating results for the patient. Likewise, superior spread of neurolytic solution can result in a permanent Horner's syndrome. The patient should be forewarned of the possibility of these complications before neurolytic stellate ganglion block using the posterior approach.

CLINICAL PEARLS

The use of CT guidance will dramatically decrease the incidence of complications associated with this technique. Raj reported a 4% pneumothorax rate, which suggests that this procedure should be performed only in a setting in which chest tube placement is practical. Given the morbidity of surgical sympathectomy at this level, this technique still has a favorable risk-to-benefit ratio despite the potential for serious complications.

CHAPTER 37

Stellate Ganglion Block: Vertebral Body Approach

CPT-2009 CODE	
Unilateral	64510
Neurolytic	64680

Relative Value Units	
Unilateral	12
Neurolytic	20

INDICATIONS

Stellate ganglion block using the vertebral body approach is indicated when considering neurolysis of the stellate ganglion. The major advantage of this approach over the traditional anterior approach is that the placement of the needle tip against the junction of the transverse process and vertebral body decreases the possibility of inadvertent lysis of the somatic nerve roots, the phrenic nerve, or the recurrent laryngeal nerve. The disadvantage of this approach when compared with the posterior approach to stellate ganglion block is the higher incidence of a permanent Horner's syndrome.

Stellate ganglion block is indicated in the treatment of acute herpes zoster in the distribution of the trigeminal nerve and cervical and upper thoracic dermatomes as well as frostbite and acute vascular insufficiency of the face and upper extremities. Stellate ganglion block is also indicated in the treatment of reflex sympathetic dystrophy of the face, neck, upper extremity, and upper thorax; Raynaud's syndrome of the upper extremities; and sympathetically mediated pain of malignant origin. There are clinical reports to suggest that stellate ganglion blocks also may be useful in the acute palliation of some atypical vascular headaches.

CLINICALLY RELEVANT ANATOMY

The stellate ganglion is located on the anterior surface of the longus colli muscle. This muscle lies just anterior to the transverse processes of the seventh cervical and first thoracic vertebrae. The stellate ganglion is made up of the fused portion of the seventh cervical and first thoracic sympathetic ganglia. The stellate ganglion lies anteromedial to the vertebral artery and is medial to the common carotid artery and jugular vein. The stellate ganglion is lateral to the trachea and esophagus.

TECHNIQUE

The patient is placed in the supine position with the cervical spine in neutral position. Three to 5 mL of local anesthetic is drawn into a 12-mL sterile syringe. For disease processes that have a component of inflammation, such as acute herpes zoster, or disease processes with associated edema, such as reflex sympathetic dystrophy, 80 mg of methylprednisolone is added for the first block, and 40 mg of methylprednisolone is added for subsequent blocks. For neurolytic blocks, 3 to 5 mL of absolute alcohol or 6.5% aqueous phenol given in incremental doses is used. Neurolytic blocks should be done under computed tomography (CT) or fluoroscopic guidance unless the clinical situation dictates that the block be done at the bedside.

If radiographic guidance is used, the junction of the C7 transverse process with the vertebral body is identified. If a blind technique is used, the medial edge of the sternocleidomastoid muscle is identified at the level of the inferior margin of the cricoid cartilage, which is at the level of C7. The sternocleidomastoid muscle is then displaced laterally with two fingers, and the tissues overlying the transverse process of C7 are compressed. The pulsations of the carotid artery are then identified under the palpating fingers. The skin medial to the carotid pulsation is prepared with antiseptic solution, and a 22-gauge, 3½-inch spinal needle is advanced in a slightly inferior and medial trajectory until contact is made with the junction of the transverse process of C7 with the vertebral body (Figs. 37-1 and 37-2). If bony contact is not made with needle insertion to a depth of 1½ inches, the needle is probably either too lateral or has slid between the transverse processes of C7 and T1. If this occurs, the needle should be withdrawn and reinserted

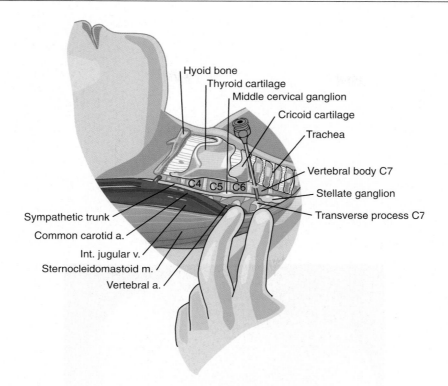

Figure 37-1.

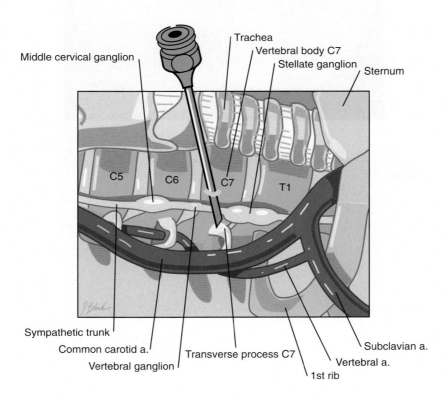

Figure 37-2.

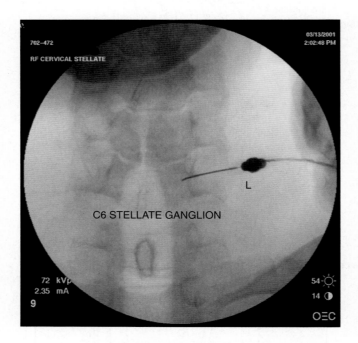

Figure 37-3.
Needle placement for stellate ganglion block using the vertebral body approach.

with a more medial and inferior trajectory. After bony contact is made, the needle is then withdrawn slightly to bring the needle tip out of the periosteum of the junction of the transverse process and the vertebral body (see Fig. 37-2). Careful aspiration is carried out, and 3 to 5 mL of local anesthetic, steroid, or both is injected. If neurolytic solution is being used, small incremental doses are injected, with time between doses given to allow for the adequate assessment of clinical response. To obtain adequate destruction of the stellate ganglion and associated sympathetic nerves, additional increments of neurolytic solution may have to be injected at the middle of the C7 transverse process and at a point 1 cm inferior on the anteromedial margin of the vertebral body. Radiofrequency lesioning and cryoneurolysis may represent safer alternatives to destruction of the stellate ganglion (Fig. 37-3).

SIDE EFFECTS AND COMPLICATIONS

This anatomic region is highly vascular, and because of the proximity of major vessels, the pain specialist should carefully observe the patient for signs of local anesthetic toxicity during injection. This vascularity and proximity to major blood vessels also give rise to an increased incidence of postblock ecchymosis and hematoma formation, and the patient should be warned of such. Despite the vascularity of this anatomic region, this technique can be performed safely in the presence of anticoagulation by using a 25- or 27-gauge needle, albeit at increased risk for hematoma, if the clinical situation dictates a favorable risk-to-benefit ratio. These complications can be decreased if manual pressure is applied to the area of the block immediately after injection. Application of cold packs for 20 minutes on, 20 minutes off, after the block also decreases the amount of postprocedure pain and bleeding the patient may experience.

Because of the proximity to the spinal column, it is also possible to inadvertently inject the local anesthetic or neurolytic solution into the epidural, subdural, or subarachnoid space. At this level, even small amounts of local anesthetic placed into the subarachnoid space may result in a total spinal anesthetic. Neurolytic solutions placed onto the neuraxis at this level can result in significant neurologic dysfunction, including quadriparesis. Because of the more inferior needle placement with the vertebral body approach to stellate ganglion block, pneumothorax is a distinct possibility. These complications can be decreased with the use of radiographic guidance.

Additional side effects that occur with sufficient frequency include inadvertent block of the recurrent laryngeal nerve with associated hoarseness and dysphagia and the sensation that there is a lump in the throat when swallowing. Horner's syndrome occurs when the superior cervical sympathetic ganglion is also blocked during stellate ganglion block. These complications can be disastrous if neurolytic solution is used. The patient should be forewarned of the possibility of these complications before stellate ganglion block using the vertebral body approach.

CLINICAL PEARLS

The use of CT or fluoroscopic guidance will dramatically decrease the incidence of complications associated with this technique. Given the possibility of pneumothorax, this procedure should be performed only in a setting where chest tube placement is practical. Given the morbidity of surgical sympathectomy at this level, this technique still has a favorable risk-to-benefit ratio despite the potential for serious complications.

CHAPTER 38

Stellate Ganglion Block: Radiofrequency Lesioning

CPT-2009 CODE

Radiofrequency—Neurolytic	64680

Relative Value Unit

Radiofrequency—Neurolytic	20

INDICATIONS

Radiofrequency lesioning of the stellate or cervicothoracic ganglion is indicated in the treatment of sympathetically mediated pain that has repeatedly responded to stellate ganglion block with local anesthetic, but the duration of pain relief with local anesthetic block is not long lasting. Pain syndromes that may be amenable to radiofrequency lesioning of the stellate ganglion include vascular insufficiency of the face and upper extremities, reflex sympathetic dystrophy of the face, neck, upper extremity, and upper thorax; Raynaud's or Berger's syndrome of the upper extremities; and sympathetically mediated pain of malignant origin.

CLINICALLY RELEVANT ANATOMY

The stellate ganglion is located on the anterior surface of the longus colli muscle. This muscle lies just anterior to the transverse processes of the seventh cervical and first thoracic vertebrae. The stellate ganglion is made up of the fused portion of the seventh cervical and first thoracic sympathetic ganglia. The stellate ganglion lies anteromedial to the vertebral artery and is medial to the common carotid artery and jugular vein. The stellate ganglion is lateral to the trachea and esophagus.

TECHNIQUE

The patient is placed in the supine position with the cervical spine in a slightly extended position. Three milliliters of local anesthetic combined with 3 mL of water-soluble contrast medium is drawn into a 12-mL sterile syringe. Using computed tomography (CT) or fluoroscopic guidance, the junction of the C7 transverse process with the vertebral body is identified, and the skin is marked with a gentian violet marker. The palpating index and ring fingers of the nondominant hand should then identify the medial edge of the sternocleidomastoid muscle at the level of the inferior margin of the cricoid cartilage, which is at the level of C7. The sternocleidomastoid muscle is then displaced laterally with two fingers, and the tissues overlying the transverse process of C7 are compressed. The pulsations of the carotid artery are then identified under the palpating fingers. The skin medial to the carotid pulsation is prepared with antiseptic solution and anesthetized with local anesthetic. Using intermittent fluoroscopic guidance, a 16-gauge introducer needle is directed toward the previously identified junction of the C7 transverse process with the vertebral body. A 20-gauge, curved, 54-cm radiofrequency needle with a 4-mm active tip is guided through the introducer and is advanced in a slightly inferior and medial trajectory until contact is made with the junction of the transverse process of C7 with the vertebral body (Figs. 38-1 and 38-2). If bony contact is not made with needle insertion to a depth of 1½ inches, the needle is probably either too lateral or has slid between the transverse processes of C7 and T1. If this occurs, the needle should be withdrawn and reinserted with a more medial and inferior trajectory. After bony contact is made, the needle is withdrawn slightly to bring the needle tip out of the periosteum of the junction of the transverse process and the vertebral body (see Fig. 38-2). Careful aspiration is carried out, and 3 to 5 mL of the mixture of local anesthetic and contrast medium is injected. The contrast medium and local anesthetic should spread anterior to the vertebra in a cephalad and caudad direction. No epidural, subdural, subarachnoid, intramuscular, or intravascular spread of contrast medium should be observed. A trial stimulation of both the sensory nerves at 50 Hz and 0.9 V and motor nerves at 2 Hz and 2 V should be carried out because of proximity of the phrenic and recurrent laryngeal nerves.

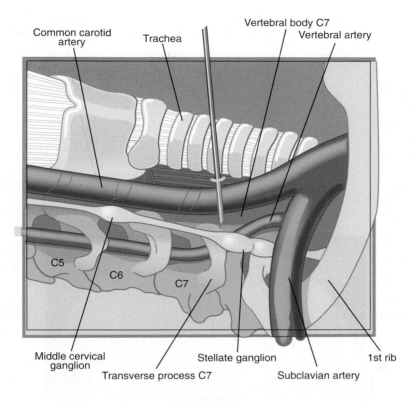

Figure 38-1.

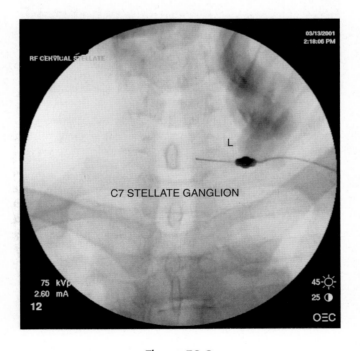

Figure 38-2.

Proper needle placement for radiofrequency lesioning of the stellate ganglion.

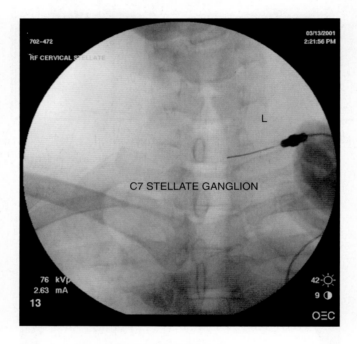

Figure 38-3.
Radiofrequency needle in position for radiofrequency lesioning of stellate ganglion.

Stimulation of the phrenic nerve suggests that the needle placement is too lateral, and stimulation of the recurrent laryngeal nerve suggests that the needle is too anterior and medial. Having the patient phonate with a prolonged "ee" during stimulation will help identify stimulation of these neural structures.

After satisfactory needle placement has been confirmed, a radiofrequency lesion is made by heating at 80°C for 60 seconds or pulsed radiofrequency at 45°C to 50°C for a longer duration. The stimulating needle is then redirected in the same plane to the most medial aspect of the transverse process, and both motor and sensory trial stimulation is repeated as described previously (Fig. 38-3). If no evidence of stimulation of motor or sensory nerves is observed, a second lesion is made. The needle is then redirected to the uppermost portion of the junction of the C7 transverse process and the vertebral body. If trial stimulation fails to reveal stimulation of motor or sensory nerves, a third lesion is made. The stimulating needle is removed, and gentle pressure is placed on the site to decrease the incidence of ecchymosis and hematoma formation.

SIDE EFFECTS AND COMPLICATIONS

Because of the proximity to the spinal canal, it is also possible to unintentionally inject the local anesthetic or neurolytic solution into the epidural, subdural, or subarachnoid space. At this level, even small amounts of local anesthetic placed into the subarachnoid space may result in a total spinal anesthetic. Radiofrequency lesioning of the neuraxial structures at this level can result in significant neurologic dysfunction, including quadriparesis. Unintentional lesioning of the phrenic nerve can result in diaphragmatic paralysis and respiratory embarrassment. Inadvertent lesioning of recurrent laryngeal nerve can result in prolonged or permanent hoarseness. A permanent Horner's syndrome may occur when the superior cervical sympathetic ganglion is damaged during this procedure.

Because of the more inferior needle placement with the vertebral body approach to stellate ganglion block, pneumothorax is a distinct possibility, especially on the right. All of these complications can be decreased with the careful use of trial stimulation and radiographic guidance.

This anatomic region is highly vascular, and because of the proximity of major vessels, the pain specialist should carefully observe the patient for signs of local anesthetic toxicity during injection. This vascularity and proximity to major blood vessels also give rise to an increased incidence of postblock ecchymosis and hematoma formation, and the patient should be warned of such. These complications can be disastrous if neurolytic solution is used. The patient should be forewarned of the possibility of all of these complications before attempting radiofrequency lesioning of the stellate ganglion.

CLINICAL PEARLS

The use of CT or fluoroscopic guidance will dramatically decrease the incidence of complications associated with this technique. Given the possibility of pneumothorax, this procedure should be performed only in a setting where chest tube placement is practical. Given the morbidity of surgical sympathectomy at this level, this technique still has a favorable risk-to-benefit ratio despite the potential for serious complications.

CHAPTER **39**

Third Occipital Nerve Block

CPT-2009 CODE	
Unilateral	64470
Bilateral	64470-50
Neurolytic	64626

Relative Value Units	
Unilateral	10
Bilateral	18
Neurolytic	20

INDICATIONS

Third occipital nerve block is useful in the diagnosis and treatment of third occipital nerve headache. This technique is also useful as a prognostic indicator of the potential efficacy of destruction of the third occipital nerve with radiofrequency lesioning or other means.

CLINICALLY RELEVANT ANATOMY

The third occipital nerve arises from superior branch fibers of the third cervical nerve at the level of the trapezius muscle (Fig. 39-1). The third occipital nerve courses dorsomedially around the superior articular process of the C3 vertebra (Fig. 39-2). Fibers from the third occipital nerve provide the primary innervation of the C2 to C3 facet joints with some contribution from the C3 medial branch and small communicating fibers from the second cervical nerve. Fibers of the third occipital nerve then course superiorly to provide sensory innervation to the ipsilateral suboccipital region (see Fig. 39-1).

TECHNIQUE

The patient is placed in a prone position with the cervical spine slightly flexed. A true lateral fluoroscopic view of the upper cervical spine including the C2-C3 facet joint is then obtained. It is important to be sure that the articular pillars on each side of the C2-C3 interspace are superimposed to ensure a true lateral view. A point midway between the opposite apex of the superior articular process of C3 and opposite base of the C2-C3 neural foramen is then identified (Fig. 39-3).

After preparation of the overlying skin with antiseptic solution, a 25-gauge, 1½-inch needle is used to inject local anesthetic to anesthetize the skin and subcutaneous tissues. A 22-gauge, 3½-inch styletted spinal needle is then inserted through the previously anesthetized area and advanced under fluoroscopic guidance toward the previously identified point that lies midway between the opposite apex of the superior articular process of C3 and opposite base of the C2-C3 neural foramen.

The needle tip will finally come to rest against the periosteum or dense facetal pericapsular fascia of the C2-C3 facet joint (Fig. 39-4). The needle is then withdrawn 2.5 to 3 mm to ensure that the needle tip is outside the facet joint. Next, 0.2 to 0.3 mL of nonionic contrast medium is injected to confirm that the needle tip is not within the facet joint, as demonstrated by pericapsular flow of contrast around the C2-C3 facet joint. A combination of 0.75 to 1.0 mL of local anesthetic and 0.25 mL of nonionic contrast medium is then gently injected under continuous fluoroscopic guidance after careful aspiration for blood and cerebrospinal fluid. Careful observation for vascular or spinal nerve root filling should be carried out during injection. Local anesthetic and contrast should be observed to spread out along the course of the third occipital nerve. Because the diameter of the third occipital nerve is greater than the other cervical medial branches, a second injection at the inferior articular process of C2 and occasionally a third injection at the superior articular facet of C3 is required to block the nerve completely.

SIDE EFFECTS AND COMPLICATIONS

This area is highly vascular, and coupled with the fact that the third occipital nerves are in close proximity to the vertebral arteries, this means that the pain specialist should carefully observe the patient undergoing third

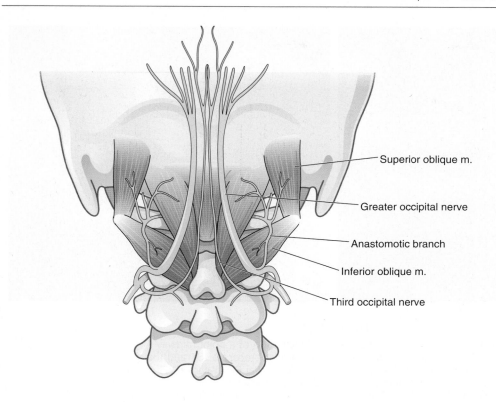

Superior oblique m.

Greater occipital nerve

Anastomotic branch

Inferior oblique m.

Third occipital nerve

Figure 39-1.
The third occipital nerve.

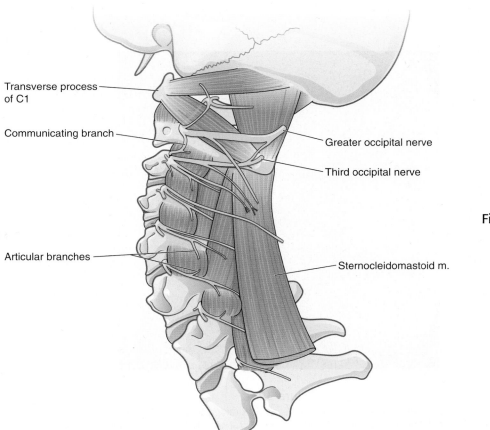

Transverse process
of C1

Communicating branch

Articular branches

Greater occipital nerve

Third occipital nerve

Sternocleidomastoid m.

Figure 39-2.

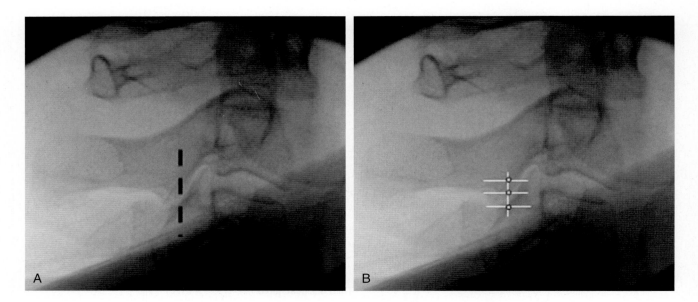

Figure 39-3.
True lateral view of the cervical spine for identification of a point midway between the opposite apex of the superior articular process of C3 and the opposite base of the C2-C3 neural foramen. (From Raj PP, Waldman SD, Erdine S, et al: Radiographic Imaging for Regional Anesthesia and Pain Management, 1st ed. New York, Churchill Livingstone, 2002, p 159.)

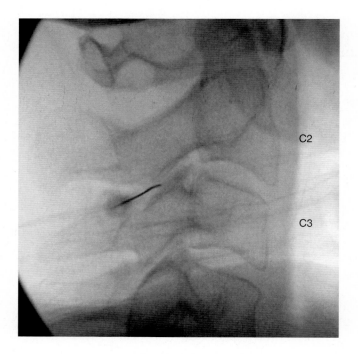

Figure 39-4.
(From Raj PP, Waldman SD, Erdine S, et al: Radiographic Imaging for Regional Anesthesia and Pain Management, 1st ed. New York, Churchill Livingstone, 2002, p 159.)

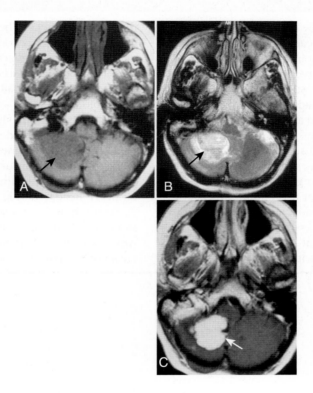

Figure 39-5.
Hemangiopericytoma in the floor of the posterior cranial fossa on the right. Axial T1-weighted (**A**) and T2-weighted (**B**) magnetic resonance images. A large, well-circumscribed, lobulated, homogeneously hypointense (T1-weighted) and hyperintense (T2-weighted) extra-axial mass (*arrows*) deeply invaginates and displaces the inferior aspect of the right cerebellar hemisphere and vermis medially across the midline and indents the right posterolateral aspect of the medulla. **C,** After intravenous administration of gadolinium, intense homogeneous contrast enhancement is noted in this lobulated tumor (*arrow*). (From Haaga JR, Lanzieri CF: CT and MR Imaging of the Whole Body, 4th ed. St. Louis, Mosby, 2002, p 172.)

occipital nerve block for inadvertent intravascular injection, which could cause significant central nervous system side effects, including ataxia, dizziness, and rarely, seizures. Proximity of the third occipital nerve to exiting spinal nerve roots makes trauma to the nerve roots and inadvertent subarachnoid, subdural, or epidural injection a distinct possibility. Care must be taken to avoid inadvertent needle placement into the foramen magnum because the subarachnoid administration of local anesthetic in this region will result in an immediate total spinal anesthetic.

CLINICAL PEARLS

Third occipital nerve headache may be an underdiagnosed type of chronic daily headache, especially after trauma to the upper cervical spine. The most common reason that third occipital nerve block fails to relieve headache pain thought to be subserved by the third occipital nerve is that the headache syndrome being treated has been misdiagnosed as third occipital nerve headache. In my experience, third occipital nerve headache is an infrequent cause of headaches in the absence of trauma. More often, the patient with headaches involving the occipital region is in fact suffering from tension-type headaches or less commonly occipital neuralgia. Tension-type headaches do not respond to third occipital nerve blocks but are amenable to treatment with antidepressant compounds such as amitriptyline in conjunction with cervical steroid epidural nerve blocks. Therefore, the pain management specialist should reconsider the diagnosis of third occipital nerve headaches in those patients whose symptoms are consistent with third occipital nerve headaches but who fail to respond to third occipital nerve block.

Any patient with headaches severe enough to require neural blockade as part of the treatment plan should undergo magnetic resonance imaging of the head to rule out unsuspected intracranial pathology that may mimic the clinical symptoms of third occipital nerve headache (Fig. 39-5).

Furthermore, cervical spine x-rays should be considered to rule out congenital abnormalities such as Arnold-Chiari malformations that may be the hidden cause of the patient's occipital headaches.

CHAPTER 40

Third Occipital Nerve Block: Radiofrequency Lesioning

CPT-2009 CODE	
Neurolytic	64626

Relative Value Units	
Neurolytic	20

INDICATIONS

Radiofrequency lesioning of the third occipital nerve block is useful in the treatment of third occipital nerve headache in patients who have responded to block of the third occipital nerve with local anesthetic but have failed to obtain long-lasting relief.

CLINICALLY RELEVANT ANATOMY

The third occipital nerve arises from superior branch fibers of the third cervical nerve at the level of the trapezius muscle (Fig. 40-1). The third occipital nerve courses dorsomedially around the superior articular process of the C3 vertebra (Fig. 40-2). Fibers from the third occipital nerve provide the primary innervation of the C2-C3 facet joints with some contribution from the C3 medial branch and small communicating fibers from the second cervical nerve. Fibers of the third occipital nerve then course superiorly to provide sensory innervation to the ipsilateral suboccipital region (see Fig. 40-1).

TECHNIQUE

The patient is placed in a prone position with the cervical spine slightly flexed. A true lateral fluoroscopic view of the upper cervical spine including the C2-C3 facet joint is then obtained (Fig. 40-3). It is important to be sure that the articular pillars on each side of the C2-C3 interspace are superimposed to ensure a true lateral view. A point midway between the opposite apex of the superior articular process of C3 and opposite base of the C2-C3 neural foramen is then identified (Fig. 40-4). After preparation of the overlying skin with antiseptic solution, a 25-gauge, 1½-inch needle is used to inject local anesthetic to anesthetize the skin and subcutaneous tissues. A 22-gauge, 15-cm insulated blunt curved needle with a 10-mm active tip is inserted through an introducer needle and is then advanced under fluoroscopic guidance as described earlier toward the previously identified point midway between the opposite apex of the superior articular process of C3 and opposite base of the C2-C3 neural foramen (Fig. 40-5). When the needle is in position, impedance is measured and should be in the range of 250 to 500 Ω.

To confirm that the needle is properly placed, motor stimulation at 2 Hz with 0.5 to 1.5 V should produce no motor stimulation of the ipsilateral muscles of the face or upper extremity. A mild paresthesia in the distribution of the third occipital nerve may be elicited by stimulating at 50 Hz with 0.1 to 0.75 V. The needle should be repositioned if the patient complains of any unpleasant paresthesias or pain in the face. Careful aspiration for blood and cerebrospinal fluid (CSF) should then be carried out and the needle repositioned until blood is not present. If no CSF or blood is present, 0.25 to 0.5 mL of 0.2% ropivacaine is then injected, and the patient is monitored closely for inadvertent intravascular or subarachnoid injection. After 60 seconds, radiofrequency lesioning is carried out at 80°C for 90 seconds. Because the diameter of the third occipital nerve is greater than the other cervical medial branches, a second radiofrequency lesion at the inferior articular process of C2 and occasionally a third radiofrequency at the superior articular facet of C3 is required to destroy the nerve completely.

SIDE EFFECTS AND COMPLICATIONS

This area is highly vascular, and coupled with the fact that the third occipital nerves are in close proximity to the vertebral arteries, this means that the pain specialist should carefully observe the patient undergoing third occipital nerve block for inadvertent intravascular injection, which could cause significant central nervous

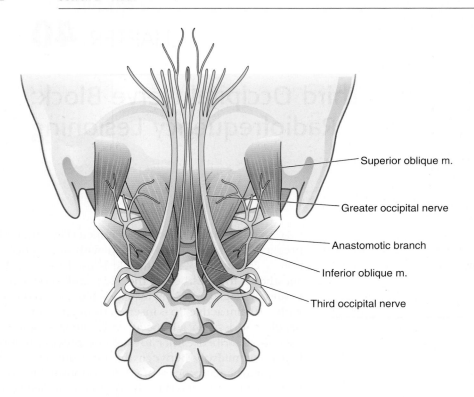

Superior oblique m.

Greater occipital nerve

Anastomotic branch

Inferior oblique m.

Third occipital nerve

Figure 40-1.
The third occipital nerve.

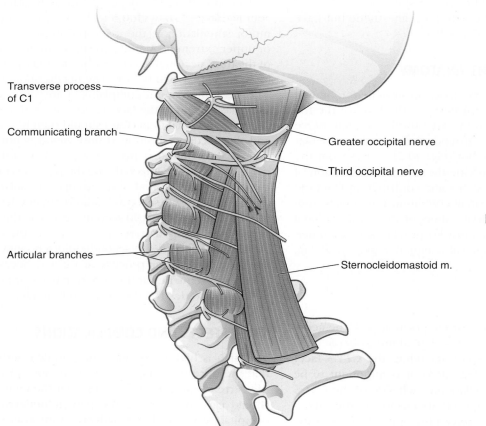

Transverse process of C1

Communicating branch

Articular branches

Greater occipital nerve

Third occipital nerve

Sternocleidomastoid m.

Figure 40-2.

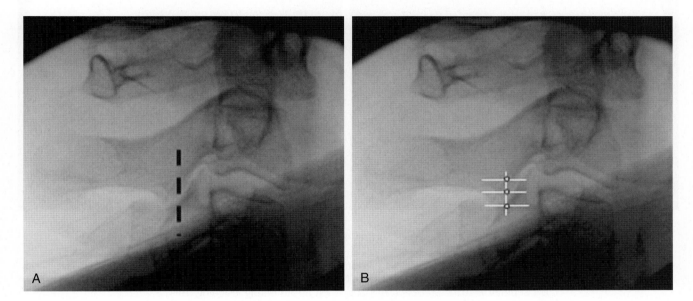

Figure 40-3.
True lateral view of the cervical spine. (From Raj PP, Waldman SD,
Erdine S, et al: Radiographic Imaging for Regional Anesthesia and Pain
Management, 1st ed. New York, Churchill Livingstone 2002, p 159.)

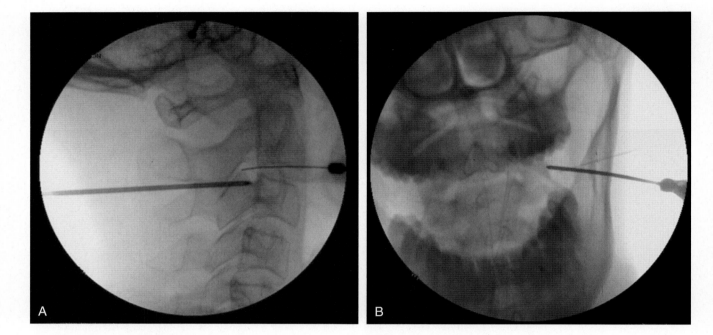

Figure 40-4.

A, Lateral cervical spine showing placement of block needle and the electrode. Note that the large RRE electrode has been inserted through the posterior muscles. The tip of the block needle depicts the superior pole of the superior articular process (SAP) and is left in situ during lesioning. This allows for the administration of supplementary local anesthetic as required. In this view, the electrode is placed to radiofrequency, the "low position" of the TON. Thereafter, lesions are created along the SAP between the trough of the intervertebral foramen and the tip of the block needle, which depicts the uppermost position of the nerve (Courtesy of Jay Govind, MD). **B,** AP or open-mouth view confirms placement of the electrode against the lateral margin (periosteum) of SAP of C3. There should be no gap between the electrode and the periosteum. Whether the electrode is too lateral and hence away from the nerve or too medial (too far inside the intervertebral foramen) will be revealed in the AP view. Both views must be secured and electrode placement confirmed prior to generating a lesion (Courtesy of Jay Govind, MD). (From Raj PP, Lou L, Erdine S, et al: Interventional Pain Management: Image-Guided Procedures, 2nd ed. Philadelphia, Saunders, 2008.)

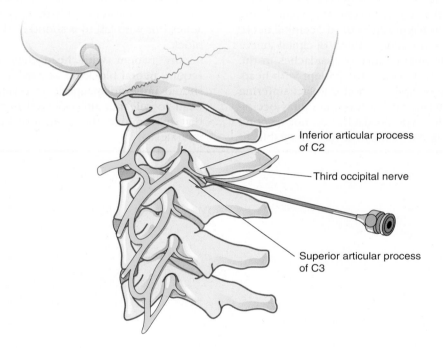

Inferior articular process
of C2

Third occipital nerve

Superior articular process
of C3

Figure 40-5.

system side effects including ataxia, dizziness, and rarely, seizures. Proximity of the third occipital nerve to exiting spinal nerve roots makes trauma to the nerve roots and inadvertent subarachnoid, subdural, or epidural injection a distinct possibility. Care must be taken to avoid inadvertent needle placement into the foramen magnum because the subarachnoid administration of local anesthetic in this region will result in an immediate total spinal anesthetic.

CLINICAL PEARLS

Third occipital nerve headache may be an underdiagnosed type of chronic daily headache, especially after trauma to the upper cervical spine. The most common reason that third occipital nerve block fails to relieve headache pain thought to be subserved by the third occipital nerve is that the headache syndrome being treated has been misdiagnosed as third occipital nerve headache. In my experience, third occipital nerve headache is an infrequent cause of headaches in the absence of trauma. More often, the patient with headaches involving the occipital region is in fact suffering from tension-type headaches or less commonly occipital neuralgia. Tension-type headaches do not respond to third occipital nerve blocks but are amenable to treatment with antidepressant compounds such as amitriptyline in conjunction with cervical steroid epidural nerve blocks. Therefore, the pain management specialist should reconsider the diagnosis of third occipital nerve headaches in patients whose symptoms are consistent with third occipital nerve headaches but who fail to respond to third occipital nerve block.

Any patient with headaches severe enough to require neural blockade as part of the treatment plan should undergo magnetic resonance imaging of the head to rule out unsuspected intracranial pathology that may mimic the clinical symptoms of occipital neuralgia.

CHAPTER 41

Cervical Facet Block: Medial Branch Technique

CPT-2009 CODE

First Joint	64470
Second Joint	64472
Neurolytic First Joint	64626
Neurolytic Second Joint	64627

Relative Value Units

First Joint	10
Second Joint	10
Neurolytic First Joint	20
Neurolytic Second Joint	20

INDICATIONS

Cervical facet block using the medial branch technique is useful in the diagnosis and treatment of painful conditions involving trauma, arthritis, or inflammation of the cervical facet joints. These problems may manifest clinically as neck pain, suboccipital headache, and occasionally shoulder and supraclavicular pain.

CLINICALLY RELEVANT ANATOMY

The cervical facet joints are formed by the articulations of the superior and inferior articular facets of adjacent vertebrae. Except for the atlanto-occipital and atlantoaxial joints, the remaining cervical facet joints are true joints in that they are lined with synovium and possess a true joint capsule. This capsule is richly innervated and supports the notion of the facet joint as a pain generator. The cervical facet joint is susceptible to arthritic changes and trauma caused by acceleration-deceleration injuries. Such damage to the joint results in pain secondary to synovial joint inflammation and adhesions.

Each facet joint receives innervation from two spinal levels. Each joint receives fibers from the dorsal ramus at the same level as the vertebra as well as fibers from the dorsal ramus of the vertebra above. This fact has clinical import in that it provides an explanation for the ill-defined nature of facet-mediated pain and also explains why the dorsal nerve from the vertebra above the offending level must often also be blocked to provide complete pain relief.

At each level, the dorsal ramus provides a medial branch that wraps around the convexity of the articular pillar of its respective vertebra. This location is constant for the C4-C7 nerves and allows a simplified approach for treatment of cervical facet syndrome.

TECHNIQUE

Cervical facet block using the medial branch technique is the preferred route of treating cervical facet syndrome. It may be done either blind or under fluoroscopic guidance. The patient is placed in a prone position. Pillows are placed under the chest to allow the cervical spine to be moderately flexed without discomfort to the patient. The forehead is allowed to rest on a folded blanket.

Blind Technique

If a blind technique is used, the spinous process at the level to be blocked is identified by palpation. A point slightly inferior and 2.5 cm lateral to the spinous process is then identified as the site of needle insertion. After preparation of the skin with antiseptic solution, a skin wheal of local anesthetic is raised at the site of needle insertion. Three milliliters of preservative-free local anesthetic is drawn up in a 5-mL sterile syringe. When treating pain thought to be secondary to an inflammatory process, a total of 80 mg of depot-steroid is added to the local anesthetic with the first block, and 40 mg of depot-steroid is added with subsequent blocks.

An 18-gauge, 1-inch needle is inserted through the skin and into the subcutaneous tissue at the previously identified insertion site to serve as an introducer. The introducer needle is then repositioned with a slightly superior and medial trajectory, pointing directly toward the posterior aspect of the articular pillar at the level to be blocked. A 25-gauge, $3\frac{1}{2}$-inch styletted spinal needle

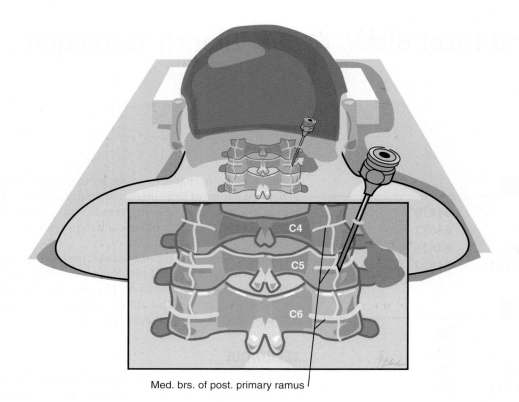

Figure 41-1.

Med. brs. of post. primary ramus

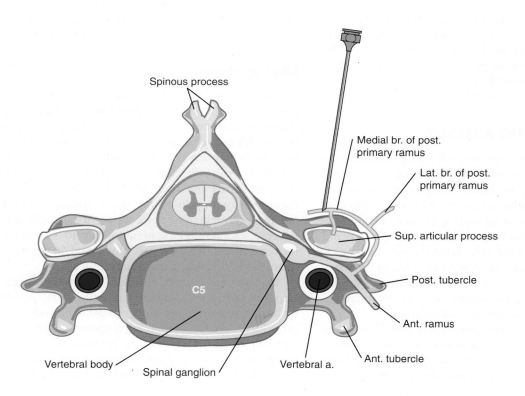

Spinous process

Medial br. of post. primary ramus

Lat. br. of post. primary ramus

Figure 41-2.

Sup. articular process

Post. tubercle

Ant. ramus

C5

Ant. tubercle

Vertebral body

Spinal ganglion

Vertebral a.

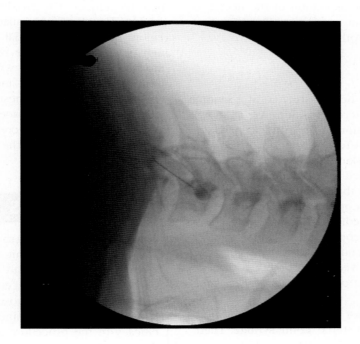

Figure 41-3.
Needle tip at the lateral-most aspect of the articular pillar.

is then inserted through the 18-gauge introducer and directed toward the articular pillar. After bony contact is made, the depth of the contact is noted, and the spinal needle is withdrawn. The introducer needle is then repositioned, aiming toward the lateral-most aspect of the articular pillar. The 25-gauge spinal needle is then readvanced until it impinges on the lateral-most aspect of the border of the articular pillar (Fig. 41-1). Should the spinal needle walk off the lateral aspect of the articular pillar, it is withdrawn and redirected slightly medially and carefully advanced to the depth of the previous bony contact (Fig. 41-2).

After the needle is felt to be in satisfactory position, the stylet is removed from the 25-gauge spinal needle, and the hub is observed for blood or cerebrospinal fluid. If neither is present, gentle aspiration of the needle is carried out. If the aspiration test is negative, 1.5 mL of solution is injected through the spinal needle.

Fluoroscopic Technique

If fluoroscopy is used, the beam is rotated in a sagittal plane from anterior to posterior position, which allows identification and visualization of the articular pillars of the respective vertebrae. After preparation of the skin with antiseptic solution, a skin wheal of local anesthetic is raised at the site of needle insertion. An 18-gauge, 1-inch needle is inserted at the insertion site to serve as an introducer. The fluoroscopy beam is aimed directly through the introducer needle, which will appear as a small point on the fluoroscopy screen. The introducer needle is then repositioned under fluoroscopic guidance until this small point is visualized pointing directly toward the posterior aspect of the articular pillar at the level to be blocked.

A total of 5 mL of contrast medium suitable for intrathecal use is drawn up in a sterile 12-mL syringe. Then, 3 mL of preservative-free local anesthetic is drawn up in a separate 5-mL sterile syringe. When treating pain thought to be secondary to an inflammatory process, a total of 80 mg of depot-steroid is added to the local anesthetic with the first block, and 40 mg of depot-steroid is added with subsequent blocks.

A 25-gauge, $3\frac{1}{2}$-inch styletted spinal needle is then inserted through the 18-gauge introducer and directed toward the articular pillar. After bony contact is made, the spinal needle is withdrawn, and the introducer needle is repositioned toward the lateral-most aspect of the articular pillar. The 25-gauge spinal needle is then readvanced until it impinges on the lateral-most aspect of the border of the articular pillar (Fig. 41-3).

After confirmation of needle placement by biplanar fluoroscopy, the stylet is removed from the 25-gauge spinal needle, and the hub is observed for blood or cerebrospinal fluid. If neither is present, gentle aspiration of the needle is carried out. If the aspiration test is negative, 1 mL of contrast medium is slowly injected under fluoroscopic guidance to reconfirm needle placement. After correct needle placement is confirmed, 1.5 mL of local anesthetic with or without steroid is injected through the spinal needle.

SIDE EFFECTS AND COMPLICATIONS

The proximity to the spinal cord and exiting nerve roots makes it imperative that this procedure be carried out only by those well versed in the regional anatomy and experienced in performing interventional pain management techniques. The proximity to the vertebral artery, combined with the vascular nature of this anatomic region, makes the potential for intravascular injection high. Even small amounts of local anesthetic injected into the vertebral arteries will result in seizures. Given the proximity of the brain and brain stem, ataxia due to vascular uptake of local anesthetic is not an uncommon occurrence after cervical facet block. Many patients also complain of a transient increase in headache and cervicalgia after injection into the joint.

CLINICAL PEARLS

Cervical facet block using the medial branch approach is the preferred technique for treatment of cervical facet syndrome. Although intra-articular placement of the needle into the facet joint is technically feasible, unless specific diagnostic information about that joint is required, such maneuvers add nothing to the efficacy of the procedure and in fact may increase the rate of complications.

Cervical facet block is often combined with atlanto-occipital block when treating pain in the previously mentioned areas. Although the atlanto-occipital joint is not a true facet joint in the anatomic sense of the word, the block is analogous to the facet joint block technique used commonly by pain practitioners and may be viewed as such. Many pain specialists believe that these techniques are currently underused in the treatment of postwhiplash cervicalgia and cervicogenic headaches. These specialists believe that both techniques should be considered when cervical epidural nerve blocks and occipital nerve blocks fail to provide palliation of these headache and neck pain syndromes.

CHAPTER 42

Cervical Facet Neurolysis: Radiofrequency Lesioning of the Cervical Medial Branch

CPT-2009 CODE

Radiofrequency Lesioning First Joint	64626
Radiofrequency Lesioning Second Joint	64627

Relative Value Units

Radiofrequency Lesioning First Joint	20
Radiofrequency Lesioning Second Joint	20

INDICATIONS

Radiofrequency neurolysis of the cervical facet joints by disrupting the medial branch of the primary posterior rami is indicated for patients who experienced significant, but short-lived, pain relief following blockade of the corresponding medial branches of the cervical facets with local anesthetic on at least two occasions.

This technique is useful in providing long-lasting pain relief for painful conditions involving trauma, arthritis, or inflammation of the cervical facet joints. These problems may manifest clinically as neck pain, occipital headache, and shoulder and supraclavicular pain.

CLINICALLY RELEVANT ANATOMY

The cervical facet joints are formed by the articulations of the superior and inferior articular process of adjacent vertebrae. Except for the atlanto-occipital and atlanto-axial joints, the remaining cervical facet joints are true joints in that they are lined with synovium and possess a true joint capsule. This capsule is richly innervated and supports the notion of the facet joint as a potential pain generator. The cervical facet joint is susceptible to arthritic changes and trauma caused by hyperextension and hyperflexion acceleration-deceleration injuries. Such damage to the joint results in pain secondary to capsular disruption, synovial joint inflammation, and adhesions.

Each facet joint receives innervation from two spinal levels. Each joint receives fibers from the dorsal ramus of the two levels comprising the articular surfaces. This fact has clinical import in that it provides an explanation for the ill-defined nature of facet-mediated pain and also explains why the dorsal nerve from the vertebra above the offending level must often also be blocked to provide complete pain relief.

At each level, the dorsal ramus provides a medial branch that wraps around the convexity of the articular pillar of its respective vertebra. This location is constant for the C3-C7 nerves and allows a simplified approach for treatment of cervical facet syndrome.

TECHNIQUE

Radiofrequency lesioning of the cervical facet joints by disrupting the corresponding medial branches of the affected cervical facet joints is the preferred route of denervating the cervical facet joints. This technique is best performed under fluoroscopic or computed tomography guidance.

Posterior Approach

The patient is placed in a prone position. Pillows are placed under the chest to allow the cervical spine to be moderately flexed without discomfort to the patient. The forehead is allowed to rest on a folded blanket (Fig. 42-1).

To properly position the radiofrequency cannula, the fluoroscopy beam is rotated to obtain a lateral view. The center of the neural arch at the targeted level is then identified. After preparation of the skin with antiseptic solution, a skin wheal of local anesthetic is raised at the site of needle insertion. A 22-gauge, 2-inch needle is then inserted using "tunnel vision" to contact bone at the centroid of the neural arch. The fluoroscope beam is then rotated to provide a clear anteroposterior (AP) view, and the waist of the articular pillar is identified.

A 22-gauge, 4-mm active-tip radiofrequency needle is then inserted through the skin and directed under AP fluoroscopic guidance toward the needle that was previously placed at the centroid of the neural arch. The needle should be noted to lie at the waist of the vertebra on the AP view, just posterior to the foramen on the

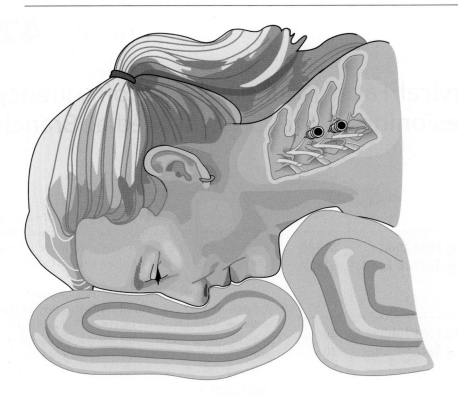

Figure 42-1.

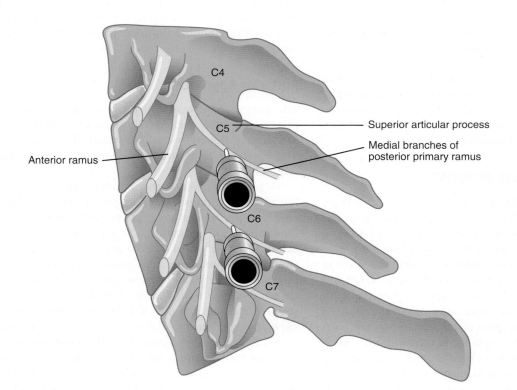

C4

C5 — Superior articular process

Medial branches of
posterior primary ramus

Anterior ramus —

C6

C7

Figure 42-2.

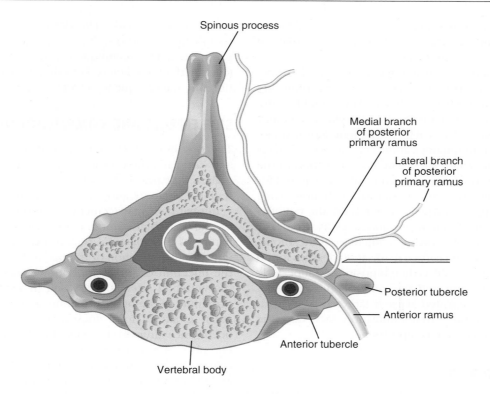

Spinous process

Medial branch
of posterior
primary ramus

Lateral branch
of posterior
primary ramus

Posterior tubercle

Anterior ramus

Anterior tubercle

Vertebral body

Figure 42-3.

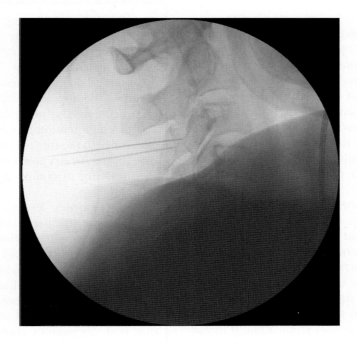

Figure 42-4.
Needles in position for radiofrequency lesioning of the medial branch.

foraminal view, and covering the centroid, and therefore in close proximity to the medial branch in the lateral view (Figs. 42-2 through 42-4).

After confirmation of proper needle placement, stimulation at 50 Hz is carried out with the patient reporting stimulation between 0.1 and 0.5 V. This should reproduce the patient's pain pattern, although the quality may not be perceived as identical by the patient. Motor stimulation of the radiofrequency cannula at 2 to 3 V at 2 Hz is increased slowly. There should be no stimulation of the upper extremity at 2½ to 3 times the voltage required for the patient to perceive sensory stimulation. If motor stimulation of the upper extremity is identified, the radiofrequency needle must be repositioned away from the cervical nerve root. After the injection of local anesthetic, a radiofrequency lesion is then made at 80 degrees for 60 to 90 seconds. The needle is then repositioned superiorly or inferiorly 2 to 3 mm, and a second lesion is repeated. This technique is repeated at each targeted level, with care taken to complete trial stimulation each time the radiofrequency electrode is repositioned.

Foraminal Approach

The patient is placed in the supine position. The skin overlying the anterior and ipsilateral region overlying the target vertebra is prepared with antiseptic solution. A lateral view is obtained with the fluoroscope and then rotated to demonstrate the foramen in its greatest diameter.

The fluoroscope beam is then moved caudally until the foramen is seen in its maximal dimension, which will place the beam parallel to the exiting nerve root. The targeted level is again confirmed, and the skin is anesthetized with local anesthetic over an area 2 times the width of the neural arch to a point even with the lower third of the foramen. A radiofrequency cannula is then inserted and advanced so as to contact bone one fourth to one third the distance between the foramen and the posterior border of the articular pillar. An AP view will confirm the cannula tip as lying at the waist of the articular column.

After confirmation of proper needle placement, stimulation at 50 Hz is carried out, with the patient reporting stimulation between 0.1 and 0.5 V. This should reproduce the patient's pain pattern, although the quality may not be perceived as identical by the patient. Motor stimulation of the radiofrequency cannula at 2 to 3 V at 2 Hz is increased slowly. There should be no stimulation of the upper extremity at 2½ to 3 times the voltage required for the patient to perceive sensory stimulation. If motor stimulation of the upper extremity is identified, the radiofrequency needle must be repositioned away from the cervical nerve root. After the injection of local anesthetic, a radiofrequency lesion is then made at 80°C

for 60 to 90 seconds. The needle is then repositioned superiorly or inferiorly 2 to 3 mm, and a second lesion is repeated. This technique is repeated at each targeted level, with care taken to complete trial stimulation each time the radiofrequency electrode is repositioned.

SIDE EFFECTS AND COMPLICATIONS

The proximity to the spinal cord, exiting nerve roots, and vascular structures makes it imperative that this procedure be carried out only by those well versed in the regional anatomy and experienced in performing interventional pain management techniques. The proximity to the vertebral artery, combined with the vascular nature of this anatomic region, makes the potential for intravascular injection or trauma to the vessel high. Even the injection of small amounts of local anesthetic into the vertebral arteries will result in seizures. Given the proximity of the brain and brain stem, ataxia due to vascular uptake of local anesthetic is not an uncommon occurrence after cervical facet block. Many patients also complain of a transient increase in headache and cervicalgia after radiofrequency lesioning of these structures, and the routine injection of methylprednisolone or other steroids during or after radiofrequency lesioning may decrease the frequency of the annoying side effect.

CLINICAL PEARLS

Radiofrequency lesioning of the cervical medial branches of the primary posterior rami is being used more frequently to provide long-lasting relief of pain emanating from the cervical facet joints. Appropriate diagnostic testing, optimization of conservative therapy, and careful patient selection will help decrease the potential for suboptimal results, and careful attention to needle placement and rigid adherence to the rule of repeat trial stimulation every time the needle is repositioned will markedly decrease the incidence of complications associated with this technique.

Radiofrequency lesioning of the C2 dorsal root ganglion (the atlantoaxial joint) of the primary posterior rami may be combined with radiofrequency lesioning of the atlantoaxial block when treating pain in the previously mentioned areas. Many pain specialists believe that these techniques are currently underused in the treatment of postwhiplash cervicalgia and cervicogenic headaches. These specialists believe that both techniques should be considered when cervical epidural nerve blocks and occipital nerve blocks fail to provide palliation of these headache and neck pain syndromes.

CHAPTER 43

Cervical Facet Block: Intra-articular Technique

CPT-2009 CODE	
First Joint	64470
Second Joint	64472
Neurolytic First Joint	64626
Neurolytic Second Joint	64627

Relative Value Units	
First Joint	10
Second Joint	10
Neurolytic First Joint	20
Neurolytic Second Joint	20

INDICATIONS

Cervical facet block using the intra-articular technique is indicated primarily as a diagnostic maneuver to prove that a specific facet joint is in fact the source of pain. The medial branch technique of facet block is suitable for most clinical applications, including the treatment of painful conditions involving trauma, arthritis, or inflammation of the cervical facet joints. These problems may manifest clinically as neck pain, suboccipital headache, and occasionally shoulder and supraclavicular pain.

CLINICALLY RELEVANT ANATOMY

The cervical facet joints are formed by the articulations of the superior and inferior articular facets of adjacent vertebrae. Except for the atlanto-occipital and atlanto-axial joints, the remaining cervical facet joints are true joints in that they are lined with synovium and possess a true joint capsule. This capsule is richly innervated and supports the notion of the facet joint as a pain generator. The cervical facet joint is susceptible to arthritic changes and trauma caused by acceleration-deceleration injuries. Such damage to the joint results in pain secondary to synovial joint inflammation and adhesions.

Each facet joint receives innervation from two spinal levels. Each joint receives fibers from the dorsal ramus at the same level as the vertebra as well as fibers from the dorsal ramus of the vertebra above. This fact has clinical import in that it provides an explanation for the ill-defined nature of facet-mediated pain and explains why the branch of the dorsal ramus arising above the offending level must often also be blocked to provide complete pain relief. At each level, the dorsal ramus provides a medial branch that wraps around the convexity of the articular pillar of its respective vertebra and provides innervation to the facet joint.

TECHNIQUE

Cervical facet block using the intra-articular technique may be performed either blind or under fluoroscopic guidance. The patient is placed in a prone position. Pillows are placed under the chest to allow the cervical spine to be moderately flexed without discomfort to the patient. The forehead is allowed to rest on a folded blanket.

Blind Technique

If a blind technique is used, the spinous process at the level to be blocked is identified by palpation. A point two spinal levels lower and 2.5 cm lateral to the spinous process is then identified as the site of needle insertion. Three milliliters of preservative-free local anesthetic is drawn up in a 5-mL sterile syringe. After preparation of the skin with antiseptic solution, a skin wheal of local anesthetic is raised at the site of needle insertion. When treating pain thought to be secondary to an inflammatory process, a total of 80 mg of depot-steroid is added to the local anesthetic with the first block, and 40 mg of depot-steroid is added with subsequent blocks.

An 18-gauge, 1-inch needle is inserted through the skin and into the subcutaneous tissues at the previously identified insertion site to serve as an introducer. The introducer needle is then repositioned with a superior and ventral trajectory, pointing directly toward the inferior margin of the facet joint at the level to be blocked. The angle of the needle from the skin is about 35 degrees. A 25-gauge, 3½-inch styletted spinal needle is then inserted through the 18-gauge introducer and directed toward the articular pillar just below the joint to be blocked. Care must be taken to be sure the trajectory of the needle does not drift either laterally or medially. Medial drift can allow the needle to enter the epidural, subdural, or subarachnoid space and to traumatize the dorsal root or spinal cord. Lateral drift can allow the needle to pass beyond the lateral border of the articular pillar and traumatize the vertebral artery or exiting nerve roots.

After bony contact is made, the depth of the contact is noted, and the spinal needle is withdrawn. The introducer needle is then redirected slightly more superiorly. The spinal needle is then advanced through the introducer needle until it impinges on the bone of the articular pillar. This maneuver is repeated until the spinal needle slides into the facet joint (Fig. 43-1). A pop is often felt as the needle slides into the joint cavity.

After the needle is felt to be in satisfactory position, the stylet is removed from the 25-gauge spinal needle, and the hub is observed for blood or cerebrospinal fluid. If neither is present, gentle aspiration of the needle is carried out. If the aspiration test is negative, 1 mL of solution is injected slowly through the spinal needle. Rapid or forceful injection may rupture the joint capsule and exacerbate the patient's pain.

Fluoroscopic Technique

If fluoroscopy is used, the beam is rotated in a sagittal plane from anterior to posterior position, which allows identification and visualization of the articular pillars of the respective vertebrae and the adjacent facet joints. After preparation of the skin with antiseptic solution, a skin wheal of local anesthetic is raised at the site of needle insertion. An 18-gauge, 1-inch needle is inserted at the insertion site to serve as an introducer. The fluoroscopy beam is aimed directly through the introducer needle, which will appear as a small point on the fluoroscopy screen. The introducer needle is then repositioned under fluoroscopic guidance until this small point is visualized pointing directly toward the inferior aspect of the facet joint to be blocked.

A total of 5 mL of contrast medium suitable for intrathecal use is drawn up in a sterile 12-mL syringe. Then, 2 mL of preservative-free local anesthetic is drawn up in a separate 5-mL sterile syringe. When treating pain thought to be secondary to an inflammatory process, a total of 80 mg of depot-steroid is added to the local anesthetic with the first block, and 40 mg of depot-steroid is added with subsequent blocks.

A 25-gauge, 3½-inch styletted spinal needle is then inserted through the 18-gauge introducer and directed toward the articular pillar just below the joint to be blocked. After bony contact is made, the spinal needle is withdrawn, and the introducer needle is repositioned superiorly, aiming toward the facet joint itself. The 25-gauge spinal needle is then readvanced through the introducer needle until it enters the target joint (Fig. 43-2).

After confirmation of needle placement by biplanar fluoroscopy, the stylet is removed from the 25-gauge spinal needle, and the hub is observed for blood or cerebrospinal fluid. If neither is present, gentle aspiration of the needle is carried out. If the aspiration test is negative, 1 mL of contrast medium is slowly injected under fluoroscopic guidance to reconfirm needle placement (Fig. 43-3). After correct needle placement is confirmed, 1 mL of local anesthetic with or without steroid is slowly injected through the spinal needle. Rapid or forceful injection may rupture the joint capsule and exacerbate the patient's pain.

SIDE EFFECTS AND COMPLICATIONS

The proximity to the spinal cord and exiting nerve roots makes it imperative that this procedure be carried out only by those well versed in the regional anatomy and experienced in performing interventional pain management techniques. The proximity to the vertebral artery, combined with the vascular nature of this anatomic region, makes the potential for intravascular injection high. Even small amounts of injection of local anesthetic into the vertebral arteries will result in seizures. Given the proximity of the brain and brain stem, ataxia due to vascular uptake of local anesthetic is not an uncommon occurrence after cervical facet block. Many patients also complain of a transient increase in headache and cervicalgia after injection of the joint.

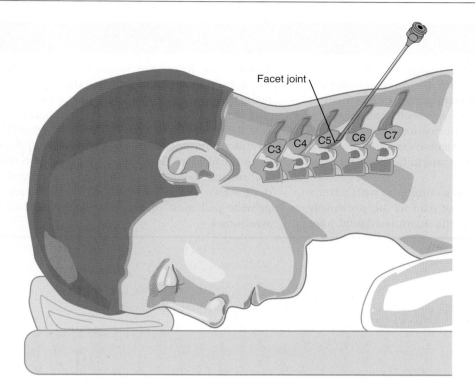

Facet joint

C3 C4 C5 C6 C7

Figure 43-1.

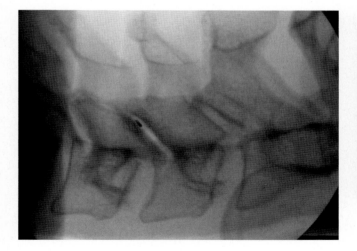

Figure 43-2.
Needle tip resting in the facet joint.

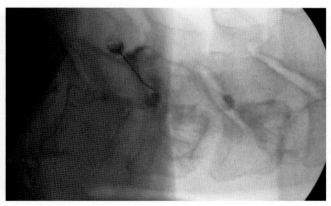

Figure 43-3.
Contrast medium with the facet joint.

CLINICAL PEARLS

Cervical facet block using the medial branch approach is the preferred technique for treatment of cervical facet syndrome. Although intra-articular placement of the needle into the facet joint is technically feasible, unless specific diagnostic information about that specific joint is required, such maneuvers add nothing to the efficacy of the procedure and in fact may increase the rate of complications.

Cervical facet block is often combined with atlanto-occipital block when treating pain in the previously mentioned areas. Although the atlanto-occipital joint is not a true facet joint in the anatomic sense of the word, the block is analogous to the facet joint block technique used commonly by pain practitioners and may be viewed as such. Many pain specialists believe that these techniques are currently underused in the treatment of postwhiplash cervicalgia and cervicogenic headaches. These specialists believe that both techniques should be considered when cervical epidural nerve blocks and occipital nerve blocks fail to provide palliation of these headache and neck pain syndromes.

CHAPTER **44**

Cervical Epidural Block: Translaminar Approach

CPT-2009 CODE	
Local Anesthetic/Narcotic	62310
Steroid	62310
Neurolytic	62281

Relative Value Units	
Local Anesthetic	10
Steroid	10
Neurolytic	20

INDICATIONS

In addition to a limited number of applications for surgical anesthesia, cervical epidural nerve block with local anesthetics can be used as a diagnostic tool when performing differential neural blockade on an anatomic basis in the evaluation of head, neck, face, shoulder, and upper extremity pain. If destruction of the cervical nerve roots is being considered, this technique is useful as a prognostic indicator of the degree of motor and sensory impairment that the patient may experience.

Cervical epidural nerve block with local anesthetics, opioids, or both may be used to palliate acute pain emergencies while waiting for pharmacologic, surgical, or antiblastic methods to become effective. This technique is useful in the management of postoperative pain as well as pain secondary to trauma. The pain of acute herpes zoster and cancer-related pain is also amenable to treatment with epidurally administered local anesthetics, steroids, or opioids. Additionally, this technique is of value in patients suffering from acute vascular insufficiency of the upper extremities secondary to vasospastic and vaso-occlusive disease, including frostbite and ergotamine toxicity. There is increasing evidence that the prophylactic or preemptive use of epidural nerve blocks in patients scheduled to undergo limb amputations for ischemia results in a decreased incidence of phantom limb pain.

The administration of local anesthetics, steroids, or both via the cervical approach to the epidural space is useful in the treatment of a variety of chronic benign pain syndromes, including cervical radiculopathy, cervicalgia, cervical spondylosis, cervical postlaminectomy syndrome, tension-type headache, phantom limb pain, vertebral compression fractures, diabetic polyneuropathy, chemotherapy-related peripheral neuropathy, postherpetic neuralgia, reflex sympathetic dystrophy, and neck and shoulder pain syndromes.

The cervical epidural administration of local anesthetics in combination with steroids, opioids, or both is also useful in the palliation of cancer-related pain of the head, face, neck, shoulder, upper extremity, and upper trunk. This technique has been especially successful in the relief of pain secondary to metastatic disease of the spine. The long-term epidural administration of opioids has become a mainstay in the palliation of cancer-related pain.

CLINICALLY RELEVANT ANATOMY

The superior boundary of the cervical epidural space is the fusion of the periosteal and spinal layers of dura at the foramen magnum. The epidural space continues inferiorly to the sacrococcygeal membrane. The cervical epidural space is bounded anteriorly by the posterior longitudinal ligament and posteriorly by the vertebral laminae and the ligamentum flavum. The vertebral pedicles and intervertebral foramina form the lateral limits of the epidural space. The cervical epidural space is 3 to 4 mm at the C7-T1 interspace with the cervical spine flexed. The cervical epidural space contains fat, veins, arteries, lymphatics, and connective tissue.

When performing cervical epidural block in the midline, after traversing the skin and subcutaneous tissues, the styletted epidural needle will impinge on the ligamentum nuchae, which runs vertically between the apices of the cervical spinous processes. The interspinous ligament, which runs obliquely between spinous processes, is next encountered, offering additional resistance to needle advancement. This ligament is dense enough to hold a needle in position even when the needle is released. Because the interspinous ligament is contiguous with the ligamentum flavum, the pain management specialist may perceive a "false" loss of resistance when the needle tip enters the space between the interspinous ligament and the ligamentum flavum. This phenomenon is more pronounced in the cervical region than in the lumbar region because the ligaments are less well defined.

A significant increase in resistance to needle advancement signals that the needle tip is impinging on the dense ligamentum flavum. Because the ligament is made up almost entirely of elastin fibers, there is a continued increase in resistance as the needle traverses the ligamentum flavum owing to the drag of the ligament on the needle. A sudden loss of resistance occurs as the needle tip enters the epidural space. There should be essentially no resistance to drugs injected into the normal epidural space.

TECHNIQUE

Cervical epidural nerve block may be carried out in the sitting, lateral, or prone position, with the sitting position being favored for simplicity of patient positioning when compared with the lateral position. The prone position should be avoided because it makes patient monitoring more difficult.

After the patient is placed in optimal sitting position with the cervical spine flexed and forehead placed on a padded bedside table, the skin is prepared with an antiseptic solution. At the C5-C6 or C6-C7 interspace, the operator's middle and index fingers are placed on each side of the spinous processes. The position of the interspace is reconfirmed with palpation using a rocking motion in the superior and inferior planes (Fig. 44-1). The midline of the selected interspace is identified by palpating the spinous processes above and below the interspace using a lateral rocking motion to ensure that the needle entry site is exactly in the midline. One milliliter of local anesthetic is used to infiltrate the skin, subcutaneous tissues, and the supraspinous and interspinous ligaments at the midline.

For experienced practitioners, a 25-gauge, 2-inch needle is preferred for this technique. For less experienced practitioners, a longer, larger, blunter needle such as the 18- or 20-gauge, $3\frac{1}{2}$-inch Hustead needle may be used. The needle chosen is inserted exactly in the midline in the previously anesthetized area through the ligamentum nuchae into the interspinous ligament (Figs. 44-2 and 44-3).

The right-handed physician holds the epidural needle firmly at the hub with his or her left thumb and index finger. The left hand is placed firmly against the patient's neck to ensure against uncontrolled needle movements should the patient unexpectedly move (Fig. 44-4). After attaching a syringe containing either preservative-free saline or the intended injectate of local anesthetic, narcotic, or steroid, with constant pressure being applied to the plunger of the syringe with the thumb of the right hand, the needle and syringe are continuously advanced in a slow and deliberate manner with the left hand. As soon as the needle bevel passes through the ligamentum flavum and enters the epidural space, there will be a sudden loss of resistance to injection, and the plunger will effortlessly surge forward (Fig. 44-5). If the practitioner is unsure about needle position, the syringe is gently removed from the needle and an air or saline acceptance test is carried out by injecting 0.5 to 1 mL of air or sterile preservative-free saline with a well-lubricated sterile glass syringe to help confirm that the needle is within the epidural space. The force required for injection should not exceed that necessary to overcome the resistance of the needle. Any significant pain or sudden increase in resistance during injection suggests incorrect needle placement, and one should *stop* injecting immediately and reassess the position of the needle.

When satisfactory needle position is confirmed, a syringe containing 5 to 7 mL of solution to be injected is carefully attached to the needle. Gentle aspiration is carried out to identify cerebrospinal fluid or blood. If cerebrospinal fluid is aspirated, the epidural block may be repeated at a different interspace. In this situation, drug dosages should be adjusted accordingly because subarachnoid migration of drugs through the dural rent can occur. If aspiration of blood occurs, the needle should be rotated slightly and the aspiration test repeated. If no blood is present, incremental doses of local anesthetic and other drugs may be administered while monitoring the patient carefully for signs of local anesthetic toxicity. Fluoroscopy is useful if surface landmarks are difficult to palpate because of patient size or previous surgery (Fig. 44-6). A small amount of contrast may be injected through the needle to confirm epidural placement (Fig. 44-7).

For diagnostic and prognostic blocks, 1.0% preservative-free lidocaine is a suitable local anesthetic. For therapeutic blocks, 0.25% preservative-free bupivacaine in combination with 80 mg of methylprednisolone is injected. Subsequent nerve blocks are carried out in a similar manner, substituting 40 mg of methylprednisolone for the initial 80-mg dose. Daily cervical epidural nerve blocks with local anesthetic or steroid may be required to treat the previously mentioned acute painful conditions. Chronic conditions such as cervical radiculopathy, tension-type headaches, and diabetic polyneuropathy are treated on an every-other-day to once-a-week basis or as the clinical situation dictates.

If the cervical epidural route is chosen for administration of opioids, 0.5 mg of preservative-free morphine

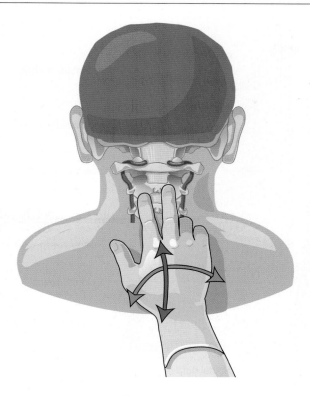

Figure 44-1.

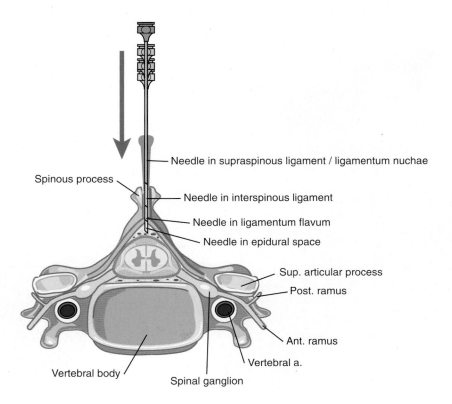

Needle in supraspinous ligament / ligamentum nuchae

Spinous process

Needle in interspinous ligament

Needle in ligamentum flavum

Needle in epidural space

Sup. articular process

Post. ramus

Ant. ramus

Vertebral a.

Spinal ganglion

Vertebral body

Figure 44-2.

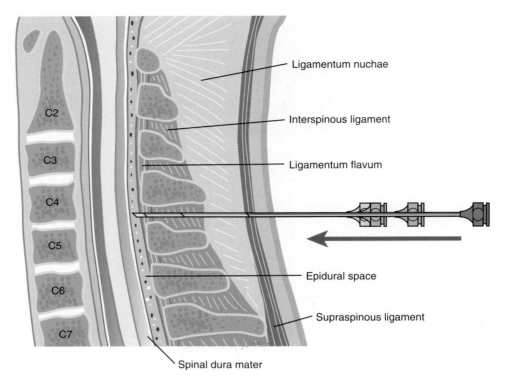

Ligamentum nuchae

Interspinous ligament

Ligamentum flavum

Epidural space

Supraspinous ligament

Spinal dura mater

C2
C3
C4
C5
C6
C7

Figure 44-3.

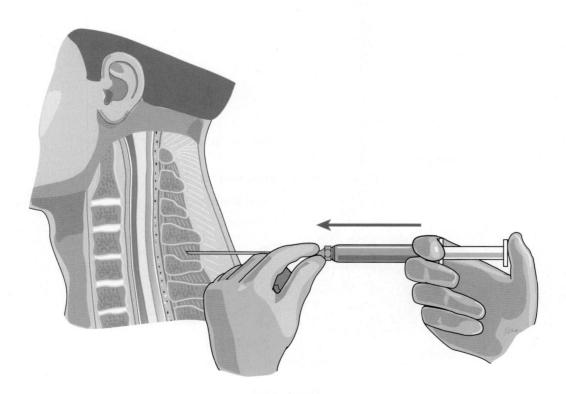

Figure 44-4.

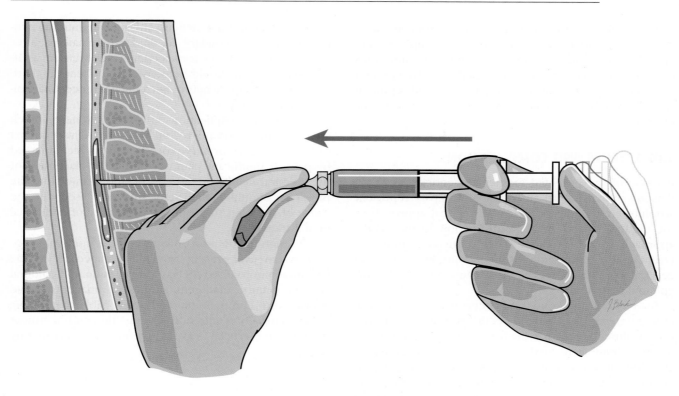

Figure 44-5.

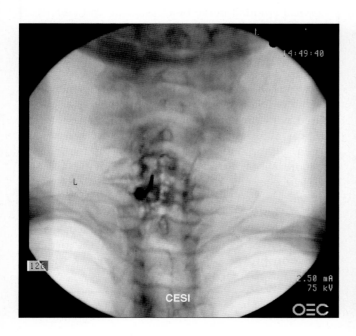

Figure 44-6.
Needle tip resting in the cervical epidural space.

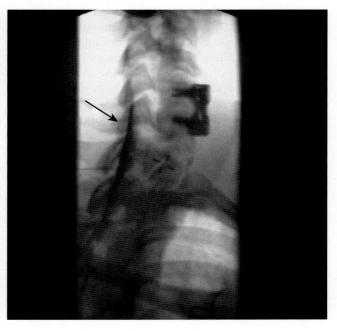

Figure 44-7.
Oblique view following injection of an additional 1.5 mL of nonionic contrast material demonstrates additional inferior flow as well as flow into the more superior cervical spinal canal (*arrow*). (From Renfrew DL: Atlas of Spine Injection, 4th ed. Philadelphia, WB Saunders, 2004, p 52.)

sulfate formulated for epidural use is a reasonable initial dose in opioid-tolerant patients. More lipid-soluble opioids such as fentanyl must be delivered by continuous infusion via a cervical epidural catheter. An epidural catheter may be placed into the cervical epidural space through a Hustead needle to allow continuous infusions.

SIDE EFFECTS AND COMPLICATIONS

Because of the potential for hematogenous spread via Batson's plexus, local infection and sepsis represent absolute contraindications to the cervical approach to the epidural space. In contradistinction to the caudal approach to the epidural space, anticoagulation and coagulopathy represent absolute contraindications to cervical epidural nerve block because of the risk for epidural hematoma.

Inadvertent dural puncture occurring during cervical epidural nerve block should occur less than 0.5% of the time. Failure to recognize inadvertent dural puncture can result in immediate total spinal anesthesia with associated loss of consciousness, hypotension, and apnea. If epidural doses of opioids are accidentally placed into the subarachnoid space, significant respiratory and central nervous system depression will result. It is also possible to inadvertently place a needle or catheter intended for the epidural space into the subdural space. If subdural placement is unrecognized and epidural doses of local anesthetics are administered, the signs and symptoms are similar to those of massive subarachnoid injection, although the resulting motor and sensory block may be spotty.

The cervical epidural space is highly vascular. The intravenous placement of the epidural needle occurs in about 0.5% to 1% of patients undergoing cervical epidural anesthesia. This complication is increased in those patients with distended epidural veins, such as the parturient and patients with a large intra-abdominal tumor mass. If the misplacement is unrecognized, injection of local anesthetic directly into an epidural vein will result in significant local anesthetic toxicity.

Needle trauma to the epidural veins may result in self-limited bleeding, which may cause postprocedure pain. Uncontrolled bleeding into the epidural space may result in compression of the spinal cord with the rapid devel-

opment of neurologic deficit. Although significant neurologic deficit secondary to epidural hematoma after cervical epidural block is exceedingly rare, this devastating complication should be considered whenever there is rapidly developing neurologic deficit after cervical epidural nerve block.

Neurologic complications after cervical nerve block are uncommon if proper technique is used. Direct trauma to the spinal cord or nerve roots is usually accompanied by pain. If significant pain occurs during placement of the epidural needle or catheter or during injection, the physician should immediately stop and ascertain the cause of the pain to avoid the possibility of additional neural trauma.

Although uncommon, infection in the epidural space remains an ever-present possibility, especially in the immunocompromised AIDS or cancer patient. If epidural abscess occurs, emergent surgical drainage to avoid spinal cord compression and irreversible neurologic deficit is usually required. Early detection and treatment of infection is crucial to avoid potentially life-threatening sequelae.

CLINICAL PEARLS

Cervical epidural nerve block is a safe and effective procedure if careful attention is paid to technique. Failure to accurately identify the midline is the most common reason for difficulty in performing cervical epidural nerve block and increases the risk for complications. It should be noted that the ligamentum flavum is relatively thin in the cervical region compared with the lumbar region. This fact has direct clinical implications in that the loss of resistance when performing cervical epidural nerve block is more subtle than when performing the loss-of-resistance technique in the lumbar or lower thoracic region.

The routine use of sedation or general anesthesia before initiation of cervical epidural nerve block is to be discouraged because it will render the patient unable to provide accurate verbal feedback should needle misplacement occur.

CHAPTER 45

Cervical Epidural Block: Transforaminal Approach

CPT-2009 CODE	
Local Anesthetic	64479
Steroid	64479
Additional Level	64480

Relative Value Units	
Local Anesthetic	10
Steroid	10
Each Additional Level	10

INDICATIONS

Cervical epidural injection via the transforaminal approach with local anesthetics, corticosteroid, or both can be used as a diagnostic tool or treatment modality when performing differential neural blockade on an anatomic basis in the evaluation of head, neck, face, shoulder, and upper extremity pain. If destruction of the cervical nerve roots is being considered, this technique is useful as a prognostic indicator of the degree of motor and sensory impairment that the patient may experience.

Although the interlaminar approach is more commonly used for routine therapeutic cervical epidural nerve injection, some interventional pain management specialists believe the transforaminal approach to the cervical epidural space is more efficacious in the treatment of painful conditions involving a single nerve root albeit with a higher incidence of potential complications (see Chapter 44 for indications for therapeutic cervical epidural nerve block). Examples of such conditions include cervical radicular pain and radiculopathy secondary to cervical disk displacement, neural foraminal stenosis, and perineural fibrosis.

CLINICALLY RELEVANT ANATOMY

The superior boundary of the cervical epidural space is the fusion of the periosteal and spinal layers of dura at the foramen magnum. The epidural space continues inferiorly to the sacrococcygeal membrane. The cervical epidural space is bounded anteriorly by the posterior longitudinal ligament and posteriorly by the vertebral laminae and the ligamentum flavum. The medial aspect of pedicles and intervertebral foramina form the lateral limits of the epidural space. The cervical epidural space is 3 to 4 mm at the C7-T1 interspace with the cervical spine flexed. The cervical epidural space contains veins, arteries, lymphatics, connective tissue, and a relative paucity of fat compared with the lumbar epidural space.

When performing cervical epidural injections using the transforaminal approach, the goal is to place the needle just inside the posterior portion of the neural foramen of the affected nerve root (Fig. 45-1). There should be essentially no resistance to drugs injected into the normal epidural space.

TECHNIQUE

Cervical epidural injection using the transforaminal approach is carried out with the patient in the supine or lateral position. Although some experienced pain practitioners perform this technique without radiographic guidance, the use of fluoroscopy is recommended to aid in needle placement and will help avoid placing the needle too deeply into the spinal canal and unintentionally injecting into the spinal cord or misplaced intervascular structures such as the vertebral or segmental arteries. With the patient in the supine or lateral position on the fluoroscopy table, the fluoroscopy beam is rotated from a lateral to an anterior oblique position to allow visualization of the affected neural foramina at its largest diameter (Figs. 45-2 and 45-3). The fluoroscopy beam is then slowly moved from a cephalad to a more caudad position to also allow visualization of the affected neural foramina. When this is accomplished, the beam should be parallel to the affected nerve root.

The skin is then prepared with an antiseptic solution, and a skin wheal of local anesthetic may be placed at a point overlying the posterior aspect of the foramen just

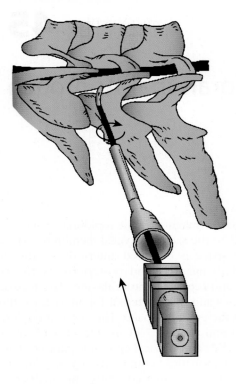

Figure 45-1.
Proper needle position for cervical transforaminal epidural block. (From Raj PP, Lou L, Erdine S, et al: Interventional Pain Management: Image-Guided Procedures, 2nd ed, Saunders, 2008.)

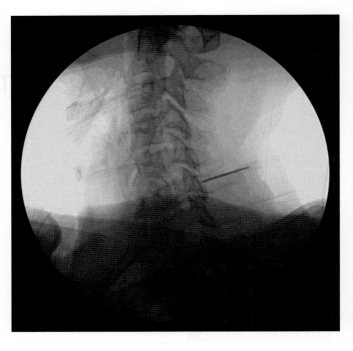

Figure 45-2.
Oblique view with introducer cannula. (From Raj PP, Lou L, Erdine S, et al: Interventional Pain Management: Image-Guided Procedures, 2nd ed, Saunders, 2008.)

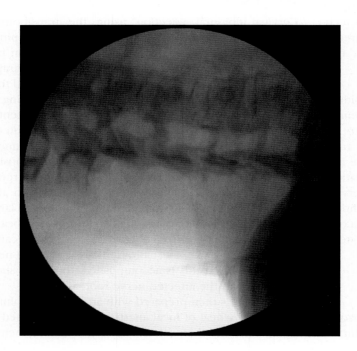

Figure 45-3.
Oblique view of the cervical neural foramina.

over the tip of the superior articular process of the level below the affected neural foramen. This point is about one third of the distance cephalad from the most posteroinferior aspect of the foramen. A 25-gauge, 2-inch needle is then placed through the previously anesthetized area and advanced until the tip rests against the posteromedial portion of the superior articular process of the targeted neural foramen (Figs. 45-4 to 45-6). Failure to impinge on bone at the point should be of grave concern and may indicate that the needle has passed through the foramen and rests within the substance of the spinal cord. Failure to identify this problem can lead to disastrous results (see "Side Effects and Complications"). After this bony landmark is identified, an anteroposterior fluoroscopic view is obtained to verify that the needle is within the nerve canal and not past the midpoint of the facetal column, to avoid placement of the needle within the dura or into the spinal cord.

After satisfactory needle position is confirmed and the needle bevel is oriented medially, 0.2 to 0.4 mL of contrast medium suitable for subarachnoid use is gently injected under active fluoroscopy. The contrast should be seen to flow into the epidural space and distal along the affected nerve root sheath (Fig. 45-7). The injection of contrast should be stopped immediately if the patient complains of significant pain on injection. After satisfactory flow of contrast is observed and there is no evidence of subdural, subarachnoid, or intravascular spread of contrast, 6 mg of betamethasone suspension or solution, 20 to 40 mg of methylprednisolone in solution, or 20 to 40 mg of triamcinolone suspension with 0.5 to 1.5 mL of 2% or 4% preservative-free lidocaine is slowly injected. Injection of the local anesthetic and steroid should be discontinued if the patient complains of any significant pain on injection. After satisfactory injection of the local anesthetic and steroid, the needle is removed, and pressure is placed on the injection site. Dr. Gabor Racz suggests that after injection, the cervical spine should be gently flexed and then gently rotated from side to side to facilitate opening of the neural foramina to reduce epidural pressure. The technique may be repeated at additional levels as a diagnostic or therapeutic maneuver.

SIDE EFFECTS AND COMPLICATIONS

Basically, all the potential side effects and complications associated with the interlaminar approach to the cervical epidural space can occur with the transforaminal approach, with the transforaminal approach having a statistically significant increase in the incidence of persistent paresthesias and trauma to neural structures including the spinal cord. As mentioned earlier, placement of the needle too far into the neural foramina when using the transforaminal approach to the cervical epi-

dural space may result in unintentional injection into the spinal cord with resultant quadriplegia or death.

Because of the potential for hematogenous spread via Batson's plexus, local infection and sepsis represent absolute contraindications to the cervical approach to the epidural space. In contradistinction to the caudal approach to the epidural space, anticoagulation and coagulopathy represent absolute contraindications to cervical epidural nerve block because of the risk for epidural hematoma.

Unintentional dural puncture occurring during cervical epidural nerve block should occur less than 0.5% of the time with the interlaminar approach and with a slightly greater frequency when using the transforaminal approach. Failure to recognize unintentional dural puncture can result in immediate total spinal anesthesia with associated loss of consciousness, hypotension, and apnea. It is also possible to unintentionally place a needle intended for the epidural space into the subdural space. If subdural placement is unrecognized and epidural doses of local anesthetics are administered, the signs and symptoms are similar to those of massive subarachnoid injection with prolonged temporal onset, although the resulting motor and sensory block may be spotty.

The cervical epidural space and spinal-nerve canals are highly vascular. The intravenous placement of the epidural needle occurs in about 0.5% to 1% of patients undergoing cervical epidural anesthesia. This complication is increased in patients with distended epidural veins, such as those with foraminal obstruction secondary to herniated nucleus pulposus or tumor as well as those with a large intra-abdominal tumor mass. If the misplacement is unrecognized, injection of local anesthetic directly into an epidural vein will result in significant local anesthetic toxicity. Damage or injection to the segmental artery can occur with increased incidence when performing the transforaminal approach to the epidural space but is more common at the C5-C7 neural foramina on the right.

Needle trauma to the epidural veins may result in self-limited bleeding, which may cause postprocedure pain. Uncontrolled bleeding into the epidural space may result in compression of the spinal cord with the rapid development of neurologic deficit. Although significant neurologic deficit secondary to epidural hematoma after cervical epidural block is exceedingly rare, this devastating complication should be considered whenever there is rapidly developing neurologic deficit after cervical epidural nerve block.

Neurologic complications after cervical nerve block are uncommon if proper technique is used and excessive sedation is avoided. Direct trauma to the spinal cord or nerve roots is usually accompanied by pain. However, the patient may experience little or no pain with needle insertion into the cord, and multiple fluoroscopic views

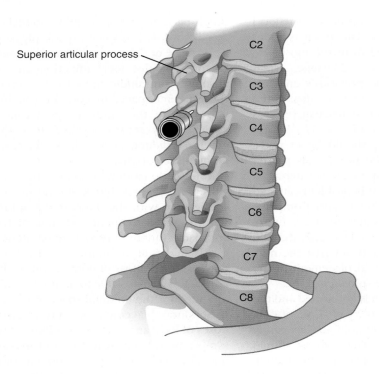

Superior articular process

C2
C3
C4
C5
C6
C7
C8

Figure 45-4.

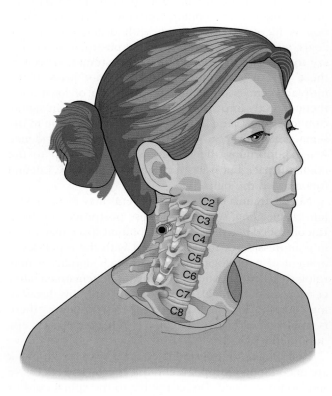

C2
C3
C4
C5
C6
C7
C8

Figure 45-5.

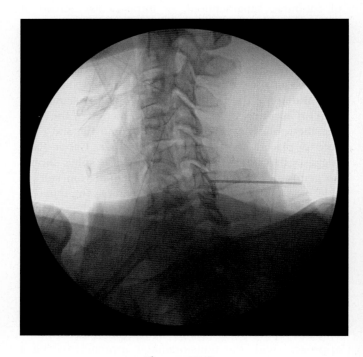

Figure 45-6.
Curved blunt needle advanced to bone. (From Raj PP, Lou L, Erdine S, et al: Interventional Pain Management: Image-Guided Procedures, 2nd ed. Saunders, 2008.)

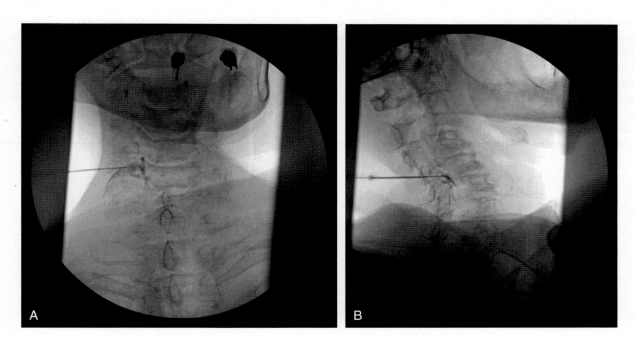

Figure 45-7.
AP (**A**) and lateral (**B**) views with contrast injection. (From Raj PP, Lou L,
Erdine S, et al: Interventional Pain Management: Image-Guided Procedures,
2nd ed, Saunders, 2008.)

are required to avoid this potentially devastating complication. If significant pain occurs during placement of the epidural needle or during the injection of contrast or local anesthetic with or without steroid, the physician should immediately stop and ascertain the cause of the pain to avoid the possibility of additional neural trauma and serious sequelae.

Although uncommon, infection in the epidural space remains an ever-present possibility, especially in the immunocompromised AIDS or cancer patient. If epidural abscess occurs, emergent surgical drainage to avoid spinal cord compression and irreversible neurologic deficit is usually required. Early detection and treatment of infection are crucial to avoid potentially life-threatening sequelae.

CLINICAL PEARLS

Some practitioners recommend the use of a blunt-tipped needle when performing the transforaminal approach to the cervical epidural space, whereas others believe a sharper needle is better suited for this technique. Any significant pain or sudden increase in resistance during injection suggests incorrect needle placement, and one should *stop* injecting immediately and reassess the position of the needle. Because pain is an important indication of improper needle place-ment, the practitioner should avoid the use of excessive sedation during transforaminal cervical injections. The use of fluoroscopy and injection of contrast to ensure correct needle placement and lack of vascular uptake will help decrease the incidence of complications associated with this procedure. As mentioned, the use of sedation in patients in the prone position requires special attention to monitoring.

CHAPTER 46

Lysis of Cervical Epidural Adhesions: Racz Technique

CPT-2009 CODE

Lysis of Adhesions–Decompression of Nerve Two Day	62263
Lysis of Adhesions–Decompression of Nerve One Day	62264

Relative Value Units

Injection Procedure Two Day	30 Units
Injection Procedure One Day	25 Units

INDICATIONS

Lysis of epidural adhesions has been used to treat a variety of painful conditions. It is postulated that the common denominator in each of these pain syndromes is the compromise of spinal nerve roots as they traverse and exit the epidural space by adhesions and scarring. It is thought that these adhesions and scar tissue not only restrict the free movement of the nerve roots as they emerge from the spinal cord and travel through the intervertebral foramina but also result in dysfunction of epidural venous blood and lymph flow. This dysfunction results in additional nerve root edema, which further compromises the affected nerves. Inflammation also may play a part in the genesis of pain as these nerves are repeatedly traumatized each time the nerve is stretched against the adhesions and scar tissue.

Diagnostic categories thought to be amenable to treatment with lysis of epidural adhesions using the Racz technique include failed cervical spine surgery with associated perineural fibrosis, herniated disk, traumatic and nontraumatic vertebral body compression fracture, metastatic carcinoma to the spine and epidural space, multilevel degenerative arthritis, facet joint pain, epidural scarring following infection, and other pain syndromes of the spine that have their basis in epidural scarring and have failed to respond to more conservative treatments.

CLINICALLY RELEVANT ANATOMY

The superior boundary of the cervical epidural space is the fusion of the periosteal and spinal layers of dura at the foramen magnum. The epidural space continues inferiorly to the sacrococcygeal membrane. The cervical epidural space is bounded anteriorly by the posterior longitudinal ligament and posteriorly by the vertebral laminae and the ligamentum flavum. The vertebral pedicles and intervertebral foramina form the lateral limits of the epidural space. The cervical epidural space is 3 to 4 mm at the C7-T1 interspace with the cervical spine flexed. The cervical epidural space contains fat, veins, arteries, lymphatics, and connective tissue. The epidural space is subject to scarring following infection, inflammation, and surgery.

TECHNIQUE

Intravenous access is obtained for administration of intravenous sedation during the injection of solutions via the catheter. Sedation during injection may be necessary because of pain produced by the distraction of the nerve roots as the solution lyses the perineural adhesions. After venous access is obtained, the patient is placed in the prone position with the cervical spine placed in a flexed position that is comfortable for the patient to allow access to the epidural space.

Preparation of a wide area of skin with antiseptic solution is then carried out so that all the landmarks can be palpated aseptically. A fenestrated sterile drape is placed to avoid contamination of the palpating fingers. At the C7-T1 interspace, the operator's middle and index fingers are placed on each side of the spinous processes. The position of the interspace is reconfirmed with palpation using a rocking motion in the superior and inferior planes. The midline of the selected interspace is identified by palpating the spinous processes above and below the interspace using a lateral rocking motion to ensure that the needle entry site is exactly in the midline. One milliliter of local anesthetic is used to infiltrate the skin, subcutaneous tissues, and supraspinous and interspinous ligaments at the midline. The interspace and midline is then confirmed with fluoroscopy.

After confirmation of the interspace and midline, a 19-gauge, 3½-inch styletted needle suitable for catheter placement is inserted through the anesthetized area. The right-handed physician holds the epidural needle firmly at the hub with his or her left thumb and index finger. The left hand is placed firmly against the patient's neck to ensure against uncontrolled needle movements should the patient unexpectedly move. After attaching a syringe containing preservative-free saline, with constant pressure being applied to the plunger of the syringe with the thumb of the right hand, the needle and syringe are continuously advanced in a slow and deliberate manner with the left hand. As soon as the needle bevel passes through the ligamentum flavum and enters the epidural space, there will be a sudden loss of resistance to injection, and the plunger will effortlessly surge forward. If the practitioner is unsure about needle position, the syringe is gently removed from the needle, and an air or saline acceptance test is carried out by injecting 0.5 to 1 mL of air or sterile preservative-free saline with a well-lubricated sterile glass syringe to help confirm that the needle is within the epidural space (Figs. 46-1 and 46-2). The force required for injection should not exceed that necessary to overcome the resistance of the needle. Any significant pain or sudden increase in resistance during injection suggests incorrect needle placement, and one should *stop* injecting immediately and reassess the position of the needle.

Needle position should be confirmed by fluoroscopy on both anteroposterior and lateral views.

After negative aspiration for blood and cerebrospinal fluid, 3 to 5 mL of a water-soluble contrast medium such as iohexol or metrizamide is slowly injected through the previously placed epidural needle under fluoroscopy (Figs. 46-3 and 46-4). The pain specialist should check closely for any evidence of contrast medium in the epidural venous plexus, which would suggest intravenous placement of the needle or subdural or subarachnoid placement and which appears as a more concentrated centrally located density. As the epidural space fills with contrast medium, a Christmas tree shape will appear as the contrast medium surrounds the perineural structures. Defects in this classic Christmas tree appearance are indicative of epidural perineural adhesions.

After confirming proper needle placement and ensuring that no blood or cerebrospinal fluid can be aspirated from the needle, 3 to 4 mL of 0.25% preservative-free bupivacaine and 40 mg of triamcinolone acetate are slowly injected through the epidural needle while observing the fluoroscope screen. The local anesthetic will force the contrast medium around the adhesions, further identifying affected nerve roots.

After the area of adhesions is identified on epidurogram, the bevel of the epidural needle is turned toward the ventrolateral aspect of the affected side. This facilitates passage of the catheter toward the affected nerves and decreases the chance of catheter breakage or shearing. The use of a wire spiral catheter such as the Racz Tun-L-Kath or Racz Brevi-XL epidural catheter will further decrease the incidence of this complication.

The catheter is then passed through the needle into the area of adhesions. Multiple attempts may be required to obtain placement of the catheter into the adhesions (Figs. 46-5 and 46-6). The Racz needle allows for the catheter to be withdrawn and repositioned and is preferred over the standard epidural needle.

After the catheter is placed within the area of adhesions, the catheter is aspirated for blood or cerebrospinal fluid. If the aspiration test is negative, an additional 3 to 4 mL of contrast medium is slowly injected through the catheter. This additional contrast medium should be seen spreading into the area of the adhesion. If the contrast material is observed to flow in satisfactory position, an additional 3 mL of 0.25% bupivacaine and 40 mg of triamcinolone are injected through the catheter to further lyse the remaining adhesions. Some investigators also recommend the addition of 200 U of hyaluronidase to facilitate the spread of solutions injected. About 3% of the population may experience some degree of allergic reaction to this drug, and this fact may limit its use.

Fifteen minutes after the second injection of bupivacaine, after negative aspiration, 5 to 6 mL of 10% saline is injected in small increments or via infusion pump over 20 to 30 minutes. The hyperosmolar properties of the hypertonic saline further shrink the nerve root and help treat the perineural edema caused by the venous obstruction secondary to the adhesions. The injection of 10% saline into the epidural space is quite painful, and intravenous sedation may be required if the saline spreads beyond the area previously anesthetized by the 0.25% bupivacaine. This pain is transient in nature and is generally gone within 10 minutes. After the final injection of 10% saline, the catheter is carefully secured, and a sterile dressing is placed. Intravenous cephalosporin antibiotics are recommended by Dr. Racz to prevent bacterial colonization of the catheter while it is in place.

This injection procedure of bupivacaine followed by 5% to 10% saline via the previously placed catheter is repeated the following day. Epidurograms are repeated only if there is a question of catheter migration because the contrast medium can be irritating to the nerve roots and is quite expensive. The catheter is removed after the last injection. The patient is instructed to keep the area clean and dry and to call at the first sign of elevated temperature or infection.

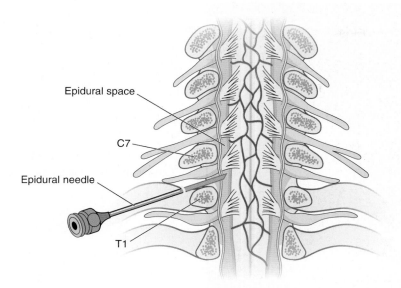

Epidural space

C7

Epidural needle

T1

Figure 46-1.

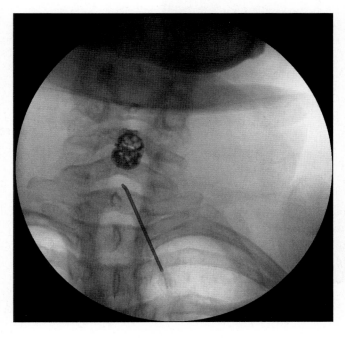

Figure 46-2.
Needle tip in the cervical epidural space.

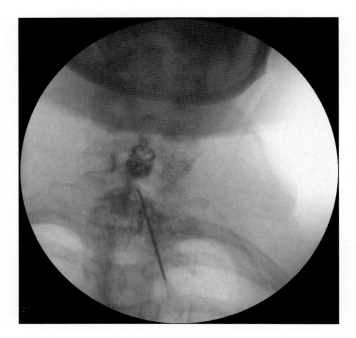

Figure 46-3.
Contrast medium within the cervical epidural space.

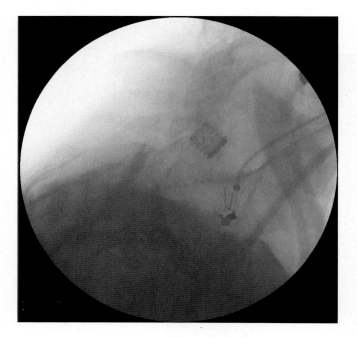

Figure 46-4.
Contrast medium within the cervical epidural space.

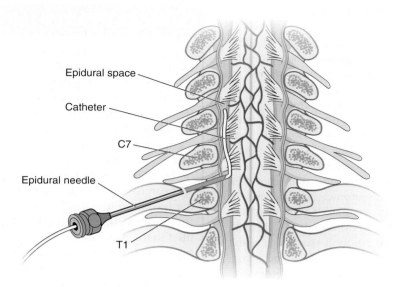

Epidural space

Catheter

C7

Epidural needle

T1

Figure 46-5.

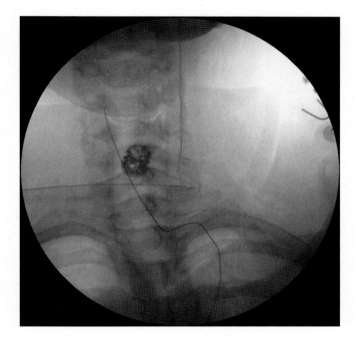

Figure 46-6.
Racz catheter within the cervical epidural space.

SIDE EFFECTS AND COMPLICATIONS

Complications directly related to epidural lysis of adhesions are generally self-limited, although occasionally, even in the best of hands, severe complications can occur. Self-limited complications include pain at the injection site, transient neck pain, ecchymosis and hematoma formation over the injection site, and unintended subdural or subarachnoid injection of local anesthetic. Severe complications of epidural lysis of adhesions include unintended subdural or subarachnoid injection of hypertonic saline, persistent sensory deficit in the lumbar and sacral dermatomes, paraparesis or paraplegia, persistent bowel or bladder dysfunction, sexual dysfunction, and infection. Although uncommon, unrecognized infection in the epidural space can result in paraplegia and death. Clinically, the signs and symptoms of epidural abscess present as a high temperature, spine pain, and progressive neurologic deficit. If epidural abscess is suspected, blood and urine cultures should be taken, antibiotics started, and emergent magnetic resonance imaging of the spine obtained to allow identification and drainage of any abscess formation before irreversible neurologic deficit.

CLINICAL PEARLS

Lysis of epidural adhesions is a straightforward technique that may provide pain relief in a carefully selected subset of patients. This technique should not be viewed as a starting point or stand-alone treatment in the continuum of pain management modalities but should be carefully integrated into a comprehensive pain management treatment plan. The identification of preexisting neurogenic bowel or bladder dysfunction by the use of urodynamics and careful neurologic examination before performing lysis of epidural adhesions is mandatory to avoid these preexisting problems being erroneously attributed to the procedure. Careful screening for preexisting sexual dysfunction is also indicated before lysis of epidural adhesions, for the same reason.

CHAPTER 47

Cervical Selective Nerve Root Block

CPT-2009 CODE	
Local Anesthetic	64479
Steroid	64479
Additional Level	64480

Relative Value Units	
Local Anesthetic	10
Steroid	10
Each Additional Level	10

INDICATIONS

Selective nerve root block of the cervical nerve roots is indicated primarily as a diagnostic maneuver designed to determine whether a specific nerve root is subserving a patient's pain. Unfortunately, there is much confusion regarding both the clinical indications and technical aspects of performing this technique, which has led to problems in assessing the clinical utility of selective nerve block. For purposes of this chapter, *selective nerve root block of the cervical nerve roots* is defined as the placement of a needle just outside the neural foramen adjacent to the target nerve root without entering the epidural, subdural, or subarachnoid space. If these conditions are met, selective spinal nerve root block is diagnostic to the specific targeted root.

However, if the needle enters the neural foramen and local anesthetic is injected, the potential to block not only the targeted nerve root but also the sinovertebral medial branch, the ramus communicans, exists. In this situation, if the local anesthetic does not enter the epidural, subdural, or subarachnoid space, the diagnostic block can be considered to be specific to that spinal segment and nerve root. However, if the local anesthetic enters the epidural, subdural, or subarachnoid space, the diagnostic block cannot be said to be specific to a given nerve root or segment and may be simply a diagnostic neuraxial block. Although these distinctions may seem minor, the implications of failing to distinguish these

subtle differences relative to technique could lead to surgical interventions that fail to benefit the patient.

CLINICALLY RELEVANT ANATOMY

The superior boundary of the cervical epidural space is the fusion of the periosteal and spinal layers of dura at the foramen magnum. The epidural space continues inferiorly to the sacrococcygeal membrane. The cervical epidural space is bounded anteriorly by the posterior longitudinal ligament and posteriorly by the vertebral laminae and the ligamentum flavum. The vertebral pedicles and intervertebral foramina form the lateral limits of the epidural space. The cervical epidural space is 3 to 4 mm at the C7-T1 interspace with the cervical spine flexed. The cervical epidural space contains a small amount of fat, veins, arteries, lymphatics, and connective tissue. The nerve roots exit their respective neural foramina and move anteriorly and inferiorly away from the cervical spine. The vertebral artery lies ventral to the neural foramen at the level of the uncinate process. Care must be taken to avoid this structure.

When performing selective nerve root block of the cervical nerve roots, the goal is to place the needle just outside the neural foramen of the affected nerve root with precise application of local anesthetic. As mentioned, placement of the needle within the neural foramina may change how the information obtained from this diagnostic maneuver should be interpreted.

TECHNIQUE

Selective nerve root block of the cervical nerve roots is carried out in a manner analogous to a cervical epidural block using the transforaminal approach. The patient is placed in the supine or lateral position. With the patient in the supine or lateral position on the fluoroscopy table, the fluoroscopy beam is rotated from a lateral to oblique position to allow visualization of the affected neural foramina at its largest diameter (Fig. 47-1). The fluoroscopy beam is then slowly moved from a cephalad to a more caudad position to also allow visualization of the

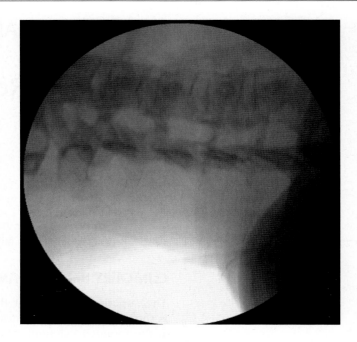

Figure 47-1.
Oblique view of the cervical neural foramina.

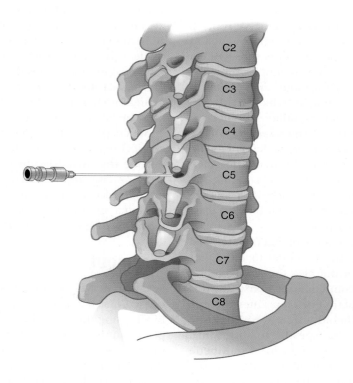

Figure 47-2.

affected neural foramina. When this is accomplished, the beam should be parallel to the targeted nerve root with the nerve in the approximate center of the inferior aspect of the foramen.

The skin is then prepared with an antiseptic solution, and a skin wheal of local anesthetic is placed at a point overlying the posterior aspect of the foramen just over the tip of the superior articular process of the level below the affected neural foramen. A 25-gauge, blunt or sharp 2-inch needle is then placed through the previously anesthetized area and advanced until the tip rests against the superior articular process of the level below the targeted neural foramen (Fig. 47-2). This contact provides the operator with an indication of the depth of the neural foramen. Failure to impinge on bone at the point may indicate that the needle has passed through the foramen and rests within the neural canal or the substance of the spinal cord. Failure to identify this problem can lead to disastrous results (see "Side Effects and Complications").

After this bony landmark is identified, the needle is withdrawn slightly and redirected caudally and ventrally to impinge on the nerve root just as it exits the neural foramen. The patient should then be warned that a paresthesia will occur and asked to say "there!" as soon as the paresthesia is felt. The needle should then be advanced very carefully because a paresthesia will be elicited as the needle touches the nerve root. Great care must be taken to stay dorsal to the uncinate process with the target being the center of the foramen.

After a paresthesia is elicited in the distribution of the targeted nerve root and the needle bevel is directed laterally, a fluoroscopic image is obtained to confirm that the needle tip is at or near the lateral margin of the lateral mass. A solution containing 0.3 mL of a contrast medium suitable for subarachnoid use is then gently injected under continuous fluoroscopic guidance. The contrast should be seen to flow around the nerve root but should not flow proximally into the epidural, subdural, or subarachnoid space. A neurogram outlining the affected nerve root should be seen (Fig. 47-3). Less than 0.5 mL of 4% lidocaine without preservative is then slowly injected under fluoroscopic guidance. The local anesthetic should be seen to flow into the nerve root canal. The injection of contrast and local anesthetic should be stopped immediately if the patient complains of significant pain on injection, although a mild pressure paresthesia is common. After satisfactory injection of the local anesthetic and contrast, the needle is removed, and pressure is placed on the injection site.

SIDE EFFECTS AND COMPLICATIONS

Basically, the potential side effects and complications associated with selective nerve root block are the same as those associated with the transforaminal approach to the cervical epidural space. As mentioned, flow of local anesthetic into the neural foramina reduces the specificity of diagnostic information obtained with selective nerve root block of the cervical nerve roots. Placement of the needle into the neural foramen may result in inadvertent injection into the spinal cord with resultant quadriplegia or death. Ventral needle placement may result in damage to the vertebral artery with the possibility of local anesthetic toxicity and, rarely, stroke.

Because of the potential for hematogenous spread via Batson's plexus, local infection and sepsis represent absolute contraindications to this technique. Anticoagulation and coagulopathy represent absolute contraindications to selective nerve root block of the cervical nerve roots because of the risk for neuraxial hematoma.

Inadvertent dural puncture occurring during selective nerve root block of the cervical nerve roots should rarely occur if attention is paid to the technical aspects of this procedure. However, failure to recognize an unintentional dural or subdural injection can result in immediate total spinal anesthesia with associated loss of consciousness, hypotension, and apnea. This can be disastrous with the patient in the prone position. It is also possible to inadvertently place the injection into the subdural or subarachnoid space with the potential for significant motor or sensory block.

This anatomic region is relatively vascular. If intravascular placement is unrecognized, injection of local anesthetic directly into a vessel could result in significant local anesthetic toxicity. Damage or injection to the segmental artery can occur with increased incidence when performing the selective nerve root block of the C5-C7 nerve roots on the right.

Needle trauma to the epidural veins may result in self-limited bleeding, which may cause postprocedure pain. Uncontrolled bleeding into the epidural space may result in compression of the spinal cord with the rapid development of neurologic deficit. Although significant neurologic deficit secondary to epidural hematoma following selective nerve root block is exceedingly rare, this devastating complication should be considered whenever there is rapidly developing neurologic deficit after cervical epidural nerve block.

Neurologic complications after selective nerve root block are uncommon if proper technique is used and excessive sedation is avoided. Direct trauma to the spinal cord or nerve roots is usually accompanied by pain. If significant pain occurs during placement of the needle or during the injection of contrast and local anesthetic, the physician should immediately stop and ascertain the cause of the pain to avoid the possibility of additional neural trauma.

Although uncommon, infection in the epidural space remains an ever-present possibility, especially in the

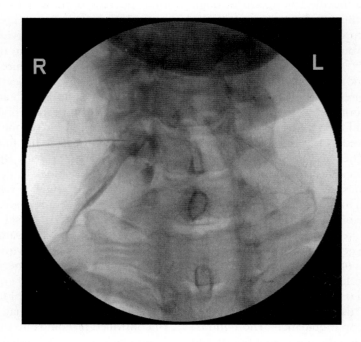

Figure 47-3.
A neurogram of a cervical nerve root.

immunocompromised AIDS or cancer patient. If epidural abscess occurs, emergent surgical drainage to avoid spinal cord compression and irreversible neurologic deficit is usually required. Early detection and treatment of infection are crucial to avoid potentially life-threatening sequelae.

CLINICAL PEARLS

Some practitioners recommend the use of a blunt-tipped needle when performing the transforaminal approach to the cervical epidural space, whereas others believe a sharper needle is better suited for this technique. Any significant pain or sudden increase in resistance during injection suggests incorrect needle placement, and one should *stop* injecting immediately and reassess the position of the needle. Because pain is an important indication of improper needle placement, the practitioner should avoid the use of excessive sedation during selective nerve root block of the cervical nerve roots. As mentioned, the use of sedation in patients in the prone position requires special attention to monitoring.

Section 3

Shoulder and Upper Extremity

Brachial Plexus Block: Interscalene Approach

INDICATIONS

The interscalene approach to the brachial plexus is the preferred technique for brachial plexus block when anesthesia or relaxation of the shoulder is required. In addition to applications for surgical anesthesia, interscalene brachial plexus nerve block with local anesthetic can be used as a diagnostic tool when performing differential neural blockade on an anatomic basis in the evaluation of shoulder and upper extremity pain. If destruction of the brachial plexus is being considered, this technique is useful as a prognostic indicator of the degree of motor and sensory impairment that the patient may experience. Interscalene brachial plexus nerve block with local anesthetic may be used to palliate acute pain emergencies, including acute herpes zoster, brachial plexus neuritis, shoulder and upper extremity trauma, and cancer pain, while waiting for pharmacologic, surgical, and antiblastic methods to become effective. Interscalene brachial plexus nerve block is also useful as an alternative to stellate ganglion block when treating reflex sympathetic dystrophy of the shoulder and upper extremity.

Destruction of the brachial plexus is indicated for the palliation of cancer pain, including invasive tumors of the brachial plexus as well as tumors of the soft tissue and bone of the shoulder and upper extremity (Fig. 48-1). Given the desperate nature of many patients suffering from aggressively invasive tumors that have invaded the brachial plexus, blockade of the brachial plexus using the interscalene approach may be carried out in the presence of coagulopathy or anticoagulation by using a 25-gauge needle, albeit with an increased risk for ecchymosis and hematoma formation.

CLINICALLY RELEVANT ANATOMY

The brachial plexus is formed by the fusion of the anterior rami of the C5, C6, C7, C8, and T1 spinal nerves. There also may be a contribution of fibers from C4 and T2 spinal nerves. The nerves that make up the plexus exit the lateral aspect of the cervical spine and pass downward and laterally in conjunction with the subclavian artery. The nerves and artery run between the anterior scalene and middle scalene muscles, passing inferiorly behind the middle of the clavicle and above the top of the first rib to reach the axilla (Figs. 48-2 and 48-3). The scalene muscles are enclosed in an extension of prevertebral fascia, which helps contain drugs injected into this region.

TECHNIQUE

The patient is placed in a supine position with the head turned away from the side to be blocked. A total of 20 to 30 mL of local anesthetic is drawn up in a 30-mL sterile syringe. When treating painful or inflammatory conditions that are mediated via the brachial plexus, a total of 80 mg of depot-steroid is added to the local anesthetic with the first block, and 40 mg of depot-steroid is added with subsequent blocks.

The patient is then asked to raise his or her head against the resistance of the pain specialist's hand to aid in identification of the posterior border of the sternocleidomastoid muscle. In most patients, a groove between the posterior border of the sternocleidomastoid muscle and the anterior scalene muscle can be palpated. Identification of the interscalene groove can be facilitated by having the patient inhale strongly against a closed glottis. The skin overlying this area is then prepared with antiseptic solution. At the level of the cricothyroid notch (C6) at the interscalene groove, a 25-gauge, 1½-inch needle is inserted with a slightly caudad and inferior

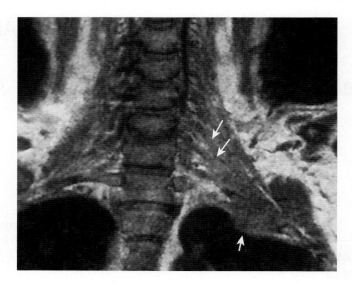

Figure 48-1.

Pancoast's tumor (adenocarcinoma) with infiltration of the brachial plexus. A 65-year-old man complained of severe pain in the shoulder radiating to the elbow, medial side of the forearm, and the fourth and fifth fingers in an ulnar nerve distribution. Screening coronal T1-weighted image shows the brachial plexus from the region of the roots (*long arrows*) to the region of the trunks and divisions, where there is tumor invasion (*short arrow*) and loss of fat planes on the left. (From Stark DD, Bradley WG: Magnetic Resonance Imaging, 3rd ed. St. Louis, Mosby, 1999, p 1824.)

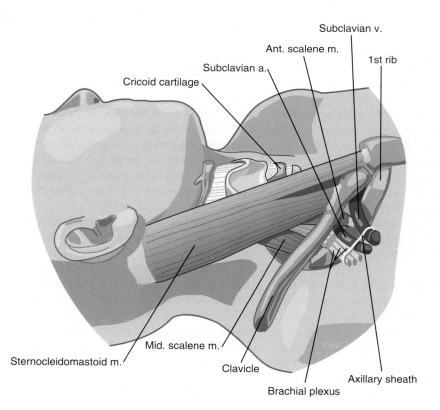

Figure 48-2.

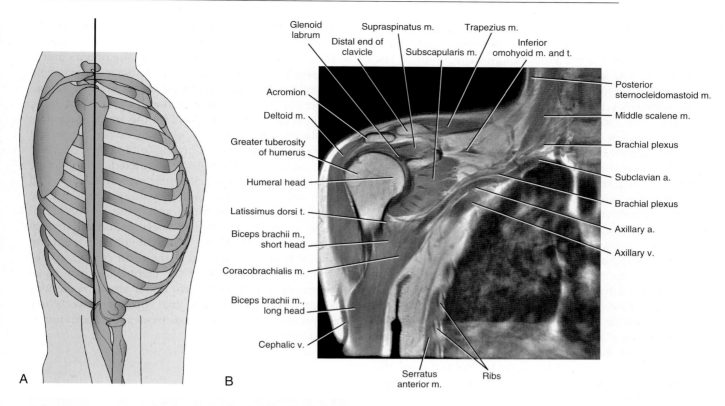

Figure 48-3.
(From El-Khoury GY, Bergman RA, Montgomery WJ: Sectional Anatomy by MRI and CT, 3rd ed. New York, Churchill Livingstone, 2007, p 27.)

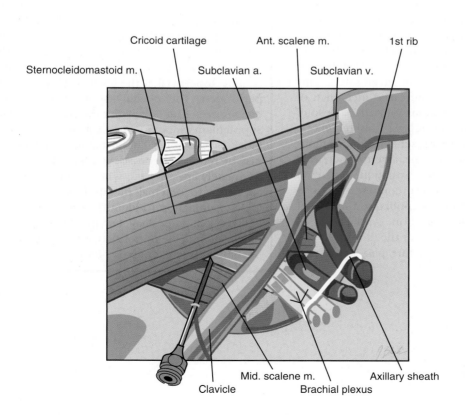

Figure 48-4.

trajectory (Fig. 48-4). If the interscalene groove cannot be identified, the needle is placed just slightly behind the posterior border of the sternocleidomastoid muscle. The needle should be advanced quite slowly because a paresthesia is almost always encountered when the needle tip impinges on the brachial plexus as it traverses the interscalene space at almost a right angle to the needle tip. The patient should be warned that a paresthesia will occur and asked to say "there!" as soon as the paresthesia is felt. Paresthesia is generally encountered at a depth of about $\frac{3}{4}$ to 1 inch.

After paresthesia is elicited, gentle aspiration is carried out to identify blood or cerebrospinal fluid. If the aspiration test is negative and no persistent paresthesia into the distribution of the brachial plexus remains, 20 to 30 mL of solution is slowly injected, with close monitoring of the patient for signs of local anesthetic toxicity or inadvertent subarachnoid injection. If surgical anesthesia is required for forearm or hand procedures, additional local anesthetic may have to be placed in a more caudad position along the brachial plexus to obtain adequate anesthesia of the lower portion of the brachial plexus. Alternatively, specific nerves may be blocked more distally if augmentation of the interscalene brachial plexus block is desired.

SIDE EFFECTS AND COMPLICATIONS

The proximity to the subclavian artery and other large vessels suggests the potential for inadvertent intravascular injection or local anesthetic toxicity from intravascular absorption. Given the large doses of local anesthetic required for interscalene brachial plexus block, the pain specialist should carefully calculate the total milligram dosage of local anesthetic that may be given safely. This vascularity also gives rise to an increased incidence of postblock ecchymosis and hematoma formation. Despite the vascularity of this anatomic region, this technique can safely be performed in the presence of anticoagulation by using a 25- or 27-gauge needle, albeit at increased risk for hematoma, if the clinical situation dictates a favorable risk-to-benefit ratio. These complications can be decreased if manual pressure is applied to the area of the block immediately after injection. Application of cold packs for 20-minute periods after the block also will decrease the amount of postprocedure pain and bleeding the patient may experience.

In addition to the potential for complications involving the vasculature, the proximity of the brachial plexus to the central neuraxial structures and the phrenic nerve can result in side effects and complications. If the needle is placed too deep, the potential for inadvertent epidural, subdural, or subarachnoid injection is a possibility. If the volume of local anesthetic used for this block is accidentally placed in any of these spaces, significant motor and sensory block will result. Unrecognized, these complications could be fatal. It should be assumed that the phrenic nerve also will be blocked when performing brachial plexus block using the interscalene approach. In the absence of significant pulmonary disease, unilateral phrenic nerve block should rarely create respiratory embarrassment. However, blockade of the recurrent laryngeal nerve with its attendant vocal cord paralysis, combined with paralysis of the diaphragm, may make the clearing of pulmonary and upper airway secretions difficult. Although less likely than with the supraclavicular approach to brachial plexus block, pneumothorax is a possibility.

CLINICAL PEARLS

The key to the safe and successful interscalene brachial plexus block is a clear understanding of the anatomy and careful identification of the anatomic landmarks necessary to perform the block. Poking around for a paresthesia without first identifying the interscalene groove is a recipe for disaster. The pain specialist should remember that the brachial plexus is quite superficial at the level at which this block is performed. The needle should rarely be inserted deeper than 1 inch in all but the most obese patients. Supplementation of interscalene brachial plexus block by more peripheral block of the ulnar nerve may be required because the C8 fibers are not always adequately anesthetized when using the interscalene approach to brachial plexus block. Careful neurologic examination to identify preexisting neurologic deficits that later may be attributed to the nerve block should be performed on all patients before beginning brachial plexus block.

CHAPTER 49

Brachial Plexus Block: Supraclavicular Approach

CPT-2009 CODE

Unilateral	64415
Neurolytic	64640

Relative Value Units

Unilateral	10
Neurolytic	20

INDICATIONS

The supraclavicular approach to brachial plexus block is an excellent choice when dense surgical anesthesia of the distal upper extremity is required. This technique is less suitable for shoulder problems because it almost always will require supplementation with cervical plexus block to provide adequate cutaneous anesthesia of the shoulder.

In addition to applications for surgical anesthesia, supraclavicular brachial plexus nerve block with local anesthetic can be used as a diagnostic tool when performing differential neural blockade on an anatomic basis in the evaluation of upper extremity pain. If destruction of the brachial plexus is being considered, this technique is useful as a prognostic indicator of the degree of motor and sensory impairment that the patient may experience. Supraclavicular brachial plexus nerve block with local anesthetic may be used to palliate acute pain emergencies, including acute herpes zoster, brachial plexus neuritis, upper extremity trauma, and cancer pain, while waiting for pharmacologic, surgical, and anti-blastic methods to become effective. Supraclavicular brachial plexus nerve block is also useful as an alternative to stellate ganglion block when treating reflex sympathetic dystrophy of the upper extremity.

Destruction of the brachial plexus via the supraclavicular approach is indicated for the palliation of cancer pain, including invasive tumors of the brachial plexus as well as tumors of the soft tissue and bone of the upper extremity. Because of the potential for intrathoracic hemorrhage, the interscalene approach to brachial plexus block should be used in patients who are receiving anticoagulant therapy only if the clinical situation dictates a favorable risk-to-benefit ratio.

CLINICALLY RELEVANT ANATOMY

The brachial plexus is formed by the fusion of the anterior rami of the C5, C6, C7, C8, and T1 spinal nerves. There is also a contribution of fibers from C4 and T2 spinal nerves in many patients. The nerves that make up the plexus exit the lateral aspect of the cervical spine and pass downward and laterally in conjunction with the subclavian artery. The nerves and artery run between the anterior scalene and middle scalene muscles, passing inferiorly behind the middle of the clavicle and above the top of the first rib to reach the axilla (Figs. 49-1 and 49-2). The scalene muscles are enclosed in an extension of prevertebral fascia, which helps contain drugs injected into this region.

TECHNIQUE

The patient is placed in a supine position with the head turned away from the side to be blocked. A total of 10 mL of local anesthetic is drawn up in a 20-mL sterile syringe. When treating painful conditions that are mediated via the brachial plexus, a total of 80 mg of depot-steroid is added to the local anesthetic with the first block, and 40 mg of depot-steroid is added with subsequent blocks.

The patient is then asked to raise his or her head against the resistance of the pain specialist's hand to aid in identification of the posterior border of the sternocleidomastoid muscle. The point at which the lateral border of the sternocleidomastoid attaches to the clavicle is then identified. At this point, just above the clavicle, after preparation of the skin with antiseptic solution, a 1½-inch needle is inserted directly perpendicular to the table top (Fig. 49-3). The needle should be advanced quite slowly because a paresthesia is almost always encountered at a depth of about ¾ to 1 inch. The patient

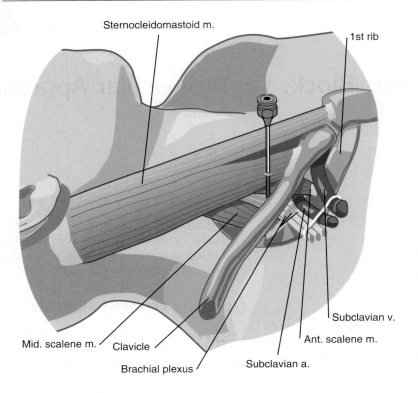

Sternocleidomastoid m.

1st rib

Figure 49-1.

Subclavian v.

Ant. scalene m.

Mid. scalene m.

Clavicle

Subclavian a.

Brachial plexus

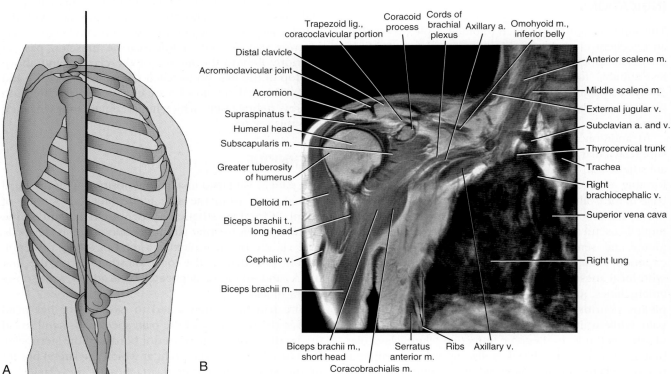

Trapezoid lig., coracoclavicular portion

Coracoid process

Cords of brachial plexus

Axillary a.

Omohyoid m., inferior belly

Distal clavicle

Anterior scalene m.

Acromioclavicular joint

Middle scalene m.

Acromion

External jugular v.

Supraspinatus t.

Subclavian a. and v.

Humeral head

Thyrocervical trunk

Subscapularis m.

Trachea

Greater tuberosity of humerus

Right brachiocephalic v.

Deltoid m.

Superior vena cava

Biceps brachii t., long head

Cephalic v.

Right lung

Biceps brachii m.

Biceps brachii m., short head

Serratus anterior m.

Ribs

Axillary v.

Coracobrachialis m.

A

B

Figure 49-2.
(El-Khoury GY, Bergman RA, Montgomery WJ: Sectional Anatomy by MRI and CT, 3rd ed. New York, Churchill Livingstone 2007, p 27.)

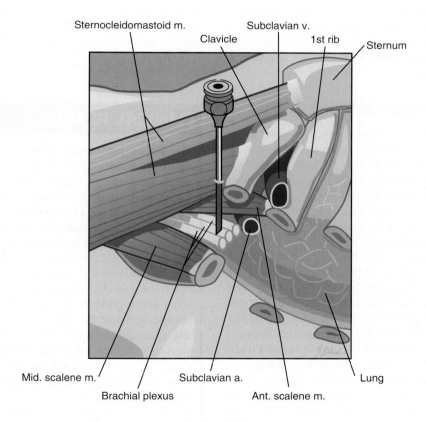

Figure 49-3.

should be warned that a paresthesia will occur and asked to say "there!" as soon as the paresthesia is felt. If a paresthesia is not elicited after the needle has been slowly advanced to a depth of 1 inch, the needle should be withdrawn and readvanced with a slightly more cephalad trajectory. This maneuver should be repeated until a paresthesia is elicited. If the first rib is encountered before obtaining a paresthesia, the needle should be walked laterally along the first rib until a paresthesia is elicited. The needle should never be directed in a more medial trajectory, or pneumothorax is likely to occur.

After paresthesia is elicited, gentle aspiration is carried out to identify blood or cerebrospinal fluid. If the aspiration test is negative and no persistent paresthesia into the distribution of the brachial plexus remains, 10 mL of solution is slowly injected, with close monitoring of the patient for signs of local anesthetic toxicity or inadvertent neuraxial injection.

SIDE EFFECTS AND COMPLICATIONS

The proximity to the subclavian artery and other large vessels suggests the potential for inadvertent intravascular injection or local anesthetic toxicity from intravascular absorption. Given the large doses of local anesthetic required for supraclavicular brachial plexus block, the pain specialist should carefully calculate the total milligram dosage of local anesthetic that may be given safely. This vascularity also gives rise to an increased incidence of postblock ecchymosis and hematoma formation. These complications can be decreased if manual pressure is applied to the area of the block immediately after injection. Application of cold packs for 20-minute periods after the block also will decrease the amount of postprocedure pain and bleeding the patient may experience.

In addition to the potential for complications involving the vasculature, the proximity of the brachial plexus to the central neuraxial structures and the phrenic nerve can result in side effects and complications. Although these complications occur less frequently than with interscalene brachial plexus block, the potential for inadvertent epidural, subdural, or subarachnoid injection remains a possibility. If the volume of local anesthetic used for this block is accidentally placed in any of these spaces, significant motor and sensory block will result. Unrecognized, these complications could be fatal. It should be assumed that the phrenic nerve also will be blocked at least 30% of the time when performing brachial plexus block using the supraclavicular approach. In the absence of significant pulmonary disease, unilateral phrenic nerve block should rarely create respiratory embarrassment. However, blockade of the recurrent laryngeal nerve with its attendant vocal cord paralysis, combined with paralysis of the diaphragm, may make the clearing of pulmonary and upper airway secretions difficult. Because of the proximity of the apex of the lung, pneumothorax is a distinct possibility, and the patient should be informed of such.

CLINICAL PEARLS

The key to performing safe and successful supraclavicular brachial plexus block is a clear understanding of the anatomy and careful identification of the anatomic landmarks necessary to perform the block. Poking around for a paresthesia without first identifying the necessary anatomic landmarks is a recipe for disaster. The pain specialist should remember that the brachial plexus is quite superficial at the level at which this block is performed. The needle should rarely be inserted deeper than 1 inch in all but the most obese patients. If strict adherence to technique is observed and the needle is never advanced medially from the lateral border of the insertion of the sternocleidomastoid muscle on the clavicle, the incidence of pneumothorax should be less than 0.5%. Careful neurologic examination to identify preexisting neurologic deficits that later may be attributed to the nerve block should be performed on all patients before beginning brachial plexus block.

CHAPTER 50

Brachial Plexus Block: Axillary Approach

CPT-2009 CODE	
Unilateral	64415
Neurolytic	64640

Relative Value Units	
Unilateral	10
Neurolytic	20

INDICATIONS

The axillary approach to the brachial plexus is the preferred technique for brachial plexus block when dense anesthesia of the forearm and hand is required. In addition to applications for surgical anesthesia, axillary brachial plexus nerve block with local anesthetic can be used as a diagnostic tool when performing differential neural blockade on an anatomic basis in the evaluation of upper extremity pain. If destruction of the brachial plexus is being considered, this technique is useful as a prognostic indicator of the degree of motor and sensory impairment that the patient may experience. Axillary brachial plexus nerve block with local anesthetic may be used to palliate acute pain emergencies, including acute herpes zoster, brachial plexus neuritis, shoulder and upper extremity trauma, and cancer pain, while waiting for pharmacologic, surgical, and antiblastic methods to become effective. Axillary brachial plexus nerve block is also useful as an alternative to stellate ganglion block when treating reflex sympathetic dystrophy of the upper extremity.

Destruction of the brachial plexus is indicated for the palliation of cancer pain, including invasive tumors of the distal brachial plexus as well as tumors of the soft tissue and bone of the upper extremity (Fig. 50-1). Given the desperate nature of many patients suffering from aggressively invasive tumors that have invaded the brachial plexus, blockade of the brachial plexus using the axillary approach may be carried out in the presence of coagulopathy or anticoagulation by using a 25-gauge needle, albeit with an increased risk for ecchymosis and hematoma formation.

CLINICALLY RELEVANT ANATOMY

The brachial plexus is formed by the fusion of the anterior rami of the C5, C6, C7, C8, and T1 spinal nerves. There also may be a contribution of fibers from C4 and T2 spinal nerves. The nerves that make up the plexus exit the lateral aspect of the cervical spine and pass downward and laterally in conjunction with the subclavian artery. The nerves and artery run between the anterior scalene and middle scalene muscles, passing inferiorly behind the middle of the clavicle and above the top of the first rib to reach the axilla. The sheath that encloses the axillary artery and nerves (the neurovascular bundle) is less consistent than that which encloses the brachial plexus at the level at which interscalene and supraclavicular brachial plexus blocks are performed, making a single injection technique less satisfactory (Fig. 50-2). The median, radial, ulnar, and musculocutaneous nerves surround the artery within this imperfect sheath.

David Brown, MD, has suggested that the position of these nerves relative to the axillary artery can best be visualized by placing them in the quadrants as represented on the face of a clock, with the axillary artery being at the center of the clock (Fig. 50-3). The median nerve is found in the 12-o'clock to 3-o'clock quadrant, the ulnar nerve is found in the 3-o'clock to 6-o'clock quadrant, the radial nerve is found in the 6-o'clock to 9-o'clock quadrant, and the musculocutaneous nerve is found in the 9-o'clock to 12-o'clock quadrant. To ensure adequate block of these nerves, drugs must be injected in each quadrant to place medication in proximity to each of these nerves.

TECHNIQUE

The patient is placed in a supine position with the arm abducted 85 to 90 degrees and the fingertips resting just behind the ear. A total of 30 to 40 mL of local anesthetic

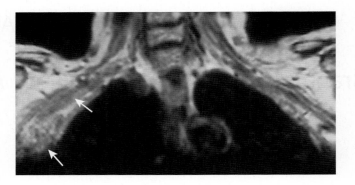

Figure 50-1.

Recurrent breast carcinoma involving the right axillary nodes and chest wall with infiltration of the cords of the brachial plexus. A 72-year-old woman with a history of bilateral mastectomies for carcinoma was seen 2 years after surgery and radiation therapy. Her chief complaint was right hand weakness. The axillary mass (*arrows*) involves the cords posterior to the brachial artery. (From Stark DD, Bradley WG: Magnetic Resonance Imaging, 3rd ed. St. Louis, Mosby, 1999, p 1826.)

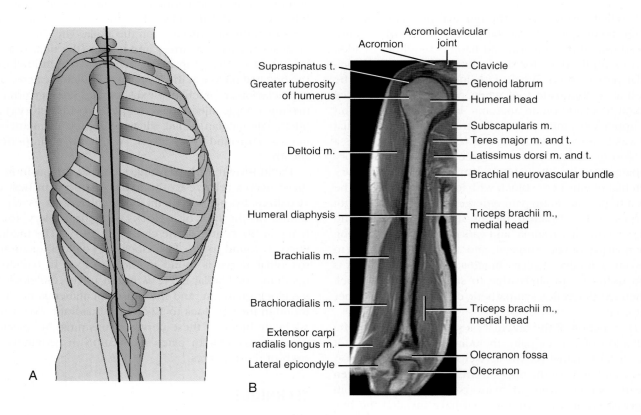

Figure 50-2.

(From El-Khoury GY, Bergman RA, Montgomery WJ: Sectional Anatomy by MRI and CT, 3rd ed. New York, 2007, p 109.)

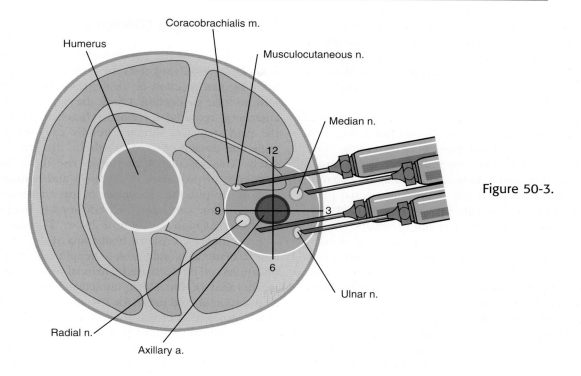

Figure 50-3.

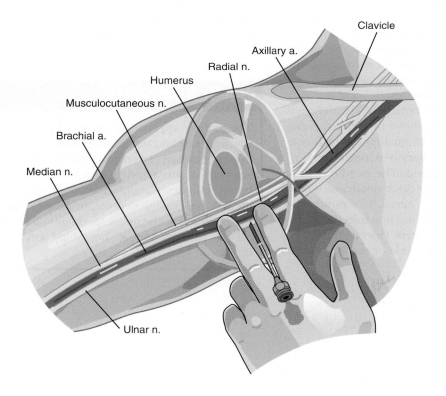

Figure 50-4.

is drawn up in a 50-mL sterile syringe. When treating painful or inflammatory conditions that are thought to be mediated via the brachial plexus, a total of 80 mg of depot-steroid is added to the local anesthetic with the first block, and 40 mg of depot-steroid is added with subsequent blocks.

The pain specialist then identifies the pulsations of the axillary artery with the middle and index fingers of the nondominant hand and then traces the course of the artery distally by following the pulsations. After preparation of the skin with antiseptic solution, a 25-gauge, 1-inch needle is inserted just below the arterial pulsations (Fig. 50-4). The needle should be advanced quite slowly because a paresthesia is almost always encountered as the needle tip impinges on the radial or ulnar nerve. The patient should be warned that a paresthesia will occur and asked to say "there!" as soon as the paresthesia is felt. Paresthesia is generally encountered at a depth of about $\frac{1}{2}$ to $\frac{3}{4}$ inch.

After paresthesia is elicited and its distribution identified, gentle aspiration is carried out to identify blood or cerebrospinal fluid. If the aspiration test is negative and no persistent paresthesia into the distribution of the brachial plexus remains, 8 to 10 mL of solution is slowly injected, with close monitoring of the patient for signs of local anesthetic toxicity or inadvertent subarachnoid injection. If a radial paresthesia was elicited, the needle is withdrawn slightly into the 3-o'clock to 6-o'clock quadrant, which contains the ulnar nerve, and after negative aspiration, an additional 8 to 10 mL of solution is injected. If an ulnar paresthesia was elicited, the needle is withdrawn and then slowly readvanced in a slightly more superior direction into the 6-o'clock to 9-o'clock quadrant, which contains the radial nerve, and the aspiration and injection technique is repeated. The needle is then withdrawn and redirected above the arterial pulsation to the 12-o'clock to 3-o'clock quadrant, which contains the median nerve. If aspiration is negative, 8 to 10 mL of solution is then injected. The needle is then directed to the 9-o'clock to 12-o'clock quadrant, which contains the musculocutaneous nerve. If aspiration is negative, the remaining local anesthetic is injected. Alternatively, the musculocutaneous nerve can be blocked by infiltrating the solution into the mass of the coracobrachialis muscle.

SIDE EFFECTS AND COMPLICATIONS

The proximity of the nerves to the axillary artery and other large vessels suggests the potential for inadvertent intravascular injection or local anesthetic toxicity from intravascular absorption. Given the large doses of local anesthetic required for axillary brachial plexus block, the pain specialist should carefully calculate the total milligram dosage of local anesthetic that may be given safely. This vascularity also gives rise to an increased incidence of postblock ecchymosis and hematoma formation. Despite the vascularity of this anatomic region, this technique can safely be performed in the presence of anticoagulation by using a 25- or 27-gauge needle, albeit at increased risk for hematoma, if the clinical situation dictates a favorable risk-to-benefit ratio. These complications can be decreased if manual pressure is applied to the area of the block immediately after injection. Application of cold packs for 20-minute periods after the block also will decrease the amount of postprocedure pain and bleeding the patient may experience.

The distance of the nerves to be blocked from the neuraxis and phrenic nerve makes the complications associated with injection of drugs onto these structures highly unlikely, which is an advantage of the axillary approach when compared with the interscalene and supraclavicular approaches to brachial plexus block. Because paresthesias are elicited, the potential for postblock persistent paresthesia is a possibility and the patient should be so advised.

CLINICAL PEARLS

The axillary approach to brachial plexus block represents a safe and simple way to anesthetize the distal upper extremity. For pain above the elbow, the interscalene or supraclavicular approach is probably a better choice. Careful neurologic examination to identify preexisting neurologic deficits that later may be attributed to the nerve block should be performed on all patients before beginning brachial plexus block.

Suprascapular Nerve Block

INDICATIONS

Suprascapular nerve block with local anesthetic can be used as a diagnostic tool when performing differential neural blockade on an anatomic basis in the evaluation of shoulder girdle and shoulder joint pain. If destruction of the suprascapular nerve is being considered, this technique is useful as a prognostic indicator of the degree of motor and sensory impairment that the patient may experience. Suprascapular nerve block with local anesthetic may be used to palliate acute pain emergencies, including postoperative pain, pain secondary to traumatic injuries of the shoulder joint and girdle, and cancer pain, while waiting for pharmacologic, surgical, and antiblastic methods to become effective. Suprascapular nerve block also is useful as an adjunctive therapy when treating the decreased range of motion of the shoulder secondary to reflex sympathetic dystrophy or adhesive capsulitis. Suprascapular nerve block also can be used to allow more aggressive physical therapy after shoulder reconstruction surgery. Suprascapular nerve block also is useful as both a diagnostic and therapeutic maneuver in the management of suprascapular nerve entrapment syndrome (Fig. 51-1).

Destruction of the suprascapular nerve is indicated for the palliation of cancer pain, including invasive tumors of the shoulder girdle. This block can be performed in patients who are receiving anticoagulant therapy if the clinical situation dictates a favorable risk-to-benefit ratio.

CLINICALLY RELEVANT ANATOMY

The suprascapular nerve is formed from fibers originating from the C5 and C6 nerve roots of the brachial plexus with some contribution of fibers from the C4 root in most patients. The nerve passes inferiorly and posteriorly from the brachial plexus to pass underneath the coracoclavicular ligament through the suprascapular notch. The suprascapular artery and vein accompany the nerve through the suprascapular notch (Fig. 51-2). The suprascapular nerve provides much of the sensory innervation to the shoulder joint and provides innervation to two of the muscles of the rotator cuff: the supraspinatus and infraspinatus.

TECHNIQUE

The patient is placed in the sitting position with the arms hanging loosely at the patient's side. A total of 10 mL of local anesthetic is drawn up in a 20-mL sterile syringe. When treating painful conditions that are mediated via the suprascapular nerve, a total of 80 mg of depot-steroid is added to the local anesthetic with the first block, and 40 mg of depot-steroid is added with subsequent blocks.

The spine of the scapula is identified, and the pain specialist then palpates along the length of the scapular spine laterally to identify the acromion. At the point at which the thicker acromion fuses with the thinner scapular spine, the skin is prepared with antiseptic solution. At this point, the skin and subcutaneous tissues are anesthetized using a 1½-inch needle. After adequate anesthesia is obtained, a 25-gauge, 3½-inch needle is inserted in an inferior trajectory toward the body of the scapula (Fig. 51-3). The needle should make contact with the body of the scapula at a depth of about 1 inch. The needle is then gently walked superiorly and medially until the needle tip walks off the scapular body into the suprascapular notch. If the notch is not identified, the same maneuver is repeated directing the needle superiorly and laterally until the needle tip walks off the scapular body into the suprascapular notch. A paresthesia often is encountered as the needle tip enters the notch,

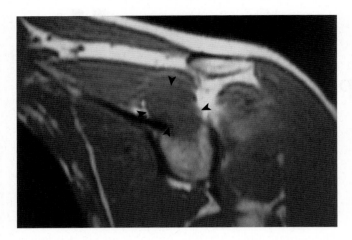

Figure 51-1.
Ganglion cyst with suprascapular nerve compromise. (From Stark DD, Bradley WG: Magnetic Resonance Imaging, 3rd ed. St. Louis, Mosby, 1999, p 723.)

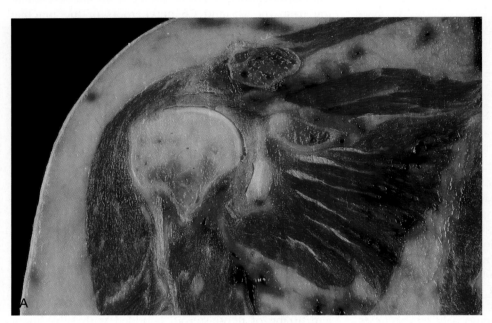

A

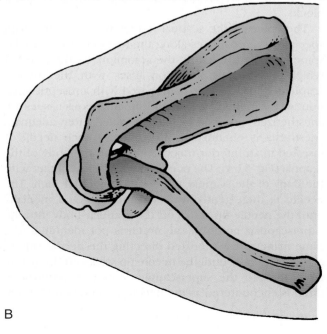

B

Figure 51-2.
(From Kang HS, Resnick D, Ahn J: MRI of the Extremities: An Anatomic Atlas, 2nd ed. Philadelphia, WB Saunders 2002, p 9.)

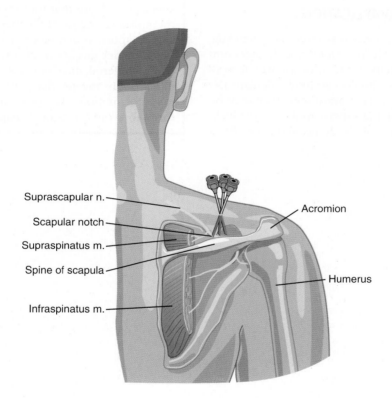

Suprascapular n.

Scapular notch

Supraspinatus m.

Spine of scapula

Infraspinatus m.

Acromion

Humerus

Figure 51-3.

and the patient should be warned of such. If a paresthesia is not elicited after the needle has entered the suprascapular notch, advance the needle an additional $\frac{1}{2}$ inch to place the needle tip beyond the substance of the coracoclavicular ligament. The needle should never be advanced deeper, or pneumothorax is likely to occur.

After paresthesia is elicited or the needle has been advanced into the notch as described here, gentle aspiration is carried out to identify blood or air. If the aspiration test is negative, 10 mL of solution is slowly injected, with close monitoring of the patient for signs of local anesthetic toxicity.

SIDE EFFECTS AND COMPLICATIONS

The proximity to the suprascapular artery and vein suggests the potential for inadvertent intravascular injection or local anesthetic toxicity from intravascular absorption. The pain specialist should carefully calculate the total milligram dosage of local anesthetic that may be given safely when performing suprascapular nerve block. Because of the proximity of the lung, if the needle is advanced too deeply through the suprascapular notch, pneumothorax is a possibility.

CLINICAL PEARLS

Suprascapular nerve block is a safe and simple regional anesthesia technique that has many pain management applications. It is probably underused in the rehabilitation of patients who have undergone shoulder reconstruction as well as those patients suffering from the "shoulder-hand" variant of reflex sympathetic dystrophy. It is important that the pain specialist be sure that the physical and occupational therapists caring for the patient who has undergone suprascapular nerve block understand that not only the shoulder girdle but also the shoulder joint have been rendered insensate after suprascapular nerve block. This means that deep-heat modalities and range of motion exercises must be carefully monitored to avoid burns or damage to the shoulder.

CHAPTER 52

Radial Nerve Block at the Humerus

CPT-2009 CODE	
Unilateral	64450
Bilateral	64450-50
Neurolytic	64640

Relative Value Units	
Unilateral	10
Bilateral	20
Neurolytic	20

INDICATIONS

Radial nerve block at the humerus is useful to supplement brachial plexus block when additional anesthesia is needed in the distribution of the radial nerve. In addition to applications for surgical anesthesia, radial nerve block at the humerus with local anesthetic can be used as a diagnostic tool when performing differential neural blockade on an anatomic basis in the evaluation of upper extremity pain. If destruction of the radial nerve is being considered, this technique is useful as a prognostic indicator of the degree of motor and sensory impairment that the patient may experience. Radial nerve block at the humerus with local anesthetic may be used to palliate acute pain emergencies subserved by the radial nerve while waiting for pharmacologic, surgical, and antiblastic methods to become effective. Radial nerve block at the humerus with local anesthetic and steroid is also useful in the diagnosis and treatment of radial tunnel syndrome.

CLINICALLY RELEVANT ANATOMY

The radial nerve is made up of fibers from C5-T1 spinal roots. The nerve lies posterior and inferior to the axillary artery in the 6-o'clock to 9-o'clock quadrant. Exiting the axilla, the radial nerve passes between the medial and long heads of the triceps muscle. As the nerve curves across the posterior aspect of the humerus, it supplies a motor branch to the triceps. Continuing its downward path, it gives off a number of sensory branches to the upper arm (Fig. 52-1). At a point between the lateral epicondyle of the humerus and the musculospiral groove, the radial nerve divides into its two terminal branches. The superficial branch continues down the arm along with the radial artery and provides sensory innervation to the dorsum of the wrist and the dorsal aspects of a portion of the thumb and index and middle fingers. The deep branch provides most of the motor innervation to the extensors of the forearm.

TECHNIQUE

The patient is placed in a supine position with the arm abducted 35 to 45 degrees and the hand resting comfortably on the abdomen. A total of 7 to 10 mL of local anesthetic is drawn up in a 12-mL sterile syringe. When treating painful or inflammatory conditions that are mediated via the radial nerve, a total of 80 mg of depot-steroid is added to the local anesthetic with the first block, and 40 mg of depot-steroid is added with subsequent blocks.

The pain specialist then identifies the lateral epicondyle of the humerus, and at a point about 3 inches above the epicondyle, the musculospiral groove is identified by deep palpation between the heads of the triceps muscle. After preparation of the skin with antiseptic solution, a 25-gauge, 1-inch needle is inserted perpendicular to the lateral aspect of the humerus and advanced slowly toward the musculospiral groove (Fig. 52-2). As the needle approaches the humerus, a strong paresthesia in the distribution of the radial nerve will be elicited. If no paresthesia is elicited and the needle contacts bone, the needle is withdrawn and redirected slightly more anterior or posterior until paresthesia is elicited. The patient should be warned that a paresthesia will occur and asked to say "there!" as soon as the paresthesia is felt. After paresthesia is elicited and its distribution iden-

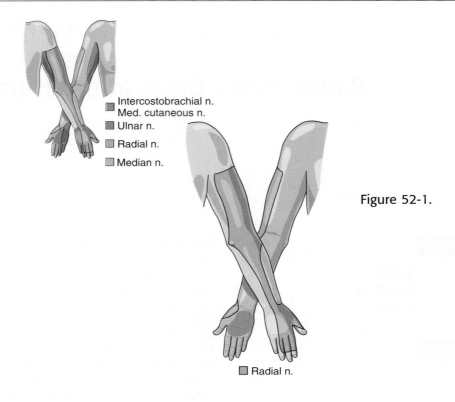

Intercostobrachial n.
Med. cutaneous n.
Ulnar n.
Radial n.
Median n.

Radial n.

Figure 52-1.

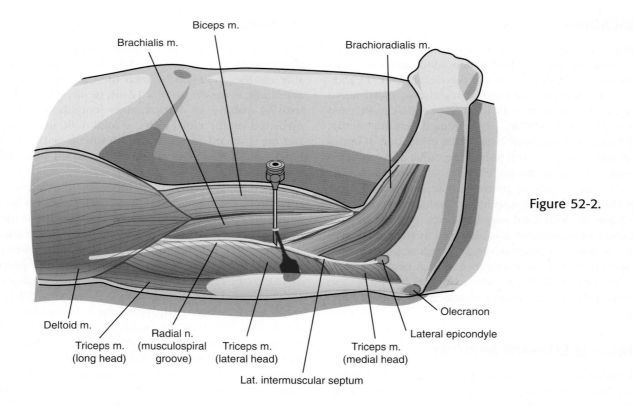

Biceps m.

Brachialis m.

Brachioradialis m.

Deltoid m.

Triceps m.
(long head)

Radial n.
(musculospiral
groove)

Triceps m.
(lateral head)

Lat. intermuscular septum

Triceps m.
(medial head)

Olecranon

Lateral epicondyle

Figure 52-2.

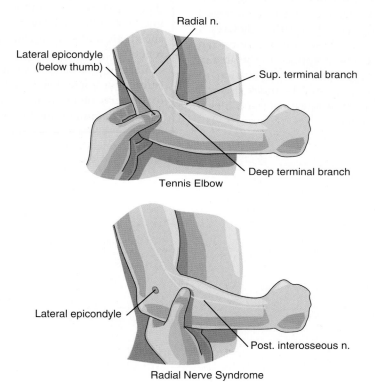

Tennis Elbow

Radial Nerve Syndrome

Figure 52-3.

tified, gentle aspiration is carried out to identify blood. If the aspiration test is negative and no persistent paresthesia into the distribution of the radial nerve remains, 7 to 10 mL of solution is slowly injected, with close monitoring of the patient for signs of local anesthetic toxicity.

SIDE EFFECTS AND COMPLICATIONS

Radial nerve block at the humerus is a relatively safe block, with the major complications being inadvertent intravascular injection and persistent paresthesia secondary to needle trauma to the nerve. This technique can safely be performed in the presence of anticoagulation by using a 25- or 27-gauge needle, albeit at increased risk for hematoma, if the clinical situation dictates a favorable risk-to-benefit ratio. These complications can be decreased if manual pressure is applied to the area of the block immediately after injection. Application of cold packs for 20-minute periods after the block also will decrease the amount of postprocedure pain and bleeding the patient may experience.

CLINICAL PEARLS

Radial nerve block at the humerus is a simple and safe technique. It is extremely useful in the management of radial tunnel syndrome. This painful condition is often misdiagnosed as tennis elbow, and this fact accounts for the many patients whose "tennis elbow" fails to respond to conservative measures. Radial tunnel syndrome can be distinguished from tennis elbow in that with radial tunnel syndrome, the maximal tenderness to palpation is over the radial nerve, whereas with tennis elbow, the maximal tenderness to palpation is over the lateral epicondyle (Fig. 52-3). If radial tunnel syndrome is suspected, injection of the radial nerve at the humerus with local anesthetic and steroid will give almost instantaneous relief.

Careful neurologic examination to identify preexisting neurologic deficits that later may be attributed to the nerve block should be performed on all patients before beginning radial nerve block at the humerus.

CHAPTER 53

Median Cutaneous and Intercostobrachial Nerve Block

CPT-2009 CODE

Unilateral	64450
Neurolytic	64640

Relative Value Units

Unilateral	10
Neurolytic	20

INDICATIONS

Median cutaneous and intercostobrachial nerve block is not commonly used as a stand-alone pain management technique but rather is used to augment brachial plexus block and to provide anesthesia of the medial cutaneous surface of the arm and axilla to decrease tourniquet pain during intravenous regional anesthesia (Fig. 53-1).

CLINICALLY RELEVANT ANATOMY

The median cutaneous nerve is formed from fibers originating from the C8 and T1 roots. These roots can be difficult to block adequately when performing brachial plexus block. The fibers of the median cutaneous nerve communicate with the fibers of the intercostobrachial nerve, which has its origin in the second intercostal nerve. These nerves exit the axilla outside the brachial plexus sheath and travel superficially parallel to the triceps muscle. The superficial location of both of these nerves makes them easily accessible for neural blockade.

TECHNIQUE

The patient is placed in the supine position with the arm abducted 85 to 90 degrees in a manner analogous to the positioning for axillary nerve block. A total of 8 mL of local anesthetic is drawn up in a 12-mL sterile syringe.

The superior margin of the biceps muscle is identified at the anterior axillary line. The skin at this point is prepared with antiseptic solution, and a bead of local anesthetic is placed subcutaneously from this point inferiorly in an arc from the biceps to the triceps continuing along the axillary surface of the arm (Fig. 53-2). This will block both the median cutaneous and intercostobrachial nerves.

SIDE EFFECTS AND COMPLICATIONS

This technique is relatively complication free as long as the pain specialist keeps the needle tip subcutaneous, thus avoiding injection into the axillary artery and vein. Bruising and injection site soreness occasionally may occur.

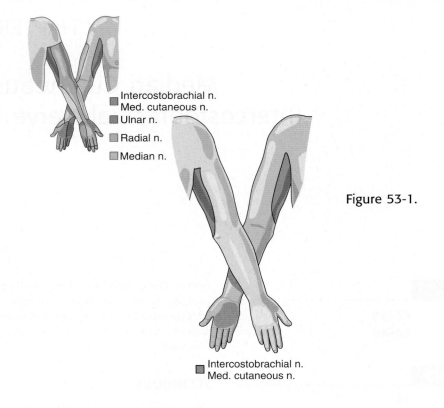

Intercostobrachial n.
Med. cutaneous n.
Ulnar n.
Radial n.
Median n.

Intercostobrachial n.
Med. cutaneous n.

Figure 53-1.

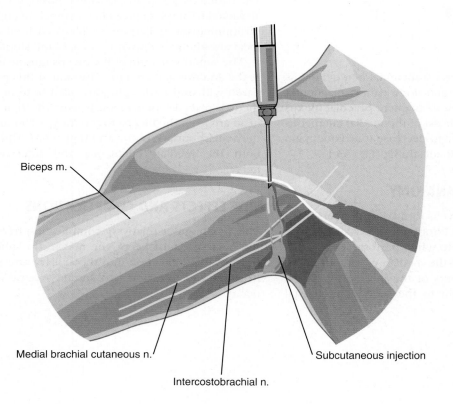

Biceps m.

Medial brachial cutaneous n.

Intercostobrachial n.

Subcutaneous injection

Figure 53-2.

CLINICAL PEARLS

Medial cutaneous and intercostobrachial nerve block can turn what appears to be a failed brachial plexus block into a success. This technique should be considered prophylactically whenever intravenous regional anesthesia with a prolonged tourniquet time is being considered to decrease the incidence of tourniquet pain.

CHAPTER **54**

Radial Nerve Block at the Elbow

CPT-2009 CODE

Unilateral	**64450**
Bilateral	**64450-50**
Neurolytic	**64640**

Relative Value Units

Unilateral	**10**
Bilateral	**20**
Neurolytic	**20**

INDICATIONS

Radial nerve block at the elbow is useful in supplementing brachial plexus block when additional anesthesia is needed in the distribution of the radial nerve. In addition to applications for surgical anesthesia, radial nerve block at the elbow with local anesthetic can be used as a diagnostic tool when performing differential neural blockade on an anatomic basis in the evaluation of upper extremity pain below the elbow. If destruction of the radial nerve is being considered, this technique is useful as a prognostic indicator of the degree of motor and sensory impairment that the patient may experience. Radial nerve block at the elbow with local anesthetic may be used to palliate acute pain emergencies subserved by the radial nerve while waiting for pharmacologic, surgical, and antiblastic methods to become effective.

CLINICALLY RELEVANT ANATOMY

The radial nerve is made up of fibers from C5-T1 spinal roots. The nerve lies posterior and inferior to the axillary artery in the 6-o'clock to 9-o'clock quadrant. Exiting the axilla, the radial nerve passes between the medial and long heads of the triceps muscle. As the nerve curves across the posterior aspect of the humerus, it supplies a motor branch to the triceps. Continuing its downward path, it gives off a number of sensory branches to the upper arm (Fig. 54-1). At a point between the lateral epicondyle of the humerus and the musculospiral groove, the radial nerve divides into its two terminal branches (Fig. 54-2). The superficial branch continues down the arm along with the radial artery and provides sensory innervation to the dorsum of the wrist and the dorsal aspects of a portion of the thumb and index and middle fingers. The deep branch provides most of the motor innervation to the extensors of the forearm.

TECHNIQUE

The patient is placed in a supine position with the arm fully abducted at the patient's side and the elbow slightly flexed with the dorsum of the hand resting on a folded towel. A total of 7 to 10 mL of local anesthetic is drawn up in a 12-mL sterile syringe. When treating painful or inflammatory conditions that are mediated via the radial nerve, a total of 80 mg of depot-steroid is added to the local anesthetic with the first block, and 40 mg of depot-steroid is added with subsequent blocks.

The pain specialist then identifies the lateral margin of the biceps tendon at the crease of the elbow. After preparation of the skin with antiseptic solution, a 25-gauge, 1½-inch needle is inserted just lateral to the biceps tendon at the crease and slowly advanced in a slightly medial and cephalad trajectory (Fig. 54-3). As the needle approaches the humerus, a strong paresthesia in the distribution of the radial nerve will be elicited. If no paresthesia is elicited and the needle contacts bone, the needle is withdrawn and redirected slightly more medial until a paresthesia is elicited. The patient should be warned that a paresthesia will occur and asked to say "there!" as soon as the paresthesia is felt. After paresthesia is elicited and its distribution identified, gentle aspiration is carried out to identify blood. If the aspiration test is negative and no persistent paresthesia into the distribution of the radial nerve remains, 7 to 10 mL of solution is slowly injected, with close monitoring of the patient for signs of local anesthetic toxicity.

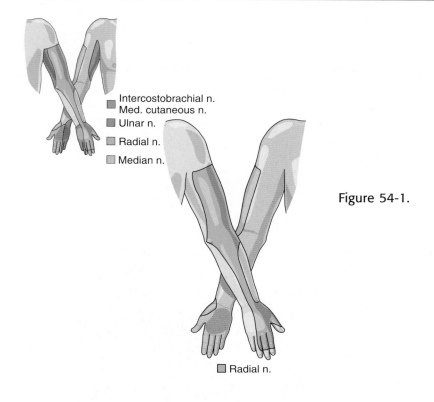

Intercostobrachial n.
Med. cutaneous n.
Ulnar n.
Radial n.
Median n.

Figure 54-1.

Radial n.

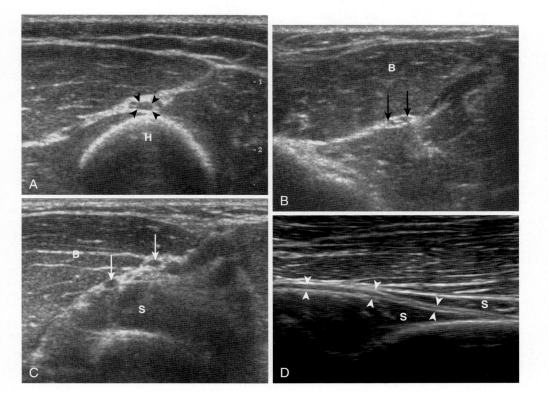

Figure 54-2.
Radial nerve evaluation.
A, Transverse imaging relative to the humerus (H) shows the radial nerve (*arrowheads*) at the level of the radial groove.
B and **C,** Transverse imaging distally shows the bifurcation of the radial nerve into the superficial and deep branches (*arrows*) deep to the brachioradialis (B) (S, supinator). **D,** Longitudinal imaging shows the deep branch of the radial nerve (*arrowheads*) between the two heads of the supinator muscle (S). (From Jacobson JA: Fundamentals of Musculoskeletal Ultrasound, 1st ed. Philadelphia, WB Saunders, 2007, p 111.)

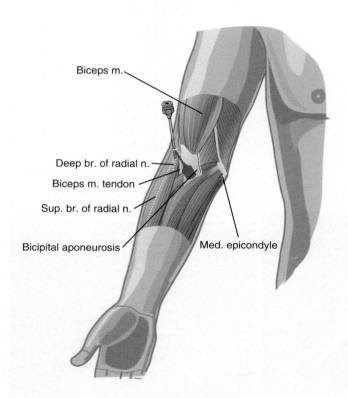

Biceps m.

Deep br. of radial n.

Biceps m. tendon

Sup. br. of radial n.

Bicipital aponeurosis

Med. epicondyle

Figure 54-3.

SIDE EFFECTS AND COMPLICATIONS

Radial nerve block at the elbow is a relatively safe block, with the major complications being inadvertent intravascular injection and persistent paresthesia secondary to needle trauma to the nerve. This technique can be performed safely in the presence of anticoagulation by using a 25- or 27-gauge needle, albeit at increased risk for hematoma, if the clinical situation dictates a favorable risk-to-benefit ratio. These complications can be decreased if manual pressure is applied to the area of the block immediately after injection. Application of cold packs for 20-minute periods after the block also will decrease the amount of postprocedure pain and bleeding the patient may experience.

CLINICAL PEARLS

Radial nerve block at the elbow is a simple and safe technique in the evaluation and treatment of the previously mentioned painful conditions. Careful neurologic examination to identify preexisting neurologic deficits that later may be attributed to the nerve block should be performed on all patients before beginning radial nerve block at the elbow.

CHAPTER 55

Median Nerve Block at the Elbow

CPT-2009 CODE	
Unilateral	**64450**
Bilateral	**64450-50**
Neurolytic	**64640**

Relative Value Units	
Unilateral	**10**
Bilateral	**20**
Neurolytic	**20**

INDICATIONS

Median nerve block at the elbow is useful in supplementing brachial plexus block when additional anesthesia is needed in the distribution of the median nerve. In addition to applications for surgical anesthesia, median nerve block at the elbow with local anesthetic can be used as a diagnostic tool when performing differential neural blockade on an anatomic basis in the evaluation of upper extremity pain below the elbow. If destruction of the median nerve is being considered, this technique is useful as a prognostic indicator of the degree of motor and sensory impairment that the patient may experience. Median nerve block at the elbow with local anesthetic may be used to palliate acute pain emergencies subserved by the median nerve while waiting for pharmacologic, surgical, and antiblastic methods to become effective. Median nerve block at the elbow with local anesthetic and steroid is also useful in the palliation of pain secondary to median nerve entrapment syndromes at the elbow, including compression by the ligament of Struthers and the pronator syndrome (Fig. 55-1).

CLINICALLY RELEVANT ANATOMY

The median nerve is made up of fibers from C5-T1 spinal roots. The nerve lies anterior and superior to the axillary artery in the 12-o'clock to 3-o'clock quadrant. Exiting the axilla, the median nerve descends into the upper arm along with the brachial artery. At the level of the elbow, the brachial artery is just medial to the biceps muscle (Fig. 55-2). At this level, the median nerve lies just medial to the brachial artery. As the median nerve proceeds downward into the forearm, it gives off numerous branches that provide motor innervation to the flexor muscles of the forearm. These branches are susceptible to nerve entrapment by aberrant ligaments, muscle hypertrophy, and direct trauma. The nerve approaches the wrist overlying the radius. It lies deep to and between the tendons of the palmaris longus muscle and the flexor carpi radialis muscle at the wrist. The terminal branches of the median nerve provide sensory innervation to a portion of the palmar surface of the hand as well as the palmar surface of the thumb, index and middle fingers, and radial portion of the ring finger (Fig. 55-3). The median nerve also provides sensory innervation to the distal dorsal surface of the index and middle fingers and the radial portion of the ring finger.

TECHNIQUE

The patient is placed in a supine position with the arm fully adducted at the patient's side and the elbow slightly flexed with the dorsum of the hand resting on a folded towel. A total of 5 to 7 mL of local anesthetic is drawn up in a 12-mL sterile syringe. When treating painful or inflammatory conditions that are mediated via the median nerve, a total of 80 mg of depot-steroid is added to the local anesthetic with the first block, and 40 mg of depot-steroid is added with subsequent blocks.

The pain specialist then identifies the pulsations of the brachial artery at the crease of the elbow. After preparation of the skin with antiseptic solution, a 25-gauge, 1½-inch needle is inserted just medial to the brachial artery at the crease and slowly advanced in a slightly medial and cephalad trajectory (Fig. 55-4). As the needle advances about ½ to ¾ inch, a strong paresthesia in the distribution of the median nerve will be elicited. If no

Text continued on p. 228

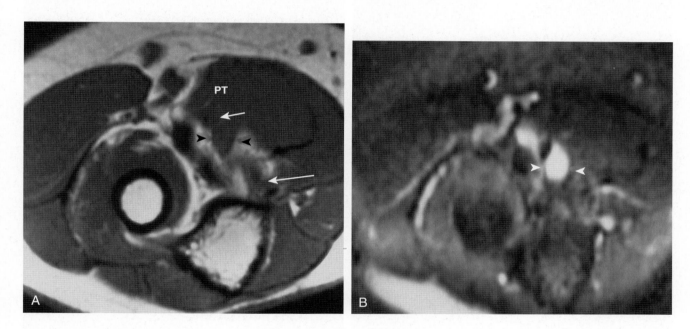

Figure 55-1.

Pronator teres syndrome in a 36-year-old woman with complaints of elbow pain and hand paresthesias in a median nerve distribution. **A,** Axial T1-weighted (700/18) image just proximal to the radial tuberosity shows fusiform enlargement of the median nerve that is isointense with muscle (*black arrowheads*). The nerve projects to just medial to the brachial artery (*short white arrow*). Enlargement is seen just proximal to the confluence of the humeral head of the pronator teres (PT) and ulnar head (*long white arrow*). **B,** Axial fast spin-echo short T1 inversion recovery (STIR) (6850/45/150/16) image shows markedly increased signal intensity within the enlarged segment of the median nerve (*white arrowheads*). (From Stark DD, Bradley WG: Magnetic Resonance Imaging, 3rd ed. St. Louis, Mosby, 1999, p 764.)

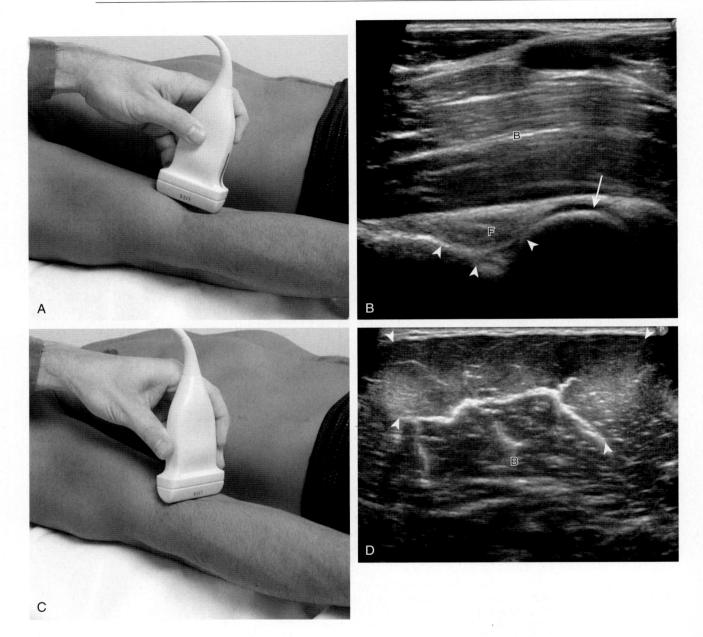

Figure 55-2.

Biceps brachii, brachialis, anterior joint recess, and median nerve evaluation. **A,** Sagittal imaging over the anterior elbow shows (**B**) the brachialis muscle (B), coronoid fossa (*arrowheads*), anterior elbow fat pad (F), and trochlea hyaline cartilage (*arrow*). **C,** Transverse imaging from superior to inferior over the anterior elbow shows (**D** to **F**) the biceps muscle (*arrowheads*) that becomes tendon lateral to the brachial artery (A), with the median artery (*arrows*) located medially (*curved arrow*, hyaline cartilage; B, brachialis; C, capitellum; T, trochlea).

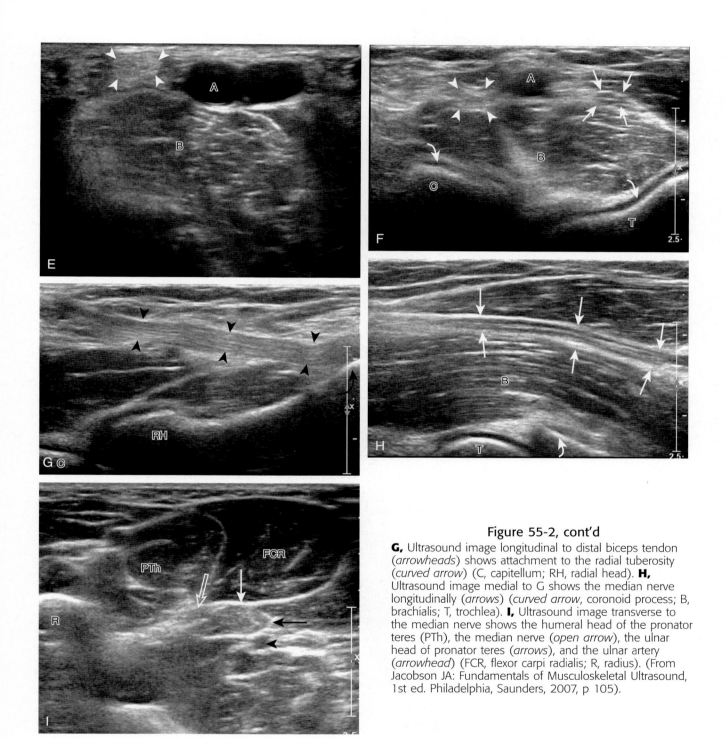

Figure 55-2, cont'd

G, Ultrasound image longitudinal to distal biceps tendon (*arrowheads*) shows attachment to the radial tuberosity (*curved arrow*) (C, capitellum; RH, radial head). **H,** Ultrasound image medial to G shows the median nerve longitudinally (*arrows*) (*curved arrow*, coronoid process; B, brachialis; T, trochlea). **I,** Ultrasound image transverse to the median nerve shows the humeral head of the pronator teres (PTh), the median nerve (*open arrow*), the ulnar head of pronator teres (*arrows*), and the ulnar artery (*arrowhead*) (FCR, flexor carpi radialis; R, radius). (From Jacobson JA: Fundamentals of Musculoskeletal Ultrasound, 1st ed. Philadelphia, Saunders, 2007, p 105).

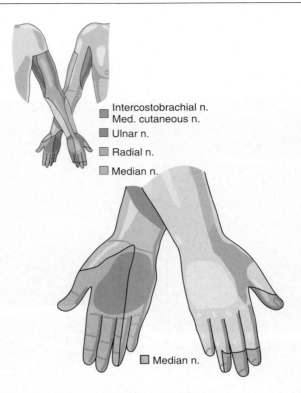

Intercostobrachial n.
Med. cutaneous n.
Ulnar n.
Radial n.
Median n.

Median n.

Figure 55-3.

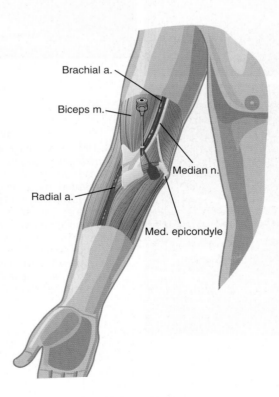

Brachial a.

Biceps m.

Median n.

Radial a.

Med. epicondyle

Figure 55-4.

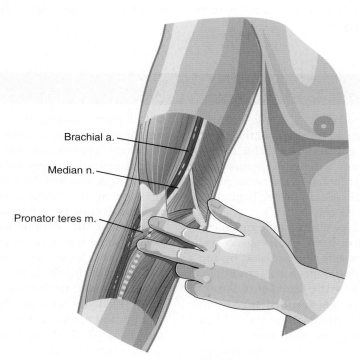

Pronator Syndrome

Figure 55-5.

paresthesia is elicited and the needle contacts bone, the needle is withdrawn and redirected slightly more medial until a paresthesia is elicited. The patient should be warned that a paresthesia will occur and asked to say "there!" as soon as the paresthesia is felt. After paresthesia is elicited and its distribution identified, gentle aspiration is carried out to identify blood.

If the aspiration test is negative and no persistent paresthesia into the distribution of the median nerve remains, 5 to 7 mL of solution is slowly injected, with close monitoring of the patient for signs of local anesthetic toxicity.

If no paresthesia can be elicited, a similar amount of solution is injected in a fanlike manner just medial to the brachial artery, with care being taken not to inadvertently inject into the artery.

SIDE EFFECTS AND COMPLICATIONS

Median nerve block at the elbow is a relatively safe block, with the major complications being inadvertent intravascular injection and persistent paresthesia secondary to needle trauma to the nerve. This technique can safely be performed in the presence of anticoagulation by using a 25- or 27-gauge needle, albeit at increased risk for hematoma, if the clinical situation dictates a favorable risk-to-benefit ratio. These complications can be decreased if manual pressure is applied to the area of the block immediately after injection. Application of cold packs for 20-minute periods after the block also will decrease the amount of postprocedure pain and bleeding the patient may experience.

CLINICAL PEARLS

Median nerve block at the elbow is a simple and safe technique in the evaluation and treatment of the previously mentioned painful conditions. Careful neurologic examination to identify preexisting neurologic deficits that later may be attributed to the nerve block should be performed on all patients before beginning median nerve block at the elbow.

This technique is especially useful in the treatment of pain secondary to median nerve compression syndromes at the elbow, including compression by the ligament of Struthers and the pronator syndrome. Median nerve compression by the ligament of Struthers presents clinically as unexplained persistent forearm pain caused by compression of the median nerve by an aberrant ligament that runs from a supracondylar process to the medial epicondyle. The diagnosis is made by electromyography and nerve conduction velocity testing, which demonstrate compression of the median nerve at the elbow, combined with the x-ray finding of a supracondylar process. The pronator syndrome is characterized by unexplained persistent forearm pain with tenderness to palpation over the pronator teres muscle (Fig. 55-5). A positive Tinel's sign also may be present. Median nerve compression by the ligament of Struthers and pronator syndrome must be differentiated from isolated compression of the anterior interosseous nerve, which occurs some 6 to 8 cm below the elbow. These syndromes also should be differentiated from cervical radiculopathy involving the C6 or C7 roots, which may at times mimic median nerve compression. Furthermore, it should be remembered that cervical radiculopathy and median nerve entrapment may coexist as the so-called double-crush syndrome. The double-crush syndrome occurs most commonly with median nerve entrapment at the wrist or carpal tunnel syndrome.

CHAPTER 56

Ulnar Nerve Block at the Elbow

CPT-2009 CODE	
Unilateral	64450
Bilateral	64450-50
Neurolytic	64640

Relative Value Units	
Unilateral	10
Bilateral	20
Neurolytic	20

INDICATIONS

Ulnar nerve block at the elbow is useful in supplementing brachial plexus block when additional anesthesia is needed in the distribution of the ulnar nerve. In addition to applications for surgical anesthesia, ulnar nerve block at the elbow with local anesthetic can be used as a diagnostic tool when performing differential neural blockade on an anatomic basis in the evaluation of upper extremity pain below the elbow. If destruction of the ulnar nerve is being considered, this technique is useful as a prognostic indicator of the degree of motor and sensory impairment that the patient may experience. Ulnar nerve block at the elbow with local anesthetic may be used to palliate acute pain emergencies subserved by the ulnar nerve while waiting for pharmacologic, surgical, and antiblastic methods to become effective. Ulnar nerve block at the elbow with local anesthetic and steroid also is useful in the palliation of pain secondary to ulnar nerve entrapment syndromes at the elbow, including cubital tunnel syndrome (Fig. 56-1).

CLINICALLY RELEVANT ANATOMY

The ulnar nerve is made up of fibers from C6-T1 spinal roots. The nerve lies anterior and inferior to the axillary artery in the 3-o'clock to 6-o'clock quadrant. Exiting the axilla, the ulnar nerve descends into the upper arm along with the brachial artery. At the middle of the upper arm, the nerve courses medially to pass between the olecranon process and medial epicondyle of the humerus (Figs. 56-2 and 56-3). The nerve then passes between the heads of the flexor carpi ulnaris muscle continuing downward, moving radially along with the ulnar artery. At a point about 1 inch proximal to the crease of the wrist, the ulnar nerve divides into the dorsal and palmar branches. The dorsal branch provides sensation to the ulnar aspect of the dorsum of the hand and the dorsal aspect of the little finger and the ulnar half of the ring finger (Fig. 56-4). The palmar branch provides sensory innervation to the ulnar aspect of the palm of the hand and the palmar aspect of the little finger and the ulnar half of the ring finger.

TECHNIQUE

The patient is placed in a supine position with the arm abducted 85 to 90 degrees and the dorsum of the hand resting against a folded towel. A total of 5 to 7 mL of local anesthetic is drawn up in a 12-mL sterile syringe. When treating painful or inflammatory conditions that are mediated via the ulnar nerve, a total of 80 mg of depot-steroid is added to the local anesthetic with the first block, and 40 mg of depot-steroid is added with subsequent blocks.

The pain specialist then identifies the olecranon process and the median epicondyle of the humerus. The ulnar nerve sulcus between these two bony landmarks is then identified. After preparation of the skin with antiseptic solution, a 25-gauge, $\frac{5}{8}$-inch needle is inserted just proximal to the sulcus and is slowly advanced in a slightly cephalad trajectory (Fig. 56-5). As the needle advances about $\frac{1}{2}$ inch, a strong paresthesia in the distribution of the ulnar nerve will be elicited. The patient should be warned that a paresthesia will occur and asked to say "there!" as soon as the paresthesia is felt. After paresthesia is elicited and its distribution identified, gentle aspiration is carried out to identify blood. If the

Text continued on p. 234

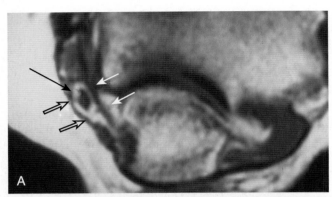

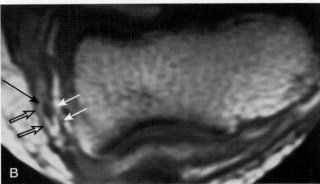

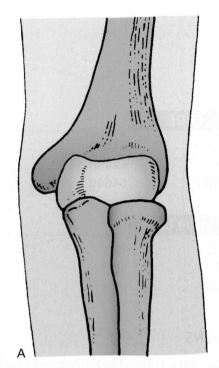

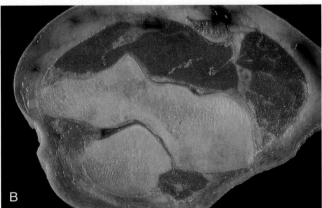

Figure 56-1.
Dynamic configuration of the cubital tunnel with elbow flexion in a cadaver elbow. **A,** Axial T1-weighted (500/15) image just distal to the medial epicondyle shows the oval configuration of the cubital tunnel defined deep by the medial capsule (*closed arrows*) and superficially by the cubital tunnel retinaculum (*open arrows*) with the elbow in extension. **B,** Radial T1-weighted image (500/15) perpendicular to the course of the ulnar nerve just distal to the medial epicondyle with the elbow flexed 90 degrees shows the taut contour of the borders of the cubital tunnel (*closed and open arrows* same as in **A**) with effaced perineural fat and a flattened configuration of the nerve. *Long black arrow,* ulnar nerve. (From Stark DD, Bradley WG: Magnetic Resonance Imaging, 3rd ed. St. Louis, Mosby, 1999, p 762.)

Figure 56-2.
(From Kang HS, Resnick D, Ahn J: MRI of the Extremities: An Anatomic Atlas, 2nd ed. Philadelphia, WB Saunders 2002, p 99.)

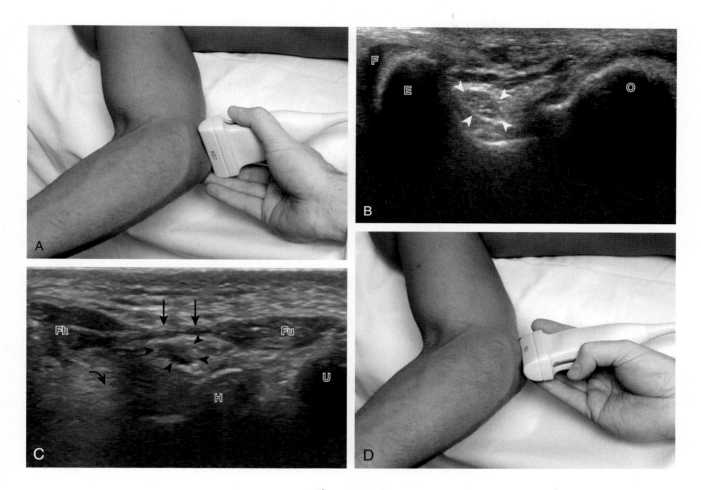

Figure 56-3.

Ulnar nerve and cubital tunnel evaluation. **A,** Transverse imaging over the medial elbow between the medial epicondyle and olecranon process (**B**) shows the ulnar nerve (*arrowheads*) posterior to the medial epicondyle (E). Note the common flexor tendon (F) and the olecranon process (O). **C,** Transverse imaging distal to **B** shows the ulnar nerve (*arrowheads*) in the cubital tunnel (*arrows,* arcuate ligament; *curved arrow,* anterior band of ulnar collateral ligament; Fh, humeral head of flexor carpi ulnaris; Fu, ulnar head of flexor carpi ulnaris; H, humerus; U, ulna). **D,** longitudinal imaging. (From Jacobson JA: Fundamentals of Musculoskeletal Ultrasound, 1st ed. Philadelphia, Saunders 2007, p 108.)

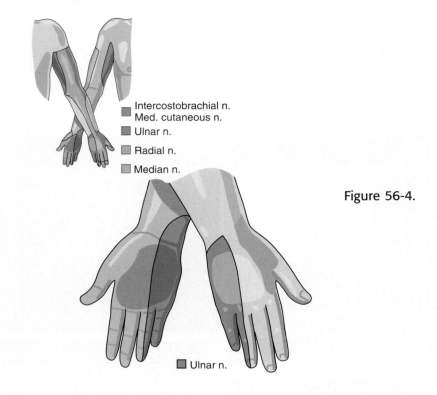

Intercostobrachial n.
Med. cutaneous n.
Ulnar n.
Radial n.
Median n.

Ulnar n.

Figure 56-4.

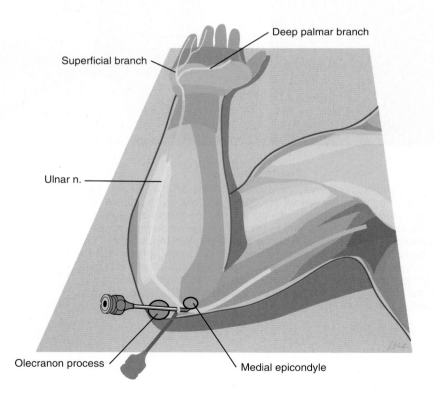

Deep palmar branch

Superficial branch

Ulnar n.

Olecranon process

Medial epicondyle

Figure 56-5.

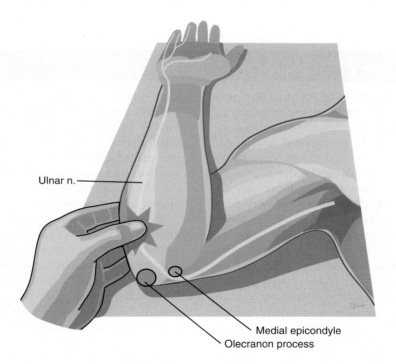

Cubital Tunnel Syndrome

Figure 56-6.

aspiration test is negative and no persistent paresthesia into the distribution of the ulnar nerve remains, 5 to 7 mL of solution is slowly injected, with close monitoring of the patient for signs of local anesthetic toxicity. If no paresthesia can be elicited, a similar amount of solution is slowly injected in a fanlike manner just proximal to the notch, with care being taken to avoid intravascular injection.

SIDE EFFECTS AND COMPLICATIONS

Ulnar nerve block at the elbow is a relatively safe block, with the major complications being inadvertent intravascular injection into the ulnar artery and persistent paresthesia secondary to needle trauma to the nerve. Because the nerve is enclosed by a dense fibrous band as it passes through the ulnar nerve sulcus, care should be taken to slowly inject just proximal to the sulcus to avoid additional compromise of the nerve. This technique can safely be performed in the presence of anticoagulation by using a 25- or 27-gauge needle, albeit at increased risk for hematoma, if the clinical situation dictates a favorable risk-to-benefit ratio. These complications can be decreased if manual pressure is applied to the area of the block immediately after injection. Application of cold packs for 20-minute periods after the block also will decrease the amount of postprocedure pain and bleeding the patient may experience.

CLINICAL PEARLS

Ulnar nerve block at the elbow is a simple and safe technique in the evaluation and treatment of the previously mentioned painful conditions. Careful neurologic examination to identify preexisting neurologic deficits that may later be attributed to the nerve block should be performed on all patients before beginning ulnar nerve block at the elbow because there appears to be a propensity for the development of persistent paresthesia when the nerve is blocked at this level. The incidence of persistent paresthesia can be decreased by blocking the nerve proximal to the ulnar nerve sulcus and injecting slowly.

Ulnar nerve block at the elbow is especially useful in the treatment of pain secondary to ulnar nerve compression syndromes at the elbow, including cubital tunnel syndrome. Cubital tunnel syndrome is often misdiagnosed as golfer's elbow, and this fact accounts for the many patients whose "golfer's elbow" fails to respond to conservative measures. Cubital tunnel syndrome can be distinguished from golfer's elbow in that in cubital tunnel syndrome, the maximal tenderness to palpation is over the ulnar nerve 1 inch below the medial epicondyle, whereas with golfer's elbow, the maximal tenderness to palpation is directly over the medial epicondyle (Fig. 56-6). If cubital tunnel syndrome is suspected, injection of the ulnar nerve at the elbow with local anesthetic and steroid will give almost instantaneous relief.

Cubital tunnel syndrome also should be differentiated from cervical radiculopathy involving the C8 spinal root, which may at times mimic ulnar nerve compression. Furthermore, it should be remembered that cervical radiculopathy and ulnar nerve entrapment may coexist in the so-called double-crush syndrome. The double-crush syndrome occurs most commonly with median nerve entrapment at the wrist or carpal tunnel syndrome. Pancoast's tumor invading the medial cord of the brachial plexus also may mimic an isolated ulnar nerve entrapment and should be ruled out with apical lordotic chest x-ray.

CHAPTER 57

Radial Nerve Block at the Wrist

CPT-2009 CODE	
Unilateral	64450
Bilateral	64450-50
Neurolytic	64640

Relative Value Units	
Unilateral	10
Bilateral	20
Neurolytic	20

INDICATIONS

In contradistinction to blockade of the median and ulnar nerves at the wrist, radial nerve block at the wrist is used primarily to supplement partial brachial plexus block when additional anesthesia is needed in the distribution of the distal radial nerve. Although less specific than the median and ulnar techniques, radial nerve block at the wrist is occasionally used as a diagnostic tool when performing differential neural blockade on an anatomic basis in the evaluation of upper extremity pain below the wrist. If destruction of the radial nerve is being considered, this technique is occasionally used as a prognostic indicator of the degree of motor and sensory impairment that the patient may experience. Radial nerve block at the wrist with local anesthetic may be used to palliate acute pain emergencies subserved by the radial nerve while waiting for pharmacologic, surgical, and antiblastic methods to become effective.

CLINICALLY RELEVANT ANATOMY

The radial nerve is made up of fibers from C5-T1 spinal roots. The nerve lies posterior and inferior to the axillary artery in the 6-o'clock to 9-o'clock quadrant. Exiting the axilla, the radial nerve passes between the medial and long heads of the triceps muscle. As the nerve curves across the posterior aspect of the humerus, it supplies a motor branch to the triceps.

Continuing its downward path, it gives off a number of sensory branches to the upper arm. At a point between the lateral epicondyle of the humerus and the musculospiral groove, the radial nerve divides into its two terminal branches. The superficial branch continues down the arm along with the radial artery and provides sensory innervation to the dorsum of the wrist and the dorsal aspects of a portion of the thumb and index and middle fingers (Fig. 57-1). The deep branch provides most of the motor innervation to the extensors of the forearm. The major portion of the superficial branch passes between the flexor carpi radialis tendon and the radial artery. However, there are a significant number of small branches that ramify to provide sensory innervation of the dorsum of the hand. These small branches also must be blocked to provide complete blockade of the radial nerve.

TECHNIQUE

The patient is placed in a supine position with the arm fully adducted at the patient's side and the elbow slightly flexed with the dorsum of the hand resting on a folded towel. A total of 7 to 8 mL of local anesthetic is drawn up in a 12-mL sterile syringe. When treating painful or inflammatory conditions that are mediated via the radial nerve, a total of 80 mg of depot-steroid is added to the local anesthetic with the first block, and 40 mg of depot-steroid is added with subsequent blocks.

The patient is instructed to flex his or her wrist to allow the pain specialist to identify the flexor carpi radialis tendon. The distal radial prominence is then identified. After preparation of the skin with antiseptic solution, a 25-gauge, $1\frac{1}{2}$-inch needle is inserted in a perpendicular trajectory just lateral to the flexor carpi radialis tendon and just medial to the radial artery at the level of the distal radial prominence (Fig. 57-2). The needle is slowly advanced. As the needle approaches the radius, a strong paresthesia in the distribution of the radial nerve will be elicited. The patient should be warned that a paresthesia will occur and asked to say "there!" as soon as the paresthesia is felt. After paresthesia is elicited and its

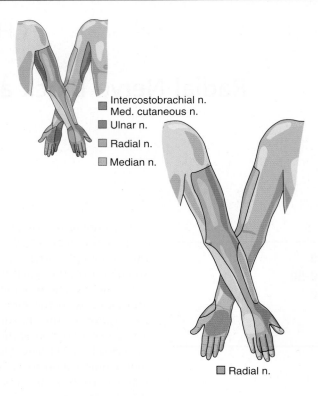

Intercostobrachial n.
Med. cutaneous n.
Ulnar n.
Radial n.
Median n.

Radial n.

Figure 57-1.

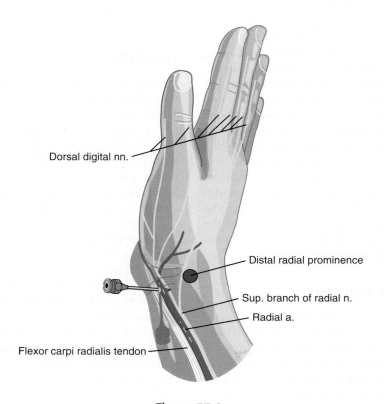

Dorsal digital nn.

Distal radial prominence

Sup. branch of radial n.

Radial a.

Flexor carpi radialis tendon

Figure 57-2.

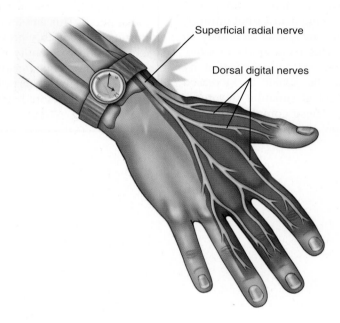

Figure 57-3.
Cheiralgia paresthetica manifests as pain, paresthesias, and numbness of the radial aspect of the dorsum of the hand to the base of the thumb. (From Waldman SD: Atlas of Uncommon Pain Syndromes, 2nd ed. Philadelphia, Saunders, 2008, Fig. 35-1.)

distribution identified, gentle aspiration is carried out to identify blood. If the aspiration test is negative and no persistent paresthesia into the distribution of the radial nerve remains, 3 to 4 mL of solution is slowly injected, with close monitoring of the patient for signs of local anesthetic toxicity.

The patient is then asked to pronate the arm, and an additional 3 to 4 mL of solution is injected in a subcutaneous bead, starting at the anatomic snuff box and carrying the injection subcutaneously to just past the midline of the dorsum of the wrist.

SIDE EFFECTS AND COMPLICATIONS

Radial nerve block at the wrist is a relatively safe block, with the major complications being inadvertent intravascular injection and persistent paresthesia secondary to needle trauma to the nerve. This technique can safely be performed in the presence of anticoagulation by using a 25- or 27-gauge needle, albeit at increased risk for hematoma, if the clinical situation dictates a favorable risk-to-benefit ratio. These complications can be decreased if manual pressure is applied to the area of the block immediately after injection. Application of cold packs for 20-minute periods after the block also will decrease the amount of postprocedure pain and bleeding the patient may experience.

CLINICAL PEARLS

Radial nerve block at the wrist is a simple and safe technique. The major limitation of radial nerve block at the wrist is the difficulty in being sure that all of the nerve fibers blocked when injecting across the dorsum of the wrist in fact have their origin in the radial nerve. This fact limits the diagnostic and prognostic utility of this procedure. Careful neurologic examination to identify preexisting neurologic deficits, including cheiralgia paresthetica, that later may be attributed to the nerve block should be performed on all patients before beginning radial nerve block at the wrist (Fig. 57-3).

CHAPTER 58

Median Nerve Block at the Wrist

CPT-2009 CODE

Unilateral	64450
Bilateral	64450-50
Neurolytic	64640

Relative Value Units

Unilateral	10
Bilateral	20
Neurolytic	20

INDICATIONS

Median nerve block at the wrist is useful to supplement brachial plexus block when additional anesthesia is needed in the distribution of the distal median nerve. In addition to applications for surgical anesthesia, median nerve block at the wrist with local anesthetic can be used as a diagnostic tool when performing differential neural blockade on an anatomic basis in the evaluation of upper extremity pain below the elbow. If destruction of the median nerve is being considered, this technique is useful as a prognostic indicator of the degree of motor and sensory impairment that the patient may experience. Median nerve block at the wrist with local anesthetic may be used to palliate acute pain emergencies subserved by the median nerve while waiting for pharmacologic, surgical, and antiblastic methods to become effective. Median nerve block at the wrist with local anesthetic and steroid also is useful in the palliation of pain secondary to median nerve entrapment syndromes at the wrist, including carpal tunnel syndrome (Figs. 58-1 and 58-2).

CLINICALLY RELEVANT ANATOMY

The median nerve is made up of fibers from C5-T1 spinal roots. The nerve lies anterior and superior to the axillary artery in the 12-o'clock to 3-o'clock quadrant. Exiting the axilla, the median nerve descends into the upper arm along with the brachial artery. At the level of the elbow, the brachial artery is just medial to the biceps muscle. At this level, the median nerve lies just medial to the brachial artery. As the median nerve proceeds downward into the forearm, it gives off numerous branches that provide motor innervation to the flexor muscles of the forearm. These branches are susceptible to nerve entrapment by aberrant ligaments, muscle hypertrophy, and direct trauma. The nerve approaches the wrist overlying the radius. It lies deep to and between the tendons of the palmaris longus muscle and the flexor carpi radialis muscle at the wrist (Fig. 58-3). The median nerve then passes beneath the flexor retinaculum and through the carpal tunnel, with the nerve's terminal branches providing sensory innervation to a portion of the palmar surface of the hand as well as the palmar surface of the thumb, index and middle fingers, and the radial portion of the ring finger (Fig. 58-4). The median nerve also provides sensory innervation to the distal dorsal surface of the index and middle fingers and the radial portion of the ring finger.

TECHNIQUE

The patient is placed in a supine position with the arm fully adducted at the patient's side and the elbow slightly flexed with the dorsum of the hand resting on a folded towel. A total of 3 to 5 mL of local anesthetic is drawn up in a 12-mL sterile syringe. When treating painful or inflammatory conditions that are mediated via the median nerve, a total of 80 mg of depot-steroid is added to the local anesthetic with the first block, and 40 mg of depot-steroid is added with subsequent blocks.

The pain specialist then has the patient make a fist and at the same time flex his or her wrist to aid in identification of the palmaris longus tendon. After preparation of the skin with antiseptic solution, a 25-gauge, ⅝-inch needle is inserted just medial to the tendon and just proximal to the crease of the wrist (Fig. 58-5). The needle is slowly advanced in a slightly cephalad trajectory. As the needle advances beyond the tendon at a depth of about ½ inch, a strong paresthesia in the

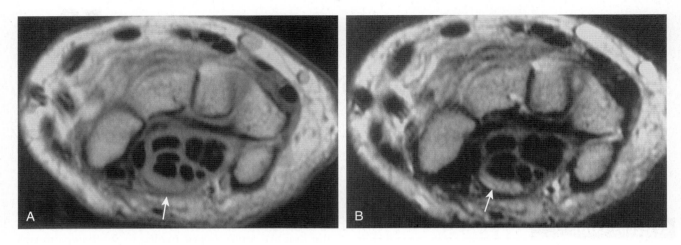

Figure 58-1.
Carpal tunnel syndrome. **A,** Axial protein density–weighted (2500/20)
image shows the bowed flexor retinaculum (*arrow*) and flattened enlarged
median nerve. **B,** Axial T2-weighted (2500/70) image shows that the
median nerve is ovoid and has increased signal (*arrow*). (From Stark DD,
Bradley WG: Magnetic Resonance Imaging, 3rd ed. St. Louis, Mosby, 1999,
p 780.)

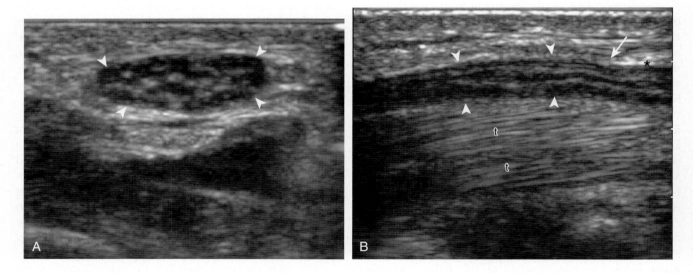

Figure 58-2.
Carpal tunnel syndrome. Ultrasound images transverse (**A**) and longitudinal
(**B**) to the median nerve show hypoechoic swelling (*arrowheads*). Note
mild deviation of the median nerve (*arrow*) as it courses beneath the
flexor retinaculum (*asterisk*) (t, flexor tendons). (From Jacobson JA:
Fundamentals of Musculoskeletal Ultrasound, 1st ed. Philadelphia,
Saunders, 2007, p 111.)

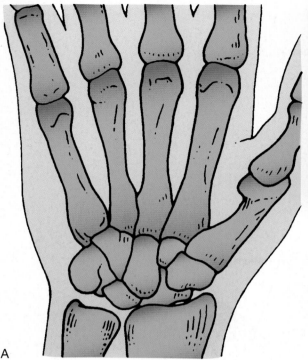

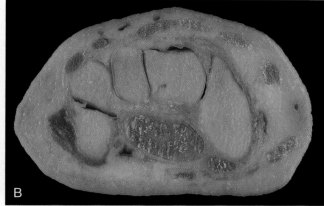

Figure 58-3.
(From Kang HS, Resnick D, Ahn J: MRI of the Extremities:
An Anatomic Atlas, 2nd ed. Philadelphia, WB Saunders, 2002,
p 177.)

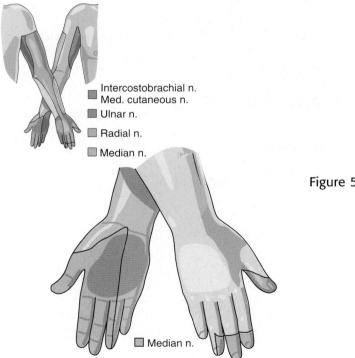

Intercostobrachial n.
Med. cutaneous n.

Ulnar n.

Radial n.

Median n.

Figure 58-4.

Median n.

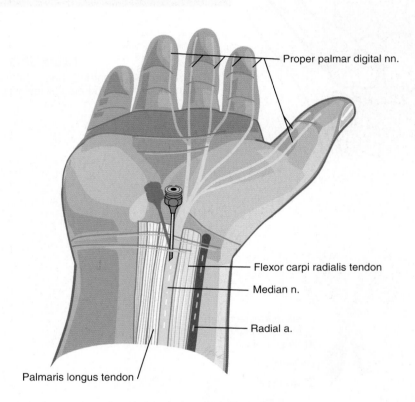

Proper palmar digital nn.

Flexor carpi radialis tendon

Median n.

Radial a.

Palmaris longus tendon

Figure 58-5.

distribution of the median nerve will be elicited. The patient should be warned that a paresthesia will occur and asked to say "there!" as soon as the paresthesia is felt.

After paresthesia is elicited and its distribution identified, gentle aspiration is carried out to identify blood. If the aspiration test is negative and no persistent paresthesia into the distribution of the median nerve remains, 3 to 5 mL of solution is slowly injected, with close monitoring of the patient for signs of local anesthetic toxicity. If no paresthesia is elicited and the needle tip hits bone, the needle is withdrawn out of the periosteum, and after careful aspiration, 3 to 5 mL of solution is slowly injected.

SIDE EFFECTS AND COMPLICATIONS

Median nerve block at the wrist is a relatively safe block, with the major complications being inadvertent intravascular injection and persistent paresthesia secondary to needle trauma to the nerve. This technique can safely be performed in the presence of anticoagulation by using a 25- or 27-gauge needle, albeit at increased risk for hematoma, if the clinical situation dictates a favorable risk-to-benefit ratio. These complications can be decreased if manual pressure is applied to the area of the block immediately after injection. Application of cold packs for 20-minute periods after the block will also decrease the amount of postprocedure pain and bleeding the patient may experience.

CLINICAL PEARLS

Median nerve block at the wrist is a simple and safe technique in the evaluation and treatment of the previously mentioned painful conditions. Careful neurologic examination to identify preexisting neurologic deficits that later may be attributed to the nerve block should be performed on all patients before beginning median nerve block at the wrist, especially in those patients with clinical symptoms to suggest carpal tunnel syndrome.

This technique is useful in the treatment of pain secondary to median nerve compression syndromes at the wrist, including carpal tunnel syndrome. Care should be taken to place the needle proximal to the flexor retinaculum and to inject slowly to allow the solution to flow easily into the carpal tunnel without further compromising the median nerve. Carpal tunnel syndrome also should be differentiated from cervical radiculopathy involving the cervical nerve roots, which may, at times, mimic median nerve compression. Furthermore, it should be remembered that cervical radiculopathy and median nerve entrapment may coexist in the so-called double-crush syndrome. The double-crush syndrome occurs most commonly with median nerve entrapment at the wrist or carpal tunnel syndrome.

CHAPTER 59

Ulnar Nerve Block at the Wrist

CPT-2009 CODE

Unilateral	64450
Bilateral	64450-50
Neurolytic	64640

Relative Value Units

Unilateral	10
Bilateral	20
Neurolytic	20

INDICATIONS

Ulnar nerve block at the wrist is useful in supplementing brachial plexus block when additional anesthesia is needed in the distribution of the ulnar nerve. In addition to applications for surgical anesthesia, ulnar nerve block at the wrist with local anesthetic can be used as a diagnostic tool when performing differential neural blockade on an anatomic basis in the evaluation of upper extremity pain below the elbow. If destruction of the ulnar nerve is being considered, this technique is useful as a prognostic indicator of the degree of motor and sensory impairment that the patient may experience. Ulnar nerve block at the wrist with local anesthetic may be used to palliate acute pain emergencies subserved by the ulnar nerve while waiting for pharmacologic, surgical, and antiblastic methods to become effective. Ulnar nerve block at the wrist with local anesthetic and steroid also is useful in the palliation of pain secondary to ulnar nerve entrapment syndromes at the wrist, including ulnar tunnel syndrome.

CLINICALLY RELEVANT ANATOMY

The ulnar nerve is made up of fibers from C6-T1 spinal roots. The nerve lies anterior and inferior to the axillary artery in the 3-o'clock to 6-o'clock quadrant. Exiting the axilla, the ulnar nerve descends into the upper arm along with the brachial artery. At the middle of the upper arm, the nerve courses medially to pass between the olecranon process and medial epicondyle of the humerus. The nerve then passes between the heads of the flexor carpi ulnaris muscle continuing downward, moving radially along with the ulnar artery (Fig. 59-1). At a point about 1 inch proximal to the crease of the wrist, the ulnar divides into the dorsal and palmar branches. The dorsal branch provides sensation to the ulnar aspect of the dorsum of the hand and the dorsal aspect of the little finger and the ulnar half of the ring finger (Fig. 59-2). The palmar branch provides sensory innervation to the ulnar aspect of the palm of the hand and the palmar aspect of the little finger and the ulnar half of the ring finger.

TECHNIQUE

The patient is placed in a supine position with the arm fully adducted at the patient's side and the wrist slightly flexed with the dorsum of the hand resting on a folded towel. A total of 5 to 7 mL of local anesthetic is drawn up in a 12-mL sterile syringe. When treating painful or inflammatory conditions that are mediated via the ulnar nerve, a total of 80 mg of depot-steroid is added to the local anesthetic with the first block, and 40 mg of depot-steroid is added with subsequent blocks.

The pain specialist then has the patient make a fist and at the same time flex his or her wrist to aid in identification of the flexor carpi ulnaris tendon. After preparation of the skin with antiseptic solution, a 25-gauge, $\frac{5}{8}$-inch needle is inserted on the radial side of the tendon at the level of the styloid process (Fig. 59-3). The needle is slowly advanced in a slightly cephalad trajectory. As the needle advances about $\frac{1}{2}$ inch, a strong paresthesia in the distribution of the ulnar nerve will be elicited. The patient should be warned that a paresthesia will occur and asked to say "there!" as soon as the paresthesia is felt.

After paresthesia is elicited and its distribution identified, gentle aspiration is carried out to identify blood. If the aspiration test is negative and no persistent

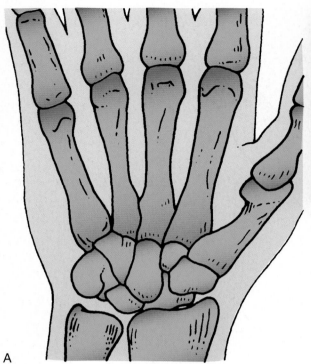

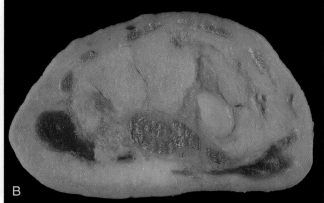

Figure 59-1.
(From Kang HS, Resnick D, Ahn J: MRI of the Extremities:
An Anatomic Atlas, 2nd ed. Philadelphia, WB Saunders, 2002,
p 178.)

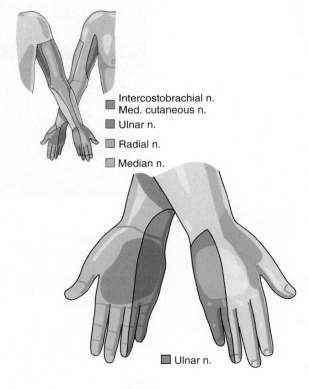

Intercostobrachial n.
Med. cutaneous n.

Ulnar n.

Radial n.

Median n.

Ulnar n.

Figure 59-2.

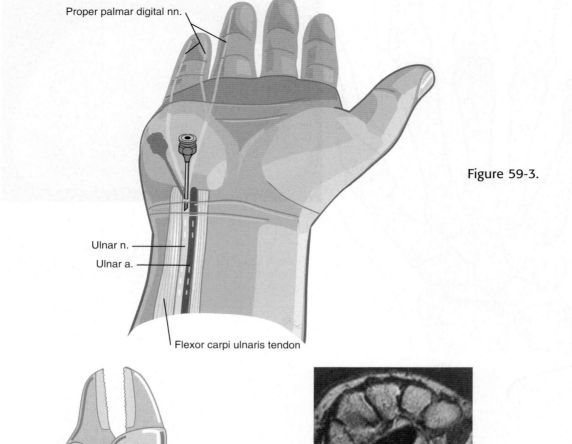

Proper palmar digital nn.

Ulnar n.

Ulnar a.

Flexor carpi ulnaris tendon

Figure 59-3.

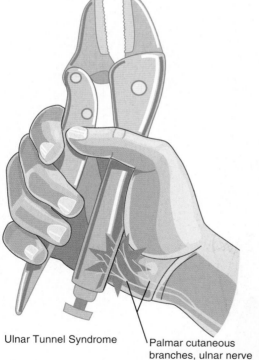

Ulnar Tunnel Syndrome

Palmar cutaneous branches, ulnar nerve

Figure 59-4.

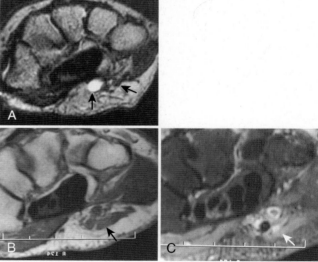

Figure 59-5.

Entrapment of the ulnar nerve: Guyon's canal syndrome (ulnar tunnel syndrome). **A,** Ganglion cyst. A transverse T2-weighted (TR/TE, 2000/80) spin-echo magnetic resonance image shows a ganglion cyst (*arrow*) adjacent to the ulnar nerve and vessels (*arrowhead*). **B** and **C,** Anomalous muscle. This accessory muscle (i.e., accessory abductor digiti minimi muscle) (*arrows*) is well shown in transverse T1-weighted (TR/TE, 550/12) spin-echo (**B**) and fat-suppressed fast spin-echo (TR/TE, 3000/11) (**C**) magnetic resonance images. Note the abnormal high signal intensity in the muscle and subjacent Guyon's canal in **C**. (Courtesy of D. Fanney, MD, Virginia Beach, Virginia; from Resnick D: Diagnosis of Bone and Joint Disorders, 4th ed. Philadelphia, WB Saunders, 2002, p 3527.)

paresthesia into the distribution of the ulnar nerve remains, 3 to 5 mL of solution is slowly injected, with close monitoring of the patient for signs of local anesthetic toxicity. If no paresthesia can be elicited, a similar amount of solution is slowly injected in a fanlike manner just proximal to the notch, with care being taken to avoid intravascular injection.

To ensure complete block of the dorsal branch of the ulnar nerve, it may be necessary to inject a bead of local anesthetic subcutaneously around the ulnar aspect of the wrist starting from the flexor carpi ulnaris tendon to the midline of the dorsum of the hand.

SIDE EFFECTS AND COMPLICATIONS

Ulnar nerve block at the wrist is a relatively safe block, with the major complications being inadvertent intravascular injection into the ulnar artery and persistent paresthesia secondary to needle trauma to the nerve. Because, like the carpal tunnel, Guyon's canal is a closed space, care should be taken to slowly inject to avoid additional compromise of the nerve. This technique can safely be performed in the presence of anticoagulation by using a 25- or 27-gauge needle, albeit at increased risk for hematoma, if the clinical situation dictates a favorable risk-to-benefit ratio. These complications can be decreased if manual pressure is applied to the area of the block immediately after injection. Application of cold packs for 20-minute periods after the block also will decrease the amount of postprocedure pain and bleeding the patient may experience.

CLINICAL PEARLS

Ulnar nerve block at the wrist is a simple and safe technique in the evaluation and treatment of the previously mentioned painful conditions. Careful neurologic examination to identify preexisting neurologic deficits that later may be attributed to the nerve block should be performed on all patients before beginning ulnar nerve block at the wrist.

Ulnar nerve block at the wrist is especially useful in the treatment of pain secondary to ulnar nerve compression syndromes at the wrist, including ulnar tunnel syndrome. Ulnar tunnel syndrome often occurs after compression of the palmar branch of the ulnar nerve proximal to Guyon's canal (Figs. 59-4 and 59-5). It often presents clinically after a long bicycle ride or after repeated use of pliers. The maximal tenderness to palpation is over the ulnar nerve just proximal to Guyon's canal. Injection of the ulnar nerve at the wrist with local anesthetic and steroid will give almost instantaneous relief.

Ulnar tunnel syndrome should be differentiated from cervical radiculopathy involving the C8 spinal root, which may, at times, mimic ulnar nerve compression. Furthermore, it should be remembered that cervical radiculopathy and ulnar nerve entrapment may coexist in the so-called double-crush syndrome. The double-crush syndrome occurs most commonly with ulnar nerve entrapment at the wrist or carpal tunnel syndrome. Pancoast's tumor invading the medial cord of the brachial plexus also may mimic an isolated ulnar nerve entrapment and should be ruled out by apical lordotic chest x-ray.

CHAPTER 60

Metacarpal and Digital Nerve Block

CPT-2009 CODE	
Unilateral	64450
Bilateral	64450-50
Neurolytic	64640

Relative Value Units	
Unilateral	7
Bilateral	14
Neurolytic	20

INDICATIONS

Metacarpal and digital nerve block is used primarily in two clinical situations: (1) to provide surgical anesthesia in the distribution of the digital nerves for laceration, tendon, and fracture repair; and (2) to provide postoperative pain relief after joint replacement or major surgical procedures on the hand.

CLINICALLY RELEVANT ANATOMY

The common digital nerves arise from fibers of the median and ulnar nerves. The thumb also has contributions from superficial branches of the radial nerve. The common digital nerves pass along the metacarpal bones and divide as they reach the distal palm. The volar digital nerves supply the majority of sensory innervation to the fingers and run along the ventrolateral aspect of the finger beside the digital vein and artery. The smaller dorsal digital nerves contain fibers from the ulnar and radial nerves and supply the dorsum of the fingers as far as the proximal joints.

TECHNIQUE

The patient is placed in a supine position with the arm fully abducted and the elbow slightly flexed with the palm of the hand resting on a folded towel. A total of 3 mL per digit of non–epinephrine-containing local anesthetic is drawn up in a 12-mL sterile syringe.

Metacarpal Nerve Block

After preparation of the skin with antiseptic solution, at a point proximal to the metacarpal head, a 25-gauge, 1½-inch needle is inserted on each side of the metacarpal bone to be blocked (Fig. 60-1). While the anesthetic is slowly injected, the needle is advanced from the dorsal surface of the hand toward the palmar surface. The common digital nerve is situated on the dorsal side of the flexor retinaculum, and thus the needle will have to be advanced almost to the palmar surface of the hand to obtain satisfactory anesthesia. The needle is removed, and pressure is placed on the injection site to avoid hematoma formation.

Digital Nerve Block

The patient is placed in a supine position with the arm fully abducted and the elbow slightly flexed with the palm of the hand resting on a folded towel.

After preparation of the skin with antiseptic solution, at a point at the base of the finger, a 25-gauge, 1½-inch needle is inserted on each side of the bone of the digit to be blocked (Fig. 60-2). While the anesthetic is slowly injected, the needle is advanced from the dorsal surface of the hand toward the palmar surface. The same technique can be used to block the thumb. The needle is removed, and pressure is placed on the injection site to avoid hematoma formation.

SIDE EFFECTS AND COMPLICATIONS

Because of the confined nature of the soft tissue surrounding the metacarpals and digits, the potential for mechanical compression of the blood supply after injection of solution must be considered. The pain specialist must avoid rapidly injecting large volumes of solution into these confined spaces, or vascular insufficiency and gangrene may occur. Furthermore, epinephrine-containing solutions should never be used to avoid ischemia and possible gangrene.

This technique can safely be performed in the presence of anticoagulation by using a 25- or 27-gauge needle, albeit at increased risk for hematoma, if the clinical

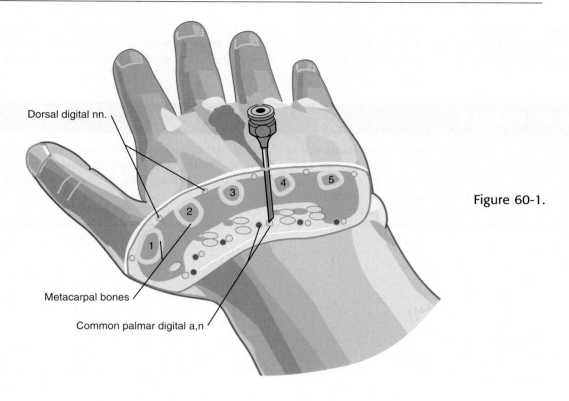

Dorsal digital nn.

Metacarpal bones

Common palmar digital a,n

Figure 60-1.

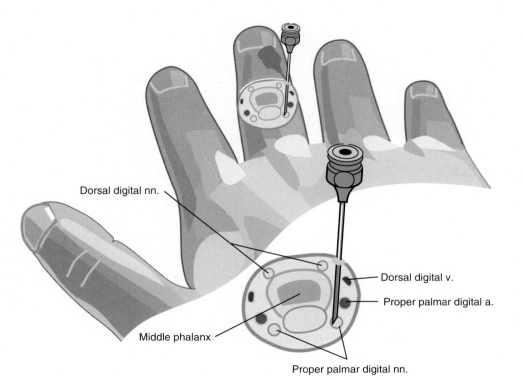

Dorsal digital nn.

Dorsal digital v.

Proper palmar digital a.

Middle phalanx

Proper palmar digital nn.

Figure 60-2.

situation dictates a favorable risk-to-benefit ratio. These complications can be decreased if manual pressure is applied to the area of the block immediately after injec- tion. Application of cold packs for 10-minute periods after the block also will decrease the amount of postpro- cedure pain and bleeding the patient may experience.

CLINICAL PEARLS

Digital nerve block is especially useful in the palliation of postoperative pain after total joint replacement in the hands. When used for pain secondary to trauma, the pain specialist must ascertain and document the status of the vascular supply before implementing digital nerve block to avoid subsequent vascular insuf- ficiency being erroneously attributed to the digital nerve block rather than preexisting trauma to the vasculature.

Intravenous Regional Anesthesia

INDICATIONS

Intravenous regional anesthesia is used primarily in two clinical situations: (1) to provide surgical anesthesia for surgical procedures on the distal extremities; and (2) to administer drugs intravenously to treat painful conditions such as reflex sympathetic dystrophy that are limited to a specific extremity.

CLINICALLY RELEVANT ANATOMY

The peripheral nerves of the extremities receive their blood supply from the blood vessels that accompany them. By administering drugs intravenously and sequestering them in the extremity by use of a tourniquet, the drugs administered can then diffuse into the soft tissues and nerves. The limiting factor for this technique is the total amount of drug administered and the length of time that the circulation of the extremity can be occluded by the tourniquet.

TECHNIQUE

The patient is placed in the supine position. An intravenous catheter is placed in the extremity to be treated. The affected extremity is elevated to drain excess blood (Fig. 61-1). The area underneath the tourniquet is wrapped with cotton cast padding, and a double tourniquet is placed tightly around the affected extremity. An Esmarch bandage is used to exsanguinate the extremity only if the surgeon requires a bloodless field. The upper portion of the double tourniquet is then inflated to a pressure of 100 mm Hg above the patient's systolic blood pressure (Fig. 61-2). Lidocaine 0.5% without preservative in a volume of 30 to 50 mL is used for surgical anesthesia. For pain management applications, water-soluble steroid methylprednisolone, reserpine, or bretylium is administered in solution with similar volumes of more dilute concentrations of preservative-free lidocaine.

After the solution has been injected for about 10 minutes, the lower tourniquet is inflated over the anesthetized area, and after ascertaining that the lower tourniquet is adequately inflated, the upper tourniquet is deflated (Fig. 61-3). The lower tourniquet is left inflated for an additional 10 to 15 minutes. The cuff is then deflated to just below the systolic pressure for a few seconds and then reinflated while the patient is observed closely for signs of local anesthetic toxicity. This maneuver is performed repeatedly while gradually decreasing the cuff pressure to allow the local anesthetic to slowly wash out. At the first sign of local anesthetic toxicity, the cuff should be reinflated for at least an additional 5 minutes or until all signs of local anesthetic toxicity have abated. After the tourniquet is completely deflated, the tourniquet and intravenous cannula are then removed.

SIDE EFFECTS AND COMPLICATIONS

The major side effect of intravenous regional anesthesia is phlebitis at the injection site and proximal vein. This problem occurs more frequently with the ester-type local anesthetics and with the administration of drugs in addition to local anesthetics. Patients taking aspirin may experience petechial hemorrhages distal to the tourniquet and should be warned of such. The major complication of intravenous regional anesthesia is local anesthetic toxicity secondary to tourniquet failure or improper technique. For this reason, intravenous regional anesthesia should never be performed unless equipment and personnel for resuscitation are available.

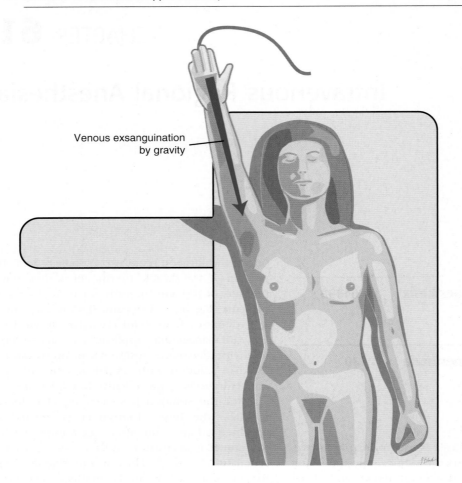

Venous exsanguination
by gravity

Figure 61-1.

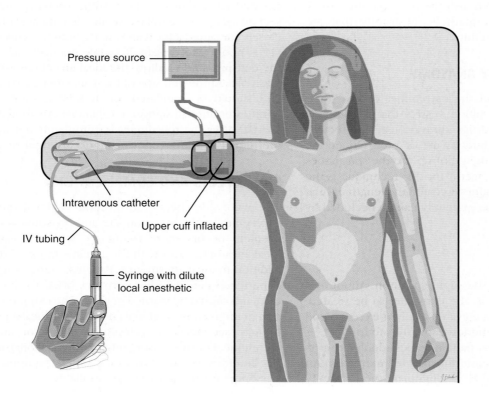

Pressure source

Intravenous catheter

Upper cuff inflated

IV tubing

Syringe with dilute
local anesthetic

Figure 61-2.

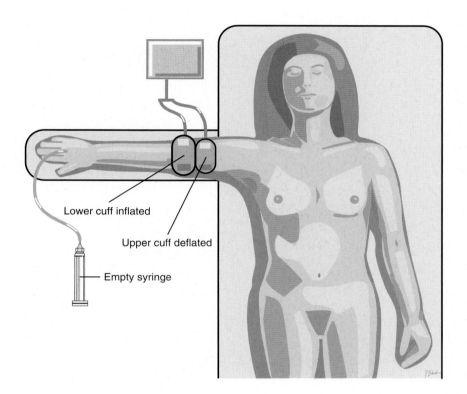

Figure 61-3.

CLINICAL PEARLS

Intravenous regional anesthesia with local anesthetic and water-soluble steroid is an especially useful technique in patients suffering from reflex sympathetic dystrophy who have a significant amount of edema of the affected extremity. If tourniquet pain is a problem, supplemental block of the intercostobrachial and median cutaneous nerves of the arm can be performed before intravenous regional anesthesia.

Section 4

Thorax and Chest Wall

CHAPTER 62

Thoracic Epidural Nerve Block: Midline Approach

CPT-2009 CODE

Local Anesthetic/Narcotic	62310
Steroid	62310
Neurolytic	62281

Relative Value Units

Local Anesthetic	10
Steroid	10
Neurolytic	20

INDICATIONS

In addition to applications for thoracic and upper abdominal surgical anesthesia, thoracic epidural nerve block with local anesthetic can be used as a diagnostic tool when performing differential neural blockade on an anatomic basis in the evaluation of chest wall and intraabdominal pain. If destruction of the thoracic nerve roots is being considered, this technique is useful as a prognostic indicator of the degree of motor and sensory impairment that the patient may experience.

Thoracic epidural nerve block with local anesthetics or opioids may be used to palliate acute pain emergencies while waiting for pharmacologic, surgical, or antiblastic methods to become effective. This technique is useful in the management of postoperative pain as well as pain secondary to trauma. The pain of acute herpes zoster, pain of acute pancreatitis, and cancer-related pain also are amenable to treatment with epidurally administered local anesthetics, steroids, or opioids. Additionally, this technique is of value in patients suffering from angina that has failed to respond to conservative measures.

The administration of local anesthetics or steroids via the thoracic approach to the epidural space is useful in the treatment of a variety of chronic benign pain syndromes, including thoracic radiculopathy, thoracic postlaminectomy syndrome, vertebral compression fractures, chronic pancreatitis, diabetic polyneuropathy, chemotherapy-related peripheral neuropathy, postherpetic neuralgia, reflex sympathetic dystrophy, and abdominal pain syndromes.

The thoracic epidural administration of local anesthetics in combination with steroids or opioids also is useful in the palliation of cancer-related pain of the chest wall and abdomen. This technique has been especially successful in the relief of pain secondary to metastatic disease of the spine. The long-term epidural administration of opioids has become a mainstay in the palliation of cancer-related pain.

CLINICALLY RELEVANT ANATOMY

The superior boundary of the epidural space is the fusion of the periosteal and spinal layers of dura at the foramen magnum. The epidural space continues inferiorly to the sacrococcygeal membrane. The thoracic epidural space is bounded anteriorly by the posterior longitudinal ligament and posteriorly by the vertebral laminae and the ligamentum flavum. The vertebral pedicles and intervertebral foramina form the lateral limits of the epidural space. The thoracic epidural space is 3 to 4 mm at the C7-T1 interspace with the cervical spine flexed and about 5 mm at the T11-T12 interspace. The thoracic epidural space contains fat, veins, arteries, lymphatics, and connective tissue.

When performing thoracic epidural block in the midline, the needle traverses the following structures. After traversing the skin and subcutaneous tissues, the styletted epidural needle impinges on the supraspinous ligament, which runs vertically between the apices of the spinous processes (Fig. 62-1). The supraspinous ligament offers some resistance to the advancing needle. This ligament is dense enough to hold a needle in position even when the needle is released.

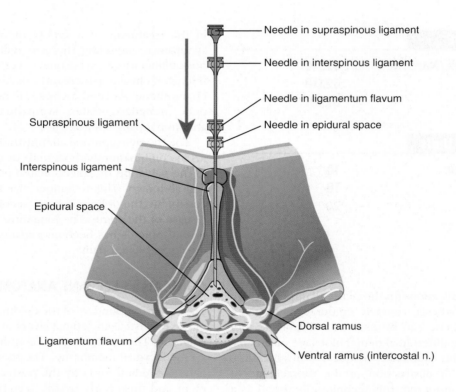

Figure 62-1.

The interspinous ligament, which runs obliquely between the spinous processes, is encountered next, offering additional resistance to needle advancement. Because the interspinous ligament is contiguous with the ligamentum flavum, the pain management specialist may perceive a "false" loss of resistance when the needle tip enters the space between the interspinous ligament and the ligamentum flavum. This phenomenon is more pronounced in the thoracic region than in the lumbar region as a result of the less well-defined ligaments.

A significant increase in resistance to needle advancement signals that the needle tip is impinging on the dense ligamentum flavum (Fig. 62-2). Because the ligament is made up almost entirely of elastin fibers, there is a continued increase in resistance as the needle traverses the ligamentum flavum owing to the drag of the ligament on the needle. A sudden loss of resistance occurs as the needle tip enters the epidural space. There should be essentially no resistance to drugs injected into the normal epidural space.

The upper thoracic vertebral interspaces from T1-T2 and the lower thoracic vertebral interspaces from T10-T12 are functionally equivalent insofar as the technique of epidural block is concerned (Fig. 62-3). The technique of performing epidural block at the level of the upper and the lower thoracic vertebral interspaces is analogous to lumbar epidural block. The thoracic vertebral interspaces between T3 and T9 are functionally unique because of the acute downward angle of the spinous processes. This downward slope means that the spinous process of any given mid-thoracic vertebra is in fact inferior to the interlaminar space of its adjacent vertebra (Fig. 62-4). Blockade of these middle thoracic interspaces requires use of the paramedian approach to the thoracic epidural space.

TECHNIQUE

Thoracic epidural nerve block may be carried out in the sitting, lateral, or prone position, with the sitting position being favored for simplicity of patient positioning when compared with the lateral position. The prone position should be avoided because it makes patient monitoring more difficult.

After the patient is placed in optimal sitting position with the thoracic spine flexed and forehead placed on a padded bedside table, the skin is prepared with an antiseptic solution. For epidural blockade at the upper T1 through T2 or lower T10 through T12 interspaces, the operator's middle and index fingers are placed on each side of the spinous processes. The position of the interspace is reconfirmed with palpation using a rocking motion in the superior and inferior planes. The midline of the selected interspace is identified by palpating the spinous processes above and below the interspace using a lateral rocking motion to ensure that the needle entry site is exactly in the midline. One milliliter of local anesthetic is used to infiltrate the skin, subcutaneous tissues, and supraspinous and interspinous ligaments at the midline.

A 2-inch, 25-gauge or an 18- or 20-gauge, 3½-inch Hustead needle is inserted exactly in the midline in the previously anesthetized area through the supraspinous ligament into the interspinous ligament. Smaller, shorter needles are being used at some centers with equally good results.

After attaching a syringe containing either preservative-free saline or the intended injectate of local anesthetic, narcotic, or steroid, with constant pressure being applied to the plunger of the syringe with the thumb of the right hand, the needle and syringe are continuously advanced in a slow and deliberate manner with the left hand. The right-handed physician holds the epidural needle firmly at the hub with his or her left thumb and index finger. The left hand is placed firmly against the patient's neck to ensure against uncontrolled needle movements should the patient unexpectedly move. With constant pressure being applied to the plunger of the syringe with the thumb of the right hand, the needle and syringe are continuously advanced in a slow and deliberate manner with the left hand. As soon as the needle bevel passes through the ligamentum flavum and enters the epidural space, there will be a sudden loss of resistance to injection, and the plunger will effortlessly surge forward. The syringe is removed gently from the needle.

An air or saline acceptance test is carried out by injecting 0.5 to 1 mL of air or sterile preservative-free saline with a well-lubricated sterile glass syringe to help confirm that the needle is within the epidural space. The force required for injection should not exceed that necessary to overcome the resistance of the needle. Any significant pain or sudden increase in resistance during injection suggests incorrect needle placement, and one should *stop* injecting immediately and reassess the position of the needle. Fluoroscopy can be a useful adjunct to this procedure, especially in obese patients in whom palpation of bony landmarks is difficult (Fig. 62-5).

When satisfactory needle position is confirmed, a syringe containing 5 to 7 mL of solution to be injected in the upper thoracic region, or 8 to 10 mL of solution to be injected in the lower thoracic region is carefully attached to the needle. Gentle aspiration is carried out to identify cerebrospinal fluid or blood. If cerebrospinal fluid is aspirated, the epidural block may be repeated at a different interspace. In this situation, drug dosages should be adjusted accordingly because subarachnoid migration of drugs through the dural rent can occur. If

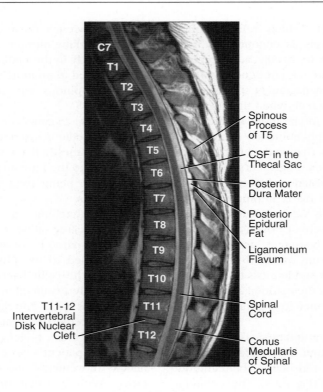

Figure 62-2.
Lateral view of the thoracic spine showing the ligamentum flavum. (From Renfrew DL: Atlas of Spine Imaging, 1st ed. Philadelphia, WB Saunders, 2002, p 6.)

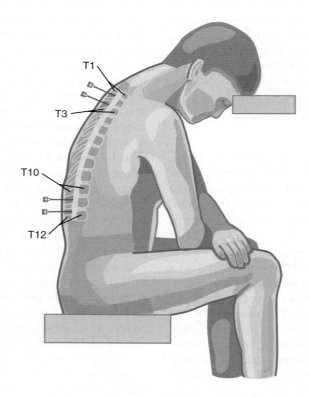

Figure 62-3.

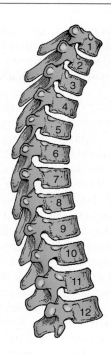

Figure 62-4.
The inclination of the spinous processes from T1-12. (From Waldman: Pain Management, 1st ed. Philadelphia, Saunders, 2006.)

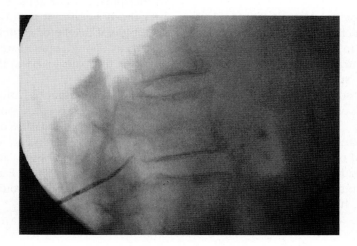

Figure 62-5.
Radiographic imaging showing lateral anterior oblique view of the spine, confirming that the needle has entered the epidural space. (From Raj PP, Lou L, Erdine S, et al: Interventional Pain Management: Image-Guided Procedures, 2nd ed. Philadelphia, Saunders, 2008.)

aspiration of blood occurs, the needle should be rotated slightly and the aspiration test repeated. If no blood is present, incremental doses of local anesthetic and other drugs may be administered while monitoring the patient carefully for signs of local anesthetic toxicity.

For diagnostic and prognostic blocks, 1.0% preservative-free lidocaine is a suitable local anesthetic. For therapeutic blocks, 0.25% preservative-free bupivacaine, in combination with 80 mg of depot methylprednisolone, is injected. Subsequent nerve blocks are carried out in a similar manner, substituting 40 mg of methylprednisolone for the initial 80-mg dose. Daily thoracic epidural nerve blocks with local anesthetic or steroid may be required to treat the previously mentioned acute painful conditions. Chronic conditions such as thoracic radiculopathy, tension-type headaches, and diabetic polyneuropathy are treated on an every-other-day to once-a-week basis or as the clinical situation dictates.

If the upper thoracic epidural route is chosen for administration of opioids, 1 mg of preservative-free morphine sulfate formulated for epidural use is a reasonable initial dose in opioid-tolerant patients. For the lower thoracic region, 4 to 5 mg of morphine is an appropriate starting dose. More lipid-soluble opioids such as fentanyl must be delivered by continuous infusion via a thoracic epidural catheter. An epidural catheter may be placed into the thoracic epidural space through a Hustead needle to allow continuous infusions.

SIDE EFFECTS AND COMPLICATIONS

Because of the potential for hematogenous spread via Batson's plexus, local infection and sepsis represent absolute contraindications to the thoracic approach to the epidural space. In contradistinction to the caudal approach to the epidural space, anticoagulation and coagulopathy represent absolute contraindications to thoracic epidural nerve block because of the risk for epidural hematoma.

Inadvertent dural puncture occurring during thoracic epidural nerve block should occur less than 0.5% of the time. Failure to recognize inadvertent dural puncture can result in immediate total spinal anesthetic with associated loss of consciousness, hypotension, and apnea. If epidural doses of opioids are accidentally placed into the subarachnoid space, significant respiratory and central nervous system depression will result. It is also possible to inadvertently place a needle or catheter intended for the epidural space into the subdural space. If subdural placement is unrecognized and epidural doses of local anesthetics are administered, the signs and symptoms are similar to those of massive subarachnoid injection, although the resulting motor and sensory block may be spotty.

The thoracic epidural space is highly vascular. The intravenous placement of the epidural needle occurs in about 0.5% to 1% of patients undergoing thoracic epidural anesthesia. This complication is increased in those patients with distended epidural veins, such as the parturient and patients with large intra-abdominal tumor mass. If the misplacement is unrecognized, injection of local anesthetic directly into an epidural vein will result in significant local anesthetic toxicity.

Needle trauma to the epidural veins may result in self-limited bleeding that may cause postprocedure pain. Uncontrolled bleeding into the epidural space may result in compression of the spinal cord with the rapid development of neurologic deficit. Although the incidence of significant neurologic deficit secondary to epidural hematoma after thoracic epidural block is exceedingly rare, this devastating complication should be considered whenever there is rapidly developing neurologic deficit after thoracic epidural nerve block.

Neurologic complications after thoracic nerve block are uncommon if proper technique is used. Direct trauma to the spinal cord or nerve roots is usually accompanied by pain. If significant pain occurs during placement of the epidural needle or catheter or during injection, the physician should immediately stop and ascertain the cause of the pain to avoid the possibility of additional neural trauma.

Although uncommon, infection in the epidural space remains an ever-present possibility, especially in the immunocompromised AIDS or cancer patient. If epidural abscess occurs, emergent surgical drainage to avoid spinal cord compression and irreversible neurologic deficit is usually required. Early detection and treatment of infection is crucial to avoid potentially life-threatening sequelae.

CLINICAL PEARLS

Thoracic epidural nerve block is a safe and effective procedure if careful attention is paid to technique. Failure to accurately identify the midline is the most common reason for difficulty in performing thoracic epidural nerve block and increases the risk for complications. It should be noted that the ligamentum flavum is relatively thin in the thoracic region when compared with the lumbar region. This fact has direct clinical implications in that the loss of resistance when performing thoracic epidural nerve block is more subtle than when performing the loss-of-resistance technique in the lumbar or lower thoracic region. Identification of the epidural space in the middle thoracic region is more difficult to accomplish and is associated with more patient discomfort and a higher complication rate and thus should be avoided whenever possible. In the rare instance when middle thoracic epidural block is deemed to be more beneficial than upper or lower thoracic epidural block, the middle epidural space should be accessed using a paramedian approach.

The routine use of sedation or general anesthesia before initiation of thoracic epidural nerve block is to be discouraged because it will render the patient unable to provide accurate verbal feedback should needle or catheter misplacement occur.

CHAPTER **63**

Thoracic Epidural Nerve Block: Paramedian Approach

CPT-2009 CODE

Local Anesthetic/Narcotic	62310
Steroid	62310
Neurolytic	62281

Relative Value Units

Local Anesthetic	10
Steroid	10
Neurolytic	20

INDICATIONS

The paramedian approach to the epidural space is used primarily for blockade of the middle thoracic vertebral interspaces in which the acute downward angulation of the spinous processes makes the midline approach to the thoracic epidural space unsatisfactory. Mid-thoracic epidural block has a limited number of applications for thoracic surgical anesthesia. Mid-thoracic epidural nerve block with local anesthetic can be used as a diagnostic tool when performing differential neural blockade on an anatomic basis in the evaluation of chest wall and thoracic pain. If destruction of the mid-thoracic nerve roots is being considered, this technique is useful as a prognostic indicator of the degree of motor and sensory impairment that the patient may experience.

Thoracic epidural nerve block with local anesthetics or opioids may be used to palliate acute pain emergencies while waiting for pharmacologic, surgical, or antiblastic methods to become effective. This technique is useful in the management of postoperative pain as well as pain secondary to trauma. The pain of acute herpes zoster and acute pancreatitis and cancer-related pain are also amenable to treatment with epidurally administered local anesthetics, steroids, or opioids.

The administration of local anesthetics or steroids via the thoracic approach to the epidural space is useful in the treatment of a variety of chronic benign pain syndromes, including thoracic radiculopathy, thoracic postlaminectomy syndrome, vertebral compression fractures, chronic pancreatitis, diabetic polyneuropathy, chemotherapy-related peripheral neuropathy, postherpetic neuralgia, and reflex sympathetic dystrophy of the chest wall.

The mid-thoracic epidural administration of local anesthetics in combination with steroids or opioids is also useful in the palliation of cancer-related pain of the chest wall and intrathoracic organs. This technique has been especially successful in the relief of pain secondary to metastatic disease of the spine. The long-term epidural administration of opioids has become a mainstay in the palliation of cancer-related pain.

CLINICALLY RELEVANT ANATOMY

The superior boundary of the epidural space is the fusion of the periosteal and spinal layers of dura at the foramen magnum. The epidural space continues inferiorly to the sacrococcygeal membrane. The thoracic epidural space is bounded anteriorly by the posterior longitudinal ligament and posteriorly by the vertebral laminae and the ligamentum flavum. The vertebral pedicles and intervertebral foramina form the lateral limits of the epidural space. The thoracic epidural space is 3 to 4 mm at the C7-T1 interspace with the cervical spine flexed and about 5 mm at the T11-T12 interspace. The thoracic epidural space contains fat, veins, arteries, lymphatics, and connective tissue.

The upper thoracic vertebral interspaces from T1-T2 and the lower thoracic vertebral interspaces from T10-T12 are functionally equivalent insofar as the technique of epidural block is concerned. The technique of performing epidural block at the level of the upper and the lower thoracic vertebral interspaces is analogous to lumbar epidural block. The thoracic vertebral interspaces between T3 and T9 are functionally unique because of the acute downward angle of the spinous processes (Fig. 63-1; see also Fig. 62-4). Blockade of these middle thoracic interspaces requires use of the paramedian or transforaminal approach to the thoracic epidural space.

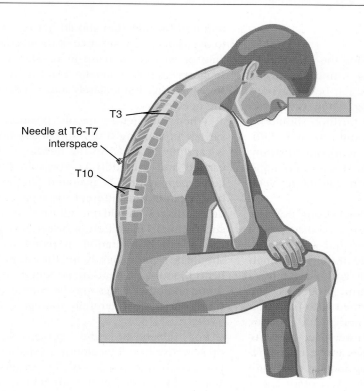

T3

Needle at T6-T7
interspace

T10

Figure 63-1.

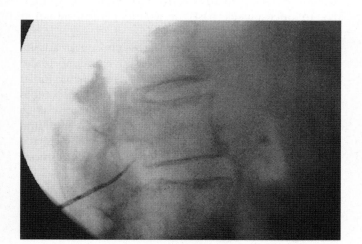

Figure 63-2.
Radiographic imaging showing lateral anterior oblique view of
the spine, confirming that the needle has entered the
epidural space. (From Raj PP, Lou L, Erdine S, et al:
Interventional Pain Management: Image-Guided
Procedures, 2nd ed. Philadelphia, Saunders, 2008.)

TECHNIQUE

Mid-thoracic epidural nerve block using the paramedian approach may be carried out in the sitting, lateral, or prone position, with the sitting position being favored for simplicity of patient positioning when compared with the lateral position. The prone position should be avoided because it makes patient monitoring more difficult. Fluoroscopy may be useful in identifying anatomy and aiding in needle placement. A lateral anterior oblique view will often clearly identify the needle target (Fig. 63-2).

After the patient is placed in optimal sitting position with the thoracic spine flexed and forehead placed on a padded bedside table, the skin is prepared with an antiseptic solution. For epidural blockade of the T3 through T9 interspaces, the operator's middle and index fingers are placed on each side of the spinous processes. The position of the interspace is reconfirmed with palpation using a rocking motion in the superior and inferior planes. The midline of the selected interspace is identified by palpating the spinous processes above and below the interspace using a lateral rocking motion to ensure accurate identification of the midline. At a point about $\frac{1}{2}$ inch lateral to the midline at the level of the inferior border of the spinous process, 1 mL of local anesthetic is used to infiltrate the skin, subcutaneous tissues, muscle, and any ligaments encountered.

The 18- or 20-gauge, $3\frac{1}{2}$-inch Hustead needle is inserted perpendicular to the skin into the subcutaneous tissues (Fig. 63-3). The needle is then redirected slightly medial and craniad and advanced about $\frac{1}{2}$ inch. The needle stylet is removed, and a well-lubricated 5-mL glass syringe filled with preservative-free sterile saline is attached.

The right-handed physician holds the epidural needle firmly at the hub with his or her left thumb and index finger. The left hand is placed firmly against the patient's neck to ensure against uncontrolled needle movements should the patient unexpectedly move. With constant pressure being applied to the plunger of the syringe with the thumb of the right hand, the needle and syringe are continuously advanced in a slow and deliberate manner with the left hand. As soon as the needle bevel passes through the ligamentum flavum and enters the epidural space, there will be a sudden loss of resistance to injection, and the plunger will effortlessly surge forward (Fig. 63-4). If bony contact is made, the needle is withdrawn and redirected in a slightly more medial and cranial trajectory. After the epidural space is identified, the syringe is gently removed from the needle.

An air or saline acceptance test is carried out by injecting 0.5 to 1 mL of air or sterile preservative-free saline with a well-lubricated sterile glass syringe to help confirm that the needle is within the epidural space. The force required for injection should not exceed that necessary to overcome the resistance of the needle. Any significant pain or sudden increase in resistance during injection suggests incorrect needle placement, and one should *stop* injecting immediately and reassess the position of the needle.

When satisfactory needle position is confirmed, a syringe containing 6 to 7 mL of solution to be injected is carefully attached to the needle. Gentle aspiration is carried out to identify cerebrospinal fluid or blood. If cerebrospinal fluid is aspirated, the epidural block may be repeated at a different interspace. In this situation, drug dosages should be adjusted accordingly because subarachnoid migration of drugs through the dural rent can occur. If aspiration of blood occurs, the needle should be rotated slightly and the aspiration test repeated. If no blood is present, incremental doses of local anesthetic and other drugs may be administered while monitoring the patient carefully for signs of local anesthetic toxicity.

For diagnostic and prognostic blocks, 1.0% preservative-free lidocaine is a suitable local anesthetic. For therapeutic blocks, 0.25% preservative-free bupivacaine, in combination with 80 mg of depot methylprednisolone, is injected. Subsequent nerve blocks are carried out in a similar manner, substituting 40 mg of methylprednisolone for the initial 80-mg dose. Daily thoracic epidural nerve blocks with local anesthetic or steroid may be required to treat the previously mentioned acute painful conditions. Chronic conditions such as thoracic radiculopathy, postherpetic neuralgia, and diabetic polyneuropathy are treated on an every-other-day to once-a-week basis or as the clinical situation dictates.

If the mid-thoracic epidural route is chosen for administration of opioids, 3 mg of preservative-free morphine sulfate formulated for epidural use is a reasonable initial dose in opioid-tolerant patients. More lipid-soluble opioids such as fentanyl must be delivered by continuous infusion via a thoracic epidural catheter. An epidural catheter may be placed into the thoracic epidural space through a Hustead needle to allow continuous infusions.

SIDE EFFECTS AND COMPLICATIONS

Because of the potential for hematogenous spread via Batson's plexus, local infection and sepsis represent absolute contraindications to the thoracic approach to the epidural space. In contradistinction to the caudal approach to the epidural space, anticoagulation and coagulopathy represent absolute contraindications to thoracic epidural nerve block because of the risk for epidural hematoma.

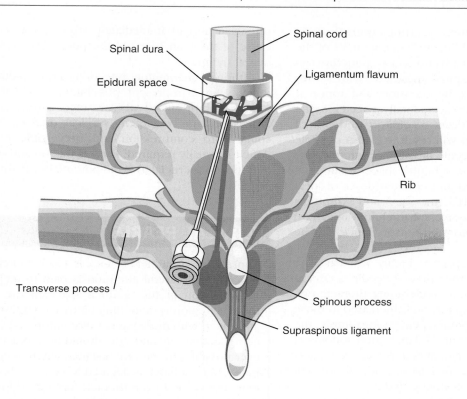

Figure 63-3.

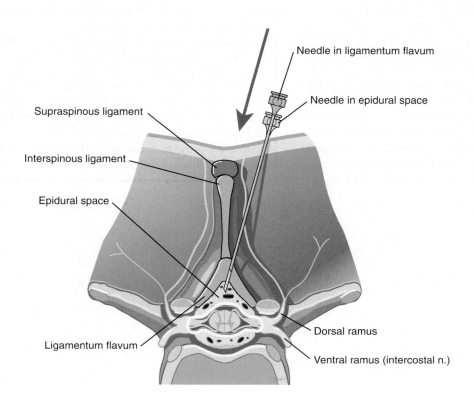

Figure 63-4.

Inadvertent dural puncture occurring during thoracic epidural nerve block should occur less than 0.5% of the time. Failure to recognize inadvertent dural puncture can result in immediate total spinal anesthetic with associated loss of consciousness, hypotension, and apnea. If epidural doses of opioids are accidentally placed into the subarachnoid space, significant respiratory and central nervous system depression will result. It is also possible to inadvertently place a needle or catheter intended for the epidural space into the subdural space. If subdural placement is unrecognized and epidural doses of local anesthetics are administered, the signs and symptoms are similar to those of massive subarachnoid injection, although the resulting motor and sensory block may be spotty.

The thoracic epidural space is highly vascular. The intravenous placement of the epidural needle occurs in about 0.5% to 1% of patients undergoing thoracic epidural anesthesia. This complication is increased in those patients with distended epidural veins, for example, the parturient and patients with a large intra-abdominal tumor mass. If the misplacement is unrecognized, injection of local anesthetic directly into an epidural vein will result in significant local anesthetic toxicity.

Needle trauma to the epidural veins may result in self-limited bleeding that may cause postprocedure pain. Uncontrolled bleeding into the epidural space may result in compression of the spinal cord with the rapid development of neurologic deficit. Although the incidence of significant neurologic deficit secondary to epidural hematoma after thoracic epidural block is exceedingly rare, this devastating complication should be considered whenever there is rapidly developing neurologic deficit after thoracic epidural nerve block.

Neurologic complications after thoracic nerve block are uncommon if proper technique is used. Direct trauma to the spinal cord or nerve roots is usually accompanied by pain. If significant pain occurs during placement of the epidural needle or catheter or during injection, the physician should immediately stop and ascertain the cause of the pain to avoid the possibility of additional neural trauma.

Although uncommon, infection in the epidural space remains an ever-present possibility, especially in the immunocompromised AIDS or cancer patient. If epidural abscess occurs, emergent surgical drainage to avoid spinal cord compression and irreversible neurologic deficit is usually required. Early detection and treatment of infection is crucial to avoid potentially life-threatening sequelae.

CLINICAL PEARLS

Thoracic epidural nerve block is a safe and effective procedure if careful attention is paid to technique. Identification of the epidural space in the middle thoracic region is more difficult to accomplish and is associated with more patient discomfort and a higher complication rate and thus should be avoided whenever possible. In the rare instance when middle thoracic epidural block is deemed to be more beneficial than upper or lower thoracic epidural block, the middle epidural space should be accessed using a paramedian approach.

It should be noted that the ligamentum flavum is relatively thin in the thoracic region when compared with the lumbar region. This fact has direct clinical implications in that the loss of resistance when performing thoracic epidural nerve block is more subtle than when performing the loss-of-resistance technique in the lumbar or lower thoracic region.

The routine use of sedation or general anesthesia before initiation of thoracic epidural nerve block is to be discouraged because it will render the patient unable to provide accurate verbal feedback should needle or catheter misplacement occur.

CHAPTER 64

Thoracic Epidural Block: Transforaminal Approach

CPT-2009 CODE	
Local Anesthetic	64479
Steroid	64479
Additional Level	64480

Relative Value Units	
Local Anesthetic	10
Steroid	10
Each Additional Level	10

INDICATIONS

Thoracic epidural injection via the transforaminal approach with local anesthetics or corticosteroid can be used as a diagnostic tool or treatment modality when performing differential neural blockade on an anatomic basis in the evaluation of pain subserved by the thoracic spinal nerve roots. If destruction of the thoracic nerve roots is being considered, this technique is useful as a prognostic indicator of the degree of motor and sensory impairment that the patient may experience.

Although the interlaminar approach is more commonly used for routine therapeutic thoracic epidural nerve injection, some interventional pain management specialists believe the transforaminal approach to the thoracic epidural space is more efficacious in the treatment of painful conditions involving a single nerve root albeit with a higher incidence of potential complications. Furthermore, because of the nature of the anatomy of the mid-thoracic spine, the paramedian or transforaminal approach to the thoracic epidural space may be required to successfully gain access to the mid-thoracic space. Common painful conditions amenable to the thoracic epidural block include thoracic radicular pain and radiculopathy secondary to thoracic disk displacement, acute herpes zoster, vertebral compression fracture, metastases to the thoracic spine, neural foraminal stenosis, and perineural fibrosis (Fig. 64-1).

CLINICALLY RELEVANT ANATOMY

The superior boundary of the epidural space is the fusion of the periosteal and spinal layers of dura at the foramen magnum. The epidural space continues inferiorly to the sacrococcygeal membrane. The thoracic epidural space is bounded anteriorly by the posterior longitudinal ligament and posteriorly by the vertebral laminae and the ligamentum flavum. The vertebral pedicles and intervertebral foramina form the lateral limits of the epidural space. The thoracic epidural space is 3 to 4 mm at the C7-T1 interspace with the cervical spine flexed and about 5 mm at the T11-T12 interspace. The thoracic epidural space contains fat, veins, arteries, lymphatics, and connective tissue. The thoracic spinal nerve roots exit via the relatively large intervertebral foramina (Fig. 64-2). In contradistinction to the cervical and lumbar vertebra, the thoracic vertebra articulates with the ribs. The head of the rib articulates with the demi-facets, which are located on the posterolateral vertebral body. The tubercle of the rib articulates with a small concavity known as the *transverse articular facet* located at the lateral border of the transverse process (Fig. 64-3).

When performing thoracic epidural block in the midline, the needle traverses the following structures. After traversing the skin and subcutaneous tissues, the styletted epidural needle impinges on the supraspinous ligament, which runs vertically between the apices of the spinous processes). The supraspinous ligament offers some resistance to the advancing needle. This ligament is dense enough to hold a needle in position even when the needle is released.

The interspinous ligament, which runs obliquely between the spinous processes, is encountered next, offering additional resistance to needle advancement. Because the interspinous ligament is contiguous with the ligamentum flavum, the pain management specialist may perceive a "false" loss of resistance when the needle tip enters the space between the interspinous ligament and the ligamentum flavum. This phenomenon is more pronounced in the thoracic region than in the lumbar region as a result of the less well-defined ligaments.

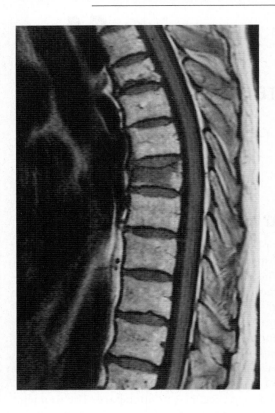

Figure 64-1.
Lateral view revealing a vertebral compression fracture. (From Haaga JR, Lanzieri CF: CT and MR Imaging of the Whole Body, 4th ed. St. Louis, Mosby 2002, p 831.)

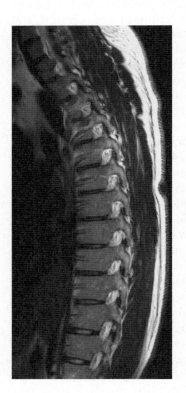

Figure 64-2.
Thoracic spine. Parasagittal T2WI. (From Renfrew DL: Atlas of Spine Imaging, 1st ed. Philadelphia, Saunders, 2002.)

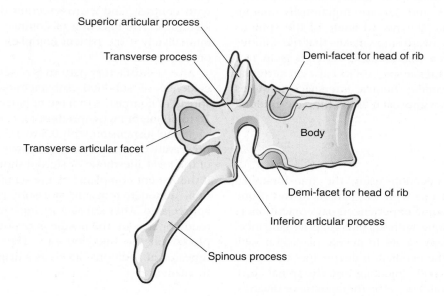

Superior articular process

Transverse process

Demi-facet for head of rib

Transverse articular facet

Body

Demi-facet for head of rib

Inferior articular process

Spinous process

Figure 64-3.

A significant increase in resistance to needle advancement signals that the needle tip is impinging on the dense ligamentum flavum (Fig. 64-4). Because the ligament is made up almost entirely of elastin fibers, there is a continued increase in resistance as the needle traverses the ligamentum flavum, owing to the drag of the ligament on the needle. A sudden loss of resistance occurs as the needle tip enters the epidural space. There should be essentially no resistance to drugs injected into the normal epidural space.

The upper thoracic vertebral interspaces from T1-T2 and the lower thoracic vertebral interspaces from T10-T12 are functionally equivalent insofar as the technique of epidural block is concerned. The technique of performing epidural block at the level of the upper and the lower thoracic vertebral interspaces is analogous to lumbar epidural block. The thoracic vertebral interspaces between T3 and T9 are functionally unique because of the acute downward angle of the spinous processes. This downward slope means that the spinous process of any given mid-thoracic vertebra is in fact inferior to the interlaminar space of its adjacent vertebra. Blockade of these middle thoracic interspaces requires use of the paramedian approach to the thoracic epidural space.

TECHNIQUE

Thoracic epidural injection using the transforaminal approach is carried out with the patient in the prone position. Although some experienced pain practitioners perform this technique without radiographic guidance, the use of fluoroscopy to aid in needle placement will help avoid placing the needle too deeply into the spinal canal and unintentionally injecting into the spinal cord. It also assumes the validity of the therapeutic or diagnostic injections. Because the procedure is usually done in the prone position, special attention to patient monitoring is mandatory.

With the patient in the prone position on the fluoroscopy table, the end plates of the affected vertebra are aligned or squared up on fluoroscopy. The fluoroscopy beam is rotated to a more ipsilateral oblique position to bring the images of the spinous process and head of the ribs medially (Fig. 64-5). A "magic box" consisting of the superior end plate, the inferior end plate, the lamina or lateral pedicle lines, and the rib head is then visualized. The magic box represents the target for needle placement.

The skin is then prepared with an antiseptic solution, and a skin wheal of local anesthetic is placed at a point overlying the magic box that corresponds to the inferior aspect of the foramen. (The foramen is not affected.) A 25-gauge or 22-gauge, 3½-inch spinal needle is then placed through the previously anesthetized area and advanced until the tip is near the level of the posterior elements (Fig. 64-6). Care must be taken to ensure the needle tip does not stray laterally (pleura) or medially (spinal cord). Failure to identify these problems can lead to disastrous results (see "Side Effects and Complications"). A lateral view is then used to advance the needle tip into the foramen (Fig. 64-7). An anteroposterior view is then obtained, and the needle tip is seen to lie just medial to the lateral laminar border. Insertion of the needle past the foramen will produce entry into the intervertebral disk.

After satisfactory needle position is confirmed, 0.2 to 0.4 mL of contrast medium suitable for subarachnoid use is gently injected under active fluoroscopy (Fig. 64-8). The contrast may be seen to flow into the epidural space, with some flow distal along the nerve root sheath. On the lateral view, the foramen can be seen to be filled with contrast, and a cross-section of the nerve root is identified. The injection of contrast should be stopped immediately if the patient complains of significant pain on injection.

After a satisfactory pattern is observed and there is no evidence of subdural, subarachnoid, or intravascular spread of contrast, 3 to 6 mg of betamethasone solution, 20 to 40 mg of methylprednisolone, or triamcinolone 20 to 40 mg suspension with 0.5 to 1.5 mL of 2.0% to 4.0% preservative-free lidocaine is slowly injected. Injection of the local anesthetic or steroid should be discontinued if the patient complains of any significant pain on injection, although transient pressure paresthesia is often appreciated. After satisfactory injection of the local anesthetic or steroid, the needle is removed, and pressure is placed on the injection site. The technique may be repeated at additional levels as a diagnostic or therapeutic maneuver.

SIDE EFFECTS AND COMPLICATIONS

Basically, all the potential side effects and complications associated with the interlaminar approach to the thoracic epidural space can occur with the transforaminal approach, with the transforaminal approach having a statistically significant increase in the incidence of persistent paresthesias and trauma to neural structures, including the spinal cord. As mentioned earlier, placement of the needle too far medial into the neural foramina when using the transforaminal approach to the thoracic epidural space may result in unintentional injection into the spinal cord with resultant quadriplegia.

Because of the potential for hematogenous spread via Batson's plexus, local infection and sepsis represent absolute contraindications to the thoracic approach to the epidural space. In contradistinction to the caudal approach to the epidural space, anticoagulation and coagulopathy represent absolute contraindications to

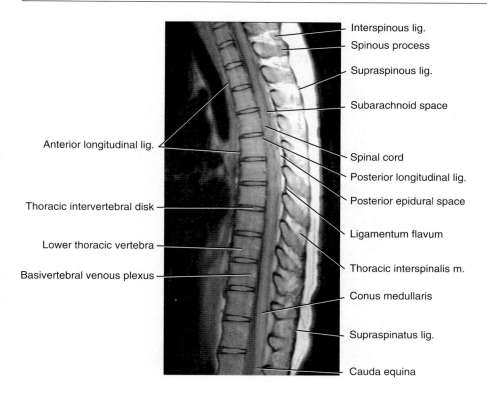

Interspinous lig.

Spinous process

Supraspinous lig.

Subarachnoid space

Anterior longitudinal lig.

Spinal cord

Posterior longitudinal lig.

Posterior epidural space

Thoracic intervertebral disk

Ligamentum flavum

Lower thoracic vertebra

Thoracic interspinalis m.

Basivertebral venous plexus

Conus medullaris

Supraspinatus lig.

Cauda equina

Figure 64-4.
Lateral view demonstrating the ligamentum flavum. (From El-Khoury GY, Bergman RA, Montgomery WJ: Sectional Anatomy by MRI and CT, 3rd ed. New York, Churchill Livingstone, 2007, p 432.)

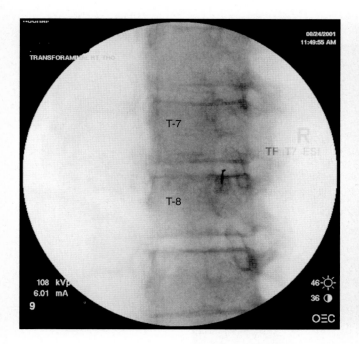

Figure 64-5.
Needle in position for thoracic transforaminal block.

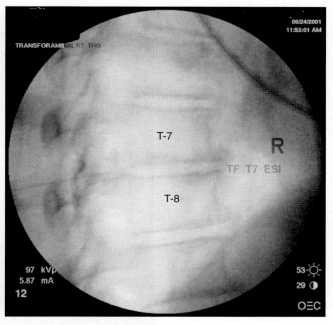

Figure 64-6.
Lateral view of needle in position for thoracic transforaminal block.

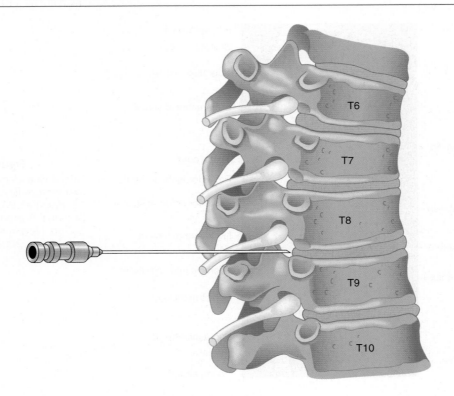

Figure 64-7.

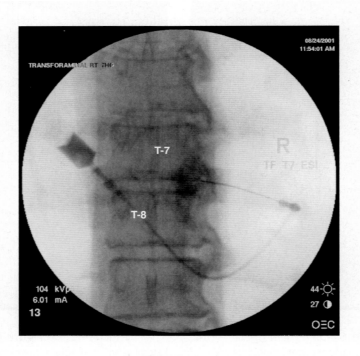

Figure 64-8.
Contrast medium outlining the epidural space and beginning to fill the nerve root.

thoracic epidural nerve block because of the risk for epidural hematoma.

Unintentional dural puncture during thoracic epidural nerve block should occur less than 0.5% of the time with the interlaminar approach and with a slightly greater frequency when using the transforaminal approach. Failure to recognize unintentional dural puncture can result in immediate total spinal anesthesia with associated loss of consciousness, hypotension, and apnea. If epidural doses of opioids are accidentally placed into the subarachnoid space, significant respiratory and central nervous system depression will result. This can be disastrous with the patient in the prone position who is not adequately monitored. It also is possible to unintentionally place a needle or catheter intended for the epidural space into the subdural space. If subdural placement is unrecognized and epidural doses of local anesthetics are administered, the signs and symptoms are similar to those of massive subarachnoid injection, although the resulting motor and sensory block may be delayed and spotty.

The thoracic epidural space is highly vascular. The intravenous placement of the epidural needle occurs in about 0.5% to 1% of patients undergoing thoracic epidural anesthesia. This complication is increased in patients with distended epidural veins, such as the parturient and patients with a large intra-abdominal tumor mass or herniated nucleus pulposis (protruding disk). If the misplacement is unrecognized, injection of local anesthetic directly into an epidural vein will result in significant local anesthetic toxicity. Damage or injection to the segmental artery can occur with increased incidence when performing the transforaminal approach to the T7-L4 neural foramen on the left.

Needle trauma to the epidural veins may result in self-limited bleeding, which may cause postprocedure pain. Uncontrolled bleeding into the epidural space may result in compression of the spinal cord with the rapid development of neurologic deficit. Although significant neurologic deficit secondary to epidural hematoma after thoracic epidural block is exceedingly rare, this devastating complication should be considered whenever there is rapidly developing neurologic deficit after thoracic epidural nerve block.

Neurologic complications after thoracic nerve block are uncommon if proper technique is used and excessive sedation is avoided. Direct trauma to the spinal cord or nerve roots is usually accompanied by pain. If significant pain occurs during placement of the epidural needle or resistance or pain during the injection of contrast or local anesthetic or steroid, the physician should immediately stop and ascertain the cause of the pain to avoid the possibility of additional neural trauma.

Although uncommon, infection in the epidural space remains an ever-present possibility, especially in the immunocompromised AIDS or cancer patient. If epidural abscess occurs, emergent surgical drainage to avoid spinal cord compression and irreversible neurologic deficit is usually required. Early detection and treatment of infection is crucial to avoid potentially life-threatening sequelae.

CLINICAL PEARLS

Some practitioners recommend the use of a blunt-tipped needle when performing the transforaminal approach to the thoracic epidural space, whereas others believe a sharper needle is better suited for this technique. Any significant pain or sudden increase in resistance during injection suggests incorrect needle placement, and one should stop injecting immediately and reassess the position of the needle. Because pain is an important indication of improper needle placement, the practitioner should avoid the use of excessive sedation during transforaminal thoracic epidural nerve block. As mentioned, the use of sedation in patients in the prone position requires special attention to monitoring.

CHAPTER **65**

Thoracic Paravertebral Nerve Block

CPT-2009 CODE

Local Anesthetic	64479
Steroid	64479
Additional Level	64480
Neurolytic	62281

Relative Value Units

Single	12
Additional Level	20
Neurolytic	25

INDICATIONS

Thoracic paravertebral nerve block is useful in the evaluation and management of pain involving the chest wall, the upper abdominal wall, and the thoracic spine. Thoracic paravertebral nerve block with local anesthetic can be used as a diagnostic tool when performing differential neural blockade on an anatomic basis in the evaluation of chest, thoracic spine, and abdominal pain. If destruction of the thoracic paravertebral nerve is being considered, this technique is useful as a prognostic indicator of the degree of motor and sensory impairment that the patient may experience. Thoracic paravertebral nerve block with local anesthetic may be used to palliate acute pain emergencies, including thoracic vertebral compression fracture, acute herpes zoster, and cancer pain, while waiting for pharmacologic, surgical, and antiblastic methods to become effective. Thoracic paravertebral nerve block with local anesthetic and steroid is also useful in the treatment of post-thoracotomy pain, posterior rib fractures, and postherpetic neuralgia.

Destruction of the thoracic paravertebral nerve is indicated for the palliation of cancer pain, including invasive tumors of the thoracic spine, posterior ribs, and the chest and upper abdominal wall. Given the desperate nature of many patients suffering from aggressively invasive malignancies, blockade of the thoracic paravertebral

nerve using a 25-gauge needle may be carried out in the presence of coagulopathy or anticoagulation, albeit with an increased risk for ecchymosis and hematoma formation.

CLINICALLY RELEVANT ANATOMY

The thoracic paravertebral nerves exit their respective intervertebral foramina just beneath the transverse process of the vertebra. After exiting the intervertebral foramen, the thoracic paravertebral nerve gives off a recurrent branch that loops back through the foramen to provide innervation to the spinal ligaments, meninges, and its respective vertebra. The thoracic paravertebral nerve also interfaces with the thoracic sympathetic chain via the myelinated preganglionic fibers of the white rami communicantes as well as the unmyelinated postganglionic fibers of the gray rami communicantes.

After providing these intercommunications with the thoracic sympathetic nervous system as well as the recurrent branch, the thoracic paravertebral nerve divides into a posterior and an anterior primary division. The posterior division courses posteriorly and, along with its branches, provides innervation to the facet joints and the muscles and skin of the back. The larger, anterior division courses laterally to pass into the subcostal groove beneath the rib to become the respective intercostal nerves. The 12th thoracic nerve courses beneath the 12th rib and is called the *subcostal nerve*. The intercostal and subcostal nerves provide the innervation to the skin, muscles, ribs, and parietal pleura and parietal peritoneum. Because blockade of the thoracic paravertebral nerve is performed at the point at which the nerve is beginning to give off its various branches, it is possible to block the anterior division and the posterior division as well as the recurrent and sympathetic components of each respective thoracic paravertebral nerve.

TECHNIQUE

The patient is placed in the prone position with a pillow under the lower chest to slightly flex the thoracic spine.

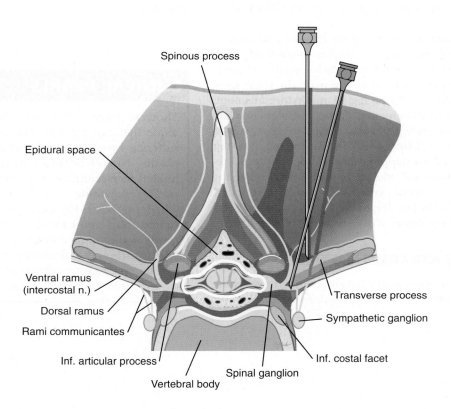

Spinous process

Epidural space

Ventral ramus
(intercostal n.)

Dorsal ramus

Rami communicantes

Inf. articular process

Vertebral body

Spinal ganglion

Inf. costal facet

Sympathetic ganglion

Transverse process

Figure 65-1.

The spinous process of the vertebra just above the nerve to be blocked is palpated. At a point just below and 1½ inches lateral to the spinous process, the skin is prepared with antiseptic solution. A 22-gauge, 3½-inch needle is attached to a 12-mL syringe and is advanced perpendicular to the skin, aiming for the middle of the transverse process. The needle should impinge on bone after being advanced about 1½ inches. After bony contact is made, the needle is withdrawn into the subcutaneous tissues and redirected inferiorly and walked off the inferior margin of the transverse process (Fig. 65-1). As soon as bony contact is lost, the needle is slowly advanced about ¾ inch deeper until a paresthesia in the distribution of the thoracic paravertebral nerve to be blocked is elicited.

Once the paresthesia has been elicited and careful aspiration reveals no blood or cerebrospinal fluid, 5 mL of 1.0% preservative-free lidocaine is injected. If there is an inflammatory component to the pain, the local anesthetic is combined with 80 mg of methylprednisolone and is injected in incremental doses. Subsequent daily nerve blocks are carried out in a similar manner, substituting 40 mg of methylprednisolone for the initial 80-mg dose. Because of overlapping innervation of the posterior elements from the medial branch of the posterior division from adjacent vertebrae, the paravertebral nerves above and below the nerve suspected of subserving the painful condition will have to be blocked.

SIDE EFFECTS AND COMPLICATIONS

The proximity to the spinal cord and exiting nerve roots makes it imperative that this procedure be carried out only by those well versed in the regional anatomy and experienced in performing interventional pain management techniques. Given the proximity of the pleural space, pneumothorax after thoracic paravertebral nerve block is a distinct possibility. Needle placement too medial may result in epidural, subdural, or subarachnoid injections or trauma to the spinal cord and exiting nerve roots. Placing the needle too deep between the transverse processes may result in trauma to the exiting thoracic nerve roots. Although uncommon, infection remains an ever-present possibility, especially in the immunocompromised cancer patient. Early detection of infection is crucial to avoid potentially life-threatening sequelae.

CLINICAL PEARLS

Thoracic paravertebral nerve block is a simple technique that can produce dramatic relief for patients suffering from the previously mentioned pain complaints. Neurolytic block with small quantities of phenol in glycerin or by cryoneurolysis or radiofrequency lesioning has been shown to provide long-term relief for patients suffering from postthoracotomy and cancer-related pain who have not responded to more conservative treatments. As mentioned earlier, the proximity of the thoracic paravertebral nerve to the neuraxis and pleural space makes careful attention to technique mandatory.

CHAPTER 66

Thoracic Facet Block: Medial Branch Technique

CPT-2009 CODE	
First Joint	64470
Second Joint	64472
Neurolytic First Joint	64626
Neurolytic Second Joint	64627

Relative Value Units	
First Joint	10
Second Joint	10
Neurolytic First Joint	20
Neurolytic Second Joint	20

INDICATIONS

Thoracic facet block using the medial branch technique is useful in the diagnosis and treatment of painful conditions involving trauma, arthritis, or inflammation of the thoracic facet joints. These problems usually occur after sudden, forceful twisting of the thoracic spine while lifting or because of acceleration-deceleration injuries. Pain secondary to thoracic facet syndrome may manifest as pain that radiates from the thoracic spine anteriorly in a nondermatomal distribution. This pain may be associated with decreased range of motion of the thoracic spine and spasm of the thoracic paraspinal musculature.

CLINICALLY RELEVANT ANATOMY

The thoracic facet joints are formed by the articulations of the superior and inferior articular facets of adjacent vertebrae. The thoracic facet joints are true joints in that they are lined with synovium and possess a true joint capsule. This capsule is richly innervated and supports the notion of the facet joint as a pain generator. The thoracic facet joint is susceptible to arthritic changes and trauma secondary to acceleration-deceleration injuries. Such damage to the joint results in pain secondary to synovial joint inflammation and adhesions.

Each facet joint receives innervation from two spinal levels. Each joint receives fibers from the dorsal ramus at the same level as the vertebra as well as fibers from the dorsal ramus of the vertebra above. This fact has clinical import in that it provides an explanation for the ill-defined nature of facet-mediated pain and explains why the dorsal nerve from the vertebra above the offending level also often must be blocked to provide complete pain relief.

At each level, the dorsal ramus provides a medial branch that exits the intertransverse space crossing over the top of the transverse process at the point where the transverse process joins the vertebra. The nerve then travels inferiorly and medially across the posterior surface of the transverse process to innervate the facet joint. In a manner analogous to lumbar facet block, the medial branch is blocked at the point at which the nerve curves around the top of the transverse process. It should be noted that in the mid-thoracic region, the medial branch of the dorsal ramus may travel superior to the point at which the transverse process joins the vertebra. This probably does not have any clinical significance unless radiofrequency lesioning or cryoneurolysis of the nerve is being considered. In this case, the needle or cryoprobe may have to be placed superior to the junction of the transverse process and vertebra.

TECHNIQUE

Thoracic facet block using the medial branch technique is the preferred route of treating thoracic facet syndrome. It may be done either blind or under fluoroscopic guidance. The patient is placed in a prone position. Pillows are placed under the chest to allow the thoracic spine to be moderately flexed without discomfort to the patient. The forehead is allowed to rest on a folded blanket.

Blind Technique

If a blind technique is used, the spinous process at the level to be blocked is identified by palpation. A point slightly inferior and 5 cm lateral to the spinous process is then identified as the site of needle insertion. After preparation of the skin with antiseptic solution, a skin wheal of local anesthetic is raised at the site of needle insertion. Three milliliters of 1% preservative-free lidocaine is drawn up in a 5-mL sterile syringe. When treating pain thought to be secondary to an inflammatory process, a total of 80 mg of depot-steroid is added to the local anesthetic with the first block, and 40 mg of depot-steroid is added with subsequent blocks.

An 18-gauge, 1-inch needle is inserted through the skin and into the subcutaneous tissue at the previously identified insertion site to serve as an introducer. The introducer needle is then repositioned with a slightly superior and medial trajectory, pointing directly toward the superior portion of the junction of the transverse process and the vertebra at the level to be blocked. A 25-gauge, 3½-inch styletted spinal needle is then inserted through the 18-gauge introducer and directed toward this junction of the transverse process and the vertebra.

After bony contact is made, the depth of the contact is noted, and the spinal needle is withdrawn. The introducer needle is then repositioned, aiming toward the most superior and medial aspect of the junction of the transverse process with the vertebra. The 25-gauge spinal needle is then readvanced until it impinges on the lateral-most aspect of the border of the articular pillar (Fig. 66-1). Should the spinal needle walk off the top of the transverse process, it is withdrawn and redirected slightly medially and inferiorly and carefully advanced to the depth of the previous bony contact.

After the needle is felt to be in satisfactory position, the stylet is removed from the 25-gauge spinal needle, and the hub is observed for blood or cerebrospinal fluid. If neither is present, gentle aspiration of the needle is carried out. If the aspiration test is negative, 1.5 mL of solution is injected through the spinal needle.

Fluoroscopic Technique

If fluoroscopy is used, the beam is rotated in a sagittal plane from anterior to posterior position, which allows identification and visualization of the junction of the transverse process and vertebra at the level to be blocked. After preparation of the skin with antiseptic solution, a skin wheal of local anesthetic is raised at a point slightly inferior and about 5 cm off the midline. An 18-gauge, 1-inch needle is inserted at the insertion site to serve as an introducer. The fluoroscopy beam is aimed directly through the introducer needle, which will appear as a small point on the fluoroscopy screen. The introducer needle is then repositioned under fluoroscopic guidance until this small point is visualized pointing directly toward the most superior and medial point at which the transverse process joins the vertebra (Figs. 66-2 and 66-3). Needle position is confirmed with a lateral fluoroscopic view (Fig. 66-4).

A total of 5 mL of contrast medium suitable for intrathecal use is drawn up in a sterile 12-mL syringe. Then, 3 mL of preservative-free local anesthetic is drawn up in a separate 5-mL sterile syringe. When treating pain thought to be secondary to an inflammatory process, a total of 80 mg of depot-steroid is added to the local anesthetic with the first block, and 40 mg of depot-steroid is added with subsequent blocks.

A 25-gauge, 3½-inch styletted spinal needle is then inserted through the 18-gauge introducer and directed toward the most superior and medial point at which the transverse process joins the vertebra. After bony contact is made, the spinal needle is withdrawn, and the introducer needle is redirected to allow the spinal needle to impinge on the most superior and medial point at which the transverse process joins the vertebra. This procedure is repeated until the tip of the 25-gauge spinal needle rests against the most superior and medial point at which the transverse process joins the vertebra.

After confirmation of needle placement by biplanar fluoroscopy, the stylet is removed from the 25-gauge spinal needle, and the hub is observed for blood or cerebrospinal fluid. If neither is present, gentle aspiration of the needle is carried out. If the aspiration test is negative, 1 mL of contrast medium is slowly injected under fluoroscopy to reconfirm needle placement. After correct needle placement is confirmed, 1.5 mL of local anesthetic with or without steroid is injected through the spinal needle.

SIDE EFFECTS AND COMPLICATIONS

The proximity to the spinal cord and exiting nerve roots makes it imperative that this procedure be carried out only by those well versed in the regional anatomy and experienced in performing interventional pain management techniques. Given the proximity of the pleural space, pneumothorax after thoracic facet block is a distinct possibility. Needle placement too medial may result in epidural, subdural, or subarachnoid injections or trauma to the spinal cord and exiting nerve roots. Placing the needle too deep between the transverse processes may result in trauma to nerve roots.

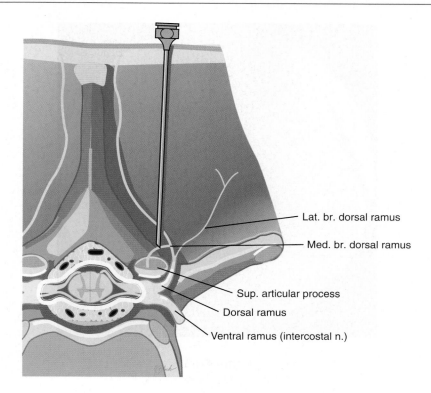

Lat. br. dorsal ramus

Med. br. dorsal ramus

Sup. articular process

Dorsal ramus

Ventral ramus (intercostal n.)

Figure 66-1.

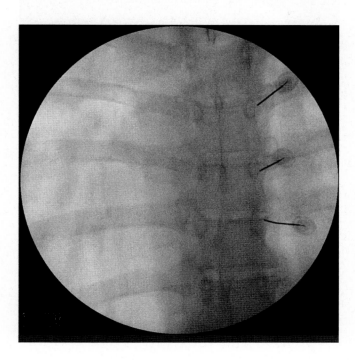

Figure 66-2.
Needles in position for thoracic medial branch block.

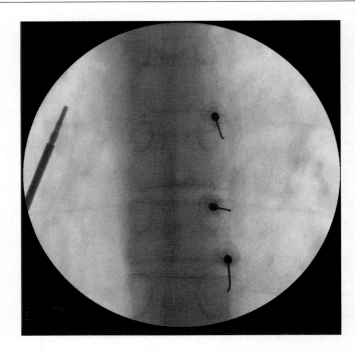

Figure 66-3.
Thoracic medial branch block.

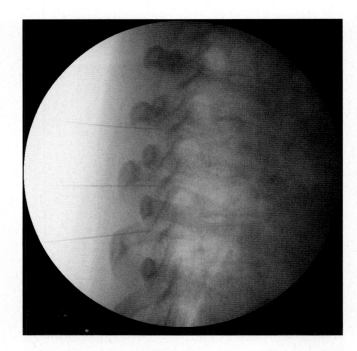

Figure 66-4.
Lateral view of needle position for thoracic medial branch block.

CLINICAL PEARLS

Thoracic facet block using the medial branch approach is the preferred technique for treatment of thoracic facet syndrome. Although intra-articular placement of the needle into the facet joint is technically feasible, unless specific diagnostic information about that specific joint is required, such maneuvers add nothing to the efficacy of the procedure and in fact may increase the rate of complications.

Thoracic facet block is often combined with pharmacotherapy and physical therapy when treating pain in the previously mentioned areas. Many pain specialists believe that thoracic facet block is currently underused in the treatment of post-traumatic thoracic spine pain. These specialists believe that thoracic facet block using the medial branch approach should be considered when thoracic epidural nerve blocks combined with conservative measures fail to provide palliation of these pain syndromes.

CHAPTER 67

Thoracic Facet Block: Radiofrequency Lesioning of the Medial Branch of the Primary Posterior Rami

CPT-2009 CODE

Radiofrequency Lesioning—First Joint	64626
Radiofrequency Lesioning—Second Joint	64627

Relative Value Units

Radiofrequency Lesioning—First Joint	20
Radiofrequency Lesioning—Second Joint	20

INDICATIONS

Radiofrequency lesioning of the thoracic facet joints is a reasonable next step for patients with chronic dorsal spine pain that is relieved by either local anesthetic block of the affected facet joints directly or local anesthetic blockade of the medial branch. Prognostic thoracic facet block with local anesthetic using the medial branch technique is useful in predicting whether radiofrequency lesioning of the affected facet joint will provide long-lasting relief of painful conditions involving trauma, arthritis, or inflammation of the thoracic facet joints.

Pain secondary to thoracic facet syndrome may manifest as pain that radiates from the middle back into the lower back, abdomen, and groin in a nondermatomal distribution. Because true radicular pain is associated with the dorsal root ganglion or spinal nerves, it will not respond to blockade of the thoracic facet joints and associated nerves. Facet joint pain may be associated with decreased range of motion of the thoracic spine and spasm of the thoracic paraspinal musculature, although no clinical test is completely valid as a prognostic indicator.

CLINICALLY RELEVANT ANATOMY

The thoracic facet joints are formed by the articulations of the superior and inferior articular facets of adjacent vertebrae. The thoracic facet joints are true joints in that they are lined with synovium and possess a true joint capsule. This capsule is richly innervated and supports the notion of the facet joint as a pain generator. The thoracic facet joint is susceptible to arthritic changes and trauma secondary to acceleration-deceleration injuries. Such damage to the joint results in pain secondary to synovial joint inflammation and adhesions.

Each facet joint receives innervation from two spinal levels. Each joint receives fibers from the dorsal ramus at the same level as the vertebra as well as fibers from the dorsal ramus of the vertebra above. This fact has clinical import in that it provides an explanation for the ill-defined nature of facet-mediated pain and explains why the dorsal nerve from the vertebra above the offending level also often must be blocked to provide complete pain relief.

At each level, the dorsal ramus provides a medial branch that exits the intertransverse space crossing over the top of the transverse process at the point at which the transverse process joins the vertebra. The nerve then travels inferiorly and medially across the posterior surface of the transverse process to innervate the facet joint. In a manner analogous to lumbar facet block, the medial branch is blocked at the point at which the nerve curves around the top of the transverse process. It should be noted that in the mid-thoracic region, the medial branch of the dorsal ramus may travel superior to the point at which the transverse process joins the vertebra (Fig. 67-1). This probably does not have clinical significance unless radiofrequency lesioning or cryoneurolysis of the nerve is being considered. In this case, the needle or cryoprobe may have to be placed superior to the junction of the transverse process and vertebra.

TECHNIQUE

Radiofrequency lesioning of the thoracic facet joints using the medial branch technique is the preferred neurodisruptive technique for pain emanating from the facet joint. It may be done under fluoroscopic or computed tomographic guidance, although a few very experienced pain management specialists will perform this technique

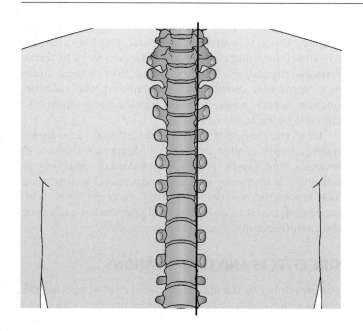

Figure 67-1.
(From El-Khoury GY, Bergman RA, Montgomery WJ. Sectional Anatomy by MRI and CT, 3rd ed. New York, Churchill Livingstone, 2007, p 431.)

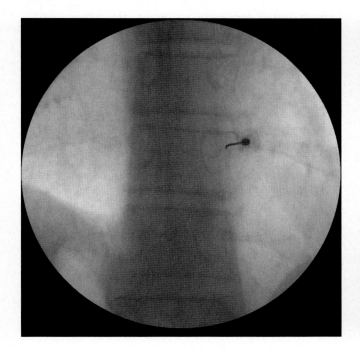

Figure 67-2.
Radiofrequency needle in position for thoracic medial branch block.

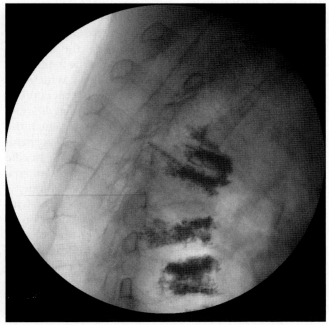

Figure 67-3.
Lateral view of radiofrequency needle in position for medial branch block.

without radiographic guidance using the blind technique and stimulation patterns to assist in safe needle placement. The patient is placed in a prone position. Pillows are placed under the upper abdomen to allow the thoracic spine to be moderately flexed without discomfort to the patient. The head rests on a folded blanket or pillow.

Fluoroscopic Technique

If fluoroscopy is used, the beam is rotated in a sagittal plane from anterior to posterior position, which allows identification and visualization of the junction of the transverse process and vertebra at the level to be blocked. After preparation of the skin with antiseptic solution, a skin wheal of local anesthetic is raised at a point slightly inferior and about 5 cm off the midline. An 18-gauge, 1-inch needle is inserted at the insertion site to serve as an introducer. The fluoroscopy beam is aimed directly through the introducer needle, which will appear as a small point on the fluoroscopy screen. The introducer needle is then repositioned under fluoroscopic guidance until this small point is visualized pointing directly toward the most superior and medial point at which the transverse process joins the vertebra.

A 22-gauge, 4-mm active tip radiofrequency needle is then inserted through the introducer needle and directed under fluoroscopic guidance toward the most superior and medial point at which the transverse process joins the vertebra. After bony contact is made, the needle is withdrawn and redirected to allow the needle to impinge on the most superior and medial point at which the transverse process joins the vertebra. This procedure is repeated until the tip of the radiofrequency needle rests against the most superior and medial point at which the transverse process joins the vertebra (Fig. 67-2). A lateral fluoroscopic view is used to confirm accurate needle placement (Fig. 67-3). Alternatively, computed tomography guidance can be used to perform this technique.

After confirmation of proper needle placement with lateral and posteroanterior fluoroscopy, stimulation at 50 Hz is carried out with the patient reporting stimulation between 0.1 and 0.5 V. This should reproduce the patient's pain pattern, although the quality may not be perceived as identical by the patient. Motor stimulation of the radiofrequency needle at 2 to 3 V at 2 Hz is increased slowly. There should be no stimulation of the chest or thoracic wall in a segmental distribution at $2\frac{1}{2}$ to 3 times the voltage required for the patient to perceive sensory stimulation. If motor stimulation of these areas in a segmental distribution is identified, the radiofrequency needle must be repositioned away from the affected thoracic nerve root.

After the injection of local anesthetic, a radiofrequency lesion is then made at 80 degrees for 60 to 90 seconds. The needle is then repositioned superiorly or inferiorly 2 to 3 mm, and a second lesion is repeated. This technique is repeated at each targeted level, with care being taken to complete trial stimulation each time the radiofrequency needle is repositioned.

SIDE EFFECTS AND COMPLICATIONS

The proximity to the spinal cord and exiting nerve roots makes it imperative that this procedure be carried out only by those well versed in the regional anatomy and experienced in performing interventional pain management techniques. Many patients also complain of a transient increase in thoracic pain after radiofrequency lesioning of the medial branch. Some advocate the use of corticosteroid injection to decrease postprocedure discomfort. Improper needle placement may lead to permanent lower extremity weakness, persistent neuritis (especially involving the genitofemoral nerve), and permanent sensory deficit. These complications can be avoided if strict adherence to the above technique is followed.

CLINICAL PEARLS

Radiofrequency lesioning of the thoracic facet using the medial branch approach is the preferred technique for providing long-lasting relief of the pain and disability associated with thoracic facet syndrome. This technique is often combined with pharmacotherapy and physical therapy when treating pain in the previously mentioned areas. Many pain specialists believe that this technique is underused in the treatment of post-traumatic thoracic spine pain.

CHAPTER 68

Thoracic Facet Block: Intra-articular Technique

CPT-2009 CODE	
First Joint	64470
Second Joint	64472
Neurolytic First Joint	64626
Neurolytic Second Joint	64627

Relative Value Units	
First Joint	10
Second Joint	10
Neurolytic First Joint	20
Neurolytic Second Joint	20

INDICATIONS

Thoracic facet block using the intra-articular technique is indicated primarily as a diagnostic maneuver to prove that a specific facet joint is in fact the source of pain. The medial branch technique of thoracic facet block is suitable for most clinical applications, including the treatment of painful conditions involving trauma, arthritis, or inflammation of the thoracic facet joints. These problems may manifest themselves clinically as ill-defined thoracic pain that radiates anteriorly in a nondermatomal pattern.

CLINICALLY RELEVANT ANATOMY

The thoracic facet joints are formed by the articulations of the superior and inferior articular facets of adjacent vertebrae. The thoracic facet joints are true joints in that they are lined with synovium and possess a true joint capsule. This capsule is richly innervated and supports the notion of the facet joint as a pain generator. The thoracic facet joint is susceptible to arthritic changes and trauma secondary to acceleration-deceleration injuries. Such damage to the joint results in pain secondary to synovial joint inflammation and adhesions.

Each facet joint receives innervation from two spinal levels. Each joint receives fibers from the dorsal ramus at the same level as the vertebra as well as fibers from the dorsal ramus of the vertebra above. This fact has clinical import in that it provides an explanation for the ill-defined nature of facet-mediated pain and explains why the dorsal nerve from the vertebra above the offending level also often must be blocked to provide complete pain relief.

At each level, the dorsal ramus provides a medial branch that exits the intertransverse space crossing over the top of the transverse process at the point at which the transverse process joins the vertebra. The nerve then travels inferiorly and medially across the posterior surface of the transverse process to innervate the facet joint. In a manner analogous to lumbar facet block, the medial branch is blocked at the point at which the nerve curves around the top of the transverse process. It should be noted that in the mid-thoracic region, the medial branch of the dorsal ramus may travel superior to the point at which the transverse process joins the vertebra. This probably does not have any clinical significance unless radiofrequency lesioning or cryoneurolysis of the nerve is being considered. In this case, the needle or cryoprobe may have to be placed superior to the junction of the transverse process and vertebra.

TECHNIQUE

Thoracic facet block using the intra-articular technique may be performed either blind or under fluoroscopic guidance. The patient is placed in a prone position. Pillows are placed under the chest to allow the thoracic spine to be moderately flexed without discomfort to the patient. The forehead is allowed to rest on a folded blanket.

Blind Technique

If a blind technique is used, the spinous process at the level to be blocked is identified by palpation. A point two spinal levels lower and 2.5 cm lateral to the spinous process is then identified as the site of needle insertion. Three milliliters of 1% preservative-free lidocaine is drawn up in a 5-mL sterile syringe. After preparation of the skin with antiseptic solution, a skin wheal of local anesthetic is raised at the site of needle insertion. When treating pain thought to be secondary to an inflammatory process, a total of 80 mg of depot-steroid is added to the local anesthetic with the first block, and 40 mg of depot-steroid is added with subsequent blocks.

An 18-gauge, 1-inch needle is inserted through the skin and into the subcutaneous tissue at the previously identified insertion site to serve as an introducer. The introducer needle is then repositioned with a superior and ventral trajectory, pointing directly toward the inferior margin of the facet joint at the level to be blocked. The angle of the needle from the skin is about 25 degrees. A 25-gauge, 3½-inch styletted spinal needle is then inserted through the 18-gauge introducer and directed toward the articular pillar just below the joint to be blocked. Care must be taken to be sure the trajectory of the needle does not drift either laterally or medially. Medial drift can allow the needle to enter the epidural, subdural, or subarachnoid space and to traumatize the dorsal root or spinal cord. Lateral drift can allow the needle to pass beyond the lateral border of the articular pillar and traumatize the exiting nerve roots.

After bony contact is made, the depth of the contact is noted, and the spinal needle is withdrawn. The introducer needle is then redirected slightly more superiorly. The spinal needle is then advanced through the introducer needle until it impinges on the bone of the articular pillar. This maneuver is repeated until the spinal needle slides into the facet joint (Fig. 68-1). A pop is often felt as the needle slides into the joint cavity.

After the needle is felt to be in satisfactory position, the stylet is removed from the 25-gauge spinal needle, and the hub is observed for blood or cerebrospinal fluid. If neither is present, gentle aspiration of the needle is carried out. If the aspiration test is negative, 1 mL of solution is injected slowly through the spinal needle. Rapid or forceful injection may rupture the joint capsule and exacerbate the patient's pain.

Fluoroscopic Technique

If fluoroscopy is used, the beam is rotated in a sagittal plane from anterior to posterior position, which allows identification and visualization of the articular pillars of the respective vertebrae and the adjacent facet joints.

After preparation of the skin with antiseptic solution, a skin wheal of local anesthetic is raised at the site of needle insertion. An 18-gauge, 1-inch needle is inserted at the insertion site to serve as an introducer. The fluoroscopy beam is aimed directly through the introducer needle, which will appear as a small point on the fluoroscopy screen. The introducer needle is then repositioned under fluoroscopic guidance until this small point is visualized pointing directly toward the inferior aspect of the facet joint to be blocked.

A total of 5 mL of contrast medium suitable for intrathecal use is drawn up in a sterile 12-mL syringe. Then, 2 mL of preservative-free local anesthetic is drawn up in a separate 5-mL sterile syringe. When treating pain thought to be secondary to an inflammatory process, a total of 80 mg of depot-steroid is added to the local anesthetic with the first block, and 40 mg of depot-steroid is added with subsequent blocks.

A 25-gauge, 3½-inch styletted spinal needle is then inserted through the 18-gauge introducer and directed toward the articular pillar just below the joint to be blocked. After bony contact is made, the spinal needle is withdrawn and the introducer needle repositioned superiorly, aiming toward the facet joint itself. The 25-gauge spinal needle is then readvanced through the introducer needle until it enters the target joint.

After confirmation of needle placement by biplanar fluoroscopy, the stylet is removed from the 25-gauge spinal needle, and the hub is observed for blood or cerebrospinal fluid. If neither is present, gentle aspiration of the needle is carried out. If the aspiration test is negative, 1 mL of contrast medium is slowly injected under fluoroscopy to reconfirm needle placement. After correct needle placement is confirmed, 1 mL of local anesthetic with or without steroid is slowly injected through the spinal needle. Rapid or forceful injection may rupture the joint capsule and exacerbate the patient's pain. This procedure also may be performed under computed tomography guidance (Fig. 68-2).

SIDE EFFECTS AND COMPLICATIONS

The proximity to the spinal cord and exiting nerve roots makes it imperative that this procedure be carried out only by those well versed in the regional anatomy and experienced in performing interventional pain management techniques. Many patients also complain of a transient increase in thoracic pain after injection of the joint.

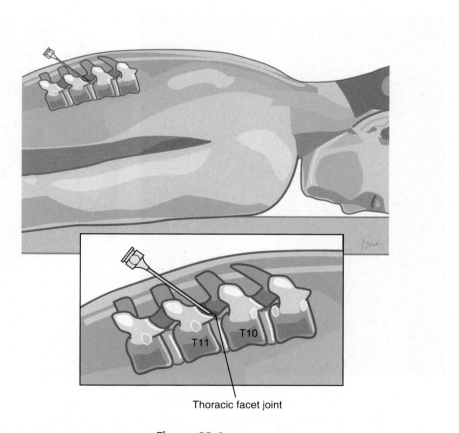

Thoracic facet joint

Figure 68-1.

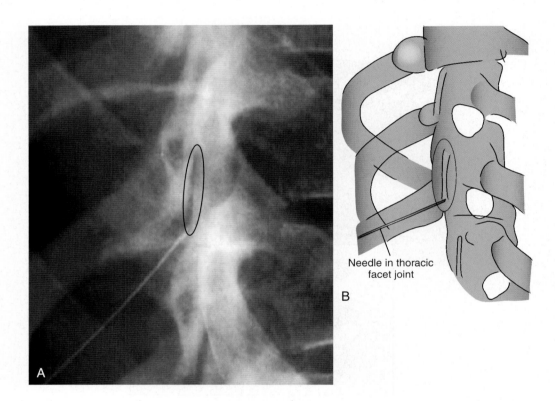

Figure 68-2.
A, This radiographic image is taken in an oblique view to optimize the thoracic facet joint. **B,** Line drawing of the same view. (From Raj PP, Lou L, Erdine S, et al: Interventional Pain Management: Image-Guided Procedures, 2nd ed. Philadelphia, Saunders, 2008.)

CLINICAL PEARLS

Thoracic facet block using the medial branch approach is the preferred technique for treatment of thoracic facet syndrome. Although intra-articular placement of the needle into the facet joint is technically feasible, unless specific diagnostic information about that specific joint is required, such maneuvers add nothing to the efficacy of the procedure and in fact may increase the rate of complications.

Thoracic facet block is often combined with pharmacotherapy and physical therapy when treating pain in the previously mentioned areas. Many pain specialists believe that thoracic facet block is currently underused in the treatment of post-traumatic thoracic spine pain. These specialists believe that thoracic facet block using the medial branch approach should be considered when thoracic epidural nerve blocks combined with conservative measures fail to provide palliation of these pain syndromes.

CHAPTER 69

Thoracic Sympathetic Ganglion Block

CPT-2009 CODE	
Unilateral	64520
Neurolytic	64640

Relative Value Units	
Unilateral	12
Neurolytic	20

INDICATIONS

Thoracic sympathetic ganglion block is useful in the evaluation and management of sympathetically mediated pain of the upper thorax, chest wall, and thoracic and upper abdominal viscera. Thoracic sympathetic ganglion block with local anesthetic can be used as a diagnostic tool when performing differential neural blockade on an anatomic basis in the evaluation of chest, thoracic, and upper abdominal pain. If destruction of the thoracic sympathetic chain is being considered, this technique is useful as a prognostic indicator of the degree of pain relief that the patient may experience. In the past, this block was used to treat intractable cardiac and abdominal angina. Thoracic sympathetic ganglion block with local anesthetic also is useful in the treatment of post-thoracotomy pain, acute herpes zoster, postherpetic neuralgia, and phantom breast pain after mastectomy. Destruction of the thoracic sympathetic chain is indicated for the palliation of pain syndromes that have temporarily responded to thoracic sympathetic blockade with local anesthetic (Fig. 69-1).

CLINICALLY RELEVANT ANATOMY

The preganglionic fibers of the thoracic sympathetics exit the intervertebral foramen along with the respective thoracic paravertebral nerves. After exiting the intervertebral foramen, the thoracic paravertebral nerve gives off a recurrent branch that loops back through the foramen to provide innervation to the spinal ligaments, meninges, and its respective vertebra. The thoracic paravertebral nerve also interfaces with the thoracic sympathetic chain via the myelinated preganglionic fibers of the white rami communicantes as well as the unmyelinated postganglionic fibers of the gray rami communicantes. At the level of the thoracic sympathetic ganglia, preganglionic and postganglionic fibers synapse. Additionally, some of the postganglionic fibers return to their respective somatic nerves via the gray rami communicantes. These fibers provide sympathetic innervation to the vasculature, sweat glands, and pilomotor muscles of the skin. Other thoracic sympathetic postganglionic fibers travel to the cardiac plexus and course up and down the sympathetic trunk to terminate in distant ganglia.

The first thoracic ganglion is fused with the lower cervical ganglion to help make up the stellate ganglion. As the chain moves caudad, it changes its position with the upper thoracic ganglia just beneath the rib and the lower thoracic ganglia, moving more anterior to rest along the posterolateral surface of the vertebral body. The pleural space lies lateral and anterior to the thoracic sympathetic chain (Fig. 69-2). Given the proximity of the thoracic somatic nerves to the thoracic sympathetic chain, the potential exists for both neural pathways to be blocked when performing blockade of the thoracic sympathetic ganglion.

TECHNIQUE

The patient is placed in the prone position with a pillow under the lower chest to slightly flex the thoracic spine. The spinous process of the vertebra just above the nerve to be blocked is palpated. At a point just below and $1\frac{1}{2}$ inches lateral to the spinous process, the skin is prepared with antiseptic solution. A 22-gauge, $3\frac{1}{2}$-inch needle is attached to a 12-mL syringe and is advanced perpendicular to the skin, aiming for the middle of the transverse process (Fig. 69-3). The needle should impinge on bone after being advanced about $1\frac{1}{2}$ inches. After bony contact is made, the needle is withdrawn into the subcutaneous tissues and redirected inferiorly and walked off the inferior margin of the transverse process. As soon as bony

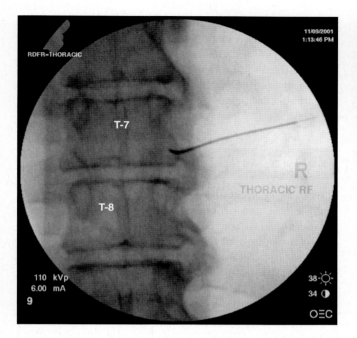

Figure 69-1.
Needle position for thoracic sympathetic block.

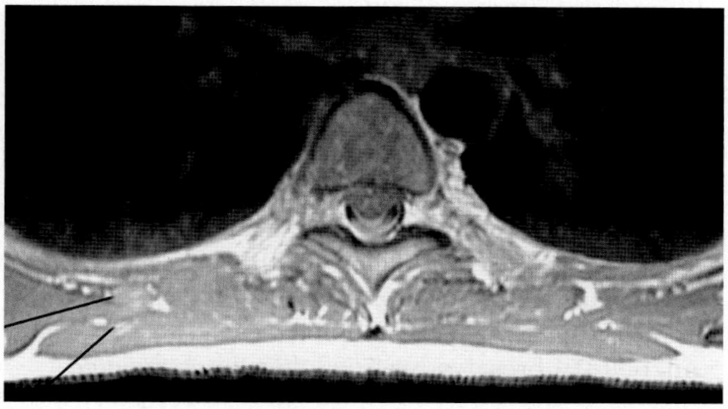

Figure 69-2.
The pleural space. (From El-Khoury GY, Bergman RA, Montgomery WJ: Sectional Anatomy by MRI and CT, 3rd ed. New York, Churchill Livingstone, 2007, p 428.)

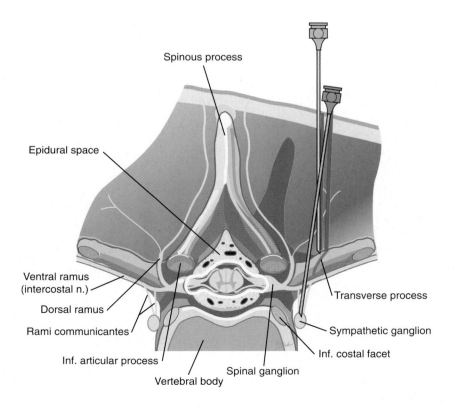

Figure 69-3.

contact is lost, the needle is slowly advanced about 1 inch deeper.

Given the proximity of the thoracic sympathetic chain to the somatic nerve, a paresthesia in the distribution of the corresponding thoracic paravertebral nerve may be elicited. If this occurs, the needle should be withdrawn and redirected slightly more cephalad, with care being taken to keep the needle close to the vertebral body to avoid pneumothorax. Once the needle is in position and careful aspiration reveals no blood or cerebrospinal fluid, 5 mL of 1.0% preservative-free lidocaine is injected.

SIDE EFFECTS AND COMPLICATIONS

The proximity to the spinal cord and exiting nerve roots makes it imperative that this procedure be carried out only by those well versed in the regional anatomy and experienced in performing interventional pain management techniques. Given the proximity of the pleural space, pneumothorax after thoracic sympathetic ganglion block is a distinct possibility. The incidence of pneumothorax will be decreased if care is taken to keep the needle placed medially against the vertebral body. Needle placement too medial may result in epidural, subdural, or subarachnoid injections or trauma to the spinal cord and exiting nerve roots. Although uncommon, infection remains an ever-present possibility, especially in the immunocompromised cancer patient. Early detection of infection is crucial to avoid potentially life-threatening sequelae.

CLINICAL PEARLS

Thoracic sympathetic ganglion block is a simple technique that can produce dramatic relief for patients suffering from the previously mentioned pain complaints. Neurolytic block with small quantities of phenol in glycerin or by cryoneurolysis or radiofrequency lesioning has been shown to provide long-term relief for patients suffering from sympathetically maintained pain that has been relieved with local anesthetics. As mentioned earlier, the proximity of the thoracic sympathetic chain to the neuraxis and pleural space makes careful attention to technique mandatory.

CHAPTER 70

Intercostal Nerve Block

CPT-2009 CODE	
Single	64420
Multiple	64421
Neurolytic	64620

Relative Value Units	
Single	8
Multiple	10
Neurolytic	20

INDICATIONS

Intercostal nerve block is useful in the evaluation and management of pain involving the chest wall and the upper abdominal wall. Intercostal nerve block with local anesthetic can be used as a diagnostic tool when performing differential neural blockade on an anatomic basis in the evaluation of chest and abdominal pain. If destruction of the intercostal nerve is being considered, this technique is useful as a prognostic indicator of the degree of motor and sensory impairment that the patient may experience. Intercostal nerve block with local anesthetic may be used to palliate acute pain emergencies, including rib fractures, acute herpes zoster, and cancer pain, while waiting for pharmacologic, surgical, and antiblastic methods to become effective (Fig. 70-1). It is also useful before placement of percutaneous thoracostomy and nephrotomy tubes. Intercostal nerve block with local anesthetic and steroid also is useful in the treatment of post-thoracotomy pain, cancer pain, rib fractures, metastatic lesions of the liver, and postherpetic neuralgia.

Destruction of the intercostal nerve is indicated for the palliation of cancer pain, including invasive tumors of the ribs and the chest and upper abdominal wall. Given the desperate nature of many patients suffering from aggressively invasive malignancies, blockade of the intercostal nerve using a 25-gauge needle may be carried out in the presence of coagulopathy or anticoagulation, albeit with an increased risk for ecchymosis and hematoma formation.

CLINICALLY RELEVANT ANATOMY

The intercostal nerves arise from the anterior division of the thoracic paravertebral nerve. A typical intercostal nerve has four major branches. The first branch is the unmyelinated postganglionic fibers of the gray rami communicantes, which interface with the sympathetic chain. The second branch is the posterior cutaneous branch, which innervates the muscles and skin of the paraspinal area. The third branch is the lateral cutaneous division, which arises in the anterior axillary line. The lateral cutaneous division provides most of the cutaneous innervation of the chest and abdominal wall. The fourth branch is the anterior cutaneous branch supplying innervation to the midline of the chest and abdominal wall. Occasionally, the terminal branches of a given intercostal nerve actually may cross the midline to provide sensory innervation to the contralateral chest and abdominal wall. The 12th nerve is called the *subcostal nerve* and is unique in that it gives off a branch to the first lumbar nerve, thus contributing to the lumbar plexus.

TECHNIQUE

The patient is placed in the prone position with the arms hanging loosely off the side of the cart. Alternatively, this block can be done in the sitting or lateral position. The rib to be blocked is identified by palpating its path at the posterior axillary line. The index and middle fingers are then placed on the rib bracketing the site of needle insertion. The skin is then prepared with antiseptic solution. A 22-gauge, $1\frac{1}{2}$-inch needle is attached to a 12-mL syringe and is advanced perpendicular to the skin, aiming for the middle of the rib between the index and middle fingers. The needle should impinge on bone after being advanced about $\frac{3}{4}$ inch.

After bony contact is made, the needle is withdrawn into the subcutaneous tissues, and the skin and subcuta-

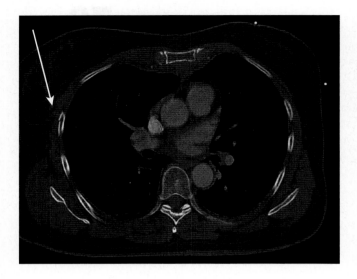

Figure 70-1.
Rib fracture (*arrow*) on CT not seen by radiography. (From Pope T, Bloem HL, Beltran J: Imaging of the Musculoskeletal System, 1st ed. Philadelphia, Saunders 2008, p 91.)

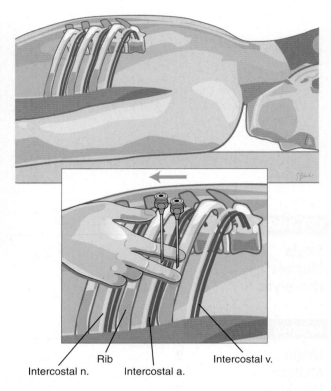

Intercostal n.   Rib   Intercostal a.   Intercostal v.

Figure 70-2.

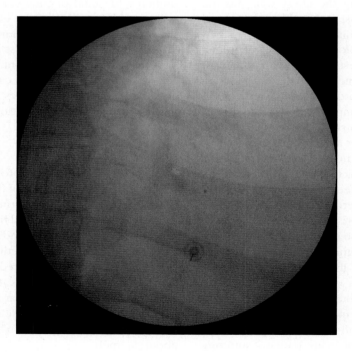

Figure 70-3.
Fluoroscopic view of posterior ribs.

neous tissues are retracted with the palpating fingers inferiorly. This allows the needle to be walked off the inferior margin of the rib (Fig. 70-2). As soon as bony contact is lost, the needle is slowly advanced about 2 mm deeper. This will place the needle in proximity to the costal grove, which contains the intercostal nerve as well as the intercostal artery and vein. After careful aspiration reveals no blood or air, 3 to 5 mL of 1.0% preservative-free lidocaine is injected. If there is an inflammatory component to the pain, the local anesthetic is combined with 80 mg of methylprednisolone and is injected in incremental doses. Subsequent daily nerve blocks are carried out in a similar manner, substituting 40 mg of methylprednisolone for the initial 80-mg dose. Because of the overlapping innervation of the chest and upper abdominal wall, the intercostal nerves above and below the nerve suspected of subserving the painful condition will have to be blocked. If surface landmarks are difficult to identify, fluoroscopy or computed tomography guidance may be helpful (Fig. 70-3).

SIDE EFFECTS AND COMPLICATIONS

Given the proximity of the pleural space, pneumothorax after intercostal nerve block is a distinct possibility. The incidence of the complication is less than 1%, but it occurs with greater frequency in patients with chronic obstructive pulmonary disease. Because of the proximity to the intercostal nerve and artery, the pain management specialist should carefully calculate the total milligram dosage of local anesthetic administered because vascular uptake via these vessels is high. Although uncommon, infection remains an ever-present possibility, especially in the immunocompromised cancer patient. Early detection of infection is crucial to avoid potentially life-threatening sequelae.

CLINICAL PEARLS

Intercostal nerve block is a simple technique that can produce dramatic relief for patients suffering from the previously mentioned pain complaints. Intercostal block with local anesthetic before placement of chest tubes provides a great degree of patient comfort and should routinely be used. Intercostal block with local anesthetic and steroid is useful in the palliation of the pleuritic pain secondary to lung tumors and liver tumors that are irritating the parietal peritoneum. Neurolytic block with small quantities of phenol in glycerin or by cryoneurolysis or radiofrequency lesioning has been shown to provide long-term relief for patients suffering from post-thoracotomy and cancer-related pain who have not responded to more conservative treatments. As mentioned earlier, the proximity of the intercostal nerve to the pleural space makes careful attention to technique mandatory.

CHAPTER **71**

Intercostal Nerve Block: Radiofrequency Lesioning

CPT-2009 CODE	
Neurolytic	64620

Relative Value Units	
Neurolytic	20 per nerve

INDICATIONS

Disruption of the intercostal nerve is indicated for the palliation of cancer pain, including invasive tumors of the ribs and the chest and upper abdominal wall. It also is used as a final step in the treatment of pain of nonmalignant origin in those patients in whom management with more conservative approaches, including adjuvant analgesics, has failed and who have experienced temporary relief with blockade of the target intercostal nerve or nerves with local anesthetic on at least two separate occasions. Disruption of the intercostal nerves can be carried out by injection with neurolytic agents, including phenol, cryoneurolysis, direct surgical sectioning at the time of thoracotomy, and destruction by radiofrequency lesioning. Most interventional pain management specialists now favor the use of radiofrequency lesioning because of its simplicity and its acceptable level of side effects and complications compared with the other modalities available.

CLINICALLY RELEVANT ANATOMY

The intercostal nerves arise from the anterior division of the thoracic spinal nerve (Fig. 71-1). A typical intercostal nerve has four major branches. The first branch is made up of the unmyelinated postganglionic fibers of the gray rami communicantes, which interface with the sympathetic chain. The second branch is the posterior cutaneous branch, which innervates the muscles and skin of the paraspinal area. The third branch is the lateral cutaneous division, which arises in the anterior axillary line. The lateral cutaneous division provides most of the cuta-

neous innervation of the chest and abdominal wall. The fourth branch is the anterior cutaneous branch supplying innervation to the midline of the chest and abdominal wall. Occasionally, the terminal branches of a given intercostal nerve actually may cross the midline to provide sensory innervation to the contralateral chest and abdominal wall. The 12th nerve is called the *subcostal nerve* and is unique in that it gives off a branch to the first lumbar nerve, thus contributing to the lumbar plexus. The nerve travels in the subcostal groove along with the intercostal artery and vein.

TECHNIQUE

The patient is placed in the prone position with the arms hanging loosely off the side of the cart. Alternatively, this block can be done in the sitting or lateral position based on the patient's ability to assume the desired position. The rib to be blocked is identified by palpating its path at the posterior axillary line or by fluoroscopy (Fig. 71-2). The index and middle fingers are then placed on the rib bracketing the site of needle insertion. The skin is then prepared with antiseptic solution. A 22-gauge, 54-mm radiofrequency needle with a 4-mm active tip is then advanced, perpendicular to the skin using a slight medial direction to lie as parallel as possible to the nerve, aiming for the middle of the rib between the index and middle fingers. The needle should impinge on bone after being advanced about $\frac{1}{2}$ inch.

After bony contact is made, the needle is withdrawn into the subcutaneous tissues, and the skin and subcutaneous tissues are retracted with the palpating fingers inferiorly. This allows the needle to be walked off the inferior margin of the rib (see Fig. 71-2). As soon as bony contact is lost, the needle is slowly advanced about 2 mm deeper. This will place the needle in proximity to the costal grove, which contains the intercostal nerve as well as the intercostal artery and vein. After confirmation of proper needle placement with fluoroscopy, trial sensory stimulation is carried out with 2 V at 50 Hz. (Fig. 71-3). If the needle is in the proper position, the patient should experience a paresthesia in the distribution of the target

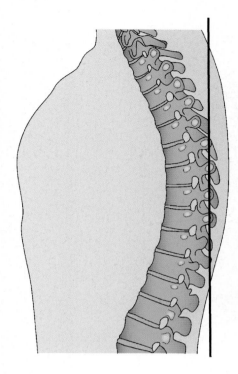

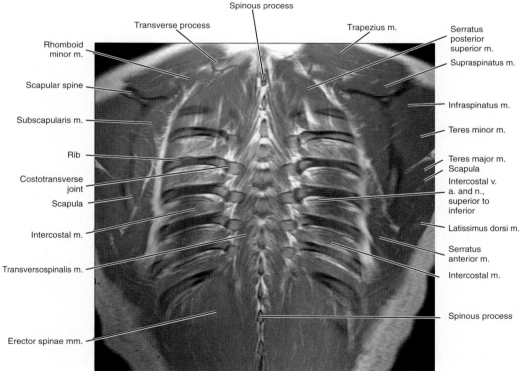

Figure 71-1.

(From El-Khoury GY, Bergman RA, Montgomery WJ: Sectional Anatomy by MRI and CT, 3rd ed. New York, Churchill Livingstone 2007, p 434.)

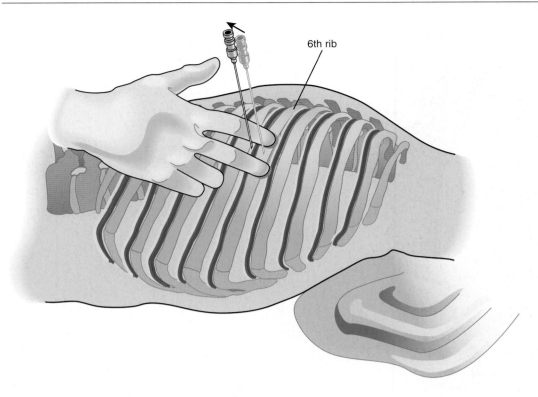

6th rib

Figure 71-2.

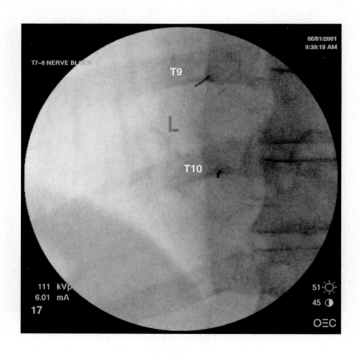

Figure 71-3.
Radiofrequency needle position for intercostal radiofrequency lesioning.

intercostal nerve. If a proper stimulation pattern is identified, a pulsed radiofrequency lesion is created by heating at 40°C to 45°C for 5 minutes or heating at 49°C to 60°C for 90 seconds. This technique is repeated for each affected nerve root.

SIDE EFFECTS AND COMPLICATIONS

Given the proximity of the pleural space, pneumothorax after intercostal nerve block is a distinct possibility. The incidence of the complication is less than 1%, but it occurs with greater frequency in patients with chronic obstructive pulmonary disease. Because of the proximity to the intercostal nerve and artery, the pain management specialist should carefully calculate the total milligram dosage of local anesthetic administered because vascular uptake via these vessels is high. Although uncommon, infection remains an ever-present possibility, especially in the immunocompromised cancer or AIDS patient. Early detection of infection is crucial to avoid potentially life-threatening sequelae. Even with perfect technique, postprocedure intercostal neuritis can occur, especially

with increasing temperatures. In most patients, this responds to the injection of 40 mg of methylprednisolone and 0.5% preservative-free bupivacaine onto the affected nerve. Occasionally, a short course of gabapentin also will be required to manage postprocedure neuritis.

CLINICAL PEARLS

Neurolytic block with small quantities of phenol in glycerin or by cryoneurolysis or radiofrequency lesioning has been shown to provide long-term relief for patients suffering from post-thoracotomy and cancer-related pain who have not responded to more conservative treatments. As mentioned earlier, the proximity of the intercostal nerve to the pleural space makes careful attention to technique mandatory. Alcohol should be avoided as a neurolytic agent because of the high incidence of postblock intercostal neuritis.

CHAPTER **72**

Interpleural Nerve Block: Percutaneous Technique

INDICATIONS

Interpleural nerve block is useful in the management of pain involving the upper extremity, chest wall, thoracic viscera, upper abdominal wall, and abdominal viscera. Interpleural nerve block with local anesthetic may be used to palliate acute pain emergencies, including rib fractures, acute herpes zoster, and cancer pain, while waiting for pharmacologic, surgical, and antiblastic methods to become effective. It also is useful before placement of percutaneous thoracostomy and nephrotomy tubes as well as percutaneous biliary drainage catheters. The technique also may be used for surgical procedures involving the breast, chest wall, and flank. Interpleural nerve block with local anesthetic and steroid also is useful in the treatment of post-thoracotomy pain, cancer pain (including pancreatic cancer), rib fractures, metastatic lesions of the lung and liver, and postherpetic neuralgia. Chronic administration of drugs into the interpleural space can be accomplished by tunneling an interpleural catheter. Administration of neurolytic solutions into the interpleural space is occasionally used for the palliation of cancer pain, including invasive tumors of the ribs and the chest and upper abdominal wall.

CLINICALLY RELEVANT ANATOMY

The pleural space extends from the apex to the base of the lung. It also envelops the anterior and posterior mediastinum. Local anesthetics placed into the interpleural space diffuse out of the interpleural space to block the thoracic somatic and lower cervical and thoracic sympathetic nerves that lie in proximity to the pleural space. Because the density and duration of the block depend on the amount and concentration of local anesthetic in contact with the nerve, it is possible to influence these variables by alterations in the patient's position during and after injection of the interpleural catheter.

TECHNIQUE

The choice of patient position is based on selection of the nerves that are to be blocked. For blockade of the lower cervical and upper thoracic sympathetic chain to treat sympathetically mediated pain, the patient is placed with the affected side up. After injection of the catheter, the patient is placed in the head down position. This position will avoid a dense block of the thoracic somatic nerves.

For a dense blockade of the thoracic somatic nerves including the thoracic spinal nerves and corresponding intercostal nerves as well as the thoracic sympathetic chain, the patient is placed in the oblique position with the affected side down and the patient's back propped against a pillow to encourage pooling of the local anesthetic into the interpleural gutter next to the thoracic spine. This will allow the maximal amount of local anesthetic to diffuse onto the somatic and sympathetic nerves. If the patient cannot lie on the affected side owing to fractured ribs, the interpleural catheter can be placed with the patient in the sitting position or with the affected side up. After injection of the catheter, the patient is then turned to the supine position with the patient tilted away from the affected side to encourage the flow of local anesthetic toward the interpleural gutter next to the thoracic spine.

After the patient is placed in the appropriate position, the eighth rib on the affected side is identified. The path of the rib is then traced posteriorly. At a point about 10 cm from the origin of the rib, the skin is marked and then prepared with antiseptic solution (Fig. 72-1A). The index and middle fingers are then placed on the rib

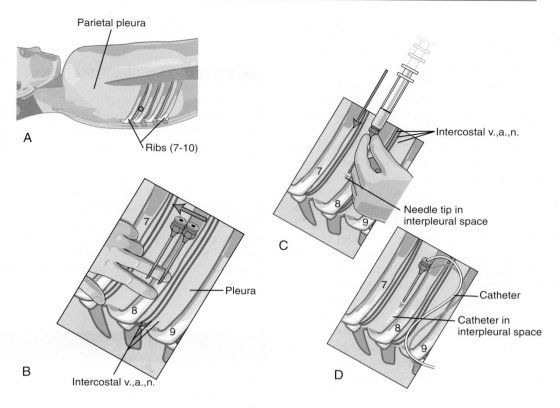

Figure 72-1.

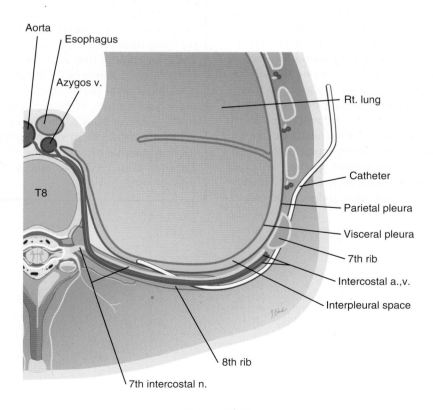

Figure 72-2.

bracketing the site of needle insertion. The skin and subcutaneous tissues are then anesthetized with local anesthetic. An 18-gauge, $3\frac{1}{2}$-inch styletted Hustead needle is then placed through the anesthetized area and is advanced perpendicular to the skin, aiming for the middle of the rib between the index and middle fingers. The needle should impinge on bone after being advanced about $\frac{1}{2}$ inch.

After bony contact is made, the needle is withdrawn into the subcutaneous tissues, and the skin and subcutaneous tissues are retracted with the palpating fingers superiorly. This allows the needle to be walked over the superior margin of the rib, avoiding trauma to the neurovascular bundle that runs beneath the rib (see Fig. 72-1B). As soon as bony contact is lost, the stylet is then removed, and the needle is attached to a well-lubricated 5-mL syringe containing air. The needle and syringe are slowly advanced toward the interpleural space. A click will be felt when the parietal pleura is penetrated with the tip of the needle bevel, and at this point the plunger of the syringe will usually advance under its own response to the negative pressure of the interpleural space (see Fig. 72-1C). The syringe is removed and a catheter is advanced 6 to 8 cm into the interpleural space (Fig. 72-2; see also Fig. 72-1D).

If no blood or air is identified after careful aspiration, the catheter is taped in place with sterile tape, and the patient is placed in the appropriate position to allow blockade of the desired nerves. From 20 to 30 mL of local anesthetic is then injected in incremental doses, with careful observation for signs of local anesthetic toxicity. If more concentrated, longer-acting local anesthetics such as 0.5% bupivacaine are used, smaller volumes on the order of 10 to 12 mL are given in incremental doses, with the total milligram dosage of drug gradually titrated upward to avoid toxic reactions. Alternatively, continuous infusions of local anesthetic can be administered by pump via the interpleural catheter. If there is an inflammatory component to the pain, the local anesthetic is combined with 80 mg of methylprednisolone and is injected in incremental doses. On subsequent days, 40 mg of methylprednisolone can be added to the local anesthetic.

SIDE EFFECTS AND COMPLICATIONS

Given the proximity of the pleural space, pneumothorax after interpleural nerve block is a distinct possibility. The incidence of clinically significant pneumothorax is probably less than 1% after interpleural catheter placement. Because of the proximity to the intercostal vein and artery, the pain management specialist should carefully calculate the total milligram dosage of local anesthetic administered because vascular uptake via these vessels is high. Although uncommon, infection remains an ever-present possibility, especially in the immunocompromised cancer patient. Early detection of infection is crucial to avoid potentially life-threatening sequelae.

CLINICAL PEARLS

Interpleural nerve block is a simple technique that can produce dramatic relief for patients suffering from the previously mentioned pain complaints. However, for most of the indications in which the pain management specialist would consider placing an interpleural catheter, other safer and less technically demanding procedures exist. In those patients suffering from pleuritic pain secondary to lung tumors and liver tumors that are irritating the parietal peritoneum who have not obtained long-lasting relief with intercostal nerve blocks containing local anesthetic and steroid, a tunneled interpleural catheter is a reasonable next step. Should a small pneumothorax occur after placement of an interpleural catheter, it may be possible to aspirate the air via the interpleural catheter and avoid placement of a thoracostomy tube.

CHAPTER 73

Interpleural Nerve Block:
Tunneled Catheter Technique

CPT-2009 CODE	
Tunneled Interpleural Catheter	64999

Relative Value Units	
Relative Value	20

INDICATIONS

Tunneling of an interpleural catheter is indicated for those patients who experience pain relief for the duration of the local anesthetic administered via intercostal or interpleural nerve block but whose pain returns when the local anesthetic wears off. In a manner analogous to epidural catheters, by tunneling the interpleural catheter, the incidence of infection including empyema is greatly decreased.

CLINICALLY RELEVANT ANATOMY

The pleural space extends from the apex to the base of the lung. It also envelops the anterior and posterior mediastinum. Local anesthetics placed into the interpleural space diffuse out of the interpleural space to block the thoracic somatic and lower cervical and thoracic sympathetic nerves that lie in proximity to the pleural space. Because the density and duration of the block depend on the amount and concentration of local anesthetic in contact with the nerve, it is possible to influence these variables by alterations in the patient's position during and after injection of the interpleural catheter.

TECHNIQUE

The choice of patient position is based on selection of the nerves that are to be blocked. For blockade of the lower cervical and upper thoracic sympathetic chain to treat sympathetically mediated pain, the patient is placed with the affected side up. After injection of the catheter, the patient is placed in the head-down position. This position will avoid a dense block of the thoracic somatic nerves.

For a dense blockade of the thoracic somatic nerves, including the thoracic spinal nerves and corresponding intercostal nerves as well as the thoracic sympathetic chain, the patient is placed in the oblique position with the affected side down and the patient's back propped against a pillow to encourage pooling of the local anesthetic into the interpleural gutter next to the thoracic spine. This will allow the maximal amount of local anesthetic to diffuse onto both the somatic and sympathetic nerves. If the patient cannot lie on the affected side owing to fractured ribs, the interpleural catheter can be placed with the patient in the sitting position or with the affected side up. After injection of the catheter, the patient is then turned to the supine position with the patient tilted away from the affected side to encourage the flow of local anesthetic toward the interpleural gutter next to the thoracic spine.

After the patient is placed in the appropriate position, the eighth rib on the affected side is identified. The path of the rib is then traced posteriorly. At a point about 10 cm from the origin of the rib, the skin is marked and then prepared with antiseptic solution (Fig. 73-1A). The index and middle fingers are then placed on the rib bracketing the site of needle insertion. The skin and subcutaneous tissues are then anesthetized with local anesthetic. An 18-gauge, $3\frac{1}{2}$-inch styletted Hustead needle is then placed through the anesthetized area and is advanced perpendicular to the skin, aiming for the middle of the rib between the index and middle fingers. The needle should impinge on bone after being advanced about $\frac{1}{2}$ inch.

After bony contact is made and with the needle still in place, a No. 15 scalpel blade is used to dissect all of the subcutaneous connective tissue away from the needle. A small curved clamp is then inserted into the incision, and a small pocket overlying the superior portion of the interspace is made by blunt dissection.

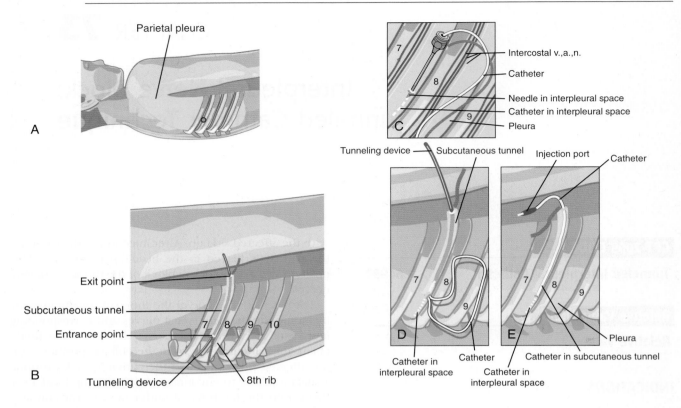

Figure 73-1.

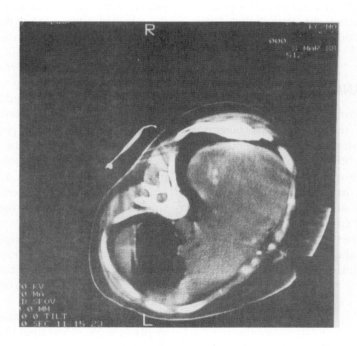

Figure 73-2.

CT scan of a patient with liver metastases demonstrating contrast media in the right interpleural space that was administered via a tunneled interpleural catheter.

This will allow the catheter to fall freely into the subcutaneous tunnel without kinking. After the pocket is made, the needle is removed, and the malleable tunneling tool is bent to match the contour of the patient's chest wall. The skin and pocket are lifted with thumb forceps, and the tunneling device is then introduced into the subcutaneous pocket and guided laterally around the chest wall (see Fig. 73-1B). When the tunneling device has reached its exit point on the anterior chest wall, it is turned away from the patient; this forces the sharp tip against the skin. The scalpel is then used to cut down on the tip. The tip of the tunneling device is then advanced through the exit incision and covered with a sterile dressing.

The styletted needle is then reintroduced into the previously made incision over the rib and advanced until contact with the rib is again made. The needle is withdrawn into the subcutaneous tissues, and the skin, subcutaneous tissues, and pocket are retracted with the palpating fingers superiorly. This allows the needle to be walked over the superior margin of the rib, avoiding trauma to the neurovascular bundle that runs beneath the rib.

As soon as bony contact is lost, the stylet is then removed, and the needle is attached to a well-lubricated 5-mL syringe containing air. The needle and syringe are slowly advanced toward the interpleural space. A click will be felt when the parietal pleura is penetrated with the tip of the needle bevel, and at this point the plunger of the syringe will usually advance under its own weight in response to the negative pressure of the interpleural space. The syringe is removed, and a catheter is advanced 6 to 8 cm into the interpleural space (see Fig. 73-1C). The needle is then removed from the interpleural space and withdrawn over the catheter. If no blood or air is identified after careful aspiration of the catheter, the distal end of the catheter is attached to the proximal end of the tunneling device (see Fig. 73-1D). The tunneling device is then withdrawn via the exit incision, bringing the catheter with it into the subcutaneous tunnel.

After the distal end of the catheter is drawn through the tunnel, the tunneling device is removed, and the remaining catheter is withdrawn until the excess catheter falls into the subcutaneous pocket. An injection port is then attached to the distal catheter, and the catheter is injected with sterile saline to ensure catheter integrity (see Fig. 73-1E). If the catheter injects easily and no leakage of saline is noted, the midline incision is closed with one or two 4-0 nylon sutures, with care taken not to damage the catheter with the suture needle. The catheter is taped in place with sterile tape, and the patient is placed in the appropriate position to allow blockade of the desired nerves. From 20 to 30 mL of local anesthetic is then injected in incremental doses, with careful observation for signs of local anesthetic toxicity. If more concentrated, longer-acting local anesthetics such as 0.5% bupivacaine are used, smaller volumes on the order of 10 to 12 mL are given in incremental doses, with the total milligram dosage of drug gradually titrated upward to avoid toxic reactions. Alternatively, continuous infusions of local anesthetic can be administered by pump via the interpleural catheter. If there is an inflammatory component to the pain, the local anesthetic is combined with 80 mg of methylprednisolone and is injected in incremental doses. On subsequent days, 40 mg of methylprednisolone can be added to the local anesthetic.

SIDE EFFECTS AND COMPLICATIONS

Care must be taken not to damage the fragile catheter during the tunneling process. Given the proximity of the pleural space, pneumothorax after interpleural nerve block is a distinct possibility. The incidence of clinically significant pneumothorax is probably less than 1% after interpleural catheter placement. Because of the proximity to the intercostal vein and artery, the pain management specialist should carefully calculate the total milligram dosage of local anesthetic administered because vascular uptake via these vessels is high. Although uncommon, infection remains an ever-present possibility, especially in the immunocompromised cancer patient. Early detection of infection is crucial to avoid potentially life-threatening sequelae.

CLINICAL PEARLS

Interpleural nerve block is a simple technique that can produce dramatic relief for patients suffering from the previously mentioned pain complaints. However, for most of the indications for which the pain management specialist would consider placing an interpleural catheter, other safer and less technically demanding procedures exist. In those patients suffering from pleuritic pain secondary to lung tumors and liver tumors that are irritating the parietal peritoneum who have not obtained long-lasting relief with intercostal nerve blocks containing local anesthetic and steroid, a tunneled interpleural catheter is a reasonable next step (Fig. 73-2). Should a small pneumothorax occur after placement of an interpleural catheter, it may be possible to aspirate the air via the interpleural catheter and avoid placement of a thoracostomy tube.

Section 5

Abdomen and Abdominal Wall

CHAPTER 74

Splanchnic Nerve Block: Classic Two-Needle Technique

CPT-2009 CODE

Local Anesthetic–With or Without Radiographic Monitoring	64530
Neurolytic–With or Without Radiographic Monitoring	64680

Relative Value Units

Local Anesthetic	18
Neurolytic	25

INDICATIONS

Although the indications for splanchnic nerve block are essentially the same as those for celiac plexus block, the higher complication rate associated with splanchnic nerve block suggests that it should be reserved for patients with upper abdominal and retroperitoneal pain that fails to respond to celiac plexus block. Most patients who fall into this category have significant preaortic adenopathy, tumor, or postoperative scarring.

Splanchnic nerve block with local anesthetic is indicated as a diagnostic maneuver to determine whether flank, retroperitoneal, or upper abdominal pain is sympathetically mediated via the splanchnic nerve. Daily splanchnic nerve block with local anesthetic also is useful in the palliation of pain secondary to acute pancreatitis and other acute pain syndromes subserved by the splanchnic nerves. Early implementation of splanchnic nerve block with local anesthetic, steroids, or both markedly reduces the morbidity and mortality associated with acute pancreatitis. Splanchnic nerve block also is used to palliate the acute pain of arterial embolization of the liver for cancer therapy as well as to treat the pain of abdominal "angina" associated with visceral arterial insufficiency. Splanchnic nerve block with local anesthetic also may be used prognostically before splanchnic nerve neurolysis.

Neurolysis of the splanchnic nerves with alcohol or phenol is indicated to treat pain secondary to malignancies of the retroperitoneum and upper abdomen. Neurolytic splanchnic nerve block also may be useful in some chronic benign abdominal pain syndromes, including chronic pancreatitis, in carefully selected patients.

CLINICALLY RELEVANT ANATOMY

The sympathetic innervation of the abdominal viscera originates in the anterolateral horn of the spinal cord. Preganglionic fibers from T5-T12 exit the spinal cord in conjunction with the ventral roots to join the white communicating rami on their way to the sympathetic chain. Rather than synapsing with the sympathetic chain, these preganglionic fibers pass through it to ultimately synapse on the celiac ganglia. The greater, lesser, and least splanchnic nerves provide the major preganglionic contribution to the celiac plexus and transmit most nociceptive information from the viscera. The splanchnic nerves are contained in a narrow compartment made up of the vertebral body and the pleura laterally, the posterior mediastinum ventrally, and the pleural attachment to the vertebra dorsally. This compartment is bounded caudally by the crura of the diaphragm. The volume of this compartment is about 10 mL on each side.

The greater splanchnic nerve has its origin from the T5-T10 spinal roots. The nerve travels along the thoracic paravertebral border through the crus of the diaphragm into the abdominal cavity, ending on the celiac ganglion of its respective side. The lesser splanchnic nerve arises from the T10-T11 roots and passes with the greater nerve to end at the celiac ganglion. The least splanchnic nerve arises from the T11-T12 spinal roots and passes through the diaphragm to the celiac ganglion.

Intrapatient anatomic variability of the celiac ganglia is significant, but the following generalizations can be drawn from anatomic studies of the celiac ganglia. The number of ganglia varies from one to five, and they range in diameter from 0.5 to 4.5 cm. The ganglia lie anterior and anterolateral to the aorta. The ganglia located on the left are uniformly more inferior than their right-sided counterparts by as much as a vertebral level, but both groups of ganglia lie below the level of the celiac artery. The ganglia usually lie about at the level of the first lumbar vertebra.

Postganglionic fibers radiate from the celiac ganglia to follow the course of the blood vessels to innervate the abdominal viscera. These organs include much of the distal esophagus, stomach, duodenum, small intestine, ascending and proximal transverse colon, adrenal glands, pancreas, spleen, liver, and biliary system. It is these postganglionic fibers, the fibers arising from the preganglionic splanchnic nerves, and the celiac ganglion that make up the celiac plexus. The celiac plexus is anterior to the crus of the diaphragm. The plexus extends in front of and around the aorta, with the greatest concentration of fibers anterior to the aorta. The relationship of the celiac plexus to the surrounding structures is as follows: The aorta lies anterior and slightly to the left of the anterior margin of the vertebral body (Fig. 74-1). The inferior vena cava lies to the right, with the kidneys posterolateral to the great vessels. The pancreas lies anterior to the celiac plexus. All these structures lie within the retroperitoneal space.

TECHNIQUE

Preblock preparation includes the administration of adequate amounts of oral or intravenous fluids to attenuate the hypotension associated with splanchnic nerve block. Evaluation for coagulopathy is indicated if the patient has undergone antiblastic therapy or has a history of significant alcohol abuse. If radiographic contrast is to be used, evaluation of the patient's renal status also is indicated.

The technique for splanchnic nerve block differs little from the classic retrocrural approach to the celiac plexus except that the needles are aimed more cephalad to ultimately rest at the anterolateral margin of the T12 vertebral body. It is imperative that both needles be placed medially against the vertebral body to reduce the incidence of pneumothorax. The patient is placed in the prone position with a pillow placed under the abdomen to flex the thoracolumbar spine. For comfort, the patient's head is turned to the side, and the arms are permitted to hang freely off each side of the table. The inferior margins of the 12th ribs are identified and traced to the T12 vertebral body. The spinous process of the L1 vertebral body is then identified and marked with a sterile marker. A point about 2 inches just inferior and lateral to each side of the spinous process of L1 is identified. The injection sites are then prepared with antiseptic solution.

The skin, subcutaneous tissues, and musculature are infiltrated with 1.0% lidocaine at the points of needle entry. Twenty-gauge, 13-cm styletted needles are inserted bilaterally through the previously anesthetized area. The needles are initially oriented 45 degrees toward the midline and about 35 degrees cephalad to ensure contact with the T12 vertebral body (Fig. 74-2). Once bony contact is made and the depth is noted, the needles are withdrawn to the level of the subcutaneous tissue and redirected slightly less mesiad (about 60 degrees from the midline) so as to walk off the lateral surface of the T12 vertebral body. The needles are replaced to the depth at which contact with the vertebral body was first noted. At this point, if no bone is contacted, the left-sided needle is gradually advanced 1.5 cm. The right-sided needle is then advanced slightly farther (i.e., 2 cm past contact with the bone). Ultimately, the tips of the needles should be just anterior to the lateral border of the vertebral body and just behind the aorta and vena cava in the retrocrural space (Fig. 74-3).

The stylets of the needles are removed, and the needle hubs are inspected for the presence of blood, cerebrospinal fluid, or urine. If radiographic guidance is being used, a small amount of contrast material is injected through each needle, and its spread is observed radiographically. On the fluoroscopic anteroposterior view, contrast is confined to the midline and concentrated near the T12 vertebral body. A smooth posterior contour can be observed that corresponds to the psoas fascia on the lateral view. Alternatively, if computed tomographic guidance is used, contrast should appear lateral to and behind the aorta. The contrast should be observed to be entirely retrocrural. If there is precrural spread, the needles are withdrawn slightly back through the crura of the diaphragm.

If radiographic guidance is not used, a rapid-onset local anesthetic is used in sufficient concentration to produce motor block (e.g., 1.5% lidocaine or 3.0% 2-chloroprocaine) before administration of neurolytic agents. If the patient experiences no motor or sensory block in the lumbar dermatomes after an adequate time, additional drugs injected through the needles probably will not reach the somatic nerve roots if given in like volumes.

For diagnostic and prognostic splanchnic nerve block, a 7 to 10 mL volume of 1.5% lidocaine or 3.0% 2-chloroprocaine is administered through the needle. For therapeutic block, 7 to 10 mL of 0.5% bupivacaine is administered. Because of the potential for local anesthetic toxicity, all local anesthetics should be administered in incremental doses. A 10-mL volume of absolute alcohol or 6.0% aqueous phenol is used for neurolytic block. After neurolytic solution is injected, each needle should be flushed with sterile saline solution because there have been anecdotal reports of neurolytic solution being tracked posteriorly with the needles as they are withdrawn.

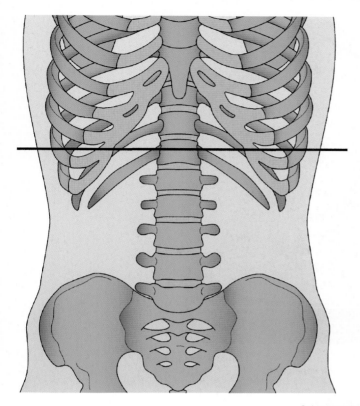

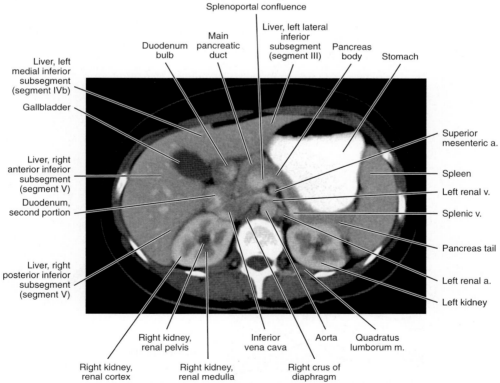

Figure 74-1.
(From El-Khoury GY, Bergman RA, Montgomery WJ: Sectional Anatomy by MRI and CT, 3rd ed. New York, Churchill Livingstone, 2007, p 490.)

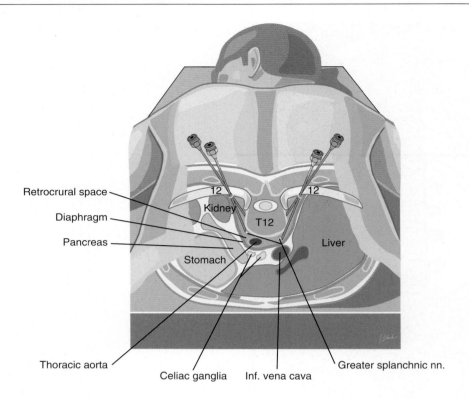

Retrocrural space

Diaphragm

Pancreas

Kidney

T12

Stomach

Liver

12   12

Thoracic aorta

Celiac ganglia

Inf. vena cava

Greater splanchnic nn.

Figure 74-2.

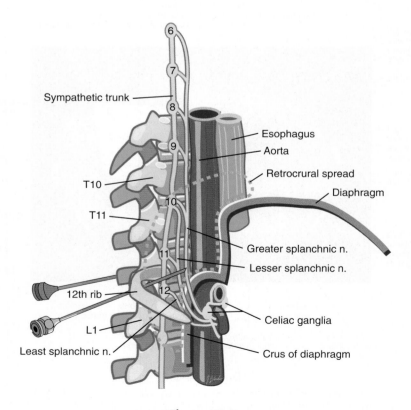

Sympathetic trunk

6

7

8

9

10

11

12

T10

T11

12th rib

L1

Least splanchnic n.

Esophagus

Aorta

Retrocrural spread

Diaphragm

Greater splanchnic n.

Lesser splanchnic n.

Celiac ganglia

Crus of diaphragm

Figure 74-3.

SIDE EFFECTS AND COMPLICATIONS

Because of the proximity to vascular structures, splanchnic nerve block is contraindicated in patients who are on anticoagulant therapy or suffer from coagulopathy secondary to antiblastic cancer therapies or liver abnormalities associated with ethanol abuse. Intravascular injection of solutions may result in thrombosis of the nutrient vessels to the spinal cord with secondary paraplegia. Local and intra-abdominal infection, as well as sepsis, are absolute contraindications to splanchnic nerve block.

Because blockade of the splanchnic nerve results in increased bowel motility, this technique should be avoided in patients with bowel obstruction. Postblock diarrhea occurs in about 50% of patients. Splanchnic nerve block should be deferred in patients who suffer from chronic abdominal pain and who are chemically dependent or exhibit drug-seeking behavior until these issues have been adequately addressed. Alcohol should not be used as a neurolytic agent in patients on disulfiram therapy for alcohol abuse.

The proximity to the spinal cord, exiting nerve roots, pleural space, and viscera makes it imperative that this procedure be performed only by those well versed in the regional anatomy and experienced in interventional pain management techniques. Needle placement that is too medial may result in epidural, subdural, or subarachnoid injections or trauma to the spinal cord and exiting nerve roots. Such incorrect needle placement can result in severe neurologic deficits, including paraplegia. Medial nerve placement also may result in intradiskal placement and resultant diskitis. Because the needle terminus is retrocrural when the classic two-needle approach to splanchnic nerve block is used, there is an increased incidence of neurologic complications, including neu-

rolysis of the lumbar nerve roots with resultant hip flexor weakness and lower extremity numbness. Techniques that result in precrural needle placement, such as the transcrural and transaortic approaches to splanchnic nerve block, have a lower incidence of this complication and should be considered by the pain management specialist.

Given the proximity of the pleural space, pneumothorax after splanchnic nerve block may occur if the needle is placed too cephalad or anterior. Trauma to the thoracic duct with resultant chylothorax also may occur. If the needles are placed too laterally, trauma to the kidneys and ureters is a distinct possibility.

CLINICAL PEARLS

Given the higher incidence of pneumothorax associated with splanchnic nerve block relative to celiac plexus block, splanchnic nerve block should be reserved for patients with upper abdominal and retroperitoneal pain that fails to respond to celiac plexus block. The incidence of pneumothorax can be decreased if the needles are kept close to the vertebral bodies during needle placement. Radiographic guidance, especially CT guidance, offers the pain specialist an added margin of safety during neurolytic splanchnic nerve block.

It should be noted that the phrenic nerve also transmits nociceptive information from the upper abdominal viscera. This information is perceived as poorly localized pain referred to the supraclavicular region; this source of pain should be considered in all patients with upper abdominal pain.

CHAPTER 75

Splanchnic Nerve Block:
Single-Needle Technique

CPT-2009 CODE

Local Anesthetic–With or Without	**64530**
Radiographic Monitoring	
Neurolytic–With or Without	**64680**
Radiographic Monitoring	

Relative Value Units

Local Anesthetic	**18**
Neurolytic	**25**

INDICATIONS

Although the indications for splanchnic nerve block are essentially the same as those for celiac plexus block, the higher complication rate associated with splanchnic nerve block suggests that it should be reserved for patients with upper abdominal and retroperitoneal pain that fails to respond to celiac plexus block. Most patients who fall into this category have significant preaortic adenopathy, tumor, or postoperative scarring.

Splanchnic nerve block with local anesthetic is indicated as a diagnostic maneuver to determine whether flank, retroperitoneal, or upper abdominal pain is sympathetically mediated via the splanchnic nerve. Daily splanchnic nerve block with local anesthetic also is useful in the palliation of pain secondary to acute pancreatitis and other acute pain syndromes subserved by the splanchnic nerves. Early implementation of splanchnic nerve block with local anesthetic, steroids, or both markedly reduces the morbidity and mortality associated with acute pancreatitis. Splanchnic nerve block also is used to palliate the acute pain of arterial embolization of the liver for cancer therapy as well as to treat the pain of abdominal "angina" associated with visceral arterial insufficiency. Splanchnic nerve block with local anesthetic also may be used prognostically before splanchnic nerve neurolysis.

Neurolysis of the splanchnic nerves with alcohol or phenol is indicated to treat pain secondary to malignancies of the retroperitoneum and upper abdomen. Neurolytic splanchnic nerve block also may be useful in some chronic benign abdominal pain syndromes, including chronic pancreatitis, in carefully selected patients.

CLINICALLY RELEVANT ANATOMY

The sympathetic innervation of the abdominal viscera originates in the anterolateral horn of the spinal cord. Preganglionic fibers from T5-T12 exit the spinal cord in conjunction with the ventral roots to join the white communicating rami on their way to the sympathetic chain. Rather than synapsing with the sympathetic chain, these preganglionic fibers pass through it to ultimately synapse on the celiac ganglia. The greater, lesser, and least splanchnic nerves provide the major preganglionic contribution to the celiac plexus and transmit most nociceptive information from the viscera. The splanchnic nerves are contained in a narrow compartment made up by the vertebral body and the pleura laterally, the posterior mediastinum ventrally, and the pleural attachment to the vertebra dorsally. This compartment is bounded caudally by the crura of the diaphragm. The volume of this compartment is about 10 mL on each side.

The greater splanchnic nerve has its origin from the T5-T10 spinal roots. The nerve travels along the thoracic paravertebral border through the crus of the diaphragm into the abdominal cavity, ending on the celiac ganglion of its respective side. The lesser splanchnic nerve arises from the T10-T11 roots and passes with the greater nerve to end at the celiac ganglion. The least splanchnic nerve arises from the T11-T12 spinal roots and passes through the diaphragm to the celiac ganglion.

Intrapatient anatomic variability of the celiac ganglia is significant, but the following generalizations can be drawn from anatomic studies of the celiac ganglia. The number of ganglia varies from one to five, and they range in diameter from 0.5 to 4.5 cm. The ganglia lie anterior and anterolateral to the aorta. The ganglia located on the left are uniformly more inferior than their right-sided counterparts by as much as a vertebral level, but both groups of ganglia lie below the level of the celiac artery. The ganglia usually lie about at the level of the first lumbar vertebra.

Postganglionic fibers radiate from the celiac ganglia to follow the course of the blood vessels to innervate the abdominal viscera. These organs include much of the distal esophagus, stomach, duodenum, small intestine, ascending and proximal transverse colon, adrenal glands, pancreas, spleen, liver, and biliary system. It is these postganglionic fibers, the fibers arising from the preganglionic splanchnic nerves, and the celiac ganglion that make up the celiac plexus. The celiac plexus is anterior to the crus of the diaphragm. The plexus extends in front of and around the aorta, with the greatest concentration of fibers anterior to the aorta. The relationship of the celiac plexus to the surrounding structures is as follows: The aorta lies anterior and slightly to the left of the anterior margin of the vertebral body (Fig. 75-1). The inferior vena cava lies to the right, with the kidneys posterolateral to the great vessels. The pancreas lies anterior to the celiac plexus. All these structures lie within the retroperitoneal space.

TECHNIQUE

Preblock preparation includes the administration of adequate amounts of oral or intravenous fluids to attenuate the hypotension associated with splanchnic nerve block. Evaluation for coagulopathy is indicated if the patient has undergone antiblastic therapy or has a history of significant alcohol abuse. If radiographic contrast is to be used, evaluation of the patient's renal status also is indicated.

The technique for single needle splanchnic nerve block differs little from the classic retrocrural approach to the celiac plexus except that the needle is aimed more cephalad to ultimately rest at the left anterolateral margin of the T12 vertebral body. It is imperative that the needle be placed medially against the vertebral body to reduce the incidence of pneumothorax. The patient is placed in the prone position with a pillow placed under the abdomen to flex the thoracolumbar spine. For comfort, the patient's head is turned to the side, and the arms are permitted to hang freely off each side of the table. The inferior margins of the 12th ribs are identified and traced to the T12 vertebral body. The spinous process of the L1 vertebral body is then identified and marked with a sterile marker. A point about 2 inches just inferior and lateral to each side of the spinous process of L1 is identified. The injection site is then prepared with antiseptic solution.

The skin, subcutaneous tissues, and musculature on the left of the midline are infiltrated with 1.0% lidocaine at the points of needle entry. A 20-gauge, 13-cm styletted needle is inserted through the previously anesthetized area. The needle is initially oriented 45 degrees toward the midline and about 35 degrees cephalad to ensure contact with the T12 vertebral body (Fig. 75-2). Once bony contact is made and the depth is noted, the needle is withdrawn to the level of the subcutaneous tissue and redirected slightly less mesiad (about 60 degrees from the midline) so as to walk off the lateral surface of the T12 vertebral body. The needle is replaced to the depth at which contact with the vertebral body was first noted. At this point, if no bone is contacted, the needle is gradually advanced 1.5 cm. Ultimately, the tip of the needle should be just anterior to the lateral border of the vertebral body and just behind the aorta and vena cava in the retrocrural space (Fig. 75-3).

The stylet of the needle is removed, and the needle hub is inspected for the presence of blood, cerebrospinal fluid, or urine. If radiographic guidance is being used, a small amount of contrast material is injected through the needle, and its spread is observed radiographically. On the fluoroscopic anteroposterior view, contrast is confined to the midline and concentrated near the T12 vertebral body. A smooth posterior contour can be observed that corresponds to the psoas fascia on the lateral view. Alternatively, if computed tomographic guidance is used, contrast should appear lateral to and behind the aorta. The contrast should be observed to be entirely retrocrural. If there is precrural spread, the needle is withdrawn slightly back through the crura of the diaphragm.

If radiographic guidance is not used, a rapid-onset local anesthetic is used in sufficient concentration to produce motor block (e.g., 1.5% lidocaine or 3.0% 2-chloroprocaine) before administration of neurolytic agents. If the patient experiences no motor or sensory block in the lumbar dermatomes after an adequate time, additional drugs injected through the needle will probably not reach the somatic nerve roots if given in like volumes.

For diagnostic and prognostic splanchnic nerve block, a 7 to 10 mL volume of 1.5% lidocaine or 3.0% 2-chloroprocaine is administered through the needle. For therapeutic block, 7 to 10 mL of 0.5% bupivacaine is administered. Because of the potential for local anesthetic toxicity, all local anesthetics should be administered in incremental doses. A 10-mL volume of absolute alcohol or 6.0% aqueous phenol is used for neurolytic block. After neurolytic solution is injected, the needle should be flushed with sterile saline solution because there have been anecdotal reports of neurolytic solution being tracked posteriorly with the needle as it is withdrawn.

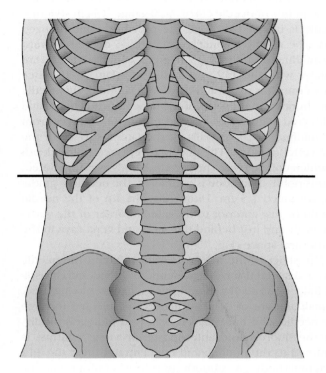

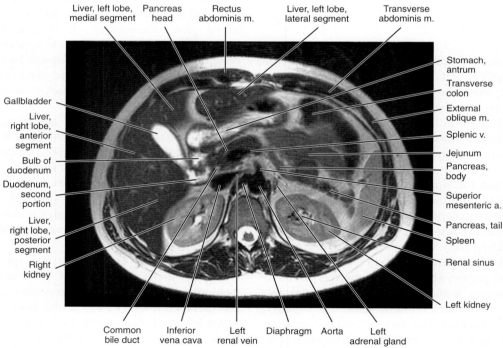

Figure 75-1.

(From El-Khoury GY, Bergman RA, Montgomery WJ: Sectional Anatomy by MRI and CT, 3rd ed. New York, Churchill Livingstone, 2007, p 510.)

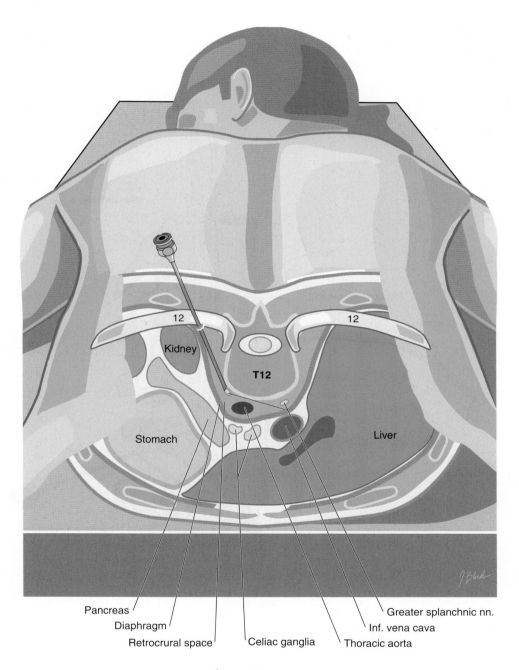

Figure 75-2.

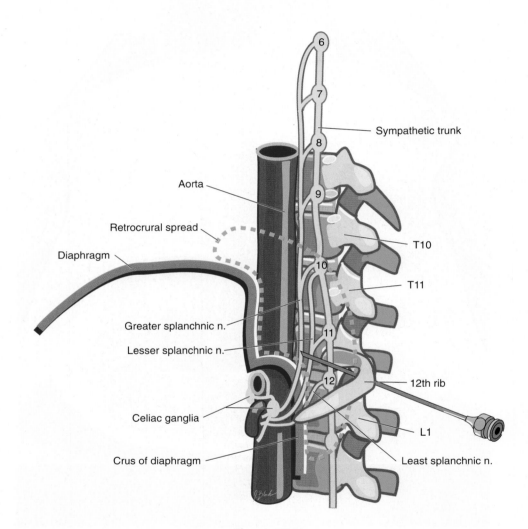

Figure 75-3.

SIDE EFFECTS AND COMPLICATIONS

Because of the proximity to vascular structures, splanchnic nerve block is contraindicated in patients who are on anticoagulant therapy or suffer from coagulopathy secondary to antiblastic cancer therapies or liver abnormalities associated with ethanol abuse. Intravascular injection of solutions may result in thrombosis of the nutrient vessels to the spinal cord with secondary paraplegia. Local and intra-abdominal infection, as well as sepsis, are absolute contraindications to splanchnic nerve block.

Because blockade of the splanchnic nerve results in increased bowel motility, this technique should be avoided in patients with bowel obstruction. Postblock diarrhea occurs in about 50% of patients. Splanchnic nerve block should be deferred in patients who suffer from chronic abdominal pain and who are chemically dependent or exhibit drug-seeking behavior until these issues have been adequately addressed. Alcohol should not be used as a neurolytic agent in patients on disulfiram therapy for alcohol abuse.

The proximity to the spinal cord, exiting nerve roots, pleural space, and viscera makes it imperative that this procedure be performed only by those well versed in the regional anatomy and experienced in interventional pain management techniques. Needle placement that is too medial may result in epidural, subdural, or subarachnoid injections or trauma to the spinal cord and exiting nerve roots. Such incorrect needle placement can result in severe neurologic deficits, including paraplegia. Medial nerve placement also may result in intradiskal placement and resultant diskitis. Because the needle terminus is retrocrural when the classic two-needle approach to splanchnic nerve block is used, there is an increased incidence of neurologic complications, including neurolysis of the lumbar nerve roots with resultant hip flexor weakness and lower extremity numbness. Techniques that result in precrural needle placement, such as the transcrural and transaortic approaches to splanchnic nerve block, have a lower incidence of this complication and should be considered by the pain management specialist.

Given the proximity of the pleural space, pneumothorax after splanchnic nerve block may occur if the needle is placed too cephalad or anterior. Trauma to the thoracic duct with resultant chylothorax also may occur. If the needle is placed too laterally, trauma to the kidneys and ureters is a distinct possibility.

CLINICAL PEARLS

Given the higher incidence of pneumothorax associated with splanchnic nerve block relative to celiac plexus block, splanchnic nerve block should be reserved for patients with upper abdominal and retroperitoneal pain that fails to respond to celiac plexus block. The incidence of pneumothorax can be decreased if the needle is kept close to the vertebral bodies during needle placement. Radiographic guidance, especially CT guidance, offers the pain specialist an added margin of safety during neurolytic splanchnic nerve block.

It should be noted that the phrenic nerve also transmits nociceptive information from the upper abdominal viscera. This information is perceived as poorly localized pain referred to the supraclavicular region; this source of pain should be considered in all patients with upper abdominal pain.

CHAPTER 76

Celiac Plexus Block: Classic Two-Needle Retrocrural Technique

CPT-2009 CODE	
Local Anesthetic–With or Without Radiographic Monitoring	**64530**
Neurolytic–With or Without Radiographic Monitoring	**64680**

Relative Value Units	
Local Anesthetic	**18**
Neurolytic	**25**

INDICATIONS

Until recently, celiac plexus block via the classic two-needle retrocrural technique has been the celiac plexus block technique most used by pain management specialists. Because the needle terminus is retrocrural with this technique, a higher incidence of neurologic complications is to be expected compared with techniques that result in precrural needle placement. However, because of the long track record of efficacy and safety enjoyed by the classic two-needle approach to celiac plexus block, this technique remains an acceptable approach to blockade of the celiac plexus.

Celiac plexus block with local anesthetic is indicated as a diagnostic maneuver to determine whether flank, retroperitoneal, or upper abdominal pain is sympathetically mediated via the celiac plexus. Daily celiac plexus block with local anesthetic also is useful in the palliation of pain secondary to acute pancreatitis and other acute pain syndromes subserved by the celiac plexus. Early implementation of celiac plexus block with local anesthetic, steroids, or both markedly reduces the morbidity and mortality associated with acute pancreatitis. Celiac plexus block also is used to palliate the acute pain of arterial embolization of the liver for cancer therapy as well as to treat the pain of abdominal "angina" associated with visceral arterial insufficiency. Celiac plexus block with local anesthetic also may be used prognostically before celiac plexus neurolysis.

Neurolysis of the celiac plexus with alcohol or phenol is indicated to treat pain secondary to malignancies of the retroperitoneum and upper abdomen. Neurolytic celiac plexus block also may be useful in some chronic benign abdominal pain syndromes, including chronic pancreatitis, in carefully selected patients.

CLINICALLY RELEVANT ANATOMY

The sympathetic innervation of the abdominal viscera originates in the anterolateral horn of the spinal cord. Preganglionic fibers from T5-T12 exit the spinal cord in conjunction with the ventral roots to join the white communicating rami on their way to the sympathetic chain. Rather than synapsing with the sympathetic chain, these preganglionic fibers pass through it to ultimately synapse on the celiac ganglia. The greater, lesser, and least splanchnic nerves provide the major preganglionic contribution to the celiac plexus. The greater splanchnic nerve has its origin from the T5-T10 spinal roots. The nerve travels along the thoracic paravertebral border through the crus of the diaphragm into the abdominal cavity, ending on the celiac ganglion of its respective side. The lesser splanchnic nerve arises from the T10-T11 roots and passes with the greater nerve to end at the celiac ganglion. The least splanchnic nerve arises from the T11-T12 spinal roots and passes through the diaphragm to the celiac ganglion.

Interpatient anatomic variability of the celiac ganglia is significant, but the following generalizations can be drawn from anatomic studies of the celiac ganglia. The number of ganglia varies from one to five, and they range in diameter from 0.5 to 4.5 cm. The ganglia lie anterior and anterolateral to the aorta. The ganglia located on the left are uniformly more inferior than their right-sided counterparts by as much as a vertebral level, but both groups of ganglia lie below the level of the celiac artery. The ganglia usually lie about at the level of the first lumbar vertebra.

Postganglionic fibers radiate from the celiac ganglia to follow the course of the blood vessels to innervate the abdominal viscera. These organs include much of the distal esophagus, stomach, duodenum, small intestine, ascending and proximal transverse colon, adrenal glands, pancreas, spleen, liver, and biliary system. It is these postganglionic fibers, the fibers arising from the preganglionic splanchnic nerves, and the celiac ganglia that make up the celiac plexus. The celiac plexus is anterior to the crus of the diaphragm. The plexus extends in front of and around the aorta, with the greatest concentration of fibers anterior to the aorta. The relationship of the celiac plexus to the surrounding structures is as follows: The aorta lies anterior and slightly to the left of the anterior margin of the vertebral body. The inferior vena cava lies to the right, with the kidneys posterolateral to the great vessels. The pancreas lies anterior to the celiac plexus. All these structures lie within the retroperitoneal space.

TECHNIQUE

Preblock preparation includes the administration of adequate amounts of oral or intravenous fluids to attenuate the hypotension associated with celiac plexus block. Evaluation for coagulopathy is indicated if the patient has undergone antiblastic therapy or has a history of significant alcohol abuse. If radiographic contrast is to be used, evaluation of the patient's renal status also is indicated.

The patient is placed in the prone position with a pillow placed under the abdomen to flex the thoracolumbar spine. For comfort, the patient's head is turned to the side, and the arms are permitted to hang freely off each side of the table. The inferior margins of the 12th ribs are identified and traced to the T12 vertebral body. The spinous process of the L1 vertebral body is then identified and marked with a sterile marker. A point about $2\frac{1}{2}$ inches just inferior and lateral to each side of the transverse process of L1 is identified. The injection sites are then prepared with antiseptic solution.

The skin, subcutaneous tissues, and musculature are infiltrated with 1.0% lidocaine at the points of needle entry. Twenty-gauge, 13-cm styletted needles are inserted bilaterally through the previously anesthetized area. The needles are initially oriented 45 degrees toward the midline and about 15 degrees cephalad to ensure contact with the L1 vertebral body. Once bone is contacted and the depth is noted, the needles are withdrawn to the level of the subcutaneous tissue and redirected slightly less mesiad (about 60 degrees from the midline) so as to walk off (Fig. 76-1) the lateral surface of the L1 vertebral body. The needles are replaced to the depth at which contact with the vertebral body was first noted. At this point, if no bone is contacted, the left-sided needle is gradually advanced 1.5 to 2 cm, or until the pulsation emanating from the aorta and transmitted to the advancing needle is noted. The right-sided needle is then advanced slightly further (i.e., 3 to 4 cm past contact with the bone). Ultimately, the tips of the needles should be just posterior to the aorta on the left and to the anterolateral aspect of the aorta on the right (Fig. 76-2).

The stylets of the needles are removed, and the needle hubs are inspected for the presence of blood, cerebrospinal fluid, or urine. If radiographic guidance is being used, a small amount of contrast material is injected through each needle, and its spread is observed radiographically. On the fluoroscopic anteroposterior view, contrast is confined to the midline and concentrated near the L1 vertebral body (Fig. 76-3). A smooth posterior contour can be observed that corresponds to the psoas fascia on the lateral view (Fig. 76-4). Alternatively, if computed tomographic guidance is used, contrast should appear lateral to and behind the aorta. If the contrast is entirely retrocrural, the needles should be advanced to the precrural space to avoid any risk for spread of local anesthetic or neurolytic agent posteriorly to the somatic nerve roots.

If radiographic guidance is not used, a rapid-onset local anesthetic is used in sufficient concentration to produce motor block (e.g., 1.5% lidocaine or 3.0% 2-chloroprocaine) before administration of neurolytic agents. If the patient experiences no motor or sensory block in the lumbar dermatomes after an adequate time, additional drugs injected through the needles will probably not reach the somatic nerve roots if given in like volumes.

For diagnostic and prognostic block using the retrocrural technique, a 12- to 15-mL volume of 1.0% lidocaine or 3.0% 2-chloroprocaine is administered through each needle. For therapeutic block, 10 to 12 mL of 0.5% bupivacaine is administered through each needle. Because of the potential for local anesthetic toxicity, all local anesthetics should be administered in incremental doses. When treating acute pancreatitis or pain of malignant origin, an 80-mg dose of depot methylprednisolone is advocated for the initial celiac plexus block, with a 40-mg dose given for subsequent blocks.

A 10- to 12-mL volume of absolute alcohol or 6.0% aqueous phenol is injected through each needle for retrocrural neurolytic block. Alternatively, 25 mL of 50% ethyl alcohol can be injected via each needle. After neurolytic solution is injected, each needle should be flushed with sterile saline solution because there have been anecdotal reports of neurolytic solution being tracked posteriorly with the needles as they are withdrawn.

SIDE EFFECTS AND COMPLICATIONS

Because of the proximity to vascular structures, celiac plexus block is contraindicated in patients who are on anticoagulant therapy or suffer from coagulopathy secondary to antiblastic cancer therapies or liver

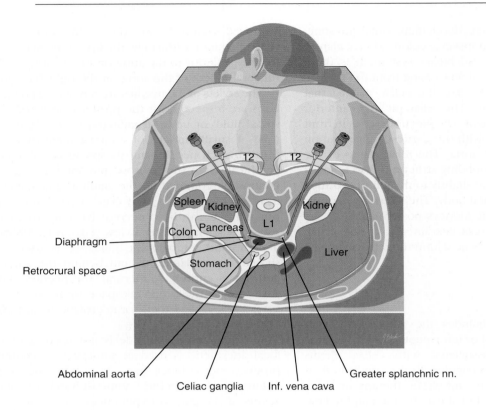

Figure 76-1.

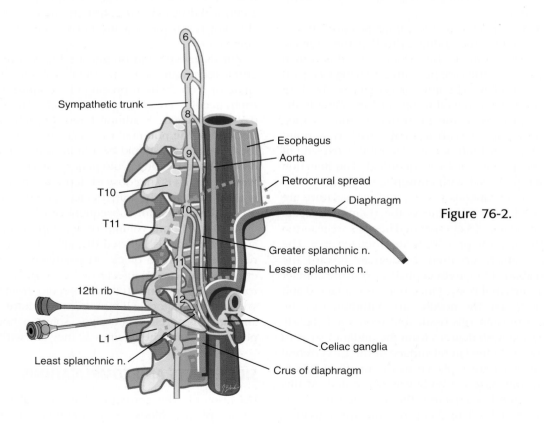

Figure 76-2.

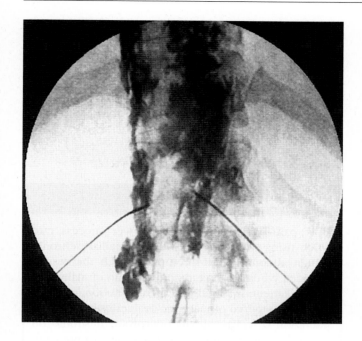

Figure 76-3.
Anteroposterior fluoroscopic view of the midline placement of contrast agent at L1. (From Waldman SD: Interventional Pain Management, 2nd ed. Philadelphia, WB Saunders, 2001, p 497.)

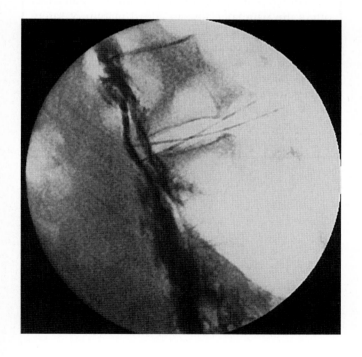

Figure 76-4.
Lateral fluoroscopic view of contrast agent bounded by psoas fascia. (From Waldman SD: Interventional Pain Management, 2nd ed. Philadelphia, WB Saunders, 2001, p 497.)

abnormalities associated with ethanol abuse. Intravascular injection of solutions may result in thrombosis of the nutrient vessels to the spinal cord with secondary paraplegia. Local and intra-abdominal infection, as well as sepsis, are absolute contraindications to celiac plexus block.

Because blockade of the celiac plexus results in increased bowel motility, this technique should be avoided in patients with bowel obstruction. Postblock diarrhea occurs in about 50% of patients. Celiac plexus block should be deferred in patients who suffer from chronic abdominal pain, who are chemically dependent, or who exhibit drug-seeking behavior until these issues have been adequately addressed. Alcohol should not be used as a neurolytic agent in patients on disulfiram therapy for alcohol abuse.

The proximity to the spinal cord, exiting nerve roots, pleural space, and viscera makes it imperative that this procedure be performed only by those well versed in the regional anatomy and experienced in interventional pain management techniques. Needle placement that is too medial may result in epidural, subdural, or subarachnoid injections or trauma to the spinal cord and exiting nerve roots. Such incorrect needle placement can result in severe neurologic deficits, including paraplegia. Medial needle placement also may result in intradiskal placement and resultant diskitis. Because the needle terminus is retrocrural when the classic two-needle approach to splanchnic nerve block is used, there is an increased incidence of neurologic complications, including neurolysis of the lumbar nerve roots with resultant hip flexor weakness and lower extremity numbness. Techniques that result in precrural needle placement, such as the transcrural and transaortic approaches to celiac plexus block, have a lower incidence of this complication and should be considered by the pain management specialist.

Given the proximity of the pleural space, pneumothorax after celiac plexus block may occur if the needle is placed too cephalad. Trauma to the thoracic duct with resultant chylothorax also may occur. If the needles are placed too laterally, trauma to the kidneys and ureters is a distinct possibility.

CLINICAL PEARLS

Most pain specialists report a lower success rate when using celiac plexus block to palliate chronic benign abdominal pain compared with the results obtained when treating abdominal pain of malignant origin. Patients with chronic benign abdominal pain should be tapered off narcotic analgesics before consideration of celiac plexus neurolysis. It should be noted that the phrenic nerve also transmits nociceptive information from the upper abdominal viscera. This information is perceived as poorly localized pain referred to the supraclavicular region; this source of pain should be considered in all patients with upper abdominal pain.

Radiographic guidance, especially CT guidance, offers the pain specialist an added margin of safety during neurolytic celiac plexus block and hence should be used routinely unless the patient's clinical status requires that celiac plexus block be performed at the bedside. Given the increased incidence of damage to the lumbar nerve roots due to the retrocrural placement of needles when the classic two-needle technique is used, the transcrural or transaortic approach to celiac plexus block is preferred.

CHAPTER **77**

Celiac Plexus Block: Single-Needle Retrocrural Technique

INDICATIONS

Until recently, celiac plexus block via the classic two-needle retrocrural technique has been the celiac plexus block technique most used by pain management specialists. Because the needle terminus is retrocrural with this technique, a higher incidence of neurologic complications is to be expected compared with techniques that result in precrural needle placement. However, because of the long track record of efficacy and safety enjoyed by the classic two-needle approach to celiac plexus block, this technique remains an acceptable approach to blockade of the celiac plexus. By using a single needle, the complications associated with the classic two-needle approach can be decreased.

Celiac plexus block with local anesthetic is indicated as a diagnostic maneuver to determine whether flank, retroperitoneal, or upper abdominal pain is sympathetically mediated via the celiac plexus. Daily celiac plexus block with local anesthetic also is useful in the palliation of pain secondary to acute pancreatitis and other acute pain syndromes subserved by the celiac plexus. Early implementation of celiac plexus block with local anesthetic, steroids, or both markedly reduces the morbidity and mortality associated with acute pancreatitis. Celiac plexus block also is used to palliate the acute pain of arterial embolization of the liver for cancer therapy as well as to treat the pain of abdominal "angina" associated

with visceral arterial insufficiency. Celiac plexus block with local anesthetic also may be used prognostically before celiac plexus neurolysis.

Neurolysis of the celiac plexus with alcohol or phenol is indicated to treat pain secondary to malignancies of the retroperitoneum and upper abdomen. Neurolytic celiac plexus block also may be useful in some chronic benign abdominal pain syndromes, including chronic pancreatitis, in carefully selected patients.

CLINICALLY RELEVANT ANATOMY

The sympathetic innervation of the abdominal viscera originates in the anterolateral horn of the spinal cord. Preganglionic fibers from T5-T12 exit the spinal cord in conjunction with the ventral roots to join the white communicating rami on their way to the sympathetic chain. Rather than synapsing with the sympathetic chain, these preganglionic fibers pass through it to ultimately synapse on the celiac ganglia. The greater, lesser, and least splanchnic nerves provide the major preganglionic contribution to the celiac plexus. The greater splanchnic nerve has its origin from the T5-T10 spinal roots. The nerve travels along the thoracic paravertebral border through the crus of the diaphragm into the abdominal cavity, ending on the celiac ganglion of its respective side. The lesser splanchnic nerve arises from the T10-T11 roots and passes with the greater nerve to end at the celiac ganglion. The least splanchnic nerve arises from the T11-T12 spinal roots and passes through the diaphragm to the celiac ganglion.

Interpatient anatomic variability of the celiac ganglia is significant, but the following generalizations can be drawn from anatomic studies of the celiac ganglia. The number of ganglia varies from one to five, and they range in diameter from 0.5 to 4.5 cm. The ganglia lie anterior and anterolateral to the aorta. The ganglia located on the left are uniformly more inferior than their right-sided counterparts by as much as a vertebral level, but both groups of ganglia lie below the level of the celiac artery. The ganglia usually lie about at the level of the first lumbar vertebra.

Postganglionic fibers radiate from the celiac ganglia to follow the course of the blood vessels to innervate the abdominal viscera. These organs include much of the distal esophagus, stomach, duodenum, small intestine, ascending and proximal transverse colon, adrenal glands, pancreas, spleen, liver, and biliary system. It is these postganglionic fibers, the fibers arising from the preganglionic splanchnic nerves, and the celiac ganglia that make up the celiac plexus. The celiac plexus is anterior to the crus of the diaphragm. The plexus extends in front of and around the aorta, with the greatest concentration of fibers anterior to the aorta. The relationship of the celiac plexus to the surrounding structures is as follows: The aorta lies anterior and slightly to the left of the anterior margin of the vertebral body. The inferior vena cava lies to the right, with the kidneys posterolateral to the great vessels. The pancreas lies anterior to the celiac plexus. All these structures lie within the retroperitoneal space.

TECHNIQUE

Preblock preparation includes the administration of adequate amounts of oral or intravenous fluids to attenuate the hypotension associated with celiac plexus block. Evaluation for coagulopathy is indicated if the patient has undergone antiblastic therapy or has a history of significant alcohol abuse. If radiographic contrast is to be used, evaluation of the patient's renal status also is indicated.

The patient is placed in the prone position with a pillow placed under the abdomen to flex the thoracolumbar spine. For comfort, the patient's head is turned to the side, and the arms are permitted to hang freely off each side of the table. The inferior margins of the 12th ribs are identified and traced to the T12 vertebral body. The spinous process of the L1 vertebral body is then identified and marked with a sterile marker. A point about 2½ inches just inferior and lateral to each side of the transverse process of L1 is identified. The injection sites are then prepared with antiseptic solution.

The skin, subcutaneous tissues, and musculature are infiltrated with 1.0% lidocaine at the points of needle entry. A 20-gauge, 13-cm styletted needle is inserted on the left of the midline through the previously anesthetized area. The needle is initially oriented 45 degrees toward the midline and about 15 degrees cephalad to ensure contact with the L1 vertebral body. Once bone is contacted and the depth is noted, the needle is withdrawn to the level of the subcutaneous tissue and redirected slightly less mesiad (about 60 degrees from the midline) so as to walk off (Fig. 77-1) the lateral surface of the L1 vertebral body. The needle is repositioned to the depth at which contact with the vertebral body was first noted. At this point, if no bone is contacted, the needle is gradually advanced 1.5 to 2 cm, or until the pulsation emanating from the aorta and transmitted to the advancing needle is noted. Ultimately, the tip of the needle should be just posterior to the aorta on the left and to the anterolateral aspect of the aorta on the right (Fig. 77-2).

The stylet of the needle is removed, and the needle hub is inspected for the presence of blood, cerebrospinal fluid, or urine. If radiographic guidance is being used, a small amount of contrast material is injected through the needle, and its spread is observed radiographically. On the fluoroscopic anteroposterior view, contrast is confined to the midline and concentrated near the L1 vertebral body. A smooth posterior contour can be observed that corresponds to the psoas fascia on the lateral view. Alternatively, if computed tomographic guidance is used, contrast should appear lateral to and behind the aorta. If the contrast is entirely retrocrural, the needle should be advanced to the precrural space to avoid any risk for spread of local anesthetic or neurolytic agent posteriorly to the somatic nerve roots.

If radiographic guidance is not used, a rapid-onset local anesthetic is used in sufficient concentration to produce motor block (e.g., 1.5% lidocaine or 3.0% 2-chloroprocaine) before administration of neurolytic agents. If the patient experiences no motor or sensory block in the lumbar dermatomes after an adequate time, additional drugs injected through the needle will probably not reach the somatic nerve roots if given in like volumes.

For diagnostic and prognostic block using the retrocrural technique, a 12- to 15-mL volume of 1.0% lidocaine or 3.0% 2-chloroprocaine is administered through the needle. For therapeutic block, 10 to 12 mL of 0.5% bupivacaine is administered through the needle. Because of the potential for local anesthetic toxicity, all local anesthetics should be administered in incremental doses. When treating acute pancreatitis or pain of malignant origin, an 80-mg dose of depot methylprednisolone is advocated for the initial celiac plexus block, with a 40-mg dose given for subsequent blocks.

A 10- to 12-mL volume of absolute alcohol or 6.0% aqueous phenol is injected through the needle for retrocrural neurolytic block. Alternatively, 25 mL of 50% ethyl alcohol can be injected via the needle. After neurolytic solution is injected, the needle should be flushed with sterile saline solution because there have been anecdotal reports of neurolytic solution being tracked posteriorly with the needle as it is withdrawn.

SIDE EFFECTS AND COMPLICATIONS

Because of the proximity to vascular structures, celiac plexus block is contraindicated in patients who are on anticoagulant therapy or suffer from coagulopathy secondary to antiblastic cancer therapies or liver

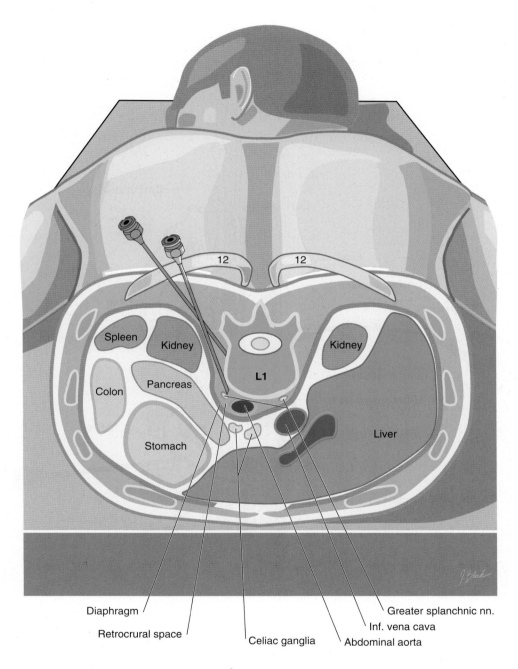

Figure 77-1.

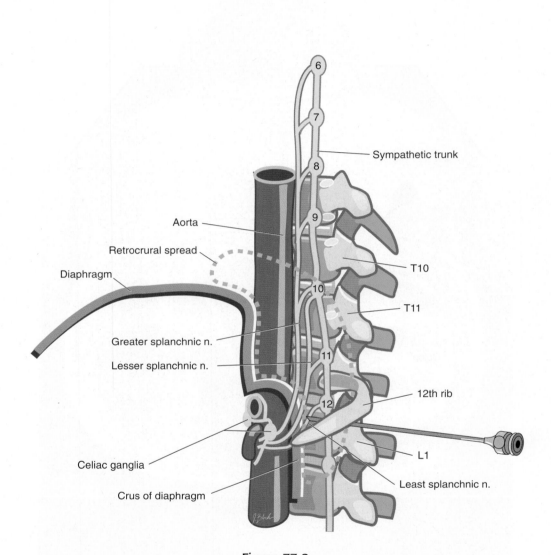

Figure 77-2.

abnormalities associated with ethanol abuse. Intravascular injection of solutions may result in thrombosis of the nutrient vessels to the spinal cord with secondary paraplegia. Local and intra-abdominal infection, as well as sepsis, are absolute contraindications to celiac plexus block.

Because blockade of the celiac plexus results in increased bowel motility, this technique should be avoided in patients with bowel obstruction. Postblock diarrhea occurs in about 50% of patients. Celiac plexus block should be deferred in patients who suffer from chronic abdominal pain, who are chemically dependent, or who exhibit drug-seeking behavior until these issues have been adequately addressed. Alcohol should not be used as a neurolytic agent in patients on disulfiram therapy for alcohol abuse.

The proximity to the spinal cord, exiting nerve roots, pleural space, and viscera makes it imperative that this procedure be performed only by those well versed in the regional anatomy and experienced in interventional pain management techniques. Needle placement that is too medial may result in epidural, subdural, or subarachnoid injections or trauma to the spinal cord and exiting nerve roots. Such incorrect needle placement can result in severe neurologic deficits, including paraplegia. Medial needle placement also may result in intradiskal placement and resultant diskitis. Because the needle terminus is retrocrural when the classic two-needle approach to splanchnic nerve block is used, there is an increased incidence of neurologic complications, including neurolysis of the lumbar nerve roots with resultant hip flexor weakness and lower extremity numbness. Techniques that result in precrural needle placement, such as the transcrural and transaortic approaches to celiac plexus block, have a lower incidence of this complication and should be considered by the pain management specialist.

Given the proximity of the pleural space, pneumothorax after celiac plexus block may occur if the needle is placed too cephalad. Trauma to the thoracic duct with resultant chylothorax also may occur. If the needle is placed too laterally, trauma to the kidneys and ureters is a distinct possibility.

CLINICAL PEARLS

Most pain specialists report a lower success rate when using celiac plexus block to palliate chronic benign abdominal pain compared with the results obtained when treating abdominal pain of malignant origin. Patients with chronic benign abdominal pain should be tapered off narcotic analgesics before consideration of celiac plexus neurolysis. It should be noted that the phrenic nerve also transmits nociceptive information from the upper abdominal viscera. This information is perceived as poorly localized pain referred to the supraclavicular region; this source of pain should be considered in all patients suffering from upper abdominal pain.

Radiographic guidance, especially CT guidance, offers the pain specialist an added margin of safety during neurolytic celiac plexus block and hence should be used routinely unless the patient's clinical status requires that celiac plexus block be performed at the bedside. Given the increased incidence of damage to the lumbar nerve roots due to the retrocrural placement of needles when the classic two-needle technique is used, the transcrural or transaortic approach to celiac plexus block is preferred.

CHAPTER 78

Celiac Plexus Block: Two-Needle Transcrural Technique

CPT-2009 CODE	
Local Anesthetic–With or Without Radiographic Monitoring	64530
Neurolytic–With or Without Radiographic Monitoring	64680

Relative Value Units	
Local Anesthetic	18
Neurolytic	20

INDICATIONS

The transcrural approach to celiac plexus block has gained increasing favor with pain management specialists. The transcrural approach to celiac plexus block has the advantage over the classic two-needle retrocrural technique in that the needle terminus is precrural, thus avoiding the higher incidence of neurologic complications associated with retrocrural needle placement. Because the transcrural approach to celiac plexus block is essentially a modification of the classic two-needle retrocrural technique that most pain specialists are familiar with, it is rapidly becoming the standard by which other approaches to celiac plexus block are judged.

Celiac plexus block using the transcrural approach with local anesthetic is indicated as a diagnostic maneuver to determine whether flank, retroperitoneal, or upper abdominal pain is sympathetically mediated via the celiac plexus. Daily transcrural celiac plexus block with local anesthetic also is useful in the palliation of pain secondary to acute pancreatitis and other acute pain syndromes subserved by the celiac plexus. Early implementation of celiac plexus block with local anesthetic, steroids, or both markedly reduces the morbidity and mortality associated with acute pancreatitis. Transcrural celiac plexus block also is used to palliate the acute pain of arterial embolization of the liver for cancer therapy as

well as to treat the pain of abdominal "angina" associated with visceral arterial insufficiency. Transcrural celiac plexus block with local anesthetic also may be used prognostically before celiac plexus neurolysis.

Neurolysis of the celiac plexus via the transcrural approach with alcohol or phenol is indicated to treat pain secondary to malignancies of the retroperitoneum and upper abdomen. Neurolytic celiac plexus block using the transcrural approach also may be useful in some chronic benign abdominal pain syndromes, including chronic pancreatitis, in carefully selected patients.

CLINICALLY RELEVANT ANATOMY

The sympathetic innervation of the abdominal viscera originates in the anterolateral horn of the spinal cord. Preganglionic fibers from T5-T12 exit the spinal cord in conjunction with the ventral roots to join the white communicating rami on their way to the sympathetic chain. Rather than synapsing with the sympathetic chain, these preganglionic fibers pass through it to ultimately synapse on the celiac ganglia. The greater, lesser, and least splanchnic nerves provide the major preganglionic contribution to the celiac plexus. The greater splanchnic nerve has its origin from the T5-T10 spinal roots. The nerve travels along the thoracic paravertebral border through the crus of the diaphragm into the abdominal cavity, ending on the celiac ganglion of its respective side. The lesser splanchnic nerve arises from the T10-T11 roots and passes with the greater nerve to end at the celiac ganglion. The least splanchnic nerve arises from the T11-T12 spinal roots and passes through the diaphragm to the celiac ganglion.

Interpatient anatomic variability of the celiac ganglia is significant, but the following generalizations can be drawn from anatomic studies of the celiac ganglia. The number of ganglia vary from one to five and range in diameter from 0.5 to 4.5 cm. The ganglia lie anterior and anterolateral to the aorta. The ganglia located on the left are uniformly more inferior than their right-sided counterparts by as much as a vertebral level, but both groups of ganglia lie below the level of the celiac artery. The ganglia usually lie about at the level of the first lumbar vertebra.

Postganglionic fibers radiate from the celiac ganglia to follow the course of the blood vessels to innervate the abdominal viscera. These organs include much of the distal esophagus, stomach, duodenum, small intestine, ascending and proximal transverse colon, adrenal glands, pancreas, spleen, liver, and biliary system. It is these postganglionic fibers, the fibers arising from the preganglionic splanchnic nerves, and the celiac ganglion that make up the celiac plexus. The diaphragm separates the thorax from the abdominal cavity while still permitting the passage of the thoracoabdominal structures, including the aorta, vena cava, and splanchnic nerves. The diaphragmatic crura are bilateral structures that arise from the anterolateral surfaces of the upper two or three lumbar vertebrae and disks. The crura of the diaphragm serve as a barrier to effectively separate the splanchnic nerves from the celiac ganglia and plexus below.

The celiac plexus is anterior to the crus of the diaphragm. The plexus extends in front of and around the aorta, with the greatest concentration of fibers anterior to the aorta. When the transcrural approach to celiac plexus block is used, the needles are placed close to this concentration of plexus fibers. The relationship of the celiac plexus to the surrounding structures is as follows: The aorta lies anterior and slightly to the left of the anterior margin of the vertebral body. The inferior vena cava lies to the right, with the kidneys posterolateral to the great vessels (Fig. 78-1). The pancreas lies anterior to the celiac plexus. All these structures lie within the retroperitoneal space.

TECHNIQUE

Preblock preparation includes the administration of adequate amounts of oral or intravenous fluids to attenuate the hypotension associated with celiac plexus block. Evaluation of the patient for coagulopathy is indicated if the patient has undergone antiblastic therapy or has a history of significant alcohol abuse. If radiographic contrast is to be used, evaluation of the patient's renal status also is indicated.

The patient is placed in the prone position with a pillow placed under the abdomen to flex the thoracolumbar spine. For comfort, the patient's head is turned to the side, and the arms are permitted to hang freely off each side of the table. The inferior margins of the 12th ribs are identified and traced to the T12 vertebral body. The spinous process of the L1 vertebral body is then identified and marked with a sterile marker. A point about 2½ inches just inferior and lateral to each side of the transverse process of L1 is identified. The injection sites are then prepared with antiseptic solution.

The skin, subcutaneous tissues, and musculature are infiltrated with 1.0% lidocaine at the points of needle entry. Twenty-gauge, 13-cm styletted needles are inserted bilaterally through the previously anesthetized area. The needles are initially oriented 45 degrees toward the midline and about 15 degrees cephalad to ensure contact with the L1 vertebral body. Once bone is contacted and the depth is noted, the needles are withdrawn to the level of the subcutaneous tissue and redirected slightly less mesiad (about 60 degrees from the midline) so as to walk off the lateral surface of the L1 vertebral body (Fig. 78-2). The needles are replaced to the depth at which contact with the vertebral body was first noted. At this point, if no bone is contacted, the left-sided needle is gradually advanced 3 to 4 cm, or until the pulsation emanating from the aorta and transmitted to the advancing needle is noted. If aortic pulsations are noted, the pain specialist may either convert the block into a transaortic celiac plexus technique or note the depth to which the needle has been placed, withdraw the needle into the subcutaneous tissues, and then redirect the needle less medially to slide laterally to the aorta in front of the crura of the diaphragm. The right-sided needle is then advanced slightly farther (i.e., 4 to 5 cm past contact with the bone). Ultimately, the tips of the needles should be just lateral and anterior to the aorta on the left and to the anterolateral aspect of the aorta on the right (Fig. 78-3). This periaortic precrural placement decreases the incidence of inadvertent spread of injected solutions onto the lumbar somatic nerve roots.

The stylets of the needles are removed and the needle hubs are inspected for the presence of blood, cerebrospinal fluid, or urine. If radiographic guidance is being used, a small amount of contrast material is injected through each needle, and its spread is observed radiographically. On the fluoroscopic anteroposterior view, contrast is confined to the midline and concentrated in the midline near the L1 vertebral body. A smooth curvilinear shadow can be observed that corresponds to the preaortic space on the lateral view. Alternatively, if computed tomographic guidance is used, contrast should appear periaortic or, if adenopathy or tumor is present, contrast should be identified lateral to the aorta bilaterally. If this occurs, one should consider redirecting the left needle more medially to pass transaortically, thus placing the needle tip just in front of the aorta. If the contrast is entirely retrocrural, the needles should be advanced to the precrural space to avoid any risk for spread of local anesthetic or neurolytic agent posteriorly to the somatic nerve roots.

If radiographic guidance is not used, a rapid-onset local anesthetic is used in sufficient concentration to produce motor block (e.g., 1.5% lidocaine or 3.0% 2-chloroprocaine) before administration of neurolytic agents. If the patient experiences no motor or sensory

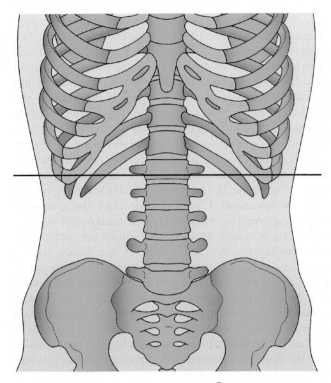

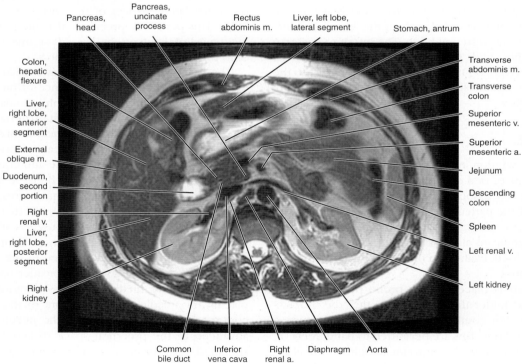

Pancreas, head

Pancreas, uncinate process

Rectus abdominis m.

Liver, left lobe, lateral segment

Stomach, antrum

Colon, hepatic flexure

Liver, right lobe, anterior segment

External oblique m.

Duodenum, second portion

Right renal v.

Liver, right lobe, posterior segment

Right kidney

Transverse abdominis m.

Transverse colon

Superior mesenteric v.

Superior mesenteric a.

Jejunum

Descending colon

Spleen

Left renal v.

Left kidney

Common bile duct

Inferior vena cava

Right renal a.

Diaphragm

Aorta

Figure 78-1.

(From El-Khoury GY, Bergman RA, Montgomery WJ: Sectional Anatomy by MRI and CT, 3rd ed. New York, Churchill Livingstone, 2007, p 511.)

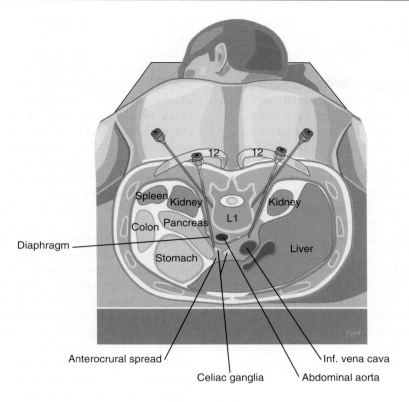

Figure 78-2.

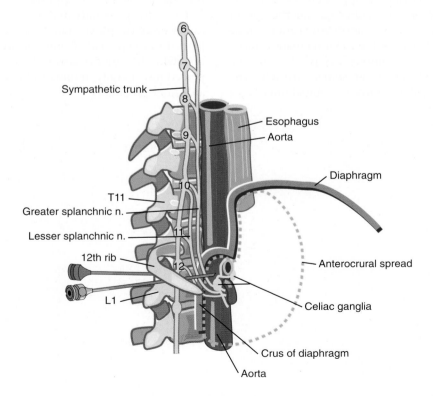

Figure 78-3.

block in the lumbar dermatomes after an adequate time, additional drugs injected through the needles will probably not reach the somatic nerve roots if given in like volumes.

For diagnostic and prognostic block via the transcrural technique, 12 to 15 mL of 1.0% lidocaine or 3.0% 2-chloroprocaine is administered through each needle. For therapeutic block, 10 to 12 mL of 0.5% bupivacaine is administered through each needle. Because of the potential for local anesthetic toxicity, all local anesthetics should be administered in incremental doses. During treatment of acute pancreatitis or pain of malignant origin, an 80-mg dose of depot methylprednisolone is advocated for the initial celiac plexus block, with a 40-mg dose given for subsequent blocks.

A 10- to 12-mL volume of absolute alcohol or 6.0% aqueous phenol is injected through each needle for transcrural neurolytic block. Alternatively, 25 mL of 50% ethyl alcohol can be injected via each needle. After neurolytic solution is injected, each needle should be flushed with sterile saline solution because there have been anecdotal reports of neurolytic solution being tracked posteriorly with the needles as they are withdrawn.

SIDE EFFECTS AND COMPLICATIONS

Because of its proximity to vascular structures, celiac plexus block via the transcrural approach is contraindicated in patients who are on anticoagulant therapy or have coagulopathy secondary to antiblastic cancer therapies or liver abnormalities associated with ethanol abuse. Intravascular injection of solutions may result in thrombosis of the nutrient vessels to the spinal cord with secondary paraplegia. Local and intra-abdominal infections, as well as sepsis, are absolute contraindications to celiac plexus block.

Because blockade of the celiac plexus results in increased bowel motility, this technique should be avoided in patients with bowel obstruction. Postblock diarrhea occurs in about 50% of patients. Celiac plexus block should be deferred in patients who suffer from chronic abdominal pain, who are chemically dependent, or who exhibit drug-seeking behavior until these issues have been adequately addressed. Alcohol should not be used as a neurolytic agent in patients on disulfiram therapy for alcohol abuse.

The proximity to the spinal cord, exiting nerve roots, pleural space, and viscera makes it imperative that this procedure be performed only by those well versed in the regional anatomy and experienced in interventional pain management techniques. Needle placement that is too medial may result in epidural, subdural, or subarachnoid injections or trauma to the spinal cord and exiting nerve roots. Such incorrect needle placement can result in severe neurologic deficits, including paraplegia. Medial needle placement also may result in intradiskal placement and resultant diskitis. Because the needle terminus is precrural when the transcrural approach to splanchnic nerve block is used, there is a decreased incidence of neurologic complications, including neurolysis of the lumbar nerve roots with resultant hip flexor weakness and lower extremity numbness, when compared with the classic two-needle approach to celiac plexus block.

Given the proximity of the pleural space, pneumothorax after celiac plexus block may occur if the needle is placed too cephalad. Trauma to the thoracic duct with resultant chylothorax also may occur. If the needles are placed too laterally, trauma to the kidneys and ureters is a distinct possibility.

CLINICAL PEARLS

When using the classic two-needle retrocrural approach to celiac plexus block, the needles will almost always be retrocrural in proximity to the splanchnic nerves rather than the celiac ganglia. That is to say, the needles and injected solution will be placed posterior and cephalad to the crura of the diaphragm.

CT and cadaver studies have given rise to the recent suggestion that the classic method of retrocrural block is more likely to produce splanchnic nerve block than blockade of the celiac plexus. This is because this approach does not result in the deposition of injected material around and anterior to the aorta and directly onto the celiac plexus at the level of the L1 vertebral body, as previously thought. Rather, the injectate appears to follow this path:

1. Concentrate posterior to the aorta and in front of and along the side of the L1 vertebral body, where it may anesthetize retroaortic celiac fibers.
2. Diffuse cephalad to anesthetize the splanchnic nerve at a site rostral to the origin of the plexus.
3. Only finally encircle the aorta at the site of the celiac plexus when enough drug is injected to transgress the diaphragm by diffusing caudad through the aortic hiatus.

Unfortunately, this larger volume of drug also is associated with an increased incidence of blockade of the lumbar somatic nerve roots.

Radiographic guidance, especially CT guidance, offers the pain specialist an added margin of safety during neurolytic celiac plexus block via the transcrural approach and hence should be used routinely unless the patient's clinical status requires that celiac plexus block be performed at the bedside. Given the increased incidence of damage to the lumbar nerve roots because of the retrocrural placement of needles with the classic two-needle technique, the transcrural, single-needle periaortic or transaortic approach to celiac plexus block is preferred.

Most pain specialists report a lower success rate when using celiac plexus block to treat chronic benign abdominal pain than when treating abdominal pain of malignant origin. Patients with chronic benign abdominal pain should be tapered off narcotic analgesics before consideration of celiac plexus neurolysis. It should be noted that the phrenic nerve also transmits nociceptive information from the upper abdominal viscera. This information is perceived as poorly localized pain referred to the supraclavicular region; this source of pain should be considered in all patients suffering from upper abdominal pain.

CHAPTER 79

Celiac Plexus Block: Single-Needle Periaortic Technique

INDICATIONS

Pain management specialists began performing celiac plexus block using a single needle after it was recognized that, when using the two-needle transcrural approach to celiac plexus block under computed tomographic guidance, contrast injected via the left-sided needle would spread around the aorta, obviating the need for injection through the second needle. The use of a single needle decreases needle-related complications as well as the pain associated with the procedure. The single-needle periaortic approach to celiac plexus block has the added advantage over the classic two-needle retrocrural technique in that the single needle is placed in the precrural space, thus avoiding the higher incidence of neurologic complications associated with retrocrural needle placement.

Celiac plexus block using the single-needle periaortic approach with local anesthetic is indicated as a diagnostic maneuver to determine whether flank, retroperitoneal, or upper abdominal pain is sympathetically mediated via the celiac plexus. Daily celiac plexus block with local anesthetic also is useful in the palliation of pain secondary to acute pancreatitis and other acute pain syndromes subserved by the celiac plexus. Early implementation of celiac plexus block with local anesthetic, steroids, or both markedly reduces the morbidity and mortality associated with acute pancreatitis. Single-

needle periaortic celiac plexus block also is used to palliate the acute pain of arterial embolization of the liver for cancer therapy as well as to treat the pain of abdominal "angina" associated with visceral arterial insufficiency. Single-needle periaortic celiac plexus block with local anesthetic also may be used prognostically before celiac plexus neurolysis.

Neurolysis of the celiac plexus via the single-needle periaortic approach with alcohol or phenol is indicated to treat pain secondary to malignancies of the retroperitoneum and upper abdomen. This approach also may be useful in some chronic benign abdominal pain syndromes, including chronic pancreatitis, in carefully selected patients.

CLINICALLY RELEVANT ANATOMY

The sympathetic innervation of the abdominal viscera originates in the anterolateral horn of the spinal cord. Preganglionic fibers from T5-T12 exit the spinal cord in conjunction with the ventral roots to join the white communicating rami on their way to the sympathetic chain. Rather than synapsing with the sympathetic chain, these preganglionic fibers pass through it to ultimately synapse on the celiac ganglia. The greater, lesser, and least splanchnic nerves provide the major preganglionic contribution to the celiac plexus. The greater splanchnic nerve has its origin from the T5-T10 spinal roots. The nerve travels along the thoracic paravertebral border through the crus of the diaphragm into the abdominal cavity, ending on the celiac ganglion of its respective side. The lesser splanchnic nerve arises from the T10-T11 roots and passes with the greater nerve to end at the celiac ganglion. The least splanchnic nerve arises from the T11-T12 spinal roots and passes through the diaphragm to the celiac ganglion.

Interpatient anatomic variability of the celiac ganglia is significant, but the following generalizations can be drawn from anatomic studies of the celiac ganglia. The number of ganglia varies from one to five, and they range in diameter from 0.5 to 4.5 cm. The ganglia lie anterior and anterolateral to the aorta. The ganglia located on the left are uniformly more inferior than their right-sided counterparts by as much as a vertebral level, but both groups of ganglia lie below the level of the celiac artery. The ganglia usually lie about at the level of the first lumbar vertebra.

Postganglionic fibers radiate from the celiac ganglia to follow the course of the blood vessels to innervate the abdominal viscera. These organs include much of the distal esophagus, stomach, duodenum, small intestine, ascending and proximal transverse colon, adrenal glands, pancreas, spleen, liver, and biliary system. It is these postganglionic fibers, the fibers arising from the preganglionic splanchnic nerves, and the celiac ganglion that make up the celiac plexus. The diaphragm separates the thorax from the abdominal cavity while still permitting the passage of the thoracoabdominal structures, including the aorta, vena cava, and splanchnic nerves. The diaphragmatic crura are bilateral structures that arise from the anterolateral surfaces of the upper two or three lumbar vertebrae and disks. The crura of the diaphragm serve as a barrier to effectively separate the splanchnic nerves from the celiac ganglia and plexus below.

The celiac plexus is anterior to the crus of the diaphragm. The plexus extends in front of and around the aorta, with the greatest concentration of fibers anterior to the aorta. With the single-needle periaortic approach to celiac plexus block, the needle is placed close to this concentration of plexus fibers. The relationship of the celiac plexus to the surrounding structures is as follows: The aorta lies anterior and slightly to the left of the anterior margin of the vertebral body. The inferior vena cava lies to the right, with the kidneys posterolateral to the great vessels. The pancreas lies anterior to the celiac plexus. All of these structures lie within the retroperitoneal space.

TECHNIQUE

Preblock preparation includes the administration of adequate amounts of oral or intravenous fluids to attenuate the hypotension associated with celiac plexus block. Evaluation of the patient for coagulopathy is indicated if the patient has undergone antiblastic therapy or has a history of significant alcohol abuse. If radiographic contrast is to be used, evaluation of the patient's renal status also is indicated.

The patient is placed in the prone position with a pillow placed under the abdomen to flex the thoracolumbar spine. For comfort, the patient's head is turned to the side, and the arms are permitted to hang freely off each side of the table. The inferior margins of the 12th ribs are identified and traced to the T12 vertebral body. The spinous process of the L1 vertebral body is then identified and marked with a sterile marker. A point about 2½ inches just inferior and lateral to the left side

of the transverse process of L1 is identified. The injection site is then prepared with antiseptic solution.

The skin, subcutaneous tissues, and musculature are infiltrated with 1.0% lidocaine at the point of needle entry. A 20-gauge, 13-cm styletted needle is inserted bilaterally through the previously anesthetized area. The needle is initially oriented 45 degrees toward the midline and about 15 degrees cephalad to ensure contact with the L1 vertebral body. Once bone is contacted and the depth noted, the needle is withdrawn to the level of the subcutaneous tissue and redirected less mesiad (about 65 degrees from the midline) so as to walk off the lateral surface of the L1 vertebral body (Fig. 79-1). The needle is reinserted to the depth at which the vertebral body was first contacted. At this point, if no bone is contacted, the needle is gradually advanced 3 to 4 cm, or until the pulsation emanating from the aorta and transmitted to the advancing needle is noted. If aortic pulsations are noted, the pain specialist may either convert the block into a transaortic celiac plexus technique or note the depth to which the needle has been placed, withdraw the needle into the subcutaneous tissues, and then redirect the needle less mesiad to slide laterally to the aorta. Ultimately, the tip of the needle should be just lateral and anterior to the side of the aorta (Fig. 79-2). This periaortic precrural placement decreases the incidence of inadvertent spread of injected solutions onto the lumbar somatic nerve roots.

The stylet of the needle is removed, and the needle hub is inspected for the presence of blood, cerebrospinal fluid, or urine. If radiographic guidance is being used, a small amount of contrast material is injected through the needle, and its spread is observed radiographically. On the fluoroscopic anteroposterior view, contrast is confined primarily to the left of the midline near the L1 vertebral body. A smooth curvilinear shadow can be observed that corresponds to contrast in the preaortic space on the lateral view. Alternatively, if computed tomographic guidance is used, contrast should appear periaortic or, if adenopathy or tumor is present, contrast should be confined to the periaortic space to the left of the aorta. If this limitation of spread of contrast occurs, one should consider redirecting the needle more medially to pass through the aorta to place the needle tip just in front of the aorta. If the contrast is entirely retrocrural, the needle should be advanced to the precrural space to avoid any risk for spread of local anesthetic or neurolytic agent posteriorly to the somatic nerve roots.

If radiographic guidance is not used, a rapid-onset local anesthetic is used in sufficient concentration to produce motor block (e.g., 1.5% lidocaine or 3.0% 2-chloroprocaine) before administration of neurolytic agents. If the patient experiences no motor or sensory block in the lumbar dermatomes after an adequate time, additional drugs injected through the needles will

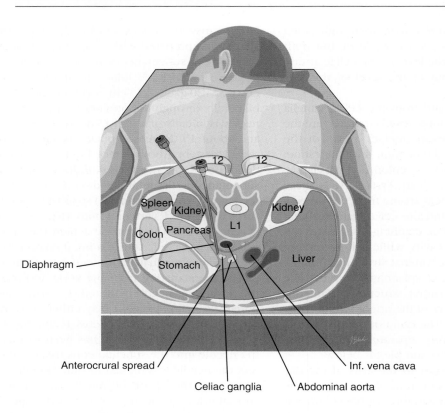

Figure 79-1.

Spleen
Kidney
Kidney
Colon
Pancreas
L1
Diaphragm
Stomach
Liver

Anterocrural spread

Celiac ganglia

Abdominal aorta

Inf. vena cava

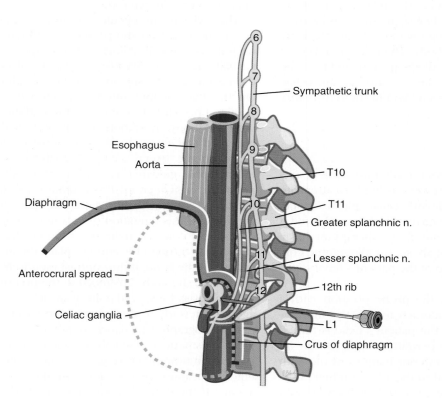

Figure 79-2.

Esophagus
Aorta
Diaphragm
Anterocrural spread
Celiac ganglia

Sympathetic trunk
T10
T11
Greater splanchnic n.
Lesser splanchnic n.
12th rib
L1
Crus of diaphragm

probably not reach the somatic nerve roots if given in like volumes.

For diagnostic and prognostic block via the single-needle periaortic technique, 12 to 15 mL of 1.0% lidocaine or 3.0% 2-chloroprocaine is administered through the needle. For therapeutic block, 10 to 12 mL of 0.5% bupivacaine is administered through the needle. Because of the potential for local anesthetic toxicity, all local anesthetics should be administered in incremental doses. When treating acute pancreatitis or pain of malignant origin, 80 mg of depot methylprednisolone is advocated for the initial celiac plexus block, with a 40-mg dose given for subsequent blocks.

A 10- to 12-mL volume of absolute alcohol or 6.0% aqueous phenol is injected through the needle for neurolytic block. Alternatively, 25 mL of 50% ethyl alcohol can be injected via the needle. After neurolytic solution is injected, the needle should be flushed with sterile saline solution because there have been anecdotal reports of neurolytic solution being tracked posteriorly with the needle as it is withdrawn.

SIDE EFFECTS AND COMPLICATIONS

Because of its proximity to vascular structures, celiac plexus block using the single-needle periaortic approach is contraindicated in patients who are on anticoagulant therapy or have coagulopathy secondary to antiblastic cancer therapies or liver abnormalities associated with ethanol abuse. Intravascular injection of solutions may result in thrombosis of the nutrient vessels to the spinal cord with secondary paraplegia. Local or intra-abdominal infection and sepsis are absolute contraindications to celiac plexus block.

Because blockade of the celiac plexus results in increased bowel motility, this technique should be avoided in patients with bowel obstruction. Postblock diarrhea occurs in about 50% of patients. Celiac plexus block should be deferred in patients who suffer from chronic abdominal pain, who are chemically dependent, or who exhibit drug-seeking behavior until these issues have been adequately addressed. Alcohol should not be used as a neurolytic agent in patients on disulfiram therapy for alcohol abuse.

The proximity to the spinal cord, exiting nerve roots, pleural space, and viscera makes it imperative that this procedure be carried out only by those well versed in the regional anatomy and experienced in interventional pain management techniques. Needle placement that is too medial may result in epidural, subdural, or subarachnoid injections or trauma to the spinal cord and exiting nerve roots. Such incorrect needle placement can result in severe neurologic deficits, including paraplegia. Medial needle placement also may result in intradiskal placement and resultant diskitis. Because the needle terminus is precrural with the single-needle periaortic approach to celiac plexus block, there is a decreased incidence of neurologic complications, including neurolysis of the lumbar nerve roots with resultant hip flexor weakness and lower extremity numbness compared with the classic two-needle approach to celiac plexus block.

Given the proximity of the pleural space, pneumothorax after celiac plexus block may occur if the needle is placed too cephalad. Trauma to the thoracic duct with resultant chylothorax also may occur. If the needle is placed too laterally, trauma to the kidneys and ureters is a distinct possibility.

CLINICAL PEARLS

When using the classic two-needle retrocrural approach to celiac plexus block, the needles will almost always be retrocrural in proximity to the splanchnic nerves rather than the celiac ganglia. That is to say, the needles and injected solution will be placed posterior and cephalad to the crura of diaphragm.

CT and cadaver studies have given rise to the recent suggestion that the classic method of retrocrural block is more likely to produce splanchnic nerve block than blockade of the celiac plexus. This is because this approach does not result in the deposition of injected material around and anterior to the aorta and directly onto the celiac plexus at the level of the L1 vertebral body, as previously thought. Rather, the injectate appears to follow this path:

1. Concentrate posterior to the aorta and in front of and along the side of the L1 vertebral body, where it may anesthetize retroaortic celiac fibers.
2. Diffuse cephalad to anesthetize the splanchnic nerve at a site rostral to the origin of the plexus.
3. Only finally encircle the aorta at the site of the celiac plexus when enough drug is injected to transgress the diaphragm by diffusing caudad through the aortic hiatus.

Unfortunately, this larger volume of drug also is associated with an increased incidence of blockade of the lumbar somatic nerve roots.

Radiographic guidance, especially CT guidance, offers the pain specialist an added margin of safety during neurolytic celiac plexus block via the single-needle periaortic approach and hence should be used routinely unless the patient's clinical status requires that celiac plexus block be performed at the bedside. Given the increased incidence of damage to the lumbar nerve roots because of the retrocrural placement of needles with the classic two-needle technique, the transcrural, single-needle periaortic, or transaortic approaches to celiac plexus block are preferred.

Most pain specialists report a lower success rate when using celiac plexus block to treat chronic benign abdominal pain than when treating abdominal pain of malignant origin. Patients with chronic benign abdominal pain should be tapered off narcotic analgesics before consideration of celiac plexus neurolysis. It should be noted that the phrenic nerve also transmits nociceptive information from the upper abdominal viscera. This information is perceived as poorly localized pain referred to the supraclavicular region; this source of pain should be considered in all patients suffering from upper abdominal pain.

CHAPTER 80

Celiac Plexus Block: Single-Needle Transaortic Technique

CPT-2009 CODE

Local Anesthetic—With or Without Radiographic Monitoring	64530
Neurolytic—With or Without Radiographic Monitoring	64680

Relative Value Units

Local Anesthetic	12
Neurolytic	25

INDICATIONS

The single-needle transaortic celiac plexus block is the safest way to perform celiac plexus block. The use of computed tomography (CT) when using this technique provides an added margin of safety by allowing the pain management physician to clearly identify the clinically relevant anatomy, including the crura of the diaphragm and aorta. This ensures accurate precrural needle placement. Furthermore, studies have suggested that the single-needle transaortic technique not only is safer but also has the highest success rate of all approaches to celiac plexus block. The single-needle transaortic approach to celiac plexus block has three additional advantages over the classic two-needle approach:

1. It avoids the risks for neurologic complications related to posterior retrocrural spread of drugs.
2. The aorta provides a definitive landmark for needle placement when radiographic guidance is unavailable.
3. Much smaller volumes of local anesthetic and neurolytic solutions are required to achieve an efficacy equal to or greater than that of the classic retrocrural approach.

As with the single-needle periaortic approach, the single-needle transaortic approach to celiac plexus block has the advantage of decreased needle-related complications as well as less pain associated with the procedure. The transaortic approach has the added advantage of placing the injectate directly in the region of the celiac ganglion, even when preaortic adenopathy or tumor is significant enough to prevent solution from spreading medially from a needle placed laterally using the periaortic approach.

Celiac plexus block via the single-needle transaortic approach with local anesthetic is indicated as a diagnostic maneuver to determine whether flank, retroperitoneal, or upper abdominal pain is sympathetically mediated via the celiac plexus. Daily celiac plexus block with local anesthetic also is useful in the palliation of pain secondary to acute pancreatitis and other acute pain syndromes subserved by the celiac plexus. Early implementation of celiac plexus block with local anesthetic, steroids, or both markedly reduces the morbidity and mortality associated with acute pancreatitis. Single-needle transaortic celiac plexus block also is used to palliate the acute pain of arterial embolization of the liver for cancer therapy as well as to treat the pain of abdominal "angina" associated with visceral arterial insufficiency. Single-needle transaortic celiac plexus block with local anesthetic also may be used prognostically before performing celiac plexus neurolysis.

Neurolysis of the celiac plexus via the single-needle transaortic approach with alcohol or phenol is indicated to treat pain secondary to malignancies of the retroperitoneum and upper abdomen. This approach also may be useful in some chronic benign abdominal pain syndromes, including chronic pancreatitis, in carefully selected patients.

CLINICALLY RELEVANT ANATOMY

The sympathetic innervation of the abdominal viscera originates in the anterolateral horn of the spinal cord. Preganglionic fibers from T5-T12 exit the spinal cord in conjunction with the ventral roots to join the white communicating rami on their way to the sympathetic chain. Rather than synapsing with the sympathetic chain, these preganglionic fibers pass through it to ultimately synapse on the celiac ganglia. The greater, lesser, and least splanchnic nerves provide the major preganglionic contribution to the celiac plexus. The greater splanchnic nerve has its origin from the T5-T10 spinal roots. The nerve travels along the thoracic paravertebral border through the crus of the diaphragm into the abdominal cavity, ending on the celiac ganglion of its respective side. The lesser splanchnic nerve arises from the T10-T11 roots and passes with the greater nerve to end at the celiac ganglion. The least splanchnic nerve arises from the T11-T12 spinal roots and passes through the diaphragm to the celiac ganglion.

Interpatient anatomic variability of the celiac ganglia is significant, but the following generalizations can be drawn from anatomic studies of the celiac ganglia. The number of ganglia varies from one to five, and they range in diameter from 0.5 to 4.5 cm. The ganglia lie anterior and anterolateral to the aorta. The ganglia located on the left are uniformly more inferior than their right-sided counterparts by as much as a vertebral level, but both groups of ganglia lie below the level of the celiac artery. The ganglia usually lie about at the level of the first lumbar vertebra.

Postganglionic fibers radiate from the celiac ganglia to follow the course of the blood vessels to innervate the abdominal viscera. These organs include much of the distal esophagus, stomach, duodenum, small intestine, ascending and proximal transverse colon, adrenal glands, pancreas, spleen, liver, and biliary system. It is these postganglionic fibers, the fibers arising from the preganglionic splanchnic nerves, and the celiac ganglia that make up the celiac plexus. The diaphragm separates the thorax from the abdominal cavity while still permitting the passage of the thoracoabdominal structures, including the aorta, vena cava, and splanchnic nerves. The diaphragmatic crura are bilateral structures that arise from the anterolateral surfaces of the upper two or three lumbar vertebrae and disks. The crura of the diaphragm serve as a barrier to effectively separate the splanchnic nerves from the celiac ganglia and plexus below.

The celiac plexus is anterior to the crus of the diaphragm. The plexus extends in front of and around the aorta, with the greatest concentration of fibers anterior to the aorta. With the single-needle transaortic approach to celiac plexus block, the needle is placed close to this concentration of plexus fibers. The relationship of the celiac plexus to the surrounding structures is as follows: The aorta lies anterior and slightly to the left of the anterior margin of the vertebral body. The inferior vena cava lies to the right, with the kidneys posterolateral to the great vessels. The pancreas lies anterior to the celiac plexus. All these structures lie within the retroperitoneal space.

TECHNIQUE

The single-needle transaortic approach to celiac plexus block is analogous to the transaxillary approach to brachial plexus block. Despite concerns about the potential for aortic trauma and subsequent occult retroperitoneal hemorrhage with the transaortic approach to celiac plexus block, it may in fact be safer than the classic two-needle posterior approach. The lower incidence of complications is thought to be due in part to the use of a single fine needle rather than two larger ones. The fact that the aorta is relatively well supported in this region by the diaphragmatic crura and prevertebral fascia also contributes to this technique's relative safety.

Preblock preparation includes the administration of adequate amounts of oral or intravenous fluids to attenuate the hypotension associated with celiac plexus block. Evaluation of the patient for coagulopathy is indicated if the patient has undergone antiblastic therapy or has a history of significant alcohol abuse. If radiographic contrast is to be used, evaluation of the patient's renal status also is indicated.

Fluoroscopically Guided Technique

The fluoroscopically guided single-needle transaortic approach uses the usual landmarks for the posterior placement of a left-sided 22-gauge, 13-cm styletted needle. Some investigators use a needle entry point 1 to 1.5 cm closer to the midline relative to the classic retrocrural approach combined with a needle trajectory closer to the perpendicular to reduce the incidence of renal trauma. The needle is advanced with the goal of passing just lateral to the anterolateral aspect of the L1 vertebral body. If the L1 vertebral body is encountered, the needle is withdrawn into the subcutaneous tissues and redirected in a manner analogous to the classic retrocrural approach. The styletted needle is gradually advanced until its tip rests in the posterior periaortic space. As the needle impinges on the posterior aortic wall, the operator feels transmitted aortic pulsations via the needle and increased resistance to needle passage.

Passing the needle through the wall of the aorta has been likened to passing a needle through a large rubber band. Free flow of arterial blood when the stylet is removed is evidence that the needle is within the aortic lumen. The stylet is replaced as the needle is advanced until it impinges on the intraluminal anterior wall of the aorta. At this point, the operator again feels an increased resistance to needle advancement. A pop is felt as the needle tip passes through the anterior aortic wall, indicating the needle tip's probable location within the preaortic fatty connective tissue and the substance of the celiac plexus (Figs. 80-1 and 80-2). A saline loss-of-

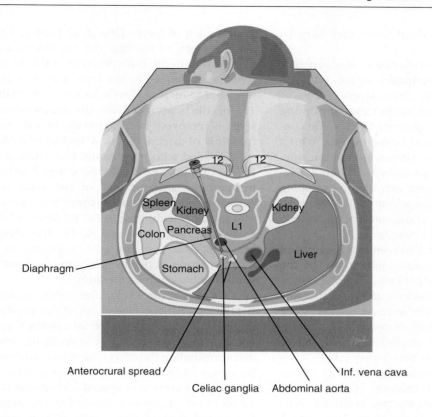

Figure 80-1.

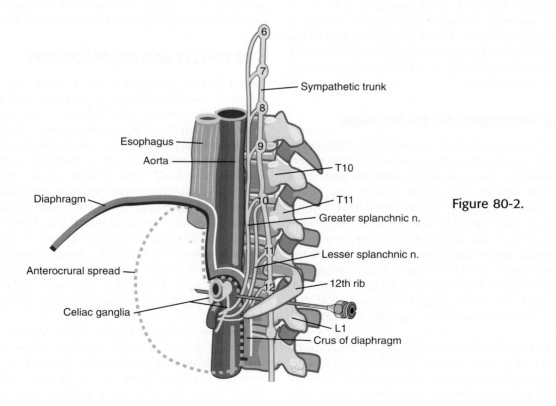

Figure 80-2.

resistance technique, as described later, may help to identify the preaortic space.

Because the needle is sometimes inadvertently advanced beyond the retroperitoneal space into the peritoneal cavity, confirmatory fluoroscopic views of injected contrast medium are advisable, especially during neurolytic blockade. On anteroposterior views, the contrast medium should be confined to the midline, with a tendency toward greater concentration around the anterolateral margins of the aorta. Lateral views should demonstrate a predominantly preaortic orientation extending from around T12-L2, sometimes accompanied by pulsations. Incomplete penetration of the anterior wall is indicated by a narrow longitudinal "line image."

The contrast medium may fail to completely surround the anterior aorta with extensive infiltration of the preaortic region by tumor or in patients who have undergone previous pancreatic surgery or radiation therapy. Experience shows that a lower success rate is to be expected when preaortic spread of contrast medium is poor. In this setting, selective alcohol neurolysis of the splanchnic nerves may provide better pain relief.

For diagnostic and prognostic block via the fluoroscopically guided transaortic technique, 10 to 12 mL of 1.5% lidocaine or 3.0% 2-chloroprocaine is administered through the needle. For therapeutic block, 10 to 12 mL of 0.5% bupivacaine is administered through the needle. Because of the potential for local anesthetic toxicity, all local anesthetics should be administered in incremental doses. For treatment of acute pancreatitis, 80 mg of depot methylprednisolone for the initial block and 40 mg for subsequent blocks is recommended. A 12- to 15-mL volume of absolute alcohol or 6.5% aqueous phenol is used for neurolytic block.

Computed Tomography–Guided Technique

The patient is prepared for CT-guided transaortic celiac plexus block in a manner analogous to the earlier mentioned techniques. After proper positioning on the CT table, a scout film is obtained to identify the T12-L1 interspace (Fig. 80-3). A CT scan is then taken through the interspace. The scan is reviewed for the position of the aorta relative to the vertebral body, the position of intra-abdominal and retroperitoneal organs, and distortion of normal anatomy due to tumor, previous surgery, or adenopathy. The aorta at this level is evaluated for significant aortic aneurysm, mural thrombus, or calcifications that would recommend against a transaortic approach.

The level at which the scan was taken is identified on the patient's skin and marked with a gentian violet marker. The skin is prepared with antiseptic solution. The skin, subcutaneous tissues, and muscle are anesthetized with 1.0% lidocaine at a point about 2½ inches

from the left of the midline. A 22-gauge, 13-cm styletted needle is placed through the anesthetized area and is advanced until the posterior wall of the aorta is encountered, as evidenced by the transmission of arterial pulsations and an increased resistance to needle advancement. The needle is advanced into the lumen of the aorta. The stylet is removed, and the needle hub is observed for a free flow of arterial blood. A well-lubricated, 5-mL glass syringe filled with preservative-free saline is attached to the needle hub. The needle and syringe are then advanced through the anterior wall of the aorta via a loss-of-resistance technique in a manner analogous to the loss-of-resistance technique used to identify the epidural space (see Figs. 80-1 and 80-2). The glass syringe is removed, and 3 mL of 1.5% lidocaine in solution is injected through the needle with an equal amount of water-soluble contrast medium.

A CT scan at the level of the needle is taken. The scan is reviewed for the placement of the needle and, most importantly, for the spread of contrast medium. The contrast medium should be seen in the preaortic area and surrounding the aorta (Fig. 80-4). No contrast should be observed in the retrocrural space. After satisfactory needle placement and spread of contrast is confirmed, 12 to 15 mL of absolute alcohol or 6% aqueous phenol is injected through the needle. The needle is flushed with a small amount of sterile saline and then removed. The patient is observed carefully for hemodynamic changes, including hypotension and tachycardia secondary to the resulting profound sympathetic blockade.

SIDE EFFECTS AND COMPLICATIONS

Because of the puncture of the aorta and the proximity of other vascular structures, including the celiac and renal arteries, celiac plexus block via the single-needle transaortic approach is contraindicated in patients who are on anticoagulant therapy or suffer from coagulopathy secondary to antiblastic cancer therapies or liver abnormalities associated with ethanol abuse. Intravascular injection of solutions may result in thrombosis of the nutrient vessels to the spinal cord with secondary paraplegia. Local and intra-abdominal infections, as well as sepsis, are absolute contraindications to celiac plexus block. Because the needle is placed through the aorta, trauma to the aortic wall or the dislodgment of atheromatous plaque is possible, although large series of patients have failed to identify either as a significant problem.

Because blockade of the celiac plexus results in increased bowel motility, this technique should be avoided in patients with bowel obstruction. Postblock diarrhea occurs in about 50% of patients. Celiac plexus block should be deferred in patients who suffer from chronic abdominal pain, who are chemically dependent,

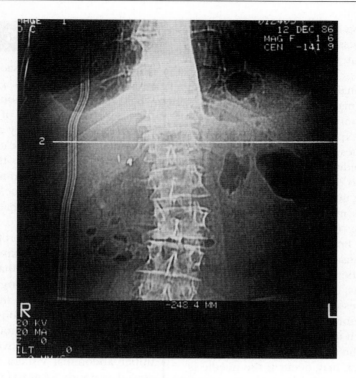

Figure 80-3.
Scout film to identify T12-L1 interspace. (From Waldman SD: Interventional Pain Management, 2nd ed. Philadelphia, WB Saunders, 2001, p 499.)

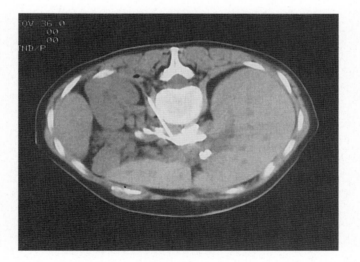

Figure 80-4.
CT demonstrating periaortic spread of contrast medium. (From Waldman SD: Interventional Pain Management, 2nd ed. Philadelphia, WB Saunders, 2001, p 500.)

or who exhibit drug-seeking behavior until these issues have been adequately addressed. Alcohol should not be used as a neurolytic agent in patients on disulfiram therapy for alcohol abuse.

The proximity to the spinal cord, exiting nerve roots, pleural space, and viscera makes it imperative that this procedure be performed only by those well versed in the regional anatomy and experienced in interventional pain management techniques. Needle placement that is too medial may result in epidural, subdural, or subarachnoid injections or trauma to the spinal cord and exiting nerve roots. Such incorrect needle placement can result in severe neurologic deficits, including paraplegia. Medial needle placement also may result in intradiskal placement and resultant diskitis. Because the needle terminus with the single-needle transaortic approach to celiac plexus block is precrural, there is a decreased incidence of neurologic complications, including neurolysis of the lumbar nerve roots with resultant hip flexor weakness and lower extremity numbness, compared with the classic two-needle approach to celiac plexus block.

Given the proximity of the pleural space, pneumothorax after celiac plexus block may occur if the needle is placed too cephalad. Trauma to the thoracic duct with resultant chylothorax also may occur. If the needle is placed too laterally, trauma to the kidneys and ureters is a distinct possibility.

CLINICAL PEARLS

The single-needle transaortic approach to celiac plexus block under CT guidance is probably the safest and most efficacious way to perform celiac plexus block. The use of CT guidance is a great advance over fluoroscopy and should be considered, especially with neurolytic celiac plexus blocks. Placement of the needle into the aorta provides a clear landmark when performing non–radiographically guided celiac plexus blocks and reassures the pain management specialist that the needle is in the right place.

Most pain specialists report a lower success rate when using celiac plexus block to treat chronic benign abdominal pain than when treating abdominal pain of malignant origin. Patients with chronic benign abdominal pain should be tapered off narcotic analgesics before consideration of celiac plexus neurolysis. It should be noted that the phrenic nerve also transmits nociceptive information from the upper abdominal viscera. This information is perceived as poorly localized pain referred to the supraclavicular region; this source of pain should be considered in all patients suffering from upper abdominal pain.

CHAPTER 81

Celiac Plexus Block: Single-Needle Lateral Technique

CPT-2009 CODE

Local Anesthetic—With or Without Radiographic Monitoring	64530
Neurolytic—With or Without Radiographic Monitoring	64680

Relative Value Units

Local Anesthetic	18
Neurolytic	25

INDICATIONS

Advantages of the single-needle lateral approach to celiac plexus block include its relative ease, speed, and potentially reduced periprocedural discomfort compared with posterior techniques. Perhaps the greatest advantage of the lateral approach is the fact that patients are spared the need to remain prone for prolonged periods. This can be a significant problem for patients suffering from intra-abdominal pain or tumor. The supine position also is advantageous for patients with ileostomies and colostomies. Less discomfort is associated with the lateral approach when compared with a classic two-needle posterior approach because only one thin needle is used. Furthermore, the needle does not impinge on the periosteum or nerve roots or pass through the bulky paraspinous musculature. Because the needle placement is precrural, there is less risk for accidental neurologic injury related to retrocrural spread of drug to somatic nerve roots or the epidural and subarachnoid space. The single-needle lateral approach to celiac plexus block can be used as an acceptable alternative to posterior or anterior approaches to celiac plexus block. Furthermore, the use of computed tomography (CT) during the lateral approach provides an added margin of safety by allowing the pain management physician to clearly identify the clinically relevant anatomy and avoid injury to the viscera.

Celiac plexus block via the single-needle lateral approach with local anesthetic is indicated as a diagnostic maneuver to determine whether flank, retroperitoneal, or upper abdominal pain is sympathetically mediated via the celiac plexus. Daily celiac plexus block with local anesthetic also is useful in the palliation of pain secondary to acute pancreatitis and other acute pain syndromes subserved by the celiac plexus. Early implementation of celiac plexus block with local anesthetic, steroids, or both markedly reduces the morbidity and mortality associated with acute pancreatitis. Single-needle lateral celiac plexus block also is used to palliate the acute pain of arterial embolization of the liver for cancer therapy as well as to treat the pain of abdominal "angina" associated with visceral arterial insufficiency. Single-needle lateral celiac plexus block with local anesthetic also may be used prognostically before celiac plexus neurolysis.

Neurolysis of the celiac plexus via the single-needle lateral approach with alcohol or phenol is indicated to treat pain secondary to malignancies of the retroperitoneum and upper abdomen. Neurolytic celiac plexus block via the single-needle lateral approach also may be useful in some chronic benign abdominal pain syndromes, including chronic pancreatitis, in carefully selected patients.

CLINICALLY RELEVANT ANATOMY

The sympathetic innervation of the abdominal viscera originates in the anterolateral horn of the spinal cord. Preganglionic fibers from T5-T12 exit the spinal cord in conjunction with the ventral roots to join the white communicating rami on their way to the sympathetic chain. Rather than synapsing with the sympathetic chain, these preganglionic fibers pass through it to ultimately synapse on the celiac ganglia. The greater, lesser, and least splanchnic nerves provide the major preganglionic contribution to the celiac plexus. The greater splanchnic nerve has its origin from the T5-T10 spinal roots. The nerve travels along the thoracic paravertebral border through the crus of the diaphragm into the abdominal cavity, ending on the celiac ganglion of its respective side. The lesser splanchnic nerve arises from the T10-T11 roots and passes with the greater nerve to end at the celiac ganglion. The least splanchnic nerve arises from the T11-T12 spinal roots and passes through the diaphragm to the celiac ganglion.

Interpatient anatomic variability of the celiac ganglia is significant, but the following generalizations can be drawn from anatomic studies of the celiac ganglia. The number of ganglia varies from one to five, and they range in diameter from 0.5 to 4.5 cm. The ganglia lie anterior and anterolateral to the aorta. The ganglia located on the left are uniformly more inferior than their right-sided counterparts by as much as a vertebral level, but both groups of ganglia lie below the level of the celiac artery. The ganglia usually lie about at the level of the first lumbar vertebra.

Postganglionic fibers radiate from the celiac ganglia to follow the course of the blood vessels to innervate the abdominal viscera. These organs include much of the distal esophagus, stomach, duodenum, small intestine, ascending and proximal transverse colon, adrenal glands, pancreas, spleen, liver, and biliary system. It is these postganglionic fibers, the fibers arising from the preganglionic splanchnic nerves, and the celiac ganglion that make up the celiac plexus. The diaphragm separates the thorax from the abdominal cavity while still permitting the passage of the thoracoabdominal structures, including the aorta, vena cava, and splanchnic nerves. The diaphragmatic crura are bilateral structures that arise from the anterolateral surfaces of the upper two or three lumbar vertebrae and disks. The crura of the diaphragm serve as a barrier to effectively separate the splanchnic nerves from the celiac ganglia and plexus below.

The celiac plexus is anterior to the crus of the diaphragm. The plexus extends in front of and around the aorta, with the greatest concentration of fibers lateral to the aorta. With the single-needle lateral approach to celiac plexus block, the needle is placed close to this concentration of plexus fibers. The relationship of the celiac plexus to the surrounding structures is as follows: The aorta lies anterior and slightly to the left of the lateral margin of the vertebral body. The inferior vena cava lies to the right, with the kidneys posterolateral to the great vessels. The pancreas lies anterior to the celiac plexus. All these structures lie within the retroperitoneal space. With the lateral approach, the needle may traverse the stomach, intestine, vessels, and pancreas.

TECHNIQUE

The lateral technique can be carried out under CT guidance. Preblock preparation includes the administration of adequate amounts of oral or intravenous fluids to attenuate the hypotension associated with celiac plexus block. Evaluation of the patient for coagulopathy is indicated if the patient has undergone antiblastic therapy or has a history of significant alcohol abuse. If radiographic contrast is to be used, evaluation of the patient's renal status also is indicated. Oral contrast medium is administered 2 hours before the procedure to allow easy identification of the stomach and bowel (Fig. 81-1).

The patient is placed in the supine position on the CT table. CT scans are taken through the T12-L1 interspace to identify the aorta, surrounding structures, and any anatomic abnormalities caused by tumor or previous surgery. The skin of the left lateral abdomen is prepared with antiseptic solution. The needle entry site is identified at a level just below the left lateral crus of the diaphragm at the mid-axillary line to avoid causing an inadvertent pneumothorax. At that point, the skin, subcutaneous tissues, and musculature are anesthetized with 1.0% lidocaine. A 22-gauge, 15-cm needle is introduced through the anesthetized area perpendicular to the skin. The needle is then advanced under CT guidance, with care taken to avoid bowel advancing the needle through the stomach to the depth of the anterior wall of the aorta as previously identified by CT (Figs. 81-2 and 81-3).

After CT scan confirms proper preaortic position of the needle tip in proximity to the celiac plexus, 4 mL of water-soluble contrast medium in solution with an equal volume of 1.0% lidocaine is injected to confirm needle placement (Fig. 81-4). After satisfactory needle placement is confirmed, diagnostic and prognostic block is performed using 15 mL of 1.5% lidocaine or 3.0% 2-chloroprocaine. Therapeutic blocks are performed with an equal volume of 0.5% bupivacaine. Because of the potential for local anesthetic toxicity, all local anesthetics should be administered in incremental doses. Good results for neurolytic blocks can be obtained by using 15 to 20 mL of absolute alcohol. Alternatively, 35 to 40 mL of 50% ethyl alcohol can be used during celiac plexus via the lateral approach.

Important precautions with use of the lateral approach to celiac plexus block include the administration of prophylactic antibiotics and the use of needles no larger than 22 gauge to minimize the risks for infection and trauma to the vasculature and viscera.

SIDE EFFECTS AND COMPLICATIONS

The lateral approach to the celiac plexus necessarily involves the passage of a fine needle through the stomach and, in some cases, the spleen, intestine, vessels, and pancreas. Surprisingly, this approach is associated with very low rates of complications as confirmed by the extensive experience with transabdominal fine-needle aspiration biopsy and the use of this approach to drain intra-abdominal abscess. The advent of fine-needle

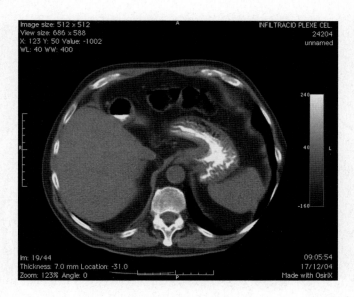

Figure 81-1.
CT demonstrating orally administered contrast medium within the stomach.
(Courtesy of Xavier Garcia-Eroles, MD.)

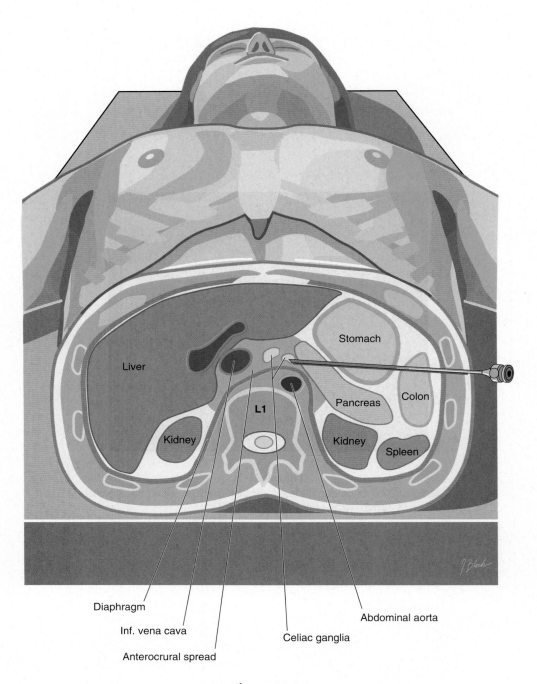

Figure 81-2.

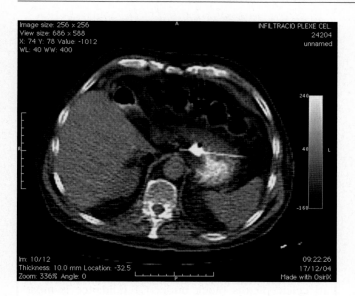

Figure 81-3.
CT scan demonstrating the needle placed through the stomach. (Courtesy of Xavier Garcia-Eroles, MD.)

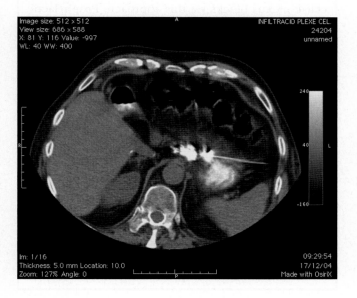

Figure 81-4.
CT scan demonstrating contrast medium in the preaortic region. (Courtesy of Xavier Garcia-Eroles, MD.)

technology and improved radiographic guidance techniques has made the lateral approach to celiac plexus block a reasonable alternative to the posterior approaches, especially when the patient is unable to remain in the prone position.

Because of the possibility of puncture of the aorta and the proximity of other vascular structures, including the celiac and renal arteries, celiac plexus block via the single-needle lateral approach is contraindicated in patients who are on anticoagulant therapy or have coagulopathy secondary to antiblastic cancer therapies or liver abnormalities associated with ethanol abuse. Intravascular injection of solutions may result in thrombosis of the nutrient vessels to the spinal cord with secondary paraplegia. Local and intra-abdominal infections, as well as sepsis, are absolute contraindications to the lateral approach to celiac plexus block. Because the needle is placed through the abdominal viscera, peritonitis and intra-abdominal abscess remain a distinct possibility. These problems with infection are decreased by the use of prophylactic antibiotics.

Because blockade of the celiac plexus results in increased bowel motility, this technique should be avoided in patients with bowel obstruction. Postblock diarrhea occurs in about 50% of patients. Celiac plexus block should be deferred in patients who have chronic abdominal pain, who are chemically dependent, or who exhibit drug-seeking behavior until these issues have been adequately addressed. Alcohol should not be used as a neurolytic agent in patients on disulfiram therapy for alcohol abuse.

The proximity to the spinal cord, exiting nerve roots, pleural space, and viscera makes it imperative that this procedure be performed only by those well versed in the regional anatomy and experienced in interventional pain management techniques. Needle placement that is too posterior may result in epidural, subdural, or subarachnoid injections or trauma to the spinal cord and exiting nerve roots. Such incorrect needle placement can result in severe neurologic deficits, including paraplegia. Medial needle placement also may result in intradiskal placement and resultant diskitis. Because the needle terminus is precrural with the single-needle lateral approach to celiac plexus, there is a decreased incidence of neurologic complications, including neurolysis of the lumbar nerve roots with resultant hip flexor weakness and lower extremity numbness compared with the classic two-needle approach to celiac plexus block.

Given the proximity of the pleural space, pneumothorax after celiac plexus block may occur if the needle is placed too cephalad. Trauma to the thoracic duct with resultant chylothorax also may occur. Even with CT guidance, trauma to the spleen, liver, kidneys, and ureters is a distinct possibility.

CLINICAL PEARLS

First described by Garcia-Eroles and associates as an alternative to the anterior and prone approaches to celiac plexus block, the single-needle lateral approach to celiac plexus block under CT guidance is most useful in patients who are unable to lie prone in order to undergo celiac plexus block via a posterior approach or in those patients in whom malignancy or previous abdominal surgery has resulted in altered anatomy, making other approaches more difficult. The use of CT guidance is a great advance over fluoroscopy and ultrasonography and should be considered, especially when one is performing neurolytic celiac plexus blocks via this approach. Prophylactic antibiotics should always be given before performing celiac plexus block using the lateral approach. After the block, the patient should be observed for early signs of peritonitis and intra-abdominal bleeding.

Most pain specialists report a lower success rate when using celiac plexus block to treat chronic benign abdominal pain than when treating abdominal pain of malignant origin. Patients with chronic benign abdominal pain should be tapered off narcotic analgesics before consideration of celiac plexus neurolysis. It should be noted that the phrenic nerve also transmits nociceptive information from the upper abdominal viscera. This information is perceived as poorly localized pain referred to the supraclavicular region; this source of pain should be considered in all patients suffering from upper abdominal pain.

CHAPTER 82

Celiac Plexus Block: Single-Needle Anterior Technique

INDICATIONS

Advantages of the single-needle anterior approach to celiac plexus block include its relative ease, speed, and reduced periprocedural discomfort compared with posterior techniques. Perhaps the greatest advantage of the anterior approach is the fact that patients are spared the need to remain prone for prolonged periods. This can be a significant problem for patients suffering from intraabdominal pain or tumor. The supine position also is advantageous for patients with ileostomies and colostomies. Less discomfort is associated with the anterior approach because only one thin needle is used. Furthermore, the needle does not impinge on the periosteum or nerve roots or pass through the bulky paraspinous musculature. Because the needle placement is precrural, there is less risk for accidental neurologic injury related to retrocrural spread of drug to somatic nerve roots or the epidural and subarachnoid space. The single-needle anterior approach to celiac plexus block can be used as an acceptable alternative to posterior approaches to celiac plexus block. Furthermore, the use of computed tomography (CT) during the anterior approach provides an added margin of safety by allowing the pain management physician to clearly identify the clinically relevant anatomy.

Celiac plexus block via the single-needle anterior approach with local anesthetic is indicated as a diagnostic maneuver to determine whether flank, retroperitoneal, or upper abdominal pain is sympathetically mediated via the celiac plexus. Daily celiac plexus block with local anesthetic also is useful in the palliation of pain secondary to acute pancreatitis and other acute pain syndromes subserved by the celiac plexus. Early implementation of celiac plexus block with local anesthetic, steroids, or both markedly reduces the morbidity and mortality associated with acute pancreatitis. Single-needle anterior celiac plexus block also is used to palliate the acute pain of arterial embolization of the liver for cancer therapy as well as to treat the pain of abdominal "angina" associated with visceral arterial insufficiency. Single-needle anterior celiac plexus block with local anesthetic also may be used prognostically before celiac plexus neurolysis.

Neurolysis of the celiac plexus via the single-needle anterior approach with alcohol or phenol is indicated to treat pain secondary to malignancies of the retroperitoneum and upper abdomen. Neurolytic celiac plexus block via the single-needle anterior approach also may be useful in some chronic benign abdominal pain syndromes, including chronic pancreatitis, in carefully selected patients.

CLINICALLY RELEVANT ANATOMY

The sympathetic innervation of the abdominal viscera originates in the anterolateral horn of the spinal cord. Preganglionic fibers from T5-T12 exit the spinal cord in conjunction with the ventral roots to join the white communicating rami on their way to the sympathetic chain. Rather than synapsing with the sympathetic chain, these preganglionic fibers pass through it to ultimately synapse on the celiac ganglia. The greater, lesser, and least splanchnic nerves provide the major preganglionic contribution to the celiac plexus. The greater splanchnic nerve has its origin from the T5-T10 spinal roots. The nerve travels along the thoracic paravertebral border through the crus of the diaphragm into the abdominal cavity, ending on the celiac ganglion of its respective side. The lesser splanchnic nerve arises from the T10-

T11 roots and passes with the greater nerve to end at the celiac ganglion. The least splanchnic nerve arises from the T11-T12 spinal roots and passes through the diaphragm to the celiac ganglion.

Interpatient anatomic variability of the celiac ganglia is significant, but the following generalizations can be drawn from anatomic studies of the celiac ganglia. The number of ganglia varies from one to five, and they range in diameter from 0.5 to 4.5 cm. The ganglia lie anterior and anterolateral to the aorta. The ganglia located on the left are uniformly more inferior than their right-sided counterparts by as much as a vertebral level, but both groups of ganglia lie below the level of the celiac artery. The ganglia usually lie about at the level of the first lumbar vertebra.

Postganglionic fibers radiate from the celiac ganglia to follow the course of the blood vessels to innervate the abdominal viscera. These organs include much of the distal esophagus, stomach, duodenum, small intestine, ascending and proximal transverse colon, adrenal glands, pancreas, spleen, liver, and biliary system. It is these postganglionic fibers, the fibers arising from the preganglionic splanchnic nerves, and the celiac ganglion that make up the celiac plexus. The diaphragm separates the thorax from the abdominal cavity while still permitting the passage of the thoracoabdominal structures, including the aorta, vena cava, and splanchnic nerves. The diaphragmatic crura are bilateral structures that arise from the anterolateral surfaces of the upper two or three lumbar vertebrae and disks. The crura of the diaphragm serve as a barrier to effectively separate the splanchnic nerves from the celiac ganglia and plexus below.

The celiac plexus is anterior to the crus of the diaphragm. The plexus extends in front of and around the aorta, with the greatest concentration of fibers anterior to the aorta. With the single-needle transaortic approach to celiac plexus block, the needle is placed close to this concentration of plexus fibers. The relationship of the celiac plexus to the surrounding structures is as follows: The aorta lies anterior and slightly to the left of the anterior margin of the vertebral body. The inferior vena cava lies to the right, with the kidneys posterolateral to the great vessels. The pancreas lies anterior to the celiac plexus. All these structures lie within the retroperitoneal space. With the anterior approach, the needle may traverse the liver, stomach, intestine, vessels, and pancreas.

TECHNIQUE

The anterior technique can be carried out under CT or ultrasonographic guidance. Preblock preparation includes the administration of adequate amounts of oral or intravenous fluids to attenuate the hypotension associated with celiac plexus block. Evaluation of the patient for coagulopathy is indicated if the patient has undergone antiblastic therapy or has a history of significant alcohol abuse. If radiographic contrast is to be used, evaluation of the patient's renal status also is indicated.

The patient is placed in the supine position on the CT or ultrasonography table. The skin of the upper abdomen is prepared with antiseptic solution. The needle entry site is identified 1.5 cm below and 1.5 cm to the left of the xiphoid process (Fig. 82-1). At that point, the skin, subcutaneous tissues, and musculature are anesthetized with 1.0% lidocaine. A 22-gauge, 15-cm needle is introduced through the anesthetized area perpendicular to the skin. The needle is then advanced to the depth of the anterior wall of the aorta as calculated by CT or ultrasound guidance.

If CT guidance is being used, 4 mL of water-soluble contrast medium in solution with an equal volume of 1.0% lidocaine is injected to confirm needle placement (Fig. 82-2). If ultrasonographic guidance is being used, 10 to 12 mL of sterile saline can be injected to help confirm needle position. After satisfactory needle placement is confirmed, diagnostic and prognostic block is performed using 15 mL of 1.5% lidocaine or 3.0% 2-chloroprocaine. Therapeutic blocks are performed with an equal volume of 0.5% bupivacaine. Because of the potential for local anesthetic toxicity, all local anesthetics should be administered in incremental doses. Good results for neurolytic blocks can be obtained by using 15 to 20 mL of absolute alcohol. Alternatively, 35 to 40 mL of 50% ethyl alcohol can be used during celiac plexus via the anterior approach.

An alternative anterior approach technique uses fluoroscopy to guide the passage of a single needle just to the right of the center of the L1 vertebral body, after which it is withdrawn 1 to 3 cm. Important precautions with use of the anterior approach to celiac plexus block include the administration of prophylactic antibiotics and the use of needles no larger than 22 gauge to minimize the risks for infection and trauma to the vasculature and viscera.

SIDE EFFECTS AND COMPLICATIONS

The anterior approach to the celiac plexus necessarily involves the passage of a fine needle through the liver, stomach, intestine, vessels, and pancreas. Surprisingly, this approach is associated with very low rates of complications, as confirmed by the extensive experience with transabdominal fine-needle aspiration biopsy. The advent of fine-needle technology and improved radiographic guidance techniques has made the anterior approach to celiac plexus block a reasonable alternative to the posterior approaches, especially when the patient is unable to remain in the prone position.

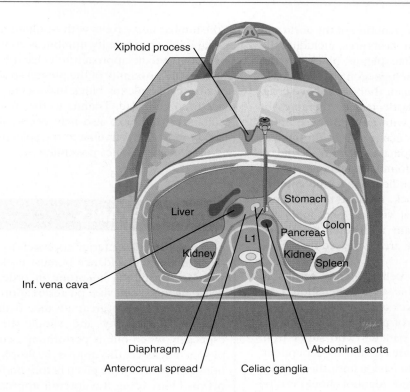

Figure 82-1.

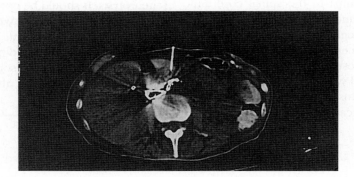

Figure 82-2.
CT scan demonstrating contrast medium surrounding the aorta. (From Waldman SD: Interventional Pain Management, 2nd ed. Philadelphia, WB Saunders, 2001, p 501.)

Because of the possibility of puncture of the aorta and the proximity of other vascular structures, including the celiac and renal arteries, celiac plexus block via the single-needle anterior approach is contraindicated in patients who are on anticoagulant therapy or have coagulopathy secondary to antiblastic cancer therapies or liver abnormalities associated with ethanol abuse. Intravascular injection of solutions may result in thrombosis of the nutrient vessels to the spinal cord with secondary paraplegia. Local and intra-abdominal infections, as well as sepsis, are absolute contraindications to the anterior approach to celiac plexus block. Because the needle is placed through the abdominal viscera, peritonitis and intra-abdominal abscess remain a distinct possibility. These problems with infection are decreased by the use of prophylactic antibiotics.

Because blockade of the celiac plexus results in increased bowel motility, this technique should be avoided in patients with bowel obstruction. Postblock diarrhea occurs in about 50% of patients. Celiac plexus block should be deferred in patients who suffer from chronic abdominal pain, who are chemically dependent, or who exhibit drug-seeking behavior until these issues have been adequately addressed. Alcohol should not be used as a neurolytic agent in patients on disulfiram therapy for alcohol abuse.

The proximity to the spinal cord, exiting nerve roots, pleural space, and viscera makes it imperative that this procedure be performed only by those well versed in the regional anatomy and experienced in interventional pain management techniques. Needle placement that is too posterior may result in epidural, subdural, or subarachnoid injections or trauma to the spinal cord and exiting nerve roots. Such incorrect needle placement can result in severe neurologic deficits, including paraplegia. Medial needle placement also may result in intradiskal placement and resultant diskitis. Because the needle terminus is precrural with the single-needle anterior approach to celiac plexus, there is a decreased incidence of neurologic complications, including neurolysis of the lumbar nerve roots with resultant hip flexor weakness and lower extremity numbness compared with the classic two-needle approach to celiac plexus block.

Given the proximity of the pleural space, pneumothorax after celiac plexus block may occur if the needle is placed too cephalad. Trauma to the thoracic duct with resultant chylothorax also may occur. If the needle is placed too laterally, trauma to the spleen, liver, kidneys, and ureters is a distinct possibility.

CLINICAL PEARLS

The single-needle anterior approach to celiac plexus block under CT guidance is most useful in patients who are unable to lie prone in order to undergo celiac plexus block via a posterior approach. The use of CT guidance is a great advance over fluoroscopy and ultrasonography and should be considered, especially when one is performing neurolytic celiac plexus blocks via this approach. Prophylactic antibiotics should always be given before performing celiac plexus block using the anterior approach. After the block, the patient should be observed for early signs of peritonitis and intra-abdominal bleeding.

Most pain specialists report a lower success rate when using celiac plexus block to treat chronic benign abdominal pain than when treating abdominal pain of malignant origin. Patients with chronic benign abdominal pain should be tapered off narcotic analgesics before consideration of celiac plexus neurolysis. It should be noted that the phrenic nerve also transmits nociceptive information from the upper abdominal viscera. This information is perceived as poorly localized pain referred to the supraclavicular region; this source of pain should be considered in all patients suffering from upper abdominal pain.

CHAPTER 83

Ilioinguinal Nerve Block

CPT-2009 CODE	
Unilateral	64425
Neurolytic	64640

Relative Value Units	
Unilateral	8
Neurolytic	20

INDICATIONS

Ilioinguinal nerve block is useful in the evaluation and management of groin pain thought to be subserved by the ilioinguinal nerve, including the pain associated with ilioinguinal neuralgia. The technique also is useful to provide surgical anesthesia for groin surgery, including inguinal herniorrhaphy when combined with iliohypogastric and genitofemoral nerve block. Ilioinguinal nerve block with local anesthetics can be used diagnostically during differential neural blockade on an anatomic basis in the evaluation of groin pain when peripheral nerve entrapment versus lumbar radiculopathy is being evaluated. If destruction of the ilioinguinal nerve is being considered, this technique is useful as a prognostic indicator of the degree of motor and sensory impairment. Ilioinguinal nerve block with local anesthetic may be used to palliate acute pain emergencies, including postoperative pain relief, while one is waiting for pharmacologic methods to become effective. Ilioinguinal nerve block with local anesthetic and steroids also is useful in the treatment of persistent pain after inguinal surgery or groin trauma when the pain is thought to be secondary to inflammation or entrapment of the ilioinguinal nerve.

Destruction of the ilioinguinal nerve is occasionally indicated for the palliation of persistent groin pain after blunt or open trauma to the groin or persistent pain mediated by the ilioinguinal nerve after groin surgery. Ilioinguinal nerve block via a 25-gauge needle may be performed in the presence of coagulopathy or anticoagu-lation, albeit with an increased risk for ecchymosis and hematoma formation.

CLINICALLY RELEVANT ANATOMY

The ilioinguinal nerve is a branch of the L1 nerve root with a contribution from T12 in some patients. The nerve follows a curvilinear course that takes it from its origin of the L1 and occasionally T12 somatic nerves to inside the concavity of the ilium. The ilioinguinal nerve continues anteriorly to perforate the transverse abdominis muscle at the level of the anterior-superior iliac spine. The nerve may interconnect with the iliohypogastric nerve as it continues to pass along its course medially and inferiorly, where it accompanies the spermatic cord through the inguinal ring and into the inguinal canal. The distribution of the sensory innervation of the ilioinguinal nerves varies from patient to patient because there may be considerable overlap with the iliohypogastric nerve. In general, the ilioinguinal nerve provides sensory innervation to the upper portion of the skin of the inner thigh and the root of the penis and upper scrotum in men or the mons pubis and lateral labia in women (Fig. 83-1).

TECHNIQUE

The patient is placed in the supine position with a pillow under the knees if extending the legs increases the patient's pain because of traction on the nerve. The anterior-superior iliac spine is identified by palpation. A point 2 inches medial and 2 inches inferior to the anterior-superior iliac spine is then identified and prepared with antiseptic solution. A 25-gauge, $1\frac{1}{2}$-inch needle is then advanced at an oblique angle toward the pubic symphysis (Fig. 83-2). From 5 to 7 mL of 1.0% preservative-free lidocaine is injected in a fanlike manner as the needle pierces the fascia of the external oblique muscle. Care must be taken not to place the needle too deep and enter the peritoneal cavity and perforate the abdominal viscera.

If the pain has an inflammatory component, the local anesthetic is combined with 80 mg of

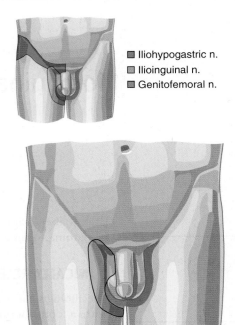

- ■ Iliohypogastric n.
- ■ Ilioinguinal n.
- ■ Genitofemoral n.

■ Ilioinguinal n.

Figure 83-1.

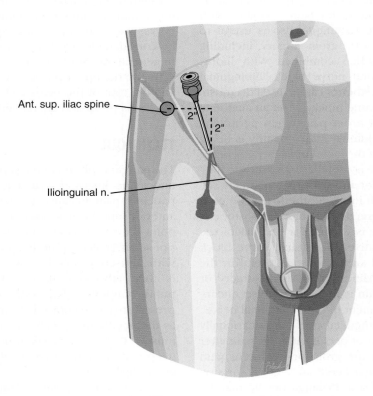

Ant. sup. iliac spine

2"

2"

Ilioinguinal n.

Figure 83-2.

methylprednisolone and is injected in incremental doses. Subsequent daily nerve blocks are performed similarly, substituting 40 mg of methylprednisolone for the initial 80-mg dose. Because of overlapping innervation of the ilioinguinal and iliohypogastric nerves, it is not unusual to block branches of each nerve when performing ilioinguinal nerve block. After the solution is injected, pressure is applied to the injection site to decrease the incidence of postblock ecchymosis and hematoma formation, which can be dramatic, especially when the patient is on anticoagulants.

SIDE EFFECTS AND COMPLICATIONS

The main side effect of ilioinguinal nerve block is postblock ecchymosis and hematoma formation. If needle placement is too deep and enters the peritoneal cavity, perforation of the colon may result in intra-abdominal abscess and fistula formation. Early detection of infection is crucial to avoid potentially life-threatening sequelae.

CLINICAL PEARLS

Ilioinguinal nerve block is a simple technique that can produce dramatic relief for patients suffering from the previously mentioned pain complaints. Neurolytic block with small quantities of phenol in glycerin or by cryoneurolysis or radiofrequency lesioning has been shown to provide long-term relief for patients suffering from chronic pain secondary to trauma to the ilioinguinal nerve in whom more conservative treatments have been ineffectual. As mentioned earlier, pressure should be maintained on the injection site after the block to avoid ecchymosis and hematoma formation.

If a patient presents with pain suggestive of ilioinguinal neuralgia and ilioinguinal nerve blocks are ineffectual, a diagnosis of lesions more proximal in the lumbar plexus or an L1 radiculopathy should be considered. Such cases often respond to epidural steroid blocks. Electromyography and magnetic resonance imaging of the lumbar plexus are indicated in these patients to help rule out other causes of ilioinguinal pain, including malignancy invading the lumbar plexus or epidural or vertebral metastatic disease at T12-L1.

CHAPTER **84**

Iliohypogastric Nerve Block

INDICATIONS

Iliohypogastric nerve block is useful in the evaluation and management of groin pain thought to be subserved by the iliohypogastric nerve, including the pain associated with iliohypogastric neuralgia. The technique also is useful to provide surgical anesthesia for groin surgery, including inguinal herniorrhaphy when combined with ilioinguinal and genitofemoral nerve block. Iliohypogastric nerve block with local anesthetic can be used diagnostically during differential neural blockade on an anatomic basis in the evaluation of groin pain when peripheral nerve entrapment versus lumbar radiculopathy is being evaluated. If destruction of the iliohypogastric nerve is being considered, this technique is useful as a prognostic indicator of the degree of motor and sensory impairment. Iliohypogastric nerve block with local anesthetic may be used to palliate acute pain emergencies, including postoperative pain relief, while one is waiting for pharmacologic methods to become effective. Iliohypogastric nerve block with local anesthetic and steroids also is useful in the treatment of persistent pain after inguinal surgery or groin trauma when the pain is thought to be secondary to inflammation or entrapment of the iliohypogastric nerve.

Destruction of the iliohypogastric nerve is occasionally indicated for the palliation of persistent groin pain after blunt or open trauma to the groin or persistent pain mediated by the iliohypogastric nerve after groin or lower abdominal surgery. Iliohypogastric nerve block via a 25-gauge needle may be performed in the presence of coagulopathy or anticoagulation, albeit with an increased risk for ecchymosis and hematoma formation.

CLINICALLY RELEVANT ANATOMY

The iliohypogastric nerve is a branch of the L1 nerve root with a contribution from T12 in some patients. The nerve follows a curvilinear course that takes it from its origin of the L1 and occasionally T12 somatic nerves to inside the concavity of the ilium. The iliohypogastric nerve continues anteriorly to perforate the transverse abdominis muscle to lie between it and the external oblique muscle (Fig. 84-1). At this point, the iliohypogastric nerve divides into an anterior and a lateral branch. The lateral branch provides cutaneous sensory innervation to the posterolateral gluteal region. The anterior branch pierces the external oblique muscle just beyond the anterior-superior iliac spine to provide cutaneous sensory innervation to the abdominal skin above the pubis (Fig. 84-2). The nerve may interconnect with the ilioinguinal nerve along its course, resulting in variation of the distribution of the sensory innervation of the iliohypogastric and ilioinguinal nerves.

TECHNIQUE

The patient is placed in the supine position with a pillow under the knees if extending the legs increases the patient's pain because of traction on the nerve. The anterior-superior iliac spine is identified by palpation. A point 1 inch medial and 1 inch inferior to the anterior-superior iliac spine is then identified and prepared with antiseptic solution. A 25-gauge, $1\frac{1}{2}$-inch needle is then advanced at an oblique angle toward the pubic symphysis (Fig. 84-3). From 5 to 7 mL of 1.0% preservative-free lidocaine is injected in a fanlike manner as the needle pierces the fascia of the external oblique muscle. Care must be taken not to place the needle too deep and enter the peritoneal cavity and perforate the abdominal viscera.

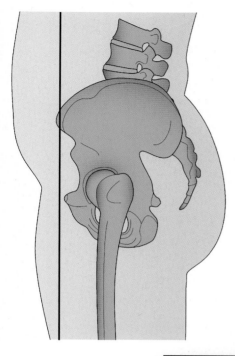

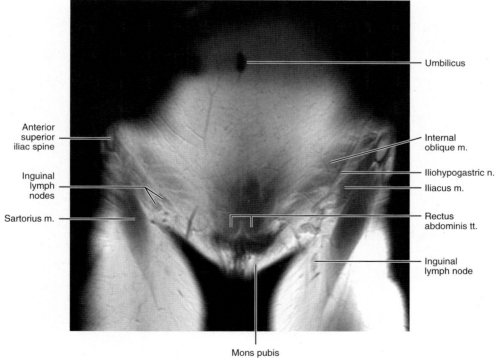

Umbilicus

Anterior
superior
iliac spine

Internal
oblique m.

Iliohypogastric n.

Inguinal
lymph
nodes

Iliacus m.

Sartorius m.

Rectus
abdominis tt.

Inguinal
lymph node

Mons pubis

Figure 84-1.
(From El-Khoury GY, Bergman RA, Montgomery WJ: Sectional Anatomy by
MRI and CT, 3rd ed. New York, Churchill Livingstone 2007, p 594.)

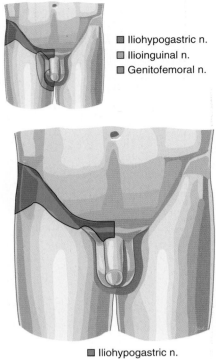

■ Iliohypogastric n.
■ Ilioinguinal n.
■ Genitofemoral n.

■ Iliohypogastric n.

Figure 84-2.

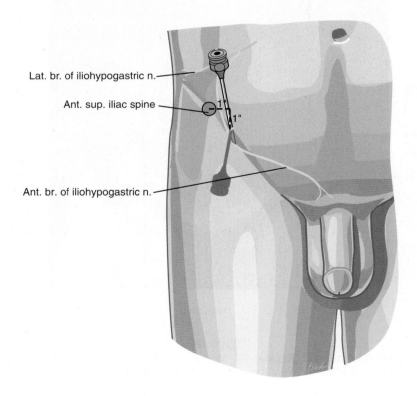

Lat. br. of iliohypogastric n.

Ant. sup. iliac spine

Ant. br. of iliohypogastric n.

Figure 84-3.

If the pain has an inflammatory component, the local anesthetic is combined with 80 mg of methylprednisolone and is injected in incremental doses. Subsequent daily nerve blocks are performed similarly, substituting 40 mg of methylprednisolone for the initial 80-mg dose. Because of overlapping innervation of the ilioinguinal and iliohypogastric nerves, it is not unusual to block branches of each nerve when performing iliohypogastric nerve block. After injection of the solution, pressure is applied to the injection site to decrease the incidence of postblock ecchymosis and hematoma formation, which can be dramatic, especially in the patient on anticoagulants.

SIDE EFFECTS AND COMPLICATIONS

The main side effect of iliohypogastric nerve block is postblock ecchymosis and hematoma formation. If needle placement is too deep and enters the peritoneal cavity, perforation of the colon may result in intra-abdominal abscess and fistula formation. Early detection of infection is crucial to avoid potentially life-threatening sequelae.

CLINICAL PEARLS

Iliohypogastric nerve block is a simple technique that can produce dramatic relief for patients suffering from the previously mentioned pain complaints. Neurolytic block with small quantities of phenol in glycerin or by cryoneurolysis or radiofrequency lesioning has been shown to provide long-term relief for patients suffering from chronic pain secondary to trauma to the ilioinguinal nerve in whom more conservative treatments have been ineffectual. As mentioned earlier, pressure should be maintained on the injection site after the block to avoid ecchymosis and hematoma formation.

If a patient presents with pain suggestive of iliohypogastric neuralgia and iliohypogastric nerve blocks are ineffectual, a diagnosis of lesions more proximal in the lumbar plexus or an L1 radiculopathy should be considered. Such patients often respond to epidural steroid blocks. Electromyography and magnetic resonance imaging of the lumbar plexus are indicated in these patients to help rule out other causes of groin pain, including malignancy invading the lumbar plexus and epidural or vertebral metastatic disease at T12-L1.

CHAPTER 85

Genitofemoral Nerve Block

CPT-2009 CODE

Unilateral	64450
Neurolytic	64640

Relative Value Units

Unilateral	8
Neurolytic	20

INDICATIONS

Genitofemoral nerve block is useful in the evaluation and management of groin pain thought to be subserved by the genitofemoral nerve, including the pain associated with genitofemoral neuralgia. The technique also is useful to provide surgical anesthesia for groin surgery, including inguinal herniorrhaphy when combined with iliohypogastric and ilioinguinal nerve block. Genitofemoral nerve block with local anesthetics can be used diagnostically during differential neural blockade on an anatomic basis in the evaluation of groin pain when peripheral nerve entrapment versus lumbar radiculopathy is being evaluated. If destruction of the genitofemoral nerve is being considered, this technique is useful as a prognostic indicator of the degree of motor and sensory impairment. Genitofemoral nerve block with local anesthetic may be used to palliate acute pain emergencies, including postoperative pain relief, while one is waiting for pharmacologic methods to become effective. Genitofemoral nerve block with local anesthetic and steroids also is useful in the treatment of persistent pain after inguinal surgery or groin trauma when the pain is thought to be secondary to inflammation or entrapment of the genitofemoral nerve.

Destruction of the genitofemoral nerve is occasionally indicated for the palliation of persistent groin pain after blunt or open trauma to the groin or persistent pain mediated by the genitofemoral nerve after groin surgery. Genitofemoral nerve block via a 25-gauge needle may be performed in the presence of coagulopathy or anticoagulation, albeit with an increased risk for ecchymosis and hematoma formation.

CLINICALLY RELEVANT ANATOMY

The genitofemoral nerve is a branch of the L1 nerve root with a contribution from T12 in some patients. The nerve follows a curvilinear course that takes it from its origin of the L1 and occasionally T12 and L2 somatic nerves to inside the concavity of the ilium. The genitofemoral nerve descends obliquely in an anterior course through the psoas major muscle to emerge on the abdominal surface opposite L3 or L4. The nerve descends subperitoneally behind the ureter and divides into a genital and femoral branch just above the inguinal ligament. In males, the genital branch travels through the inguinal canal passing inside the deep inguinal ring to innervate the cremaster muscle and skin of the scrotum. In females, the genital branch follows the course of the round ligament and provides innervation to the ipsilateral mons pubis and labia majora. In males and females, the femoral branch descends lateral to the external iliac artery to pass behind the inguinal ligament. The nerve enters the femoral sheath lateral to the femoral artery to innervate the skin of the anterior superior femoral triangle (Fig. 85-1).

TECHNIQUE

The patient is placed in the supine position with a pillow under the knees if extending the legs increases the patient's pain because of traction on the nerve. The anterior-superior iliac spine, femoral artery, femoral crease, and pubic tubercle are identified by palpation. To block the genital branch of the genitofemoral nerve, the pubic tubercle and the inguinal ligament are identified. A point just lateral to the pubic tubercle just below the inguinal ligament is then identified and prepared with antiseptic solution. A 25-gauge, $1\frac{1}{2}$-inch needle is then advanced through the skin and subcutaneous tissues (Fig. 85-2). Five milliliters of 1.0% preservative-free lidocaine is injected after careful aspiration. Care must be

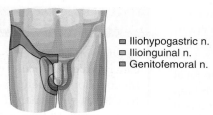

- Iliohypogastric n.
- Ilioinguinal n.
- Genitofemoral n.

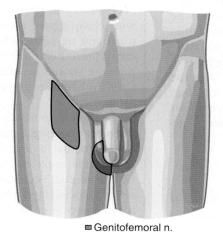

Figure 85-1.

- Genitofemoral n.

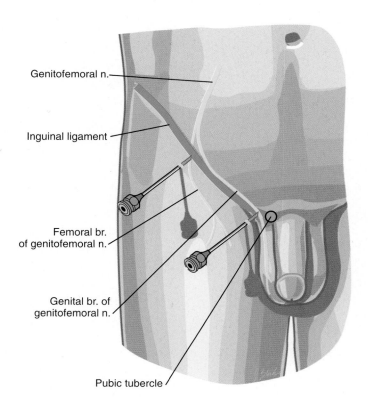

Genitofemoral n.

Inguinal ligament

Femoral br.
of genitofemoral n.

Genital br. of
genitofemoral n.

Pubic tubercle

Figure 85-2.

taken not to place the needle too deep and enter the peritoneal cavity and perforate the abdominal viscera or to inadvertently inject the local anesthetic into the femoral artery.

If the pain has an inflammatory component, the local anesthetic for the above blocks is combined with 80 mg of methylprednisolone and is injected in incremental doses. Subsequent daily nerve blocks are performed similarly, substituting 40 mg of methylprednisolone for the initial 80-mg dose. Because of overlapping innervation of the genitofemoral, ilioinguinal, and iliohypogastric nerves, it is not unusual to block branches of each nerve when performing genitofemoral nerve block. After the solution is injected, pressure is applied to the injection site to decrease the incidence of postblock ecchymosis and hematoma formation, which can be dramatic, especially when the patient is on anticoagulants.

SIDE EFFECTS AND COMPLICATIONS

The main side effect of genitofemoral nerve block is postblock ecchymosis and hematoma formation. If needle placement is too deep and enters the peritoneal cavity, perforation of the colon may result in intra-abdominal abscess and fistula formation. Early detection of infection is crucial to avoid potentially life-threatening sequelae.

CLINICAL PEARLS

Genitofemoral nerve block is a simple technique that can produce dramatic relief for patients who have the previously mentioned pain complaints. Neurolytic block with small quantities of phenol in glycerin or by cryoneurolysis or radiofrequency lesioning has been shown to provide long-term relief for patients with chronic pain secondary to trauma to the genitofemoral nerve in whom more conservative treatments have been ineffectual. As mentioned earlier, pressure should be maintained on the injection site after the block to avoid ecchymosis and hematoma formation.

If a patient presents with pain suggestive of genitofemoral neuralgia and genitofemoral nerve blocks are ineffectual, a diagnosis of lesions more proximal in the lumbar plexus or an L1 radiculopathy should be considered. Such cases often respond to epidural steroid blocks. Electromyography and magnetic resonance imaging of the lumbar plexus are indicated in this patient population to help rule out other causes of genitofemoral pain, including malignancy invading the lumbar plexus or epidural or vertebral metastatic disease at T12-L1.

Section 6

Back and Pelvis

CHAPTER **86**

Lumbar Sympathetic Ganglion Block

INDICATIONS

Lumbar sympathetic ganglion block is useful in the evaluation and management of sympathetically mediated pain of the kidneys, ureters, genitalia, and lower extremities. Included in this category are phantom limb pain, reflex sympathetic dystrophy, causalgia, and a variety of peripheral neuropathies. Lumbar sympathetic ganglion block also is useful in the palliation of pain secondary to vascular insufficiency of the lower extremity, including pain secondary to frostbite, atherosclerosis, Buerger's disease, and arteritis secondary to collagen vascular disease and to maximize blood flow after vascular procedures on the lower extremities.

Lumbar sympathetic ganglion block with local anesthetic can be used as a diagnostic tool when performing differential neural blockade on an anatomic basis in the evaluation of flank, pelvis, and lower extremity pain. If destruction of the lumbar sympathetic chain is being considered, this technique is useful as a prognostic indicator of the degree of pain relief that the patient may experience. Lumbar sympathetic ganglion block with local anesthetic also is useful in the treatment of acute herpes zoster and postherpetic neuralgia involving the lumbar and sacral dermatomes. Destruction of the lumbar sympathetic chain is indicated for the palliation of pain syndromes that have responded to lumbar sympathetic blockade with local anesthetic.

CLINICALLY RELEVANT ANATOMY

The preganglionic fibers of the lumbar sympathetics exit the intervertebral foramina along with the lumbar paravertebral nerves. After exiting the intervertebral foramen, the lumbar paravertebral nerve gives off a recurrent branch that loops back through the foramen to provide innervation to the spinal ligaments, meninges, and its respective vertebra. The upper lumbar paravertebral nerve also interfaces with the lumbar sympathetic chain via the myelinated preganglionic fibers of the white rami communicantes. All five of the lumbar nerves interface with the unmyelinated postganglionic fibers of the gray rami communicantes. At the level of the lumbar sympathetic ganglia, preganglionic and postganglionic fibers synapse. Additionally, some of the postganglionic fibers return to their respective somatic nerves via the gray rami communicantes. Other lumbar sympathetic postganglionic fibers travel to the aortic and hypogastric plexus and course up and down the sympathetic trunk to terminate in distant ganglia.

In many patients, the first and second lumbar ganglia are fused. These ganglia and the remainder of the lumbar chain and ganglia lie at the anterolateral margin of the lumbar vertebral bodies. The peritoneal cavity lies lateral and anterior to the lumbar sympathetic chain. Given the proximity of the lumbar somatic nerves to the lumbar sympathetic chain, the potential exists for both neural pathways to be blocked when performing blockade of the lumbar sympathetic ganglion.

TECHNIQUE

The patient is placed in the prone position with a pillow under the abdomen to gently flex the lumbar spine. The spinous process of the vertebra just above the nerve to be blocked is palpated. At a point just below and 3 inches lateral to the spinous process, the skin is prepared with antiseptic solution. A 22-gauge, $3\frac{1}{2}$-inch needle is attached to a 12-mL syringe and is advanced at a 35- to 45-degree angle to the skin, aiming for the lateral aspect of the vertebral body. The needle should impinge on

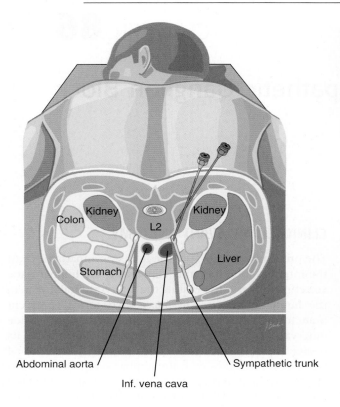

Abdominal aorta

Inf. vena cava

Sympathetic trunk

Figure 86-1.

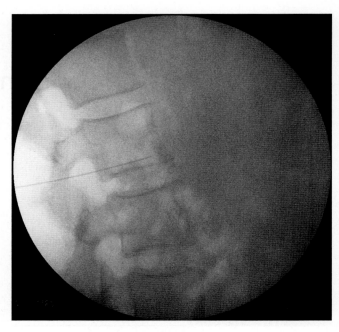

Figure 86-2.
Needle tip resting at the anterolateral border of the vertebral body.

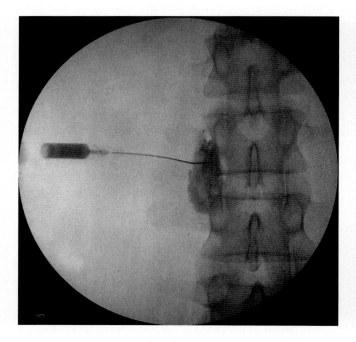

Figure 86-3.
PA view of contrast medium lateral to the vertebral body.

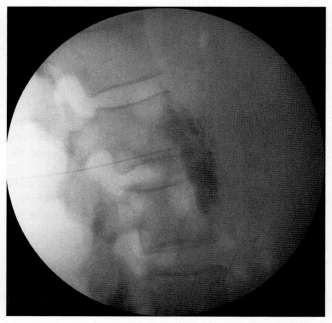

Figure 86-4.
Lateral view of contrast medium just anterior to the vertebral body.

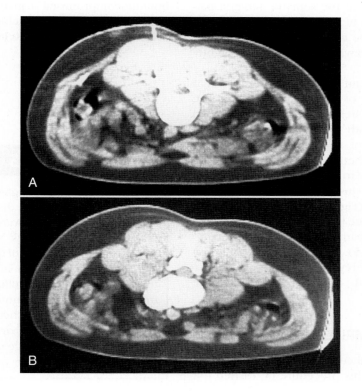

Figure 86-5.
A, CT–guided needle placement for lumbar sympathetic block. **B,** Proper spread of contrast medium outlining the sympathetic chain. (From Waldman SD: Interventional Pain Management, 2nd ed. Philadelphia, WB Saunders, 2001, p 501.)

bone after being advanced about 2 inches. If the needle comes into contact with bone at a shallower depth, it has probably impinged on the transverse process. If this occurs, the needle should be directed in a slightly more cephalad trajectory to pass above the transverse process to impinge on the lateral aspect of the vertebral body. After bony contact is made with the vertebral body, the needle is withdrawn into the subcutaneous tissues and redirected at a slightly steeper angle and walked off the lateral margin of the vertebral body. As soon as bony contact is lost, the needle is slowly advanced about $\frac{1}{2}$ inch deeper (Fig. 86-1). Given the proximity of the lumbar sympathetic chain to the somatic nerve, a paresthesia in the distribution of the corresponding lumbar paravertebral nerve may be elicited. If this occurs, the needle should be withdrawn and redirected slightly more cephalad.

The needle is then again slowly advanced until it passes the lateral border of the vertebral body. The needle should ultimately rest at the anterior lateral margin of the vertebral body (Fig. 86-2). If fluoroscopy is used, a small amount of contrast medium may be added to the local anesthetic. The contrast medium should appear just anterior to the vertebral body on the posteroanterior view and just lateral to the vertebral body on the lateral view (Figs. 86-3 and 86-4). If computed tomographic guidance is used, the contrast can be seen surrounding the sympathetic chain anterolateral to the vertebral body (Fig. 86-5). Once the needle is in position and careful aspiration reveals no blood or cerebrospinal fluid, 12 to 15 mL of 1.0% preservative-free lidocaine is injected.

SIDE EFFECTS AND COMPLICATIONS

The proximity to the spinal cord and exiting nerve roots makes it imperative that this procedure be carried out only by those well versed in the regional anatomy and experienced in performing interventional pain management techniques. Given the proximity of the peritoneal cavity, damage to the abdominal viscera during lumbar sympathetic ganglion block is a distinct possibility. The incidence of this complication is decreased when care is taken to place the needle just beyond the anterolateral margin vertebral body. Needle placement too medial may result in epidural, subdural, or subarachnoid injections or trauma to the intervertebral disk, spinal cord, and exiting nerve roots. Although uncommon, infection remains an ever-present possibility, especially in the immunocompromised cancer or AIDS patient. Early detection of infection, including diskitis, is crucial to avoid potentially life-threatening sequelae.

CLINICAL PEARLS

Lumbar sympathetic ganglion block is a simple technique that can produce dramatic relief for patients suffering from the previously mentioned pain complaints. Neurolytic block with small quantities of absolute alcohol or phenol in glycerin, or by cryoneurolysis or radiofrequency lesioning, has been shown to provide long-term relief for patients suffering from sympathetically maintained pain that has been relieved with local anesthetic. As mentioned earlier, the proximity of the lumbar sympathetic chain to the neuraxis and pleural space makes careful attention to technique mandatory.

CHAPTER 87

Lumbar Sympathetic Ganglion Block: Radiofrequency Lesioning

CPT-2009 CODE

Radiofrequency Lesioning	64680

Relative Value Units

Neurolytic	20

INDICATIONS

Radiofrequency lesioning of the lumbar sympathetic chain is indicated for patients who have experienced short-term pain relief following lumbar sympathetic blockade with local anesthetic but have failed to experience long-term relief. Pain syndromes amenable to treatment with lumbar sympathetic ganglion block include sympathetically mediated pain of the kidneys, ureters, genitalia, and lower extremities. Included in this category are phantom limb pain, reflex sympathetic dystrophy, causalgia, and a variety of peripheral neuropathies. Lumbar sympathetic ganglion radiofrequency lesioning also may be considered in patients suffering from pain secondary to vascular insufficiency of the lower extremity, including pain secondary to frostbite, atherosclerosis, Buerger's disease, and arteritis secondary to collagen vascular disease and to maximize blood flow after vascular procedures on the lower extremities.

CLINICALLY RELEVANT ANATOMY

The preganglionic fibers of the lumbar sympathetics exit the intervertebral foramina along with the lumbar paravertebral nerves. After exiting the intervertebral foramen, the lumbar paravertebral nerve gives off a recurrent branch that loops back through the foramen to provide innervation to the spinal ligaments, meninges, and its respective vertebra. The upper lumbar paravertebral nerve also interfaces with the lumbar sympathetic chain via the myelinated preganglionic fibers of the white rami communicantes. All five of the lumbar nerves interface with the unmyelinated postganglionic fibers of the gray rami communicantes. At the level of the lumbar sympathetic ganglia, preganglionic and postganglionic fibers synapse. Additionally, some of the postganglionic fibers return to their respective somatic nerves via the gray rami communicantes. Other lumbar sympathetic postganglionic fibers travel to the aortic and hypogastric plexus and course up and down the sympathetic trunk to terminate in distant ganglia.

In many patients, the first and second lumbar ganglia are fused. These ganglia and the remainder of the lumbar chain and ganglia lie at the anterolateral margin of the lumbar vertebral bodies. The peritoneal cavity lies lateral and anterior to the lumbar sympathetic chain. Given the proximity of the lumbar somatic nerves to the lumbar sympathetic chain, the potential exists for both neural pathways to be blocked when performing blockade of the lumbar sympathetic ganglion.

TECHNIQUE

The patient is placed in the prone position with a pillow under the abdomen to gently flex the lumbar spine. The spinous process of the vertebra just above the nerve to be blocked is palpated. At a point just below and 3 inches lateral to the spinous process, the skin is prepared with antiseptic solution. A 20-gauge, 150-mm radiofrequency needle with a 10-mm active tip is advanced at a 35- to 45-degree angle to the skin, aiming for the lateral aspect of the L2 vertebral body. The needle should impinge on bone after being advanced about 2 inches. If the needle comes into contact with bone at a shallower depth, it has probably impinged on the transverse process. If this occurs, the needle should be directed in a slightly more cephalad trajectory to pass above the transverse process to impinge on the lateral aspect of the vertebral body.

After bony contact is made with the vertebral body, the needle is withdrawn into the subcutaneous tissues and redirected at a slightly steeper angle and walked off the lateral margin of the vertebral body. As soon as bony contact is lost, the needle is slowly advanced about ½ inch deeper (Fig. 87-1; see also Fig. 86-1). Given the

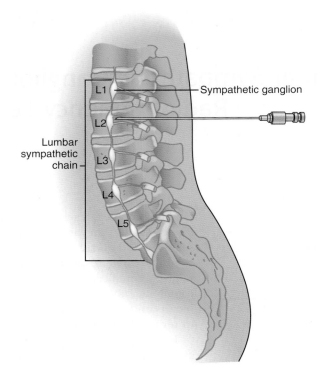

L1
L2
L3
L4
L5

Lumbar
sympathetic
chain

Sympathetic ganglion

Figure 87-1.

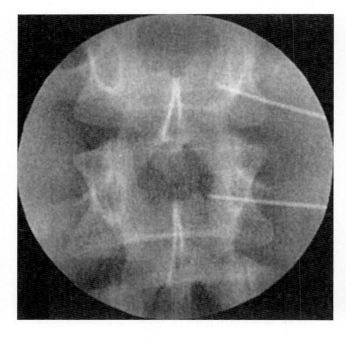

Figure 87-2.

PA radiograph shows the radiofrequency cannula positions during lesioning of the lumbar sympathetic chain. Note that the tips of the radiofrequency cannulas are directly behind the facet joint line. (From Waldman SD: Interventional Pain Management, 2nd ed. Philadelphia, WB Saunders, 2001, p 285.)

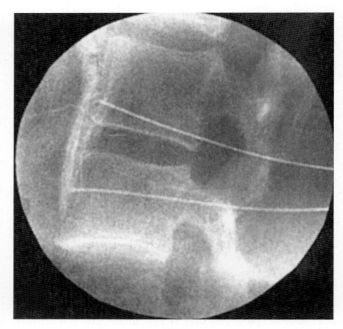

Figure 87-3.

Lateral radiograph shows the radiofrequency cannula positions at the L2 and L3 levels for lesioning of the lumbar sympathetic chain. (From Waldman SD: Interventional Pain Management, 2nd ed. Philadelphia, WB Saunders, 2001, p 285.)

proximity of the lumbar sympathetic chain to the somatic nerve, a paresthesia in the distribution of the corresponding lumbar paravertebral nerve may be elicited. If this occurs, the needle should be withdrawn and redirected slightly more cephalad. The needle is then again slowly advanced until it passes the lateral border of the vertebral body. The needle should ultimately rest at the anterior lateral margin of the vertebral body (Figs. 87-2 and 87-3; see also Fig. 86-2). A small amount of contrast medium is then injected through the needle. The contrast medium should appear just anterior to the vertebral body on the posteroanterior view and just lateral to the vertebral body on the lateral view (see Figs. 86-1 and 86-2). If computed tomographic guidance is used, the contrast can be seen surrounding the sympathetic chain anterolateral to the vertebral body (see Fig. 86-5).

Once the needle is in position and careful aspiration reveals no blood or cerebrospinal fluid, trial stimulation at 50 Hz at 1 V is carried out. The patient should experience pain localized to the low back. If pain is felt in the groin, the needle is in proximity of the genitofemoral nerve or L1 or L2 nerve roots and must be repositioned. If pain is felt in the lower extremity, the needle is in proximity to the lower lumbar nerve roots and must be repositioned. Motor stimulation should be negative with 3 V at 2 Hz. If stimulation trials are satisfactory, a lesion is created for 60 seconds at 80°C. Based on the patient's clinical response, additional lesions below the initial lesions may be required to provide long-lasting pain relief.

SIDE EFFECTS AND COMPLICATIONS

The proximity to the spinal cord and exiting nerve roots makes it imperative that this procedure be carried out only by those well versed in the regional anatomy and experienced in performing interventional pain management techniques. Given the proximity of the peritoneal cavity, damage to the abdominal viscera during lumbar sympathetic ganglion radiofrequency lesioning is a distinct possibility. The incidence of this complication is decreased when care is taken to place the needle just beyond the anterolateral margin vertebral body. Needle placement that is too medial may result in epidural, subdural, or subarachnoid injections or trauma to the intervertebral disk, spinal cord, and exiting nerve roots. Lesioning with the needle in proximity to the genitofemoral nerve may result in persistent genitofemoral neuritis that can be difficult to treat. Although uncommon, infection remains an ever-present possibility, especially in the immunocompromised cancer or AIDS patient. Early detection of infection, including diskitis, is crucial to avoid potentially life-threatening sequelae.

CLINICAL PEARLS

Lumbar sympathetic ganglion radiofrequency lesioning is a straightforward technique that can produce long-lasting relief for patients suffering from the previously mentioned pain complaints who have responded temporarily to blockade with local anesthetics. Neurolytic block with small quantities of absolute alcohol or phenol in glycerin, or by cryoneurolysis or radiofrequency lesioning, also has been shown to provide long-term relief for patients suffering from sympathetically maintained pain that has been relieved with local anesthetic and represents reasonable alternatives to radiofrequency lesioning of the lumbar sympathetic ganglion. Spinal cord stimulation is also an appropriate intervention in many of the patients suffering from the previously mentioned pain complaints. As mentioned earlier, the proximity of the lumbar sympathetic chain to the neuraxis, genitofemoral nerve, and peritoneal and pleural space makes careful attention to technique mandatory.

CHAPTER 88

Lumbar Paravertebral Nerve Block

CPT-2009 CODE

Unilateral Single	64483
Additional Nerve	64484
Neurolytic	64640

Relative Value Units

Unilateral Single	12
Each Additional Level	8
Neurolytic	20

INDICATIONS

Lumbar paravertebral nerve block is useful in the evaluation and management of pain involving the upper abdominal wall, groin, lower extremity, and lumbar spine. Lumbar paravertebral nerve block with local anesthetic can be used as a diagnostic tool when performing differential neural blockade on an anatomic basis in the evaluation of lower extremity, lumbar spine, abdominal, and groin pain. If destruction of the lumbar paravertebral nerve is being considered, this technique is useful as a prognostic indicator of the degree of motor and sensory impairment that the patient may experience. Lumbar paravertebral nerve block with local anesthetic may be used to palliate acute pain emergencies, including lumbar vertebral compression fracture, acute herpes zoster, and cancer pain while waiting for pharmacologic, surgical, and antiblastic methods to become effective. Lumbar paravertebral nerve block with local anesthetic and steroid also is useful in the treatment of postlaparotomy pain, the pain of vertebral fractures, and postherpetic neuralgia. For less localized pain syndromes, either lumbar plexus block or lumbar epidural block is used.

Destruction of the lumbar paravertebral nerve is indicated for the palliation of cancer pain, including invasive tumors of the lumbar spine, posterior elements of the lumbar vertebra and the groin, and upper abdominal wall. Given the desperate nature of many patients suffer-ing from aggressively invasive malignancies, blockade of the lumbar paravertebral nerve using a 25-gauge needle may be carried out in the presence of coagulopathy or anticoagulation, albeit with an increased risk for ecchymosis and hematoma formation.

CLINICALLY RELEVANT ANATOMY

The lumbar paravertebral nerves exit their respective intervertebral foramina just beneath the transverse process of the vertebra. After exiting the intervertebral foramen, the lumbar paravertebral nerve gives off a recurrent branch that loops back through the foramen to provide innervation to the spinal ligaments, meninges, and its respective vertebra. The lumbar paravertebral nerve then divides into posterior and anterior primary divisions. The posterior division courses posteriorly and, along with its branches, provides innervation to the facet joints and the muscles and skin of the back. The larger anterior division courses laterally and inferiorly to enter the body of the psoas muscle. Within the muscle, the first four lumbar paravertebral nerves join to form the lumbar plexus. The lumbar plexus also receives a contribution from the 12th thoracic paravertebral nerve. The lumbar plexus provides innervation to the lower abdominal wall, groin, portions of the external genitalia, and portions of the lower extremity.

TECHNIQUE

The patient is placed in the prone position with a pillow under the abdomen to slightly flex the lumbar spine. The spinous process of the vertebra at the level to be blocked is palpated. At a point 1½ inches lateral to the spinous process, the skin is prepared with antiseptic solution. A 22-gauge, 3½-inch needle is attached to a 12-mL syringe and is advanced perpendicular to the skin aiming for the middle of the transverse process (Fig. 88-1). The needle should impinge on bone after being advanced about 1½ inches. After bony contact is made, the needle is withdrawn into the subcutaneous tissues and redirected inferiorly and walked off the inferior margin of the transverse

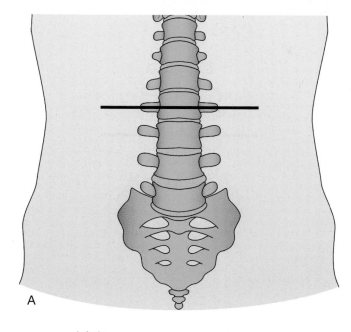

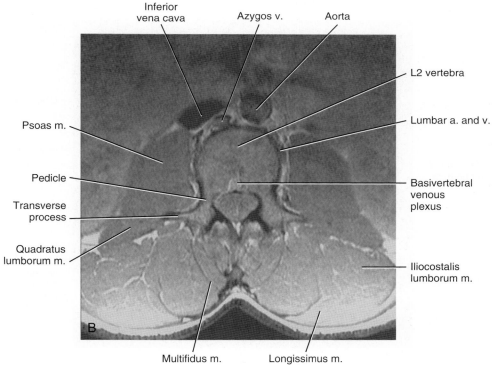

Figure 88-1.
(From: El-Khoury GY, Bergman RA, Montgomery WJ: Sectional Anatomy by MRI and CT, 3rd ed. New York, Churchill Livingstone, 2007, p 438.)

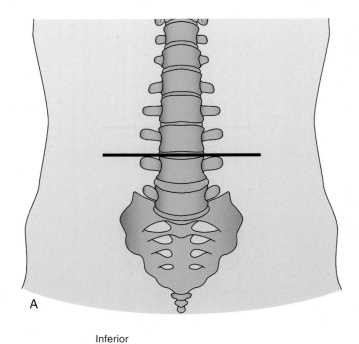

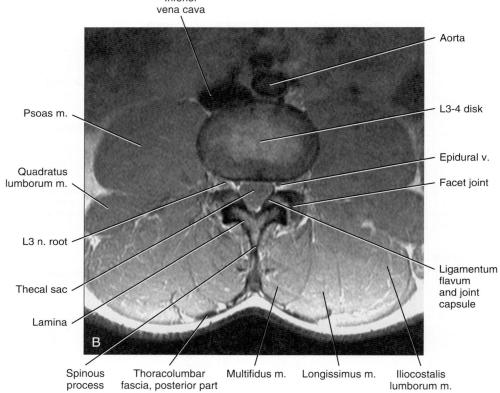

Figure 88-2.
(From El-Khoury GY, Bergman RA, Montgomery WJ: Sectional Anatomy by MRI and CT, 3rd ed. New York, Churchill Livingstone, 2007, p 438.)

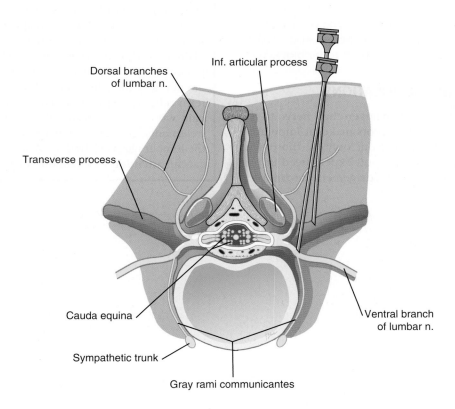

Figure 88-3.

process. As soon as bony contact is lost, the needle is slowly advanced ½ to ¾ inch deeper until a paresthesia in the distribution of the lumbar paravertebral nerve to be blocked is elicited (Figs. 88-2 and 88-3).

Once the paresthesia has been elicited and careful aspiration reveals no blood or cerebrospinal fluid, 3 mL of 1.0% preservative-free lidocaine is injected. If there is an inflammatory component to the pain, the local anesthetic is combined with 80 mg of methylprednisolone and is injected in incremental doses. Subsequent daily nerve blocks are carried out in a similar manner, substituting 40 mg of methylprednisolone for the initial 80-mg dose. Because of overlapping innervation of the posterior elements from the medial branch of the posterior division from the vertebra above, the lumbar paravertebral nerves above and below the nerve suspected of subserving the painful condition have to be blocked.

SIDE EFFECTS AND COMPLICATIONS

The proximity of the lumbar paravertebral nerve to the spinal cord and exiting nerve roots makes it imperative that this procedure be carried out only by those well versed in the regional anatomy and experienced in performing interventional pain management techniques.

Needle placement too medial may result in epidural, subdural, or subarachnoid injections or trauma to the spinal cord and exiting nerve roots. Placing the needle too deep between the transverse processes may result in trauma to the exiting lumbar nerve roots. Although uncommon, infection remains an ever-present possibility, especially in the immunocompromised cancer patient. Early detection of infection is crucial to avoid potentially life-threatening sequelae.

CLINICAL PEARLS

Lumbar paravertebral nerve block is a simple technique that can produce dramatic relief for patients suffering from the previously mentioned pain complaints. Neurolytic block with small quantities of phenol in glycerin or by cryoneurolysis or radiofrequency lesioning has been shown to provide long-term relief for patients suffering from cancer-related pain who have not responded to more conservative treatments. As mentioned earlier, the proximity of the lumbar paravertebral nerve to the neuraxis makes careful attention to technique mandatory.

CHAPTER 89

Lumbar Facet Block: Medial Branch Technique

CPT-2009 CODE	
First Joint	64475
Second Joint	64476
Neurolytic First Joint	64622
Neurolytic Second Joint	64623

Relative Value Units	
First Joint	10
Second Joint	10
Neurolytic First Joint	20
Neurolytic Second Joint	20

INDICATIONS

Lumbar facet block using the medial branch technique is useful in the diagnosis and treatment of painful conditions involving trauma, arthritis, or inflammation of the lumbar facet joints. These problems usually occur after sudden, forceful twisting of the lumbar spine while lifting or after acceleration-deceleration injuries. Pain secondary to lumbar facet syndrome may present as pain that radiates from the low back into the hips, buttocks, and thighs in a nondermatomal distribution. This pain may be associated with decreased range of motion of the lumbar spine and spasm of the lumbar paraspinal musculature.

CLINICALLY RELEVANT ANATOMY

The lumbar facet joints are formed by the articulations of the superior and inferior articular facets of adjacent vertebrae. The lumbar facet joints are true joints in that they are lined with synovium and possess a true joint capsule. This capsule is richly innervated and supports the notion of the facet joint as a pain generator. The lumbar facet joint is susceptible to arthritic changes and trauma secondary to acceleration-deceleration injuries.

Such damage to the joint results in pain secondary to synovial joint inflammation and adhesions.

Each facet joint receives innervation from two spinal levels. Each joint receives fibers from the dorsal ramus at the same level as the vertebra as well as fibers from the dorsal ramus of the vertebra above. This fact has clinical importance in that it provides an explanation for the ill-defined nature of facet-mediated pain and explains why the dorsal nerve from the vertebra above the offending level often also must be blocked to provide complete pain relief.

At each level, the dorsal ramus provides a medial branch that exits the intertransverse space crossing over the top of the transverse process in a groove at the point where the transverse process joins the vertebra. The nerve then travels inferiorly and medially across the posterior surface of the vertebral lamina where it gives off branches to innervate the facet joint. The medial branch is blocked at the point at which the nerve curves around the top of the transverse process (Fig. 89-1).

At the L5 level, it is the dorsal ramus of L5 rather than the medial branch that crosses the sacral ala at the junction of the superior articular process. After crossing the sacral ala, the dorsal ramus then gives off a medial branch that provides innervation for the lumbosacral facet joint. During performance of lumbar facet block using the medial branch approach, the L5 nerve is blocked at this point rather than at the superomedial junction of the transverse process with the vertebra, as is done when blocking the L1-L4 medial branches (Fig. 89-2).

TECHNIQUE

Lumbar facet block using the medial branch technique is the preferred route of treating lumbar facet syndrome. It may be done either blind or under fluoroscopic guidance.

The patient is placed in a prone position. Pillows are placed under the chest to allow the lumbar spine to be moderately flexed without discomfort to the patient. The forehead is allowed to rest on a folded blanket.

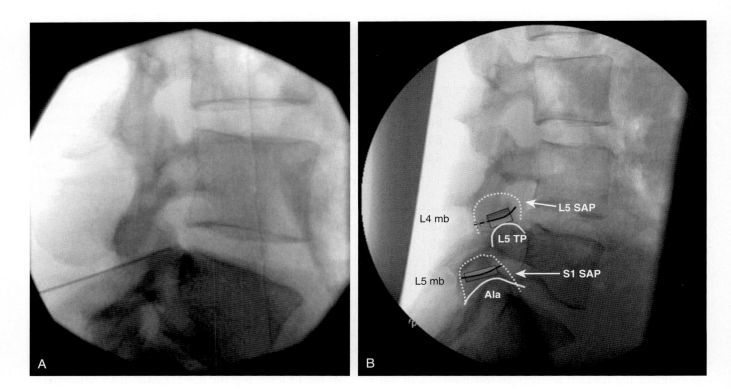

Figure 89-1.
A, In the lateral view the active tip should lie across the middle two fourths of the neck of the SAP for L1-L4 and across the posterior three fourths of the SAP for the L5 dorsal ramus, where there is no mammalo-accessory ligament that shields the nerve from the radiofrequency lesion. **B,** In the lateral view, the needle should lie along the neck of the SAP. Bone should be visible between the needle tip and the neuroforamen. SAP, superior articular process. (From Raj PP, Lou L, Erdine S, et al: Interventional Pain Management: Image-Guided Procedures, 2nd ed. Philadelphia, Saunders, 2008.)

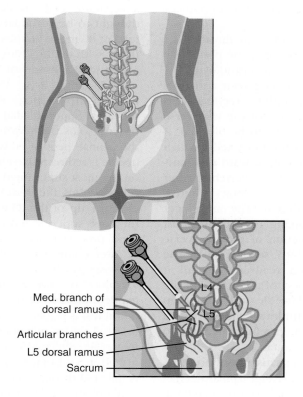

Figure 89-2.
(From Waldman: Atlas of Interventional Pain Management, 2nd ed. Philadelphia, Saunders, 2004.)

Blind Technique

To block the L1-L4 facets using a blind technique, the spinous process at the level to be blocked is identified by palpation. A point slightly inferior and 5 cm lateral to the spinous process is then identified as the site of needle insertion. After preparation of the skin with antiseptic solution, a skin wheal of local anesthetic is raised at the site of needle insertion. Three milliliters of preservative-free local anesthetic is drawn up in a 5-mL sterile syringe. When treating pain believed to be secondary to an inflammatory process, a total of 80 mg of depot-steroid is added to the local anesthetic with the first block, and 40 mg of depot-steroid is added with subsequent blocks.

An 18-gauge, 1-inch needle is inserted through the skin and into the subcutaneous tissue at the previously identified insertion site to serve as an introducer. The introducer needle is then repositioned with a slightly superior and medial trajectory, pointing directly toward the superior portion of the junction of the transverse process and the vertebra at the level to be blocked. A 25-gauge, 2- to 3½-inch needle is then inserted through the 18-gauge introducer and directed toward this junction of the transverse process and the vertebra. After bony contact is made, the depth of the contact is noted, and the spinal needle is withdrawn. The introducer needle is then repositioned, aiming toward the most superomedial aspect of the junction of the transverse process with the vertebra (Fig. 89-3; see Fig. 89-1). The 25-gauge spinal needle is then readvanced until it impinges on the lateral-most aspect of the border of the articular pillar. Should the spinal needle walk off the top of the transverse process, it is withdrawn and redirected slightly medially and inferiorly and carefully advanced to the depth of the previous bony contact.

After the needle is felt to be in satisfactory position, the stylet is removed from the 25-gauge spinal needle, and the hub is observed for blood or cerebrospinal fluid. If neither is present, gentle aspiration of the needle is carried out. If the aspiration test is negative, 1.5 mL of solution is injected through the spinal needle.

For blockade of the dorsal ramus of L5, this same technique is used, but the needle tip is placed more laterally to block the nerve as it passes through the groove between the sacral ala and the superior articular process of the sacrum (see Fig. 89-2).

Fluoroscopic Technique

If fluoroscopy is used to block the L1-L4 facets, the beam is rotated in a sagittal plane from an anterior to a posterior position, which allows identification and visualization of the junction of the transverse process and vertebra at the level to be blocked. After preparation of the skin with antiseptic solution, a skin wheal of local anesthetic is raised at a point slightly inferior and about 5 cm off the midline. An 18-gauge, 1-inch needle is inserted at the insertion site to serve as an introducer. The fluoroscopy beam is aimed directly through the introducer needle, which will appear as a small point on the fluoroscopy screen. The introducer needle is then repositioned under fluoroscopic guidance until this small point is visualized pointing directly toward the most superomedial point at which the transverse process joins the vertebra.

A total of 5 mL of contrast medium suitable for intrathecal use is drawn up in a sterile 12-mL syringe. Then, 3 mL of preservative-free local anesthetic is drawn up in a separate 5-mL sterile syringe. When treating pain thought to be secondary to an inflammatory process, a total of 80 mg of depot-steroid is added to the local anesthetic with the first block, and 40 mg of depot-steroid is added with subsequent blocks.

A 25-gauge, 2- to 3½-inch needle is then inserted through the 18-gauge introducer and directed toward the most superomedial point at which the transverse process joins the vertebra. After bony contact is made, the spinal needle is withdrawn, and the introducer needle is redirected to allow the spinal needle to impinge on the most superomedial point at which the transverse process joins the vertebra. This procedure is repeated until the tip of the 25-gauge spinal needle rests against the most superior and medial point at which the transverse process joins the vertebra (Fig. 89-4).

After confirmation of needle placement by biplanar fluoroscopy, the hub of the 25-gauge needle is observed for blood or cerebrospinal fluid. If neither is present, gentle aspiration of the needle is carried out. If the aspiration test is negative, 1 mL of contrast medium is slowly injected under fluoroscopy to reconfirm needle placement (Fig. 89-5). After correct needle placement is confirmed, 1.5 mL of local anesthetic with or without steroid is injected through the spinal needle.

To block the L5 facet, the needle tip is placed under fluoroscopic guidance to rest in the groove between the sacral ala and the superior articular process of the sacrum (see Fig. 89-2). A foam wedge placed under the pelvis helps rotate the posterior-superior iliac crest out of the way. After confirmation of needle placement by biplanar fluoroscopy, the hub of the 25-gauge needle is observed for blood or cerebrospinal fluid. If neither is present, gentle aspiration of the needle is carried out. If the aspiration test is negative, 1 mL of contrast medium is slowly injected under fluoroscopy to reconfirm needle placement (Fig. 89-6).

SIDE EFFECTS AND COMPLICATIONS

The proximity to the spinal cord and exiting nerve roots makes it imperative that this procedure be carried out

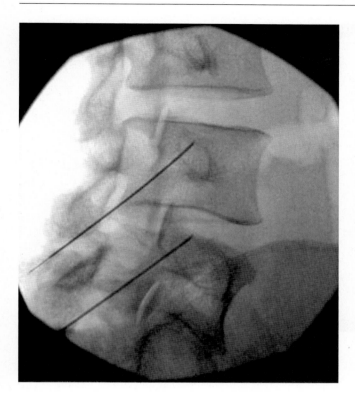

Figure 89-3.
Oblique view showing needle tips at the superior aspect of the transverse process–superior articular process junction. (From Raj PP, Lou L, Erdine S, et al: Interventional Pain Management: Image-Guided Procedures, 2nd ed. Philadelphia, Saunders, 2008.)

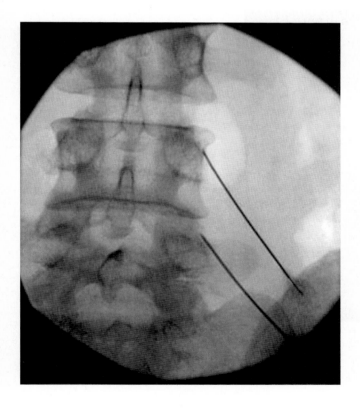

Figure 89-4.
PA view shows needle tips snug against the superior articular process and above the transverse process. (From Raj PP, Lou L, Erdine S, et al: Interventional Pain Management: Image-Guided Procedures, 2nd ed. Philadelphia, Saunders, 2008.)

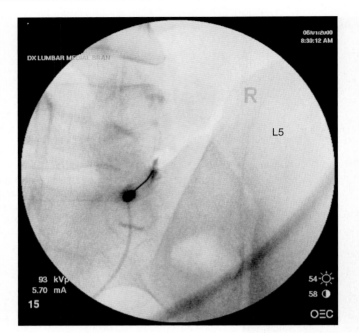

Figure 89-5.

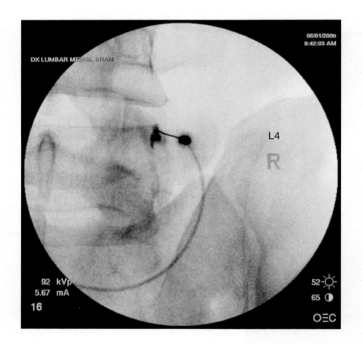

Figure 89-6.

only by those well versed in the regional anatomy and experienced in performing interventional pain management techniques. Many patients also complain of a transient increase in lumbar pain after injection into the joint.

CLINICAL PEARLS

Lumbar facet block using the medial branch approach is the preferred technique for the treatment of lumbar facet syndrome. Although intra-articular placement of the needle into the facet joint is technically feasible, unless specific diagnostic information about that specific joint is required, such maneuvers add nothing to the efficacy of the procedure and, in fact, may increase the rate of complications. Lumbar facet block is often combined with pharmacotherapy and physical therapy when treating pain in the previously mentioned areas. Many pain specialists believe that lumbar facet block is underused in the treatment of posttraumatic lumbar spine pain. These specialists believe that lumbar facet block using the medial branch approach should be considered when lumbar or caudal epidural nerve blocks, combined with conservative measures, fail to provide palliation of these pain syndromes.

CHAPTER 90

Lumbar Facet Block: Radiofrequency Lesioning of the Medial Branch of the Primary Posterior Rami

INDICATIONS

Radiofrequency lesioning of the lumbar facet joints is a reasonable next step for patients with chronic back pain that is relieved by either local anesthetic block of the affected facet joints directly or local anesthetic blockade of the medial branch. Prognostic lumbar facet block with local anesthetic using the medial branch technique is useful in predicting whether radiofrequency lesioning of the affected facet joint will provide long-lasting relief of painful conditions involving trauma, arthritis, or inflammation of the lumbar facet joints. Pain secondary to lumbar facet syndrome may manifest as pain that radiates from the low back into the hips, buttocks, thighs, and groin in a nondermatomal distribution. Because true radicular pain is associated with the dorsal root ganglion or spinal nerves, it will not respond to blockade of the lumbar facet joints and associated nerves. Facet joint pain may be associated with decreased range of motion of the lumbar spine and spasm of the lumbar paraspinal musculature, although no clinical test is completely valid as a prognostic indicator.

CLINICALLY RELEVANT ANATOMY

The lumbar facet joints are formed by the articulations of the superior and inferior articular facets of adjacent vertebrae. The lumbar facet joints are true joints in that they are lined with synovium and possess a true joint capsule. This capsule is richly innervated and supports the notion of the facet joint as a pain generator. The lumbar facet joint is susceptible to arthritic changes and trauma secondary to flexion-extension and torsion injuries. Such damage to the joint results in pain secondary to synovial joint inflammation and adhesions.

Each facet joint receives innervation from two spinal levels involving branches from the dorsal ramus at the same segmental level as well as fibers from the dorsal ramus of the suprasegmental level above. This fact has clinical importance in that it provides an explanation for the ill-defined nature of facet-mediated pain and explains why contribution from the dorsal nerve from the suprasegmental level also must be blocked to provide complete pain relief.

At each level, the dorsal ramus provides a medial branch that exits within the lateral aspect of the spinal cord coursing under the mammaloaccessory ligament (MAL) at the junction of the transverse and superior articular processes. The nerve then travels inferiorly and medially across the posterior surface of the vertebral lamina, where it gives off branches to innervate the segmental facet joint and the joint one level below. The medial branch is blocked either at the point where the nerve emerges under the MAL or at the "eye of the Scotty dog" (Fig. 90-1). At the L5 level, it is the actual dorsal ramus of L5 rather than the medial branch that crosses the sacral ala at the junction of the superior articular process. After crossing the sacral ala, the dorsal ramus courses medially and then gives off a medial branch that provides innervation for the lumbosacral facet joint. During performance of lumbar facet block using the medial branch approach, the L5 dorsal ramus is blocked at this point rather than at the superomedial junction of the transverse process with the superior articular process, as is done when blocking the L1-L4 medial branches (Fig. 90-2). Diagnostic injections must be performed twice using either the direct intra-articular or indirect medial branch approach with 75% relief of dis-

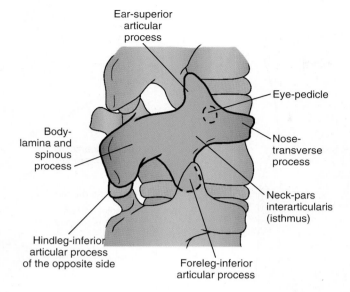

Figure 90-1.

Oblique "Scottie dog" view. (From Raj PP, Lou L, Erdine S, et al: Interventional Pain Management: Image-Guided Procedures, 2nd ed. Philadelphia, Saunders, 2008.)

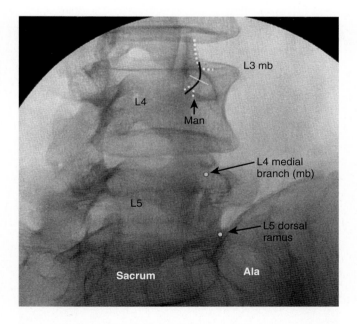

Figure 90-2.

Oblique view of the lumbar spine. Dots show targets for medial branch block. The target is midway between the mammalo-accessory notch (Man) and the superior border of the transverse process–superior articular process junction. (From Raj PP, Lou L, Erdine S, et al: Interventional Pain Management: Image-Guided Procedures, 2nd ed. Philadelphia, Saunders, 2008.)

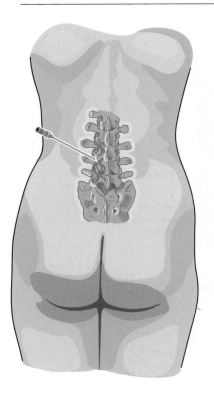

Figure 90-3.

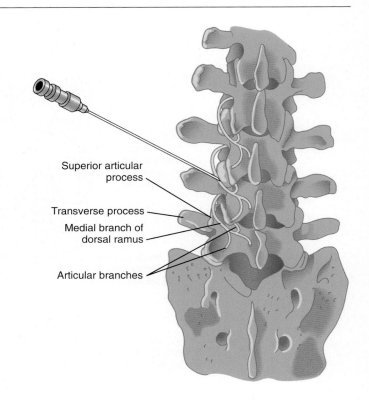

Superior articular process

Transverse process

Medial branch of dorsal ramus

Articular branches

Figure 90-4.

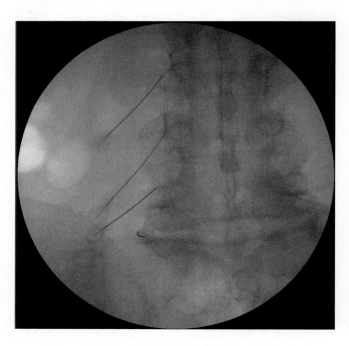

Figure 90-5.
Needle tips in position for radiofrequency lesioning.

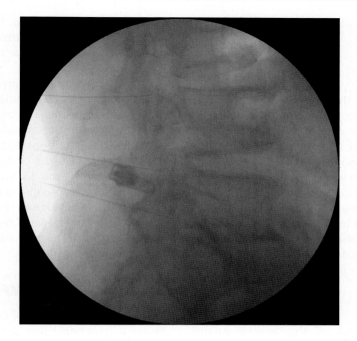

Figure 90-6.
Lateral view of needles in position for radiofrequency lesioning of the medial branch.

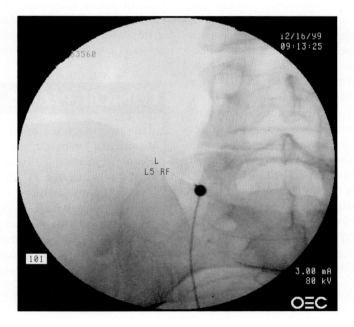

Figure 90-7.
Needle tip resting in groove between the sacral ala and the superior articular process of S1.

comfort with provocative movement before radiofrequency lesioning.

TECHNIQUE

Radiofrequency lesioning of the lumbar facet joints using the medial branch technique is the preferred neurodisruptive technique for pain emanating from the facet joint. It may be done under fluoroscopic or computed tomographic guidance, although a few very experienced pain management specialists will perform this technique without radiographic guidance using the blind technique and stimulation patterns to assist in safe needle placement. The patient is placed in a prone position. Pillows are placed under the upper abdomen to allow the lumbar spine to be moderately flexed without discomfort to the patient. The head rests on a folded blanket or pillow.

Fluoroscopic Technique

When performing neurolysis of the lumbar medial branches, the fluoroscopy beam is positioned in an anterior to posterior position with up to 15 degrees of ipsilateral obliquity, which allows identification and visualization of the transverse process, the superior articular process, and the pedicle, at the level to be blocked. After preparation of the skin with antiseptic solution, a skin wheal of local anesthetic is raised at a point inferior and medial to the junction of the transverse process and superior articular process.

A 20-gauge, 100-mm radiofrequency needle with a 10-mm curved active tip is then inserted through a puncture made with an 18-gauge needle point just inferior and medial to the junction of the transverse and superior articular processes) (Figs. 90-3 and 90-4). After bony contact is made, the radiofrequency cannula is walked over to the point where the medial branch courses under the MAL (Figs. 90-5 and 90-6). The cannula is then simulated at 5 Hz. The patient should experience stimulation described as pressure or discomfort in the low back, hip, or buttocks area at less than 0.4 V. There should be no stimulation in a radicular pattern below the knee. This stimulation pattern suggests improper needle placement in proximity to the segmental spinal nerve. Motor stimulation of the radiofrequency cannula is then performed at 2 Hz up to 2 to 2.5 V. Fasciculations of the multifidus

muscle should be observed. No motor stimulation of the muscles of the lower extremity should be noted. If present, the needle must be repositioned away from the segmental nerve root.

After confirmation of correct needle placement with both fluoroscopy and stimulation of the radiofrequency needle, local anesthetic is injected, and a lesion is made at 80°C for 60 to 90 seconds. A second lesion is often made after slight repositioning of the cannula either medial or lateral to its original position. To lesion the medial branch of the L5 facet joint, the needle tip is placed under fluoroscopic guidance to rest in the groove between the sacral ala and the superior articular process of S1 (Fig. 90-7). The same technique as described previously is then used to perform radiofrequency lesioning of the dorsal rami of L5.

SIDE EFFECTS AND COMPLICATIONS

The proximity to the spinal cord and exiting nerve roots makes it imperative that this procedure be carried out only by those well versed in the regional anatomy and experienced in performing interventional pain management techniques. Many patients also complain of a transient increase in lumbar pain after radiofrequency lesioning of the medial branch. Some advocate the use of corticosteroid injection to decrease postprocedure discomfort. Improper needle placement may lead to permanent lower extremity weakness, persistent neuritis, especially involving the genitofemoral nerve, and permanent sensory deficit. These complications can be avoided by strict adherence to the previous technique.

CLINICAL PEARLS

Radiofrequency lesioning of the lumbar facet using the medial branch approach is the preferred technique for providing long-lasting relief of the pain and disability associated with lumbar facet syndrome. This technique is often combined with pharmacotherapy and physical therapy when treating pain in the previously mentioned areas. Many pain specialists believe that this technique is underused in the treatment of post-traumatic lumbar spine pain.

CHAPTER 91

Lumbar Facet Block: Intra-articular Technique

CPT-2009 CODE	
First Joint	64475
Second Joint	64476
Neurolytic First Joint	64622
Neurolytic Second Joint	64623

Relative Value Units	
First Joint	10
Second Joint	10
Neurolytic First Joint	20
Neurolytic Second Joint	20

INDICATIONS

Lumbar facet block using the intra-articular technique is indicated primarily as a diagnostic maneuver to prove that a specific facet joint is in fact the source of pain. The medial branch technique of lumbar facet block is suitable for most clinical applications, including the treatment of painful conditions involving trauma, arthritis, or inflammation of the lumbar facet joints. These problems may manifest clinically as ill-defined back pain that radiates into the hips, buttocks, and thighs in a nondermatomal pattern.

CLINICALLY RELEVANT ANATOMY

The lumbar facet joints are formed by the articulations of the superior and inferior articular facets of adjacent vertebrae. The lumbar facet joints are true joints in that they are lined with synovium and possess a true joint capsule. This capsule is richly innervated and supports the notion of the facet joint as a pain generator. The lumbar facet joint is susceptible to arthritic changes and trauma secondary to acceleration-deceleration injuries.

Such damage to the joint results in pain secondary to synovial joint inflammation and adhesions.

Each facet joint receives innervation from two spinal levels. Each joint receives fibers from the dorsal ramus at the same level as the vertebra as well as fibers from the dorsal ramus of the vertebra above. This fact has clinical importance in that it provides an explanation for the ill-defined nature of facet-mediated pain and explains why the dorsal nerve from the vertebra above the offending level often also must be blocked to provide complete pain relief.

At each level, the dorsal ramus provides a medial branch that exits the intertransverse space crossing over the top of the transverse process in a groove at the point where the transverse process joins the vertebra. The nerve then travels inferiorly and medially across the posterior surface of the vertebral lamina where it gives off branches to innervate the facet joint. The medial branch is blocked at the point at which the nerve curves around the top of the transverse process. At the L5 level, it is the actual dorsal ramus of L5 rather than the medial branch that crosses the sacral ala at the junction of the superior articular process. After crossing the sacral ala, the dorsal ramus then gives off a medial branch that provides innervation for the lumbosacral facet joint. During performance of lumbar facet block using the medial branch approach, the L5 nerve is blocked at this point, rather than at the superomedial junction of the transverse process with the vertebra, as is done when blocking the L1-L4 medial branches.

TECHNIQUE

Lumbar facet block using the intra-articular technique may be performed either blind or under fluoroscopic guidance. The patient is placed in a prone position. Pillows are placed under the chest to allow the lumbar spine to be moderately flexed without discomfort to the patient. The forehead is allowed to rest on a folded blanket.

Blind Technique

To block the L1-L4 facet joints using the blind technique, the spinous process at the level to be blocked is identified by palpation. A point one spinal level lower and 3.5 cm lateral to the spinous process is then identified as the site of needle insertion. Three milliliters of preservative-free local anesthetic is drawn up in a 5-mL sterile syringe. After preparation of the skin with antiseptic solution, a skin wheal of local anesthetic is raised at the site of needle insertion. When treating pain believed to be secondary to an inflammatory process, a total of 80 mg of depot-steroid is added to the local anesthetic with the first block, and 40 mg of depot-steroid is added with subsequent blocks.

An 18-gauge, 1-inch needle is inserted through the skin and into the subcutaneous tissue at the previously identified insertion site to serve as an introducer. The introducer needle is then repositioned with a superior and ventral trajectory, pointing directly toward the inferior margin of the facet joint at the level to be blocked. The angle of the needle from the skin is about 35 degrees. A 25-gauge, 3½-inch styletted spinal needle is then inserted through the 18-gauge introducer and directed toward the bone just below the joint to be blocked. Care must be taken to be sure the trajectory of the needle does not drift either laterally or medially. Medial drift can allow the needle to enter the epidural, subdural, or subarachnoid space and to traumatize the dorsal root or spinal cord. Lateral drift can allow the needle to pass beyond the lateral border of the vertebra and traumatize the exiting nerve roots.

After bony contact is made, the depth of the contact is noted, and the spinal needle is withdrawn. The introducer needle is then redirected slightly more superiorly. The spinal needle is then advanced through the introducer needle until it either enters the facet joint or again impinges on bone. If the needle again impinges on bone, the maneuver is repeated until the spinal needle slides into the facet joint (Fig. 91-1). A pop is often felt as the needle slides into the joint cavity.

After the needle is believed to be in satisfactory position, the stylet is removed from the 25-gauge spinal needle, and the hub is observed for blood or cerebrospinal fluid. If neither is present, gentle aspiration of the needle is carried out. If the aspiration test is negative, 1 mL of solution is injected slowly through the spinal needle. Rapid or forceful injection may rupture the joint capsule and exacerbate the patient's pain.

To block the lumbosacral (L5) facet joint using the intra-articular technique, the previously discussed technique is used, but it may be necessary to move the needle insertion point slightly more inferior and lateral to avoid the posterior-superior iliac crest. Placing a foam wedge under the pelvis to rotate the iliac crest may also help.

Fluoroscopic Technique

If fluoroscopy is used to block the L1-L4 joints, the beam is rotated in a sagittal plane from an anterior to posterior position, which allows identification and visualization of the articular pillars of the respective vertebrae and the adjacent facet joints. After preparation of the skin with antiseptic solution, a skin wheal of local anesthetic is raised at the site of needle insertion. An 18-gauge, 1-inch needle is inserted at the insertion site to serve as an introducer. The fluoroscopy beam is aimed directly through the introducer needle, which will appear as a small point on the fluoroscopy screen. The introducer needle is then repositioned under fluoroscopic guidance until this small point is visualized pointing directly toward the inferior aspect of the facet joint to be blocked.

A total of 5 mL of contrast medium suitable for intrathecal use is drawn up in a sterile 12-mL syringe. Then, 2 mL of preservative-free local anesthetic is drawn up in a separate 5-mL sterile syringe. When treating pain believed to be secondary to an inflammatory process, a total of 80 mg of depot-steroid is added to the local anesthetic with the first block, and 40 mg of depot-steroid is added with subsequent blocks.

A 25-gauge, 2- to 3½-inch needle is then inserted through the 18-gauge introducer and directed toward the articular pillar just below the joint to be blocked. After bony contact is made, the spinal needle is withdrawn and the introducer needle repositioned superiorly, aiming toward the facet joint. The 25-gauge spinal needle is then readvanced through the introducer needle until it enters the target joint (Figs. 91-2 and 91-3).

To block the lumbosacral (L5) facet joint using the intra-articular technique, the just-discussed technique is used, but it may be necessary to move the needle insertion point slightly more inferior and lateral to avoid the posterior-superior iliac crest (Fig. 91-4). Placing a foam wedge under the pelvis to rotate the iliac crest may also help.

After confirmation of needle placement by biplanar fluoroscopy, the stylet is removed from the 25-gauge spinal needle, and the hub is observed for blood or cerebrospinal fluid. If neither is present, gentle aspiration of the needle is carried out. If the aspiration test is negative, 1 mL of contrast medium is slowly injected under fluoroscopy to reconfirm needle placement (Figs. 91-5 and 91-6). After correct needle placement is confirmed, 1 mL of local anesthetic with or without steroid is slowly injected through the spinal needle. Rapid or forceful injection may rupture the joint capsule and exacerbate the patient's pain.

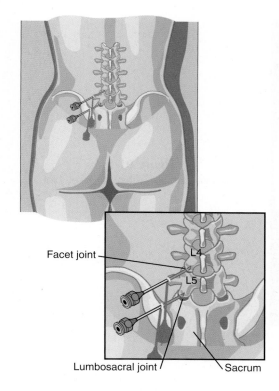

Facet joint

L4

L5

Lumbosacral joint

Sacrum

Figure 91-1.

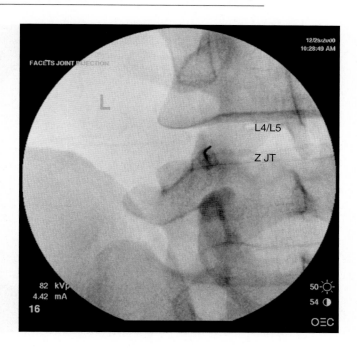

Figure 91-2.
Introducer needle in facet joint.

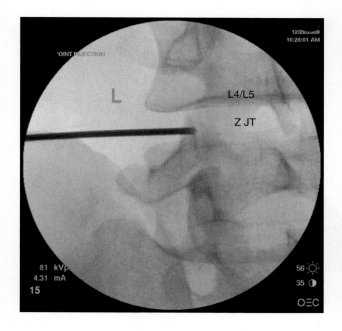

Figure 91-3.
Introducer needle in facet joint.

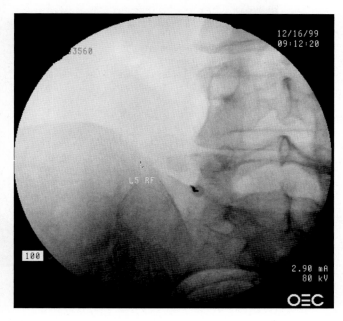

Figure 91-4.
Needle in position for L5 injection.

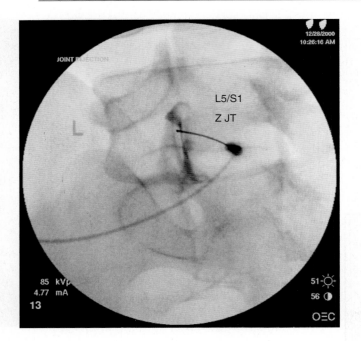

Figure 91-5.
Contrast medium within the facet joint.

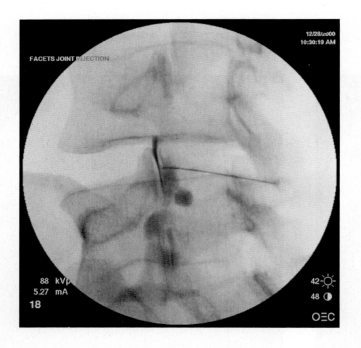

Figure 91-6.
Contrast medium within the facet joint.

SIDE EFFECTS AND COMPLICATIONS

The proximity to the spinal cord and exiting nerve roots makes it imperative that this procedure be carried out only by those well versed in the regional anatomy and experienced in performing interventional pain management techniques. Many patients also complain of a transient increase in lumbar pain after injection into the joint.

CLINICAL PEARLS

Lumbar facet block using the medial branch approach is the preferred technique for treatment of lumbar facet syndrome. Although intra-articular placement of the needle into the facet joint is technically feasible, unless specific diagnostic information about that specific joint is required, such maneuvers add nothing to the efficacy of the procedure and may, in fact, increase the rate of complications. Lumbar facet block is often combined with pharmacotherapy and physical therapy when treating pain in the previously mentioned areas. Many pain specialists believe that lumbar facet block is underused in the treatment of post-traumatic lumbar spine pain. These specialists believe that lumbar facet block using the medial branch approach should be considered when lumbar or caudal epidural nerve blocks, combined with conservative measures, fail to provide palliation of these pain syndromes.

CHAPTER 92

Lumbar Epidural Nerve Block

CPT-2009 CODE

Local Anesthetic/Narcotic	62311
Steroid	62311
Neurolytic	62282

Relative Value Units

Local Anesthetic	8
Steroid	8
Neurolytic	20

INDICATIONS

In addition to a limited number of applications for surgical anesthesia, lumbar epidural nerve block with local anesthetic can be used as a diagnostic tool when performing differential neural blockade on an anatomic basis in the evaluation of lower abdominal, back, groin, pelvic, bladder, perineal, genital, rectal, anal, and lower extremity pain. If destruction of the lumbar nerve roots is being considered, this technique is useful as a prognostic indicator of the degree of motor and sensory impairment that the patient may experience.

Lumbar epidural nerve block with local anesthetic, opioids, or both may be used to palliate acute pain emergencies while waiting for pharmacologic, surgical, or antiblastic methods to become effective. This technique is useful in the management of postoperative pain as well as pain secondary to trauma involving the lower abdomen, back, retroperitoneum, pelvis, and lower extremity. The pain of acute herpes zoster, ureteral calculi, and cancer also is amenable to treatment with epidurally administered local anesthetic and opioids. Additionally, this technique is of value in patients suffering from acute vascular insufficiency of the lower extremities secondary to vasospastic and vaso-occlusive disease, including frostbite and ergotamine toxicity. There is increasing evidence that the prophylactic or preemptive use of lumbar epidural nerve blocks in patients scheduled to undergo lower extremity amputations for ischemia will result in a decreased incidence of phantom limb pain.

The administration of local anesthetic, steroids, or both via the lumbar approach to the epidural space is useful in the treatment of a variety of chronic benign pain syndromes, including lumbar radiculopathy, low back syndrome, spinal stenosis, postlaminectomy syndrome, phantom limb pain, vertebral compression fractures, diabetic polyneuropathy, chemotherapy-related peripheral neuropathy, postherpetic neuralgia, reflex sympathetic dystrophy, orchalgia, proctalgia, and pelvic pain syndromes.

The lumbar epidural administration of local anesthetic in combination with steroids, opioids, or both is useful in the palliation of cancer-related lower abdominal, groin, back, pelvic, perineal, and rectal pain. This technique has been especially successful in the relief of pain secondary to metastatic disease of the spine caused by breast and prostate cancer as well as other malignancies. The long-term epidural administration of opioids has become a mainstay in the palliation of cancer-related pain. The role of epidural opioids in the management of chronic benign pain syndromes is being evaluated.

CLINICALLY RELEVANT ANATOMY

The superior boundary of the epidural space is the fusion of the periosteal and spinal layers of dura at the foramen magnum. The epidural space continues inferiorly to the sacrococcygeal membrane. The lumbar epidural space is bounded anteriorly by the posterior longitudinal ligament and posteriorly by the vertebral laminae and the ligamentum flavum (Fig. 92-1). The vertebral pedicles and intervertebral foramina form the lateral limits of the epidural space. The lumbar epidural space is 5 to 6 mm at the L2-L3 interspace with the lumbar spine flexed. The lumbar epidural space contains fat, veins, arteries, lymphatics, and connective tissue (Fig. 92-2).

During performance of lumbar epidural block in the midline, the needle will traverse the following structures (Figs. 92-3 and 92-4). After traversing the skin and subcutaneous tissues, the stylleted epidural needle will

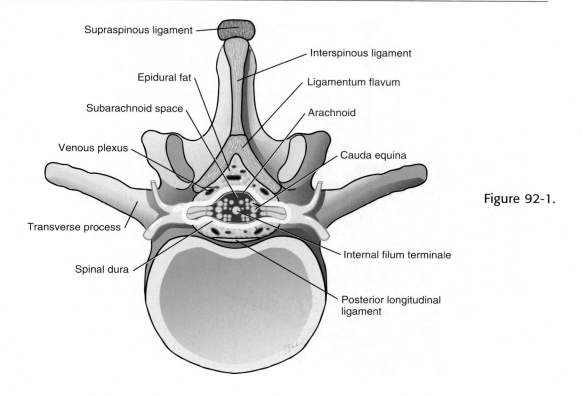

Figure 92-1.

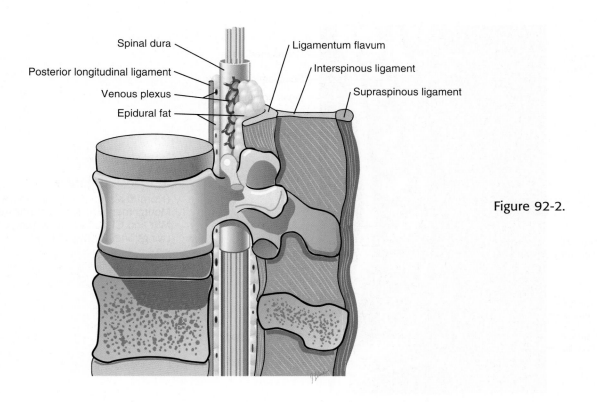

Figure 92-2.

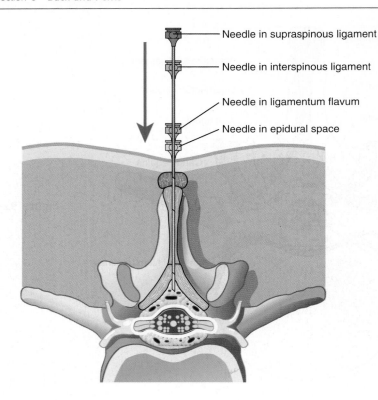

Needle in supraspinous ligament

Needle in interspinous ligament

Needle in ligamentum flavum

Needle in epidural space

Figure 92-3.

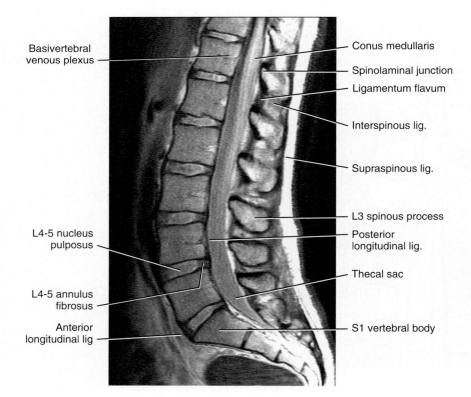

Basivertebral
venous plexus

Conus medullaris

Spinolaminal junction

Ligamentum flavum

Interspinous lig.

Supraspinous lig.

L3 spinous process

Posterior
longitudinal lig.

L4-5 nucleus
pulposus

Thecal sac

L4-5 annulus
fibrosus

Anterior
longitudinal lig

S1 vertebral body

Figure 92-4.
(From El-Khoury GY, Bergman RA,
Montgomery WJ: Sectional Anatomy by
MRI and CT, 3rd ed. New York, Churchill
Livingstone, 2007, p 444.)

impinge on the supraspinous ligament, which runs vertically between the apices of the spinous processes. The supraspinous ligament offers some resistance to the advancing needle. This ligament is dense enough to hold a needle in position even when the needle is released.

The interspinous ligament that runs obliquely between the spinous processes is next encountered, offering additional resistance to needle advancement. Because the interspinous ligament is contiguous with the ligamentum flavum, the pain management specialist may perceive a "false" loss of resistance when the needle tip enters the space between the interspinous ligament and the ligamentum flavum.

A significant increase in resistance to needle advancement signals that the needle tip is impinging on the dense ligamentum flavum. Because the ligament is made up almost entirely of elastin fibers, there is a continued increase in resistance as the needle traverses the ligamentum flavum, owing to the drag of the ligament on the needle. A sudden loss of resistance occurs as the needle tip enters the epidural space. There should be essentially no resistance to drugs injected into the normal epidural space.

TECHNIQUE

Lumbar epidural nerve block may be carried out with the patient in a sitting, lateral, or prone position.

The sitting position is easier for both the patient and the pain management specialist. This position enhances the ability to identify the midline and also avoids the problem of rotation of the spine inherent in the use of the lateral position, which may make identification of the epidural space difficult. Some investigators believe that the effects of gravity on local anesthetics is enhanced in the sitting position, improving the ability to block the S1 nerve roots, which can be difficult because of their larger size.

After the patient is placed in optimal position with the lumbar spine flexed and forearms resting on a padded bedside table, the skin is prepared with an antiseptic solution. At the L3-L4 interspace, the operator's middle and index fingers are placed on each side of the spinous processes (Fig. 92-5). The position of the interspace is reconfirmed with palpation using a rocking motion in the superior and inferior planes. The midline of the selected interspace is identified by palpating the spinous processes above and below the interspace using a lateral rocking motion to ensure that the needle entry site is exactly in the midline. One milliliter of local anesthetic is used to infiltrate the skin, subcutaneous tissues, and supraspinous and interspinous ligament at the midline.

The 25-gauge, 2- to 2½-inch needle or an 18- or 20-gauge, 3½-inch Hustead needle is inserted exactly in the midline in the previously anesthetized area through the supraspinous ligament into the interspinous ligament. Smaller, shorter needles are being used more frequently with equally good results. The needle stylet is removed and a well-lubricated 5-mL glass syringe filled with preservative-free sterile saline is attached. Alternatively, the physician can simply use a 12-mL plastic syringe filled with the intended injectate for the following loss of resistance maneuver. This approach has the advantage of not attaching and removing the glass syringe with the attendant risk for inadvertently moving the needle out of the epidural space.

The right-handed physician holds the epidural needle firmly at the hub with his or her left thumb and index finger. The left hand is placed firmly against the patient's back to ensure against uncontrolled needle movements should the patient unexpectedly move. With constant pressure being applied to the plunger of the syringe with the thumb of the right hand, the needle and syringe are continuously advanced in a slow and deliberate manner with the left hand. As soon as the needle bevel passes through the ligamentum flavum and enters the epidural space, there will be a sudden loss of resistance to injection, and the plunger will effortlessly surge forward (Fig. 92-6). The syringe is gently removed from the needle. If there is a question regarding needle placement, fluoroscopy may be useful (Figs. 92-7 and 92-8).

An air or saline acceptance test is carried out by injecting 0.5 to 1 mL of air or sterile preservative-free saline with a well-lubricated sterile glass syringe to help confirm that the needle is within the epidural space. The force required for injection should not exceed that necessary to overcome the resistance of the needle. Any significant pain or sudden increases in resistance during injection suggest incorrect needle placement, and one should *stop* injecting immediately and reassess the position of the needle. A small amount of contrast medium also may be injected through the needle to confirm placement within the epidural space (Figs. 92-9 and 92-10). Most experienced pain management specialists do not require the added step to correctly place the needle into the epidural space.

When satisfactory needle position is confirmed, a syringe containing 10 to 12 mL of solution to be injected is carefully attached to the needle. Gentle aspiration is carried out to identify cerebrospinal fluid or blood. If cerebrospinal fluid is aspirated, the epidural block may be repeated at a different interspace. In this situation, drug dosages should be adjusted accordingly because subarachnoid migration of drugs through the dural rent can occur. If aspiration of blood occurs, the needle should be rotated slightly and the aspiration test repeated. If no blood is present, incremental doses of local anesthetic and other drugs may be administered while monitoring the patient carefully for signs of local anesthetic toxicity.

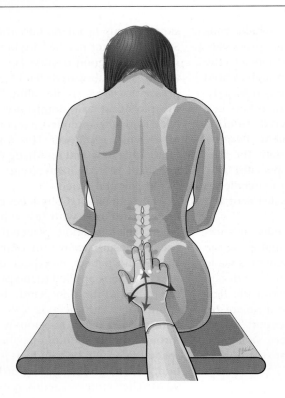

Figure 92-5.

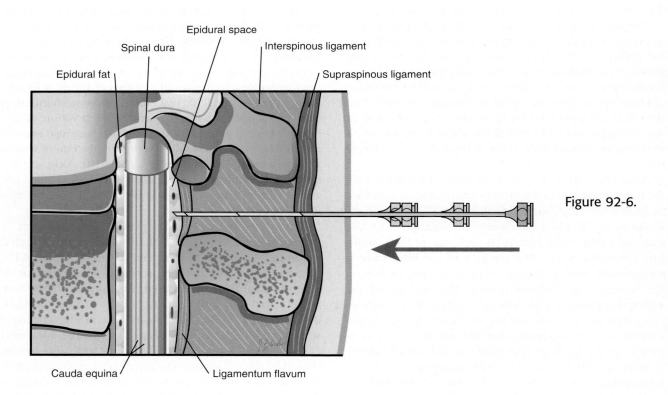

Epidural space

Spinal dura

Interspinous ligament

Epidural fat

Supraspinous ligament

Cauda equina

Ligamentum flavum

Figure 92-6.

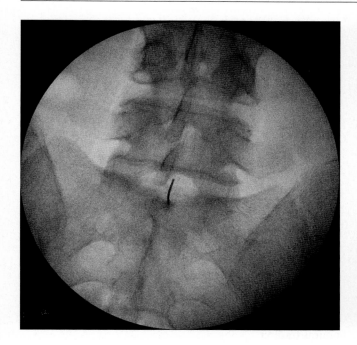

Figure 92-7.
PA view of needle tip within the epidural space.

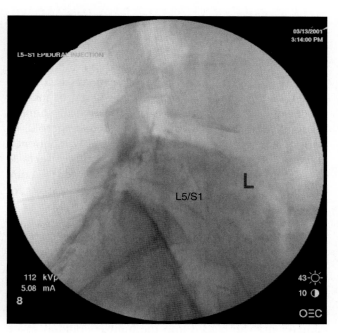

Figure 92-8.
Lateral view of needle tip within the epidural space.

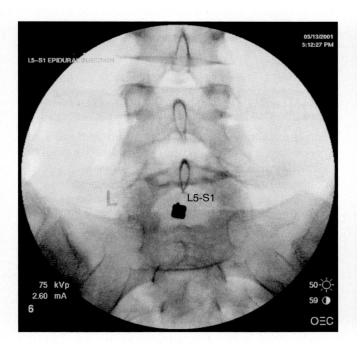

Figure 92-9.
Needle tip within the epidural space.

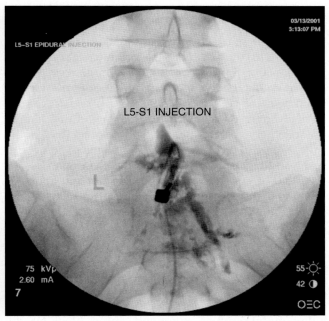

Figure 92-10.
Contrast medium within the epidural space.

For diagnostic and prognostic blocks, 1.0% preservative-free lidocaine is a suitable local anesthetic. For therapeutic blocks, 0.25% preservative-free bupivacaine in combination with 80 mg of depot methylprednisolone is injected. Subsequent nerve blocks are carried out in a similar manner, substituting 40 mg of methylprednisolone for the initial 80-mg dose. Daily lumbar epidural nerve blocks with local anesthetic, steroid, or both may be required to treat the previously mentioned acute painful conditions. Chronic conditions such as lumbar radiculopathy, spinal stenosis, vertebral compression fractures, and diabetic polyneuropathy are treated on an every-other-day to once-a-week basis or as the clinical situation dictates.

If the lumbar epidural route is chosen for administration of opioids, 5 to 7 mg of preservative-free morphine sulfate formulated for epidural use is a reasonable initial dose in opioid-tolerant patients. More lipid-soluble opioids such as fentanyl must be delivered by continuous infusion via a lumbar epidural catheter. An epidural catheter may be placed into the lumbar epidural space through a Hustead needle to allow continuous infusions.

SIDE EFFECTS AND COMPLICATIONS

Because of the potential for hematogenous spread via Batson's plexus, local infection and sepsis represent absolute contraindications to the lumbar approach to the epidural space. In contradistinction to the caudal approach to the epidural space, anticoagulation and coagulopathy represent absolute contraindications to lumbar epidural nerve block because of the risk for epidural hematoma.

Inadvertent dural puncture occurring during lumbar epidural nerve block should occur less than 0.5% of the time. Failure to recognize inadvertent dural puncture can result in immediate total spinal anesthetic with associated loss of consciousness, hypotension, and apnea. If epidural doses of opioids are accidentally placed into the subarachnoid space, significant respiratory and central nervous system depression will result. It is also possible to inadvertently place a needle or catheter intended for the epidural space into the subdural space. If subdural placement is unrecognized and epidural doses of local anesthetic are administered, the signs and symptoms are similar to those of massive subarachnoid injection, although the resulting motor and sensory block may be spotty.

The lumbar epidural space is highly vascular. The intravenous placement of the epidural needle occurs in 0.5% to 1% of patients undergoing lumbar epidural anesthesia. This complication is increased in patients with distended epidural veins (i.e., the parturient and patients with a large intra-abdominal tumor mass). If the

misplacement is unrecognized, injection of local anesthetic directly into an epidural vein will result in significant local anesthetic toxicity.

Needle trauma to the epidural veins may result in self-limited bleeding, which may cause postprocedural pain. Uncontrolled bleeding into the epidural space may result in compression of the spinal cord, with the rapid development of neurologic deficit. Although the incidence of significant neurologic deficit secondary to epidural hematoma after lumbar epidural block is exceedingly rare, this devastating complication should be considered whenever there is rapidly developing neurologic deficit after lumbar epidural nerve block.

Neurologic complications after lumbar nerve block are uncommon if proper technique is used. Direct trauma to the spinal cord or nerve roots is usually accompanied by pain. If significant pain occurs during placement of the epidural needle or catheter or during injection, the physician should immediately stop and ascertain the cause of the pain to avoid the possibility of additional neural trauma.

Although uncommon, infection in the epidural space remains an ever-present possibility, especially in the immunocompromised AIDS or cancer patient. If epidural abscess occurs, emergent surgical drainage to avoid spinal cord compression and irreversible neurologic deficit is usually required. Early detection and treatment of infection is crucial to avoid potentially life-threatening sequelae.

CLINICAL PEARLS

Lumbar epidural nerve block is a safe and effective procedure if careful attention is paid to technique. Failure to accurately identify the midline is the most common reason for difficulty in performing lumbar epidural nerve block and increases the risk for complications. The routine use of sedation or general anesthesia before initiation of lumbar epidural nerve block is to be discouraged because it will render the patient unable to provide accurate verbal feedback should needle misplacement occur.

Many pain centers have begun using caudal block for most pain management indications for which in the past a lumbar epidural block would have routinely been used. The advantages of the caudal approach to the epidural space include the fact that it may be used in the presence of anticoagulation, that the incidence of inadvertent dural puncture is almost nonexistent, that smaller needles may be used that enhance patient comfort, and that patient positioning is easier.

CHAPTER 93

Lumbar Epidural Nerve Block: Transforaminal Approach

CPT-2009 CODE

Local Anesthetic	64483
Steroid	64483
Additional Level	64484
Neurolytic	62281

Relative Value Units

Local Anesthetic	10
Steroid	10
Each Additional Level	10
Neurolytic	20

INDICATIONS

Lumbar epidural nerve block using the transforaminal approach with local anesthetics and corticosteroids can be a diagnostic tool when performing differential neural blockade on an anatomic basis in the evaluation of back, pelvic, and lower extremity pain as well as a therapeutic modality. If disruption of the lumbar nerve roots or dorsal root ganglion is being considered, this technique is useful as a prognostic indicator of the degree of motor and sensory impairment that the patient may experience. Although the interlaminar approach is more commonly used for routine therapeutic lumbar epidural nerve block, some interventional pain management specialists believe the transforaminal approach to the lumbar epidural space is more efficacious in the treatment of painful conditions involving a single nerve root with a higher incidence of complications (see Chapter 92 for indications for therapeutic lumbar epidural nerve block). Examples of such conditions include lumbar radiculopathy secondary to displaced intervertebral disk, neural foraminal stenosis, and perineural fibrosis.

CLINICALLY RELEVANT ANATOMY

The superior boundary of the epidural space is the fusion of the periosteal and spinal layers of dura at the foramen magnum. The epidural space continues inferiorly to the sacrococcygeal membrane. The lumbar epidural space is bounded anteriorly by the posterior longitudinal ligament and posteriorly by the vertebral laminae and the ligamentum flavum (Fig. 93-1). The lateral margin of the vertebral pedicles and intervertebral foramina form the lateral limits of the epidural space. The lumbar epidural space is 5 to 6 mm at the L2-L3 interspace with the lumbar spine flexed. The lumbar epidural space contains fat, veins, arteries, lymphatics, and connective tissue.

TECHNIQUE

Lumbar epidural injection using the transforaminal approach is carried out with the patient in the prone position. Although some experienced pain practitioners perform this technique without radiographic guidance, many pain practitioners use fluoroscopy to aid in needle placement, which helps to avoid placing the needle too deeply into the spinal canal and inadvertently injecting into the intrathecal space, subdural space, or the spinal cord. Because the procedure is usually done in the prone position, special attention to patient monitoring is mandatory.

With the patient in the prone position on the fluoroscopy table, the end plates of the affected vertebra are aligned. The fluoroscopy beam is then rotated ipsilaterally to align the superior articular process of the vertebra below with the 6-o'clock position of the pedicle above (Fig. 93-2).

The skin is then prepared with an antiseptic solution, and a skin wheal of local anesthetic is placed at a point overlying or just lateral to the tip of the superior articular process of the level below the indicated neural foramen. A 22- or 25-gauge, $3\frac{1}{2}$-inch needle is then placed through the previously anesthetized area and advanced until the tip impinges on bone over the pedicle lateral to the 6-o'clock position (Figs. 93-3 and 93-4). Failure to impinge on bone at the point may indicate that the needle has passed into and through the spinal canal and rests within the intrathecal space. Failure to identify this problem can lead to disastrous results (see Side Effects and Complications).

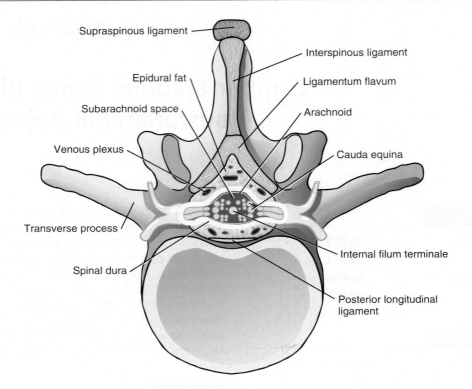

Figure 93-1.

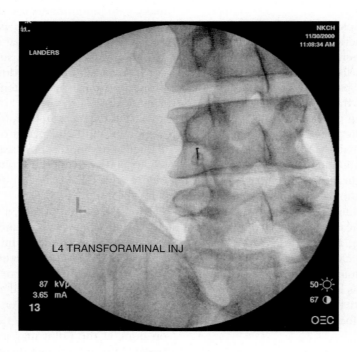

Figure 93-2.
Proper alignment of the superior articular process.

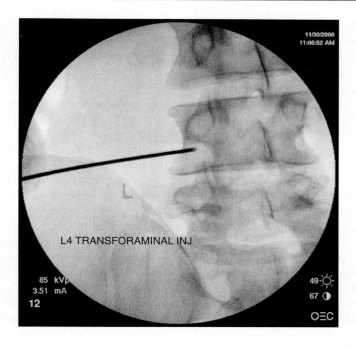

Figure 93-3.
Needle tip impinging on bone over the pedicle lateral to the 6-o'clock position of the pedicle above.

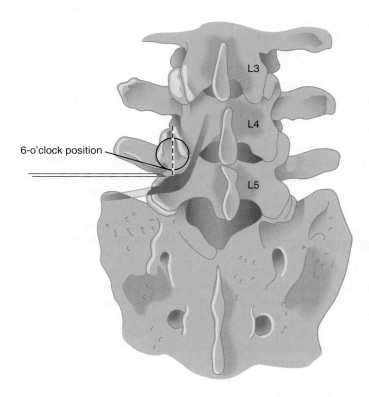

Figure 93-4.

After this bony landmark is identified, the needle is redirected inferiorly into the targeted spinal nerve canal. An anteroposterior fluoroscopic view is obtained to verify that the needle is not medial to the 6-o'clock position on the pedicle to avoid placement of the needle too deeply into the spinal nerve canal with its attendant risk for entry into the dural sleeve or spinal canal. A lateral view is then used to verify needle position. Special care should be taken when performing left upper lumbar transforaminal blocks to avoid advancing the needle beyond the halfway point of the foramen on the lateral view, to avoid damage to the segmental artery of Adamkiewicz, which lies in the superior ventral aspect of the foramen, with its attendant risk for spinal cord ischemia and paraplegia.

After satisfactory needle position is confirmed, 0.2 to 0.4 mL of contrast medium suitable for subarachnoid use is gently injected under fluoroscopic guidance. The contrast should be seen to flow proximally around the pedicle into the epidural space (Fig. 93-5). Flow distal along the nerve root sheath is usually appreciated. The injection of contrast should be stopped immediately if the patient complains of significant pain on injection. After satisfactory flow of contrast is observed and there is no evidence of subdural, subarachnoid, or intravascular spread of contrast, 6 mg of betamethasone suspension or solution, or 20 to 40 mg of methylprednisolone, or triamcinolone suspension 20 or 40 mg with 0.5 to 2.0 mL of 2.0% to 4.0% preservative-free lidocaine or 0.5% to 0.75% bupivacaine is slowly injected to a total volume of 1 to 3 mL. Injection of the local anesthetic with or without steroid should be discontinued if the patient complains of any significant pain on injection. Transient mild pressure paresthesia is often noted. After satisfactory injection of the local anesthetic with or without steroid, and washed of contrast by the local anesthetic and steroid solution is noted, the needle is removed, and pressure is placed on the injection site. The technique may be repeated at additional levels as a diagnostic or therapeutic maneuver.

SIDE EFFECTS AND COMPLICATIONS

Basically, all the potential side effects and complications associated with the interlaminar approach to the lumbar epidural space can occur with the transforaminal approach. The transforaminal approach also is associated with a statistically significant increase in the incidence of persistent paresthesias and trauma to neural structures, including the spinal cord. As mentioned earlier, placement of the needle too far into the neural foramina when using the transforaminal approach to the lumbar epidural space may result in unintentional injection into the spinal cord with resultant paraplegia. As noted earlier, injection into the segmental artery can lead to disastrous morbidity owing to spinal cord ischemia.

Because of the potential for hematogenous spread via Batson's plexus, local infection and sepsis represent absolute contraindications to the lumbar approach to the epidural space. In contradistinction to the caudal approach to the epidural space, anticoagulation and coagulopathy represent absolute contraindications to lumbar epidural nerve block because of the risk for epidural hematoma.

Unintentional dural puncture occurring during lumbar epidural nerve block should occur less than 0.5% of the time with the interlaminar approach and with a slightly greater frequency when using the transforaminal approach. Failure to recognize unintentional dural puncture can result in immediate total spinal anesthesia with associated loss of consciousness, hypotension, and apnea. If epidural doses of opioids are accidentally placed into the subarachnoid space, significant respiratory and central nervous system depression will result. This can be disastrous with the patient in the prone position. It also is possible to unintentionally place a needle or catheter intended for the epidural space into the subdural space. If subdural placement is unrecognized, and epidural doses of local anesthetics are administered, the signs and symptoms are similar to those of massive subarachnoid injection, although this temporal course may be altered, and the resulting motor and sensory block may be spotty.

The ventral lumbar epidural space and foramen are highly vascular. The intravenous placement of the epidural needle occurs in about 0.5% to 1% of patients undergoing lumbar epidural anesthesia. This complication is increased in patients with distended epidural veins, such as congestion from 2-degree obstruction from protruding disks, spinal stenosis in the parturient, and patients with a large intra-abdominal or spinal canal tumor mass. If the misplacement is unrecognized, injection of local anesthetic directly into an epidural vein may result in significant local anesthetic toxicity.

Needle trauma to the epidural veins may result in self-limited bleeding, which may cause postprocedure pain. Uncontrolled bleeding into the epidural space may result in compression of the spinal cord with the rapid development of neurologic deficit. Although significant neurologic deficit secondary to epidural hematoma after lumbar epidural block is exceedingly rare, this devastating complication should be considered whenever there is rapidly developing neurologic deficit after lumbar epidural nerve block.

Neurologic complications after lumbar nerve block are uncommon if proper technique is used and excessive sedation is avoided. Although unintentional placement of a needle within the substance of the spinal cord is nonpainful, injection into the spinal cord or nerve roots

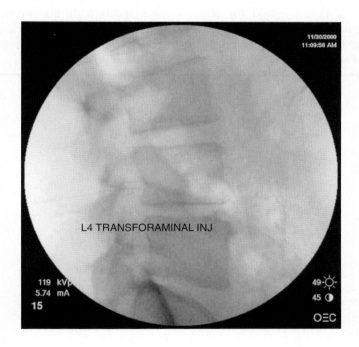

Figure 93-5.
Contrast medium flowing into the epidural space.

is usually accompanied by severe pain. If significant pain occurs during placement of the needle or during the injection of contrast or local anesthetic with or without steroid, the physician should immediately stop and ascertain the cause of the pain to avoid the possibility of additional neural trauma. Although uncommon, infection in the epidural space remains an ever-present pos-sibility, especially in the immunocompromised AIDS or cancer patient. If epidural abscess occurs, emergent surgical drainage to avoid spinal cord compression and irreversible neurologic deficit is usually required. Early detection and treatment of infection are crucial to avoid potentially life-threatening sequelae.

CLINICAL PEARLS

Some practitioners recommend the use of a blunt-tipped needle when performing the transforaminal approach to the lumbar epidural space, whereas others believe a sharper needle is better suited for this technique. Any significant pain or sudden increase in resistance during injection suggests incorrect needle placement, and one should stop injecting immediately and reassess the position of the needle. Because pain is an important indication of improper needle placement, the practitioner should avoid the use of excessive sedation during transforaminal lumbar epidural nerve block. As mentioned, the use of sedation in patients in the prone position requires special attention to monitoring.

CHAPTER 94

Lumbar Selective Spinal Nerve Block

CPT-2009 CODE	
Local Anesthetic	64483
Steroid	64483
Additional Level	64484
Neurolytic	2281

Relative Value Units	
Local Anesthetic	10
Steroid	10
Each Additional Level	10
Neurolytic	20

INDICATIONS

Selective spinal nerve block of the lumbar nerve roots is indicated as a diagnostic maneuver designed to determine whether a specific nerve root is subserving a patient's pain. Unfortunately, there is much confusion regarding both the nomenclature for this procedure and the clinical indications and technical aspects of performing this technique, which has led to problems in assessing the clinical utility of selective spinal nerve block. For purposes of this chapter, *selective spinal nerve block of the lumbar nerve roots* is defined as the placement of a needle just outside the neural foramen adjacent to the target nerve root without entering the nerve root canal or the epidural, subdural, or subarachnoid space.

If these conditions are met, a selective spinal nerve block may be said to be diagnostic to the specific targeted segmental nerve. However, if the needle enters the neural foramen, that is, the spinal nerve canal, and local anesthetic is injected, the potential to block not only the targeted nerve root but also the sinuvertebral nerve, the medial branch, and the ramus communicans, with anesthesia of the structures innervated by these neural elements exists. In this situation, if the local anesthetic does not enter the spinal canal or the epidural, subdural, or subarachnoid space, the diagnostic block can be con-

sidered to be specific as to structure and spinal segment. However, if the local anesthetic enters the spinal nerve canal and the epidural, subdural, or subarachnoid space, the diagnostic block cannot be said to be specific to a specific given spinal nerve root, although a pain generator limited to a structure below a specific level might be assumed. Although these distinctions may seem minor, the implications of failing to distinguish these subtle differences relative to technique could lead to surgical interventions at a nonpathologic level that ultimately fail to benefit the patient.

CLINICALLY RELEVANT ANATOMY

The superior boundary of the lumbar epidural space is the fusion of the periosteal and spinal layers of dura at the foramen magnum. The epidural space continues inferiorly to the sacrococcygeal membrane. The lumbar epidural space is bounded anteriorly by the posterior longitudinal ligament and posteriorly by the vertebral laminae and the ligamentum flavum. The medial aspect of the vertebral pedicles and spinal nerve canal form the lateral limits of the epidural space. The lumbar epidural space is 5 to 6 mm at L1-3 and widens at the S1 level with the lumbar spine flexed. The lumbar epidural space contains fat, veins, arteries, lymphatics, and connective tissue. The nerve roots exit their respective neural foramina and move anteriorly and inferiorly away from the lumbar spine.

When performing selective spinal nerve block of the lumbar spinal nerve, the goal is to place the needle just outside the neural foramen of the affected nerve root. As mentioned, placement of the needle within the neural foramina changes how the information obtained from this diagnostic maneuver should be interpreted.

TECHNIQUE

Lumbar selective spinal nerve block is carried out with the patient in the prone position. Although some experienced pain practitioners may perform this technique without radiographic guidance using a paresthesia into the targeted dermatome and segmental sensory deficit as the end point, the use of fluoroscopy or computed tomographic guidance is recommended to ensure the validity of the diagnostic aspect of this injection and prevention of unintentional misplacement of the needle with possibly serious consequences. Because the procedure is usually done in the prone position, special attention to patient monitoring is mandatory.

With the patient in the prone position on the fluoroscopy table, the end plates of the targeted vertebra are aligned. The fluoroscopy beam is then rotated slightly ipsilateral to align the superior articular process of the vertebra below with the 4-o'clock position of the pedicle above on the right or the 8-o'clock position on the left when looking at the pedicle as a clock face (Figs. 94-1 to 94-3). At levels above L4, a direct anteroposterior orientation may provide a more optimal view.

The skin is then prepared with an antiseptic solution, and a skin wheal of local anesthetic is placed just cephalad to a point overlying the appropriate junction of the middle and lateral third portion of the transverse process of the level below. A 22- or 25-gauge, 2- to 3½-inch needle is then inserted through the previously anesthetized area and advanced toward a point delineated at the junction of a lateral line from the tip of the superior articular process and a cephalad to caudad line from the 4-o'clock to 8-o'clock position at the pedicle (Fig. 94-4). The needle must pass lateral and ventral to the nerve root canal (see "Side Effects and Complications"). The needle should come in close proximity to the spinal nerve as it exits the foramen with a resultant mild paresthesia. The patient should be warned that a paresthesia may occur and to say "there!" immediately when he or she feels it. Care must be taken not to transfix the nerve by aggressive insertion of the needle. As mentioned earlier, the needle should not enter the neural foramen if maximal diagnostic information is expected.

After satisfactory needle position is confirmed, 0.2 to 0.4 mL of nonionic water-soluble contrast medium suitable for subarachnoid use is gently injected under fluoroscopic guidance. The contrast should be seen to flow distally along the neural sheath without flowing medially into the nerve root canal or epidural space (Fig. 94-5). The injection of contrast should be stopped immediately if the patient complains of significant pain on injection. However, mild transient pressure paresthesia is often appreciated by the patient. After satisfactory flow of contrast is observed and there is no evidence of epidural, subdural, subarachnoid, or intravascular spread of contrast, 0.5 to 1.0 mL of 4.0% preservative-free lidocaine is slowly injected. Because the injectate will not contact the dorsal root ganglion or other possible inflamed structures, corticosteroid is not required. After satisfactory injection of the local anesthetic, steroid, or both, the needle is removed, and pressure is placed on the injection site.

SIDE EFFECTS AND COMPLICATIONS

Basically, the potential side effects and complications associated with lumbar selective spinal nerve block are the same as those associated with the transforaminal approach to the lumbar epidural space. As mentioned earlier, placement of the needle into the neural foramina invalidates the specificity of the injection and lessens the diagnostic information. Unintentional placement of the needle into or through the neural canal may result in unintentional injection into the spinal cord or sequential artery with resultant paraplegia.

Because of the potential for hematogenous spread via Batson's plexus, local infection and sepsis represent absolute contraindications to this technique. Anticoagulation and coagulopathy represent absolute contraindications to selective spinal nerve block because of the risk for neuroaxial hematoma.

Unintentional dural puncture occurring during lumbar selective spinal nerve block should rarely occur if attention is paid to the technical aspects of this procedure. Failure to recognize unintentional dural puncture can result in significant motor or sensory block and the possibility of total spinal anesthetic with associated loss of consciousness, hypotension, and apnea. This can be disastrous with the patient in the prone position. It also is possible to inadvertently place the needle into the subdural or epidural space with the potential for significant motor or sensory block.

The space within the spinal nerve canal is highly vascular. If intravascular placement is unrecognized, injection of local anesthetic directly into a vessel could result in significant local anesthetic toxicity. Damage or injection to the segmental artery can occur with increased incidence when performing the selective spinal nerve block of the upper lumbar level, especially on the right.

Needle trauma to the epidural veins may result in self-limited bleeding, which may cause postprocedure pain. Uncontrolled bleeding into the epidural space may result in compression of the spinal cord with the rapid development of neurologic deficit. Although significant neurologic deficit secondary to epidural hematoma following selective spinal nerve block should be exceedingly rare, this devastating complication should be considered whenever there is rapidly developing neurologic deficit after lumbar epidural nerve block.

Neurologic complications after selective spinal nerve block are uncommon if proper technique is used and excessive sedation is avoided. Direct trauma to the spinal cord or nerve roots is usually accompanied by pain. If significant pain occurs during placement of the needle

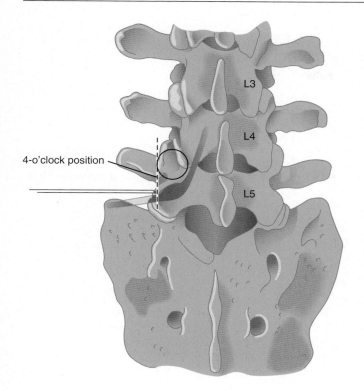

4-o'clock position

Figure 94-1.

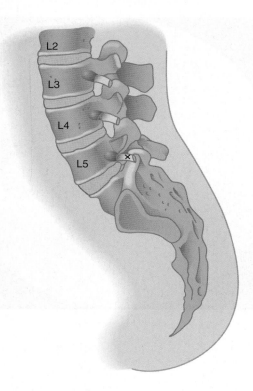

L2

L3

L4

L5

Figure 94-2.

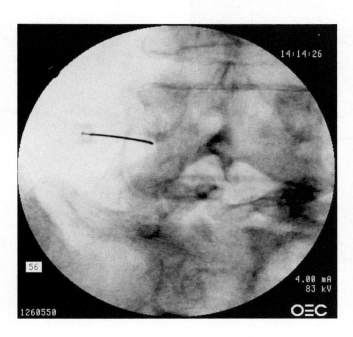

Figure 94-3.
Proper position for lumbar selective spinal nerve block.

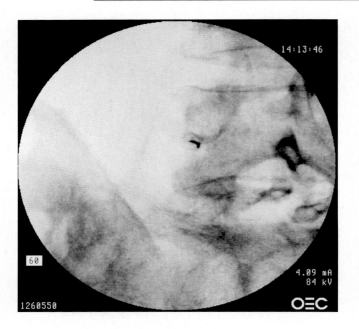

Figure 94-4.
Needle tip in position for lumbar selective spinal nerve block.

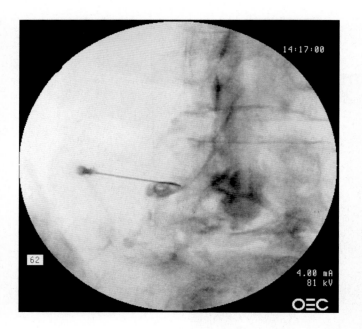

Figure 94-5.
Contrast medium flowing distally along the nerve sheath.

or during the injection of contrast and local anesthetic, the physician should immediately stop and ascertain the cause of the pain to avoid the possibility of additional neural trauma.

Although uncommon, infection in the epidural space remains an ever-present possibility, especially in the immunocompromised AIDS or cancer patient. If epidural abscess occurs, emergent surgical drainage to avoid spinal cord compression and irreversible neurologic deficit is usually required. Early detection and treatment of infection are crucial to avoid potentially life-threatening sequelae.

CLINICAL PEARLS

Some practitioners recommend the use of a blunt-tipped needle when performing the selective spinal nerve block or transforaminal approach to the lumbar epidural space, whereas others believe a sharper needle is better suited for this technique. Any significant pain or sudden increase in resistance during injection suggests incorrect needle placement, and one should stop injecting immediately and reassess the position of the needle. Because pain is an important indication of improper needle placement, the practitioner should avoid the use of excessive sedation during selective spinal nerve block of the lumbar nerve roots. As mentioned earlier, the use of sedation in patients in the prone position requires special attention to monitoring.

CHAPTER 95

Lumbar Subarachnoid Nerve Block: Midline Approach

CPT-2009 CODE

Local Anesthetic/Antispasmodic	62311
Narcotic	62311
Differential Spinal	62311
Continuous Spinal	62319
Neurolytic	62280

Relative Value Units

Local Anesthetic/Antispasmodic	10
Narcotic	10
Differential Spinal	12
Continuous Spinal	14
Neurolytic	20

INDICATIONS

Lumbar subarachnoid nerve block is used primarily for surgical and obstetric anesthesia. It is unique among regional anesthesia techniques in that the small amounts of drugs used to perform a successful lumbar subarachnoid nerve block exert essentially no systemic pharmacologic effects. Lumbar subarachnoid nerve block with local anesthetic is occasionally used as a diagnostic tool when performing differential neural blockade on a pharmacologic basis in the evaluation of lower abdominal, back, groin, pelvic, bladder, perineal, genital, rectal, anal, and lower extremity pain. If destruction of the spinal cord or nerve roots is being considered, this technique is occasionally used as a prognostic indicator of the degree of motor and sensory impairment that the patient may experience. The administration of opioids and other drugs such as clonidine and baclofen into the lumbar subarachnoid space may be used as both a diagnostic and prognostic maneuver when considering placement of an implantable drug delivery system.

Lumbar subarachnoid nerve block with local anesthetic, opioids, or both may be used to palliate acute pain emergencies while waiting for pharmacologic, surgical, or antiblastic methods to become effective. This technique is useful in the management of postoperative pain as well as pain secondary to trauma involving the lower abdomen, back, retroperitoneum, pelvis, and lower extremity. Pain due to impacted ureteral calculi and cancer-related pain also are amenable to treatment with the subarachnoid administration of local anesthetic and opioids. Additionally, this technique is of value in patients suffering from acute vascular insufficiency of the lower extremities secondary to vasospastic and vaso-occlusive disease, including frostbite and ergotamine toxicity. A catheter may be placed into the subarachnoid space to allow continuous administration of local anesthetic for this indication. There is increasing evidence that the prophylactic or preemptive use of lumbar subarachnoid nerve blocks in patients scheduled to undergo lower extremity amputations for ischemia will result in a decreased incidence of phantom limb pain.

The administration of local anesthetic, steroids, or both via the lumbar subarachnoid nerve block has been advocated in the past for the treatment of a variety of chronic benign pain syndromes, including lumbar radiculopathy and pain secondary to multiple sclerosis. Concerns about the potential for steroid-induced arachnoiditis have led to a decreased use of this technique, although many pain experts believe there is no scientific basis for these concerns. Many pain centers use the subarachnoid administration of steroids to palliate a rapidly progressive case of transverse myelitis associated with an exacerbation of multiple sclerosis.

The lumbar subarachnoid administration of local anesthetic in combination with opioids is useful in the palliation of cancer-related lower abdominal, groin, back, pelvic, perineal, and rectal pain. The long-term subarachnoid administration of opioids via implantable drug delivery systems has become a mainstay in the palliation of cancer-related pain. The role of chronic subarachnoid opioid administration in the management of chronic benign pain syndromes is being evaluated.

CLINICALLY RELEVANT ANATOMY

The spinal cord ends at about L2 in most adults and at about L4 in most infants. Therefore, in most settings, lumbar subarachnoid nerve block should be performed below these levels to avoid the potential for trauma to the spinal cord. The spinal cord is surrounded by three layers of protective connective tissue: the dura, the arachnoid, and the pia mater. The dura is the outermost layer and is composed of tough fibroelastic fibers that form a mechanical barrier to protect the spinal cord. The next layer is the arachnoid. The arachnoid is separated from the dura by only a small potential space, which is filled with serous fluid. The arachnoid is a barrier to the diffusion of substances and effectively serves to limit the spread of drugs administered into the epidural space from diffusing into the spinal fluid. The innermost layer is the pia, a vascular structure that helps provide lateral support to the spinal cord.

To reach the subarachnoid space, a needle placed in the midline at the L3-L4 interspace will pass through the skin, subcutaneous tissues, supraspinous ligament, interspinous ligament, ligamentum flavum, epidural space, dura, subdural space, and arachnoid (Fig. 95-1). Drugs administered into the subarachnoid space are placed between the arachnoid and pia, although inadvertent subdural injection is possible. Subdural injection of local anesthetic is characterized by a spotty, incomplete block.

TECHNIQUE

Lumbar subarachnoid nerve block may be carried out in the sitting, lateral, or prone position. The sitting position is easier for both the patient and the pain management specialist. This position enhances the ability to identify the midline and avoids the problem of rotation of the spine inherent in the use of the lateral position (Fig. 95-2). Such rotation may make placement of the needle into the subarachnoid space difficult. If the lateral position is chosen, careful attention to patient positioning, including identifying the midline, avoiding rotation of the spine, and maximizing flexion of the lumbar spine, is essential to successfully completing subarachnoid nerve block. The prone position is best used with the patient in the jackknife position to maximize flexion of the lumbar spine (Fig. 95-3). It is occasionally used for administration of hypobaric solutions for midline procedures such as hemorrhoidectomy. Although this position limits the amount of rotation of the spine possible and simplifies midline identification, the inherent dangers of the prone position, including difficulty in monitoring the patient and problems with airway management, militate against the routine use of the prone position for lumbar subarachnoid nerve block.

After the patient is placed in optimal position with the lumbar spine flexed and without rotation, the iliac crests are identified. The spinous process of L4 is approximately on an imaginary line drawn between the two iliac crests. The skin is then prepared with an antiseptic solution. At the L3-L4 interspace, the operator's middle and index fingers are placed on each side of the spinous processes. The position of the interspace is reconfirmed with palpation using a rocking motion in the superior and inferior planes. The midline of the selected interspace is identified by palpating the spinous processes above and below the interspace using a lateral rocking motion to ensure that the needle entry site is exactly in the midline. Failure to accurately identify the midline is the number one reason for failed lumbar subarachnoid nerve block. One milliliter of local anesthetic is used to infiltrate the skin, subcutaneous tissues, and the supraspinous and interspinous ligaments at the midline.

The choice of needle for lumbar subarachnoid block is based in part on the experience of the operator and in part on the desire to decrease the incidence of postdural puncture headache. In general, use of smaller-gauge needles with points that separate, rather than cut, dural fibers results in a decreased incidence of postdural puncture headaches, all other things being equal. The use of an introducer needle facilitates the successful use of smaller-gauge needles. The chosen styletted spinal needle is inserted exactly in the midline in the previously anesthetized area and advanced with a 10- to 15-degree cephalad trajectory.

The needle is advanced through the subcutaneous tissues and supraspinous ligament into the interspinous ligament. The operator will perceive an increase in resistance to needle advancement as the needle passes through the interspinous ligament and the dense ligamentum flavum. The needle will then traverse the epidural space, and the operator will feel a pop as the needle pierces the dura. The needle is slowly advanced an additional 1 mm, and the stylet is removed. A free flow of spinal fluid should be observed; or if a smaller spinal needle has been used, cerebrospinal fluid should appear in the hub. If no spinal fluid is observed, the stylet is replaced, and the needle is advanced slightly and then rotated 90 degrees. The stylet is again removed, and the hub is again observed for spinal fluid. If no spinal fluid appears, the needle should be removed and the midline reidentified before attempting to repeat the previous technique. After spinal fluid is observed, the needle is fixed in position by the operator placing his or her hand against the patient's back. A drug suitable for subarachnoid administration is chosen, and the addition of glucose to make a hyperbaric solution or vasoconstrictors such as epinephrine or phenylephrine to prolong the duration of spinal block is considered. The solution is slowly injected,

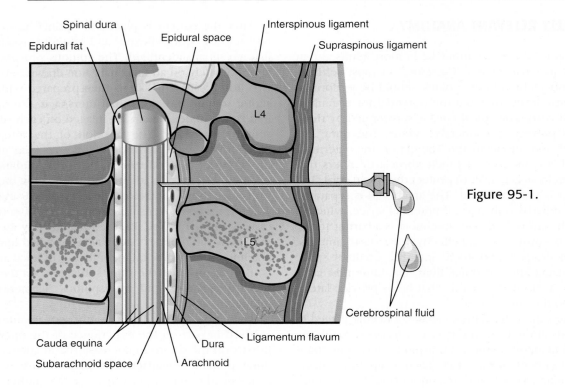

Spinal dura

Epidural fat

Epidural space

Interspinous ligament

Supraspinous ligament

L4

L5

Cerebrospinal fluid

Cauda equina

Subarachnoid space

Dura

Arachnoid

Ligamentum flavum

Figure 95-1.

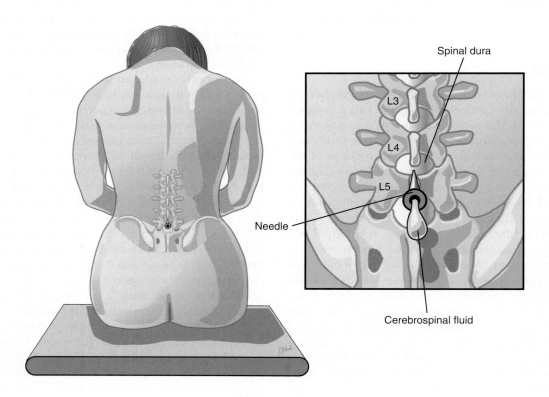

Spinal dura

L3

L4

L5

Needle

Cerebrospinal fluid

Figure 95-2.

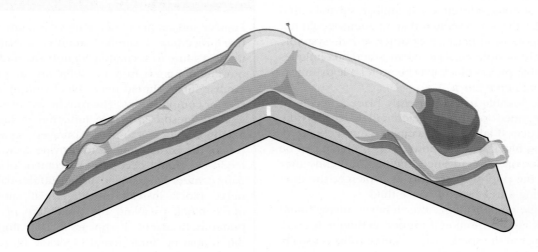

Figure 95-3.

and the injection is immediately discontinued if the patient reports any pain. The needle is then removed.

SIDE EFFECTS AND COMPLICATIONS

Because of the potential for hematogenous spread via Batson's plexus, local infection and sepsis represent absolute contraindications to the midline approach to the lumbar subarachnoid space. In contradistinction to the caudal approach to the epidural space, anticoagulation and coagulopathy represent absolute contraindications to lumbar subarachnoid nerve block because of the risk for epidural and subarachnoid hematoma.

Hypotension is a common side effect of lumbar subarachnoid nerve block and is the result of the profound sympathetic blockade attendant with this procedure. Prophylactic intramuscular or intravenous administration of vasopressors and fluid loading may help avoid this potentially serious side effect of lumbar subarachnoid nerve block. If it is ascertained that a patient would not tolerate hypotension because of other serious systemic disease, more peripheral regional anesthetic techniques such as lumbar plexus block may be preferable to lumbar subarachnoid nerve block.

It also is possible to inadvertently place a needle or catheter intended for the subarachnoid space into the subdural space. If subdural placement is unrecognized, the resulting block will be spotty. This problem can be avoided if the operator advances the needle slightly after perceiving the pop of the needle as it pierces the dura and observing a free flow of spinal fluid.

Neurologic complications after lumbar subarachnoid nerve block are uncommon if proper technique is used. Direct trauma to the spinal cord or nerve roots is usually accompanied by pain. If significant pain occurs during placement of the spinal needle or catheter or during injection, the physician should immediately stop and ascertain the cause of the pain to avoid the possibility of additional neural trauma. Delayed neurologic complications due to chemical irritation of the spinal cord and the coverings of the spinal cord and nerves have been reported. Most severe complications have been attrib-

uted to contaminants to the local anesthetic, although the addition of steroids and vasopressors and the use of concentrated hyperbaric solutions also have been implicated.

Although uncommon, infection in the subarachnoid space remains an ever-present possibility, especially in the immunocompromised AIDS or cancer patient. If epidural abscess occurs, emergent surgical drainage to avoid spinal cord compression and irreversible neurologic deficit is usually required. Meningitis occurring after lumbar subarachnoid nerve block may require subarachnoid administration of antibiotics. Early detection and treatment of infection is crucial to avoid potentially life-threatening sequelae.

CLINICAL PEARLS

Lumbar subarachnoid nerve block is a safe and effective procedure if careful attention is paid to technique. Failure to accurately identify the midline is the most common reason for difficulty in performing lumbar subarachnoid nerve block and increases the risk for complications. The routine use of sedation or general anesthesia before initiation of lumbar subarachnoid block is to be discouraged because it will render the patient unable to provide accurate verbal feedback should needle misplacement occur. Many pain centers have begun using differential epidural nerve block instead of differential subarachnoid nerve block to avoid the possibility of postdural puncture headache. It appears that the findings with differential epidural neural blockade correlate with those of differential subarachnoid neural blockade. This correlation may not hold true when administering test doses of opioids or other drugs before placement of an implantable drug delivery system. If a subarachnoid terminus for the catheter is intended, subarachnoid rather than epidural test doses should be administered.

CHAPTER 96

Lumbar Subarachnoid Nerve Block: Paramedian Approach

CPT-2009 CODE

Local Anesthetic/Antispasmodic	62311
Narcotic	62311
Differential Spinal	62311
Continuous Spinal	62319
Neurolytic	62280

Relative Value Units

Local Anesthetic/Antispasmodic	10
Narcotic	10
Differential Spinal	12
Continuous Spinal	14
Neurolytic	20

INDICATIONS

Lumbar subarachnoid nerve block via the paramedian approach is used primarily in three clinical settings:

1. In patients with significant osteophyte formation and degenerative changes of the lumbar spine that make the midline approach more difficult
2. In patients who are unable to maximally flex the lumbar spine to open the intervertebral space
3. For the placement of subarachnoid catheters for implantable drug delivery systems

The paramedian and Taylor's approaches to the subarachnoid space are preferred for this last indication because they allow the catheter to enter the subarachnoid space at a less acute angle than with the midline approach. This results in less catheter kinking and breakage.

Lumbar subarachnoid block is used primarily for surgical and obstetric anesthesia. It is unique among regional anesthesia techniques in that the small amounts of drugs used to perform a successful lumbar subarachnoid nerve block exert essentially no systemic pharmacologic effects. Lumbar subarachnoid nerve block with local anesthetic is occasionally used as a diagnostic tool when performing differential neural blockade on a pharmacologic basis in the evaluation of lower abdominal, back, groin, pelvic, bladder, perineal, genital, rectal, anal, and lower extremity pain. If destruction of the spinal cord or nerve roots is being considered, this technique is occasionally used as a prognostic indicator of the degree of motor and sensory impairment that the patient may experience. The administration of opioids and other drugs such as clonidine and baclofen into the lumbar subarachnoid space may be used as both a diagnostic and prognostic maneuver when considering placement of an implantable drug delivery system for the long-term treatment of pain or spasticity.

Lumbar subarachnoid nerve block with local anesthetic, opioids, or both may be used to palliate acute pain emergencies while waiting for pharmacologic, surgical, or antiblastic methods to become effective. This technique is useful in the management of postoperative pain as well as pain secondary to trauma involving the lower abdomen, back, retroperitoneum, pelvis, and lower extremity. The pain of impacted ureteral calculi and cancer-related pain also are amenable to treatment with the subarachnoid administration of local anesthetic and opioids. Additionally, this technique is of value in patients suffering from acute vascular insufficiency of the lower extremities secondary to vasospastic and vaso-occlusive disease, including frostbite and ergotamine toxicity. A catheter may be placed into the subarachnoid space to allow continuous administration of local anesthetic for this indication. There is increasing evidence that the prophylactic or preemptive use of lumbar subarachnoid nerve blocks in patients scheduled to undergo lower extremity amputations for ischemia will result in a decreased incidence of phantom limb pain.

The administration of local anesthetic, steroids, or both via the lumbar subarachnoid nerve block has been advocated in the past for the treatment of a variety of chronic benign pain syndromes, including lumbar radiculopathy and pain secondary to multiple sclerosis. Concerns about the potential for steroid-induced arachnoiditis have led to a decreased use of this technique, although many pain experts believe there is no scientific basis for the concerns raised. Many pain centers use the subarachnoid administration of steroids to palliate a rapidly progressive case of transverse myelitis associated with an exacerbation of multiple sclerosis.

The lumbar subarachnoid administration of local anesthetic in combination with opioids is useful in the palliation of cancer-related lower abdominal, groin, back, pelvic, perineal, and rectal pain. The long-term subarachnoid administration of opioids via implantable drug delivery systems has become a mainstay in the palliation of cancer-related pain. The role of chronic subarachnoid opioid administration in the management of chronic benign pain syndromes is being evaluated.

CLINICALLY RELEVANT ANATOMY

The spinal cord ends at about L2 in most adults and at about L4 in most infants. Therefore, in most settings, lumbar subarachnoid nerve block should be performed below these levels to avoid the potential for trauma to the spinal cord. The spinal cord is surrounded by three layers of protective connective tissue: the dura, the arachnoid, and the pia mater. The dura is the outermost layer and is composed of tough fibroelastic fibers that form a mechanical barrier to protect the spinal cord. The next layer is the arachnoid. The arachnoid is separated from the dura by only a small potential space, which is filled with serous fluid. The arachnoid is a barrier to the diffusion of substances and effectively serves to limit the spread of drugs administered into the epidural space from diffusing into the spinal fluid. The innermost layer is the pia, a vascular structure that helps provide lateral support to the spinal cord.

To reach the subarachnoid space, a needle placed via the paramedian approach at the L3-L4 interspace will pass through the skin, subcutaneous tissues, inner margin of the interspinous ligament, ligamentum flavum, epidural space, dura, subdural space, and arachnoid. Drugs administered into the subarachnoid space are placed between the arachnoid and pia, although inadvertent subdural injection is possible. Subdural injection of local anesthetic is characterized by a spotty, incomplete block.

TECHNIQUE

Lumbar subarachnoid nerve block via the paramedian approach may be carried out in the sitting, lateral, or prone position. The sitting position is easier for both the patient and the pain management specialist. This position enhances the ability to identify the midline and avoids the problem of rotation of the spine inherent in the use of the lateral position. Such rotation may make placement of the needle into the subarachnoid space difficult. If the lateral position is chosen, careful attention to patient positioning, including identification of the midline, avoiding rotation of the spine, and maximizing flexion of the lumbar spine, is essential to successfully complete subarachnoid nerve block. The prone position is best used with the patient in the jackknife position to maximize flexion of the lumbar spine. It is occasionally used for administration of hypobaric solutions for midline procedures such as hemorrhoidectomy. Although this position limits the amount of rotation of the spine possible and simplifies midline identification, the inherent dangers of the prone position, including difficulty in monitoring the patient and problems with airway management, militate against the routine use of the prone position for lumbar subarachnoid nerve block.

After the patient is placed in optimal position with the lumbar spine flexed and without rotation, the iliac crests are identified. The spinous process of L4 is approximately on an imaginary line drawn between the two iliac crests. The skin is then prepared with an antiseptic solution. At the L3-L4 interspace, the operator's middle and index fingers are placed on each side of the spinous processes. The position of the interspace is reconfirmed with palpation using a rocking motion in the superior and inferior planes. The midline of the selected interspace is identified by palpating the spinous processes above and below the interspace using a lateral rocking motion. Failure to accurately identify the midline is the number one reason for failed lumbar subarachnoid nerve block. At a point 1 cm lateral and 1 cm below the midline of the L4-L5 interspace, local anesthetic is used to infiltrate the skin, subcutaneous tissues, and edge of the interspinous ligament, aiming toward the center of the interspace (Fig. 96-1).

The choice of needle for lumbar subarachnoid block is based in part on the experience of the operator and in part on the desire to decrease the incidence of postdural puncture headache. In general, smaller-gauge needles with points that separate, rather than cut, dural fibers will result in a decreased incidence of postdural puncture headaches, all other things being equal. The use of an introducer needle facilitates the successful use of smaller-gauge needles. A longer 5- or 6-inch needle is often needed to reach the subarachnoid space when using the paramedian approach, especially in larger individuals. The chosen styletted spinal needle is inserted through the previously anesthetized area and advanced with a 10- to 15-degree cephalomedial trajectory. It is advanced through the subcutaneous tissues and supraspinous ligament into the interspinous ligament. The operator will perceive an increase in resistance to needle advancement as the needle passes through the edge of the interspinous ligament and the dense ligamentum flavum. Should the needle impinge on bone, the needle

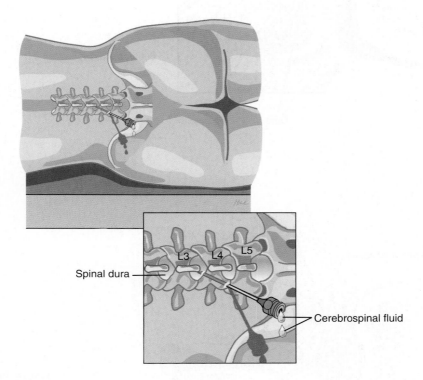

Figure 96-1.

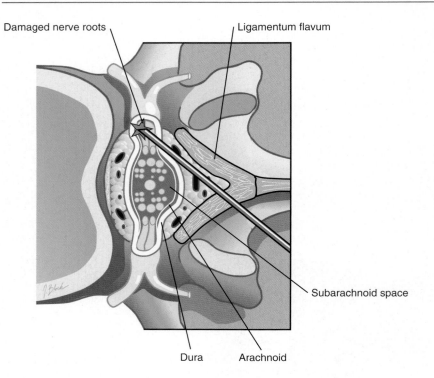

Figure 96-2.

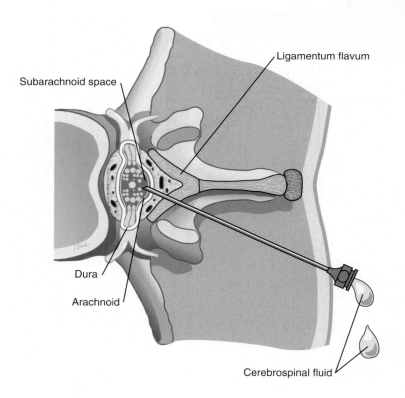

Figure 96-3.

is withdrawn and readvanced with a slightly more cephalad trajectory. Care must be taken not to allow the needle to cross the midline by directing the needle too laterally, or trauma to the spinal cord or exiting nerve roots on the side opposite needle placement may result (Fig. 96-2).

The needle will then traverse the epidural space, and the operator will feel a pop as the needle pierces the dura (Fig. 96-3). The needle is slowly advanced an additional 1 mm, and the stylet is removed. A free flow of spinal fluid should be observed; or if a smaller spinal needle has been used, cerebrospinal fluid should appear in the hub. If no spinal fluid is observed, the stylet is replaced, and the needle is advanced slightly and then rotated 90 degrees. The stylet is again removed, and the hub is again observed for spinal fluid. If no spinal fluid appears, the needle should be removed and the midline reidentified before attempting to repeat the previous technique. After spinal fluid is observed, the needle is fixed in position by the operator placing his or her hand against the patient's back. A drug suitable for subarachnoid administration is chosen, and the addition of glucose to make a hyperbaric solution with or without vasoconstrictors such as epinephrine or phenylephrine to prolong the duration of spinal block is considered. The solution is slowly injected, and the injection is immediately discontinued if the patient reports any pain. The needle is then removed.

SIDE EFFECTS AND COMPLICATIONS

Because of the potential for hematogenous spread via Batson's plexus, local infection and sepsis represent absolute contraindications to the paramedian approach to the subarachnoid space. In contradistinction to the caudal approach to the epidural space, anticoagulation and coagulopathy represent absolute contraindications to lumbar subarachnoid nerve block owing to the risk for epidural and subarachnoid hematoma.

Hypotension is a common side effect of lumbar subarachnoid nerve block and is the result of the profound sympathetic blockade attendant with this procedure. Prophylactic intramuscular or intravenous administration of vasopressors and fluid loading may help avoid this potentially serious side effect of lumbar subarachnoid nerve block. If it is ascertained that a patient would not tolerate hypotension because of other serious systemic disease, more peripheral regional anesthetic techniques such as lumbar plexus block may be preferable to lumbar subarachnoid nerve block.

It is also possible to inadvertently place a needle or catheter intended for the subarachnoid space into the subdural space. If subdural placement is unrecognized, the resulting block will be spotty. This problem can be avoided if the operator advances the needle slightly after perceiving the pop of the needle as it pierces the dura and observing a free flow of spinal fluid.

Neurologic complications after lumbar subarachnoid nerve block are uncommon if proper technique is used. Direct trauma to the spinal cord or nerve roots is usually accompanied by pain. If significant pain occurs during placement of the spinal needle or catheter or during injection, the physician should immediately stop and ascertain the cause of the pain to avoid the possibility of additional neural trauma. Delayed neurologic complications due to chemical irritation of the spinal cord and the coverings of the spinal cord and nerves have been reported. Most severe complications have been attributed to contaminants to the local anesthetic, although the addition of steroids and vasopressors and the use of concentrated hyperbaric solutions also have been implicated.

Although uncommon, infection in the subarachnoid space remains an ever-present possibility, especially in the immunocompromised AIDS or cancer patient. If epidural abscess occurs, emergent surgical drainage to avoid spinal cord compression and irreversible neurologic deficit is usually required. Meningitis occurring after lumbar subarachnoid nerve block may require subarachnoid administration of antibiotics. Early detection and treatment of infection is crucial to avoid potentially life-threatening sequelae.

CLINICAL PEARLS

Lumbar subarachnoid nerve block via the paramedian approach is a safe and effective procedure if careful attention is paid to technique. The three most common reasons for failure to reach the subarachnoid space when using the paramedian approach to achieve lumbar subarachnoid nerve block are listed:

1. Failure to identify the midline before needle placement
2. Underestimating the added depth of needle insertion necessary to reach the subarachnoid space from a paramedian entry site
3. Allowing the needle to cross the midline by using too lateral a trajectory

The first two reasons will ordinarily result only in failure to complete the block. The third reason not only will result in failed block but also may result in significant trauma to the contralateral spinal cord or nerve roots. For this reason, it is crucial to first identify the midline and then ensure that the needle never crosses the midline on its path toward the subarachnoid space. The routine use of sedation or general anesthesia before initiation of lumbar subarachnoid block is to be discouraged because it will render the patient unable to provide accurate verbal feedback should needle misplacement occur.

Many pain centers have begun using differential epidural nerve block instead of differential subarachnoid nerve block to avoid the possibility of postdural puncture headache. It appears that the findings with differential epidural neural blockade correlate with those of differential subarachnoid neural blockade. This correlation may not hold true when administering test doses of opioids or other drugs before placement of an implantable drug delivery system. If a subarachnoid terminus for the catheter is intended, subarachnoid rather than epidural test doses should be administered.

CHAPTER 97

Lumbar Subarachnoid Nerve Block: Lumbosacral Approach of Taylor

CPT-2009 CODE	
Local Anesthetic/Antispasmodic	62311
Narcotic	62311
Differential Spinal	62311
Continuous Spinal	62319
Neurolytic	62280

Relative Value Units	
Local Anesthetic/Antispasmodic	10
Narcotic	10
Differential Spinal	12
Continuous Spinal	14
Neurolytic	20

INDICATIONS

Lumbar subarachnoid nerve block via the lumbosacral approach of Taylor is used primarily in four clinical settings:

1. In patients with significant osteophyte formation and degenerative changes of the lumbar spine that make the midline or paramedian approach at more cephalad interspaces more difficult
2. In patients who are unable to maximally flex the lumbar spine to open the intervertebral space
3. In patients in whom dense block of the larger S1 nerves is desired
4. For the placement of subarachnoid catheters for implantable drug delivery systems

The paramedian and Taylor's approaches to the subarachnoid space are preferred for this last indication because they allow the catheter to enter the subarachnoid space at a less acute angle than with the midline approach. This results in less catheter kinking and breakage.

Lumbar subarachnoid block is used primarily for surgical and obstetric anesthesia. It is unique among regional anesthesia techniques in that the small amounts of drugs used to perform a successful lumbar subarachnoid nerve block exert essentially no systemic pharmacologic effects. The lumbosacral approach of Taylor is especially useful for those surgical procedures that require dense block of the lower lumbar and sacral nerve roots because the small amounts of drugs injected are in close proximity to these nerves.

Lumbar subarachnoid nerve block with local anesthetic is occasionally used as a diagnostic tool when performing differential neural blockade on a pharmacologic basis in the evaluation of lower abdominal, back, groin, pelvic, bladder, perineal, genital, rectal, anal, and lower extremity pain. If destruction of the spinal cord or nerve roots is being considered, this technique is occasionally used as a prognostic indicator of the degree of motor and sensory impairment that the patient may experience. The administration of opioids and other drugs such as clonidine and baclofen into the lumbar subarachnoid space may be used as both a diagnostic and prognostic maneuver when considering placement of an implantable drug delivery system for the long-term treatment of pain or spasticity.

Lumbar subarachnoid nerve block with local anesthetic, opioids, or both may be used to palliate acute pain emergencies while waiting for pharmacologic, surgical, or antiblastic methods to become effective. This technique is useful in the management of postoperative pain as well as pain secondary to trauma involving the lower abdomen, back, retroperitoneum, pelvis, and lower extremity. Pain of impacted ureteral calculi and cancer-related pain also are amenable to treatment with the subarachnoid administration of local anesthetic and opioids. Additionally, this technique is of value in patients suffering from acute vascular insufficiency of the lower extremities secondary to vasospastic and vaso-occlusive disease, including frostbite and ergotamine toxicity. A catheter may be placed into the subarachnoid space to allow continuous administration of local anesthetic for this indication. There is increasing evidence that the prophylactic or preemptive use of lumbar subarachnoid nerve blocks in patients scheduled to undergo lower extremity amputations for ischemia will result in a decreased incidence of phantom limb pain.

The administration of local anesthetic, steroids, or both via the lumbar subarachnoid nerve block has been advocated in the past for the treatment of a variety of chronic benign pain syndromes, including lumbar radiculopathy and pain secondary to multiple sclerosis. Concerns about the potential for steroid-induced arachnoiditis have led to a decreased use of this technique, although many pain experts believe there is no scientific basis for these concerns. Many pain centers use the subarachnoid administration of steroids to palliate a rapidly progressive case of transverse myelitis associated with an exacerbation of multiple sclerosis.

The lumbar subarachnoid administration of local anesthetic in combination with opioids is useful in the palliation of cancer-related lower abdominal, groin, back, pelvic, perineal, and rectal pain. The long-term subarachnoid administration of opioids via implantable drug delivery systems has become a mainstay in the palliation of cancer-related pain. The role of chronic subarachnoid opioid administration in the management of chronic benign pain syndromes is being evaluated.

CLINICALLY RELEVANT ANATOMY

The spinal cord ends at about L2 in most adults and at about L4 in most infants. Therefore, in most settings, lumbar subarachnoid nerve block should be performed below these levels to avoid the potential for trauma to the spinal cord. The spinal cord is surrounded by three layers of protective connective tissue: the dura, the arachnoid, and the pia mater. The dura is the outermost layer and is composed of tough fibroelastic fibers that form a mechanical barrier to protect the spinal cord. The next layer is the arachnoid. The arachnoid is separated from the dura by only a small potential space, which is filled with serous fluid. The arachnoid is a barrier to the diffusion of substances and effectively serves to limit the spread of drugs administered into the epidural space from diffusing into the spinal fluid. The innermost layer is the pia, a vascular structure that helps provide lateral support to the spinal cord.

The lumbosacral interspace is the largest of the spinal column. However, a midline approach to the subarachnoid space at this level is precluded, owing to the extension of the spinous process of L5 over the lumbosacral interspace. To reach the subarachnoid space at this level, the entry point for a spinal needle will have to be lateral to and inferior to the space to allow the needle to slide

under the overhanging spinous process of L5. A needle placed via the lumbosacral approach of Taylor at the L5-S1 interspace will pass through the skin, subcutaneous tissues, ligamentum flavum, epidural space, dura, subdural space, and arachnoid. Drugs administered into the subarachnoid space are placed between the arachnoid and pia, although inadvertent subdural injection is possible. Subdural injection of local anesthetic is characterized by a spotty, incomplete block.

TECHNIQUE

Lumbar subarachnoid nerve block via the lumbosacral approach of Taylor may be carried out in the sitting, lateral, or prone position. The sitting position is easier for both the patient and pain management specialist. This position enhances the ability to identify the midline and avoids the problem of rotation of the spine inherent in the use of the lateral position. Such rotation may make placement of the needle into the subarachnoid space difficult.

If the lateral position is chosen, careful attention to patient positioning, including identifying the midline, avoiding rotation of the spine, and maximizing flexion of the lumbar spine, is essential to successfully completing subarachnoid nerve block.

The prone position is best used with the patient in the jackknife position to maximize flexion of the lumbar spine. It is occasionally used for administration of hypobaric solutions for midline procedures such as hemorrhoidectomy. Although this position limits the amount of rotation of the spine possible and simplifies midline identification, the inherent dangers of the prone position, including difficulty in monitoring the patient and problems with airway management, militate against the routine use of the prone position for lumbar subarachnoid nerve block.

After the patient is placed in optimal position with the lumbar spine flexed and without rotation, the iliac crests are identified. The spinous process of L4 is approximately on an imaginary line drawn between the two iliac crests. The skin is then prepared with an antiseptic solution.

The L5 spinous process is then identified, and at the L5-S1 interspace, the operator's middle and index fingers are placed on each side of the spinous processes. The position of the interspace is reconfirmed with palpation using a rocking motion in the superior and inferior planes. The midline of this interspace is then identified by palpating the spinous processes above and below the interspace using a lateral rocking motion. Failure to accurately identify the midline is the number one reason for failed lumbar subarachnoid nerve block. At a point 1

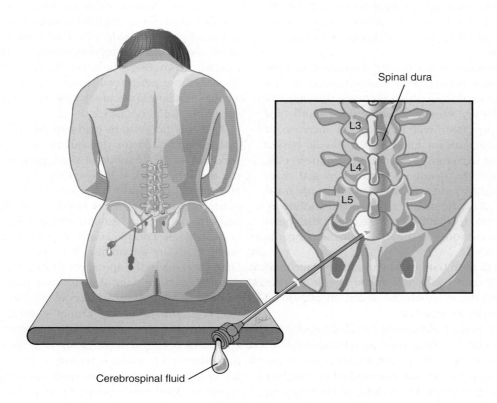

Figure 97-1.

inch lateral and 1 inch below the midline of the L5-S1 interspace, local anesthetic is used to infiltrate the skin and subcutaneous tissues down to the ligamentum flavum with a medial and cephalad trajectory aiming directly for the center of the interspace (Fig. 97-1).

The choice of needle for lumbar subarachnoid block is based in part on the experience of the operator and in part on the desire to decrease the incidence of postdural puncture headache. In general, smaller-gauge needles with points that separate, rather than cut, dural fibers will result in a decreased incidence of postdural puncture headaches, all other things being equal. The use of an introducer needle will facilitate the successful use of smaller-gauge needles. A longer 5- or 6-inch needle is often needed to reach the subarachnoid space when using the lumbosacral approach of Taylor, especially in larger individuals.

The chosen styletted spinal needle is inserted through the previously anesthetized area and advanced with a 10- to 15-degree cephalomedial trajectory through the subcutaneous tissues into the ligamentum flavum (see Fig. 97-1). The operator will perceive an increase in resistance to needle advancement as the needle passes through the dense ligamentum flavum. Should the needle impinge on bone, the needle is withdrawn and readvanced with a slightly more caudad trajectory. Care must be taken not to allow the needle to cross the midline by directing the needle too laterally, or trauma to the spinal cord or exiting nerve roots on the side opposite of needle placement may result.

The needle will then traverse the epidural space, and the operator will then feel a pop as the needle pierces the dura. The needle is slowly advanced an additional 1 mm, and the stylet is removed.

A free flow of spinal fluid should be observed; or if a smaller spinal needle has been used, cerebrospinal fluid should appear in the hub. If no spinal fluid is observed, the stylet is replaced, and the needle is advanced slightly and then rotated 90 degrees. The stylet is again removed, and the hub is again observed for spinal fluid. If no spinal fluid appears, the needle should be removed and the midline reidentified before attempting to repeat the above technique.

After spinal fluid is observed, the needle is fixed in position by the operator placing his or her hand against the patient's back. A drug suitable for subarachnoid administration is chosen, and the addition of glucose to make a hyperbaric solution with or without vasoconstrictors such as epinephrine or phenylephrine to prolong the duration of spinal block is considered. The solution is slowly injected, and the injection is immediately discontinued if the patient reports any pain. The needle is then removed.

SIDE EFFECTS AND COMPLICATIONS

Because of the potential for hematogenous spread via Batson's plexus, local infection and sepsis represent absolute contraindications to the lumbosacral approach of Taylor to the subarachnoid space. In contradistinction to the caudal approach to the epidural space, anticoagulation and coagulopathy represent absolute contraindications to lumbar subarachnoid nerve block because of the risk for epidural and subarachnoid hematoma.

Hypotension is a common side effect of lumbar subarachnoid nerve block and is the result of the profound sympathetic blockade attendant with this procedure. Prophylactic intramuscular or intravenous administration of vasopressors and fluid loading may help avoid this potentially serious side effect of lumbar subarachnoid nerve block. If it is ascertained that a patient would not tolerate hypotension because of other serious systemic disease, more peripheral regional anesthetic techniques such as lumbar plexus block may be preferable to lumbar subarachnoid nerve block.

It also is possible to inadvertently place a needle or catheter intended for the subarachnoid space into the subdural space. If subdural placement is unrecognized, the resulting block will be spotty. This problem can be avoided if the operator advances the needle slightly after perceiving the pop of the needle as it pierces the dura and observing a free flow of spinal fluid.

Neurologic complications after lumbar subarachnoid nerve block are uncommon if proper technique is used. Direct trauma to the spinal cord or nerve roots is usually accompanied by pain. If significant pain occurs during placement of the spinal needle or catheter or during injection, the physician should immediately stop and ascertain the cause of the pain to avoid the possibility of additional neural trauma. Delayed neurologic complications due to chemical irritation of the spinal cord and the coverings of the spinal cord and nerves have been reported. Most severe complications have been attributed to contaminants to the local anesthetic, although the addition of steroids and vasopressors and the use of concentrated hyperbaric solutions also have been implicated.

Although uncommon, infection in the subarachnoid space remains an ever-present possibility, especially in the immunocompromised AIDS or cancer patient. If epidural abscess occurs, emergent surgical drainage to avoid spinal cord compression and irreversible neurologic deficit is usually required. Meningitis after lumbar subarachnoid nerve block may require subarachnoid administration of antibiotics. Early detection and treatment of infection is crucial to avoid potentially life-threatening sequelae.

CLINICAL PEARLS

Lumbar subarachnoid nerve block via the lumbosacral approach of Taylor is a safe and effective procedure if careful attention is paid to technique. The three most common reasons for failure to reach the subarachnoid space when using the lumbosacral approach of Taylor to achieve lumbar subarachnoid nerve block are as follows:

1. Failure to identify the midline before needle placement
2. Underestimating the added depth of needle insertion necessary to reach the subarachnoid space from a paramedian entry site
3. Allowing the needle to cross the midline by using too lateral a trajectory

The first two reasons ordinarily result only in failure to complete the block. The third reason not only results in failed block but also may result in significant trauma to the contralateral spinal cord or nerve roots.

For this reason, it is crucial to first identify the midline and then ensure that the needle never crosses the midline on its path toward the subarachnoid space. The routine use of sedation or general anesthesia before initiation of lumbar subarachnoid block is to be discouraged because it will render the patient unable to provide accurate verbal feedback should needle misplacement occur.

Many pain centers have begun using differential epidural nerve block instead of differential subarachnoid nerve block to avoid the possibility of postdural puncture headache. It appears that the findings with differential epidural neural blockade correlate with those of differential subarachnoid neural blockade. This correlation may not hold true when administering test doses of opioids or other drugs before placement of an implantable drug delivery system. If a subarachnoid terminus for the catheter is intended, subarachnoid rather than epidural test doses should be administered.

CHAPTER 98

Lumbar Myelography

INDICATIONS

Lumbar myelography is indicated to assess the structure and integrity of the spinal canal. As an adjunct to magnetic resonance imaging (MRI) and computed tomography (CT) of the lumbar spine, lumbar myelography may provide the clinician with additional valuable information not obtained from these noninvasive imaging modalities. Myelography is particularly useful in the assessment of the following:

1. Herniated nucleus propulsus
2. Spinal stenosis
3. Space-occupying lesions such as tumor or arteriovenous malformation that may be compressing the spinal cord or exiting nerve roots

Lumbar myelography is most often performed with water-soluble iodinated contrast medium and occasionally with gadolinium. Postmyelography CT following the injection of water-soluble iodinated contrast medium, or MRI following subarachnoid injection of gadolinium, increases the diagnostic accuracy of simple myelography.

CLINICALLY RELEVANT ANATOMY

The spinal cord ends at about L2 in most adults and at about L4 in most infants. Therefore, in most settings, lumbar subarachnoid nerve block should be performed below these levels to avoid the potential for trauma to the spinal cord. The spinal cord is surrounded by three layers of protective connective tissue: the dura, the arachnoid, and the pia mater. The dura is the outermost layer and is composed of tough fibroelastic fibers that form a mechanical barrier to protect the spinal cord. The next layer is the arachnoid. The arachnoid is separated from the dura by only a small potential space, which is filled with serous fluid. The arachnoid is a barrier to the diffusion of substances and effectively serves to limit the spread of drugs administered into the epidural space from diffusing into the spinal fluid. The innermost layer is the pia, a vascular structure that helps provide lateral support to the spinal cord.

To reach the subarachnoid space, a needle placed in the midline at the L3-L4 interspace will pass through the skin, subcutaneous tissues, supraspinous ligament, interspinous ligament, ligamentum flavum, epidural space, dura, subdural space, and arachnoid (Fig. 98-1). Drugs administered into the subarachnoid space are placed between the arachnoid and pia, although inadvertent subdural injection is possible (Fig. 98-2). Subdural injection of contrast is characterized by a dense-appearing column of contrast that is confined to the posterior aspect of the spinal canal with the anterior margin of the column, which is bounded by the arachnoid, appearing irregular and the posterior column, bounded by the dura mater, appearing more linear (Fig. 98-3).

TECHNIQUE

Access to the lumbar subarachnoid space may be obtained with the patient in the sitting, lateral, or prone position, although the imaging required for lumbar myelography requires the patient be in the lateral or prone position. If the lateral position is chosen, careful attention to patient positioning, including identifying the

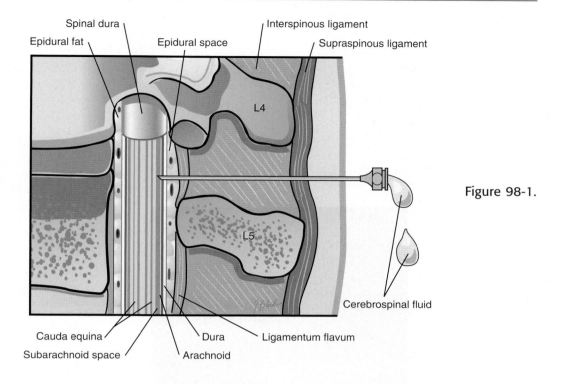

Spinal dura

Epidural fat

Epidural space

Interspinous ligament

Supraspinous ligament

L4

L5

Figure 98-1.

Cerebrospinal fluid

Cauda equina

Subarachnoid space

Dura

Arachnoid

Ligamentum flavum

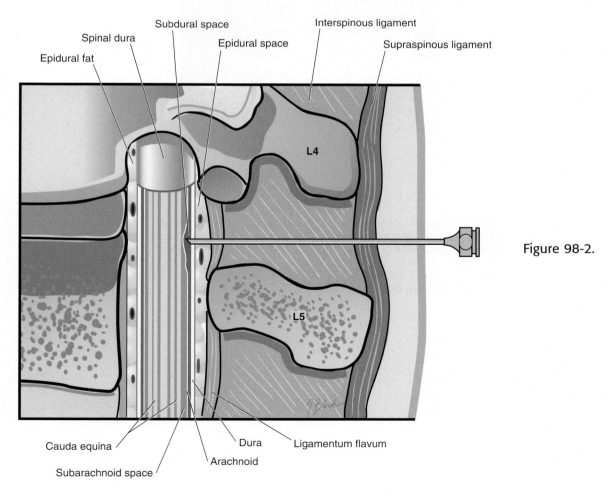

Subdural space

Spinal dura

Epidural space

Epidural fat

Interspinous ligament

Supraspinous ligament

L4

L5

Figure 98-2.

Cauda equina

Subarachnoid space

Dura

Arachnoid

Ligamentum flavum

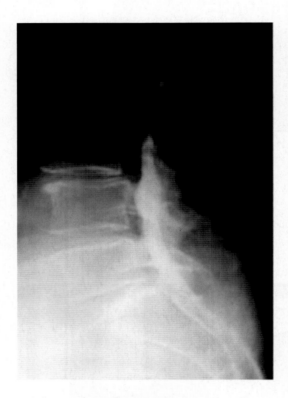

Figure 98-3.
Lateral radiograph of the lumbar spine with subdural contrast media. The dense collection of contrast media is confined to the posterior aspect of the spinal canal. The posterior border of the fluid collection is linear (the dura mater), whereas the anterior border is somewhat more irregular (the arachnoid mater). (From Ajar AH, Rathmell JP, Mukherji SK: The subdural compartment. Reg Anesth Pain Med 27:72-76, 2002.)

midline, avoiding rotation of the spine, and maximizing flexion of the lumbar spine, is essential to successfully completing subarachnoid nerve block. The prone position is best used with the patient's lumbar spine moderately flexed by placing a pillow underneath the lumbar spine. Although this position limits the amount of rotation of the spine possible and simplifies midline identification, the inherent dangers of the prone position, including difficulty in monitoring the patient and problems with airway management, require careful monitoring of the patient when performing lumbar myelography.

After the patient is placed in optimal position with the lumbar spine flexed and without rotation, the iliac crests are identified. The spinous process of L4 is approximately on an imaginary line drawn between the two iliac crests. The skin is then prepared with an antiseptic solution. At the L3-L4 interspace, the operator's middle and index fingers are placed on each side of the spinous processes. The position of the interspace is reconfirmed with palpation using a rocking motion in the superior and inferior planes. The midline of the selected interspace is identified by palpating the spinous processes above and below the interspace using a lateral rocking motion to ensure that the needle entry site is exactly in the midline. Failure to accurately identify the midline is the number one reason for failed lumbar subarachnoid nerve block. One milliliter of local anesthetic is used to infiltrate the skin, subcutaneous tissues, and supraspinous and interspinous ligaments at the midline. Fluoroscopy will aid the clinician in accurate identification of the previously mentioned landmarks and with subsequent needle placement.

The choice of needle for lumbar subarachnoid block is based in part on the experience of the operator and in part on the desire to decrease the incidence of postdural puncture headache. In general, smaller-gauge needles with points that separate, rather than cut, dural fibers will result in a decreased incidence of postdural puncture headaches, all other things being equal. The use of an introducer needle facilitates the successful use of smaller-gauge needles. The chosen styletted spinal needle is inserted exactly in the midline in the previously anesthetized area and advanced with a 10- to 15-degree cephalad trajectory. The needle is advanced through the subcutaneous tissues and supraspinous ligament into the interspinous ligament. The operator will perceive an increase in resistance to needle advancement as the needle passes through the interspinous ligament and the dense ligamentum flavum.

The needle will then traverse the epidural space, and the operator will feel a pop as the needle pierces the dura. The needle is slowly advanced an additional 1 mm, and the stylet is removed. A free flow of spinal fluid should be observed; or if a smaller spinal needle has been used, cerebrospinal fluid should appear in the hub. If no spinal fluid is observed, the stylet is replaced, and the needle is advanced slightly and then rotated 90 degrees. The stylet is again removed, and the hub is again observed for spinal fluid. If no spinal fluid appears, the needle should be removed and the midline reidentified before attempting to repeat the previous technique. After spinal fluid is observed, the needle is fixed in position by the operator placing his or her hand against the patient's back. A water-soluble iodinated contrast agent such as iopamidol or iohexol in a volume of 10 to 12 mL is then drawn up using sterile technique. A 0.5-mL test dose is then slowly injected through the previously placed needle, and the position of contrast within the subarachnoid space is then confirmed with both posteroanterior and lateral fluoroscopy. The injection should be immediately discontinued if the patient reports any pain. If satisfactory position of contrast is confirmed, 10-12 mL of contrast is then slowly injected under continuous fluoroscopic guidance. The injection should be immediately discontinued if the patient reports any pain. The flow of contrast into the subarachnoid space is observed in both the posteroanterior and lateral views (Figs. 98-4 and 98-5). The patient may be moved into a gentle head-down position to aid in the flow of contrast into the upper lumbar segments. After satisfactory spread of contrast to include the T12-L1 interspace and conus, the stylet is replaced, and the needle is then removed (Fig. 98-6). Postmyelography CT often adds diagnostic information that may help clarify the pathology responsible for the patient's symptomatology (Figs. 98-7 to 98-9).

SIDE EFFECTS AND COMPLICATIONS

Because of the potential for hematogenous spread via Batson's plexus, local infection and sepsis represent absolute contraindications to the midline approach to the lumbar subarachnoid space. In contradistinction to the caudal approach to the epidural space, anticoagulation and coagulopathy represent absolute contraindications to lumbar myelography because of the risk for epidural and subarachnoid hematoma.

It also is possible to inadvertently place a needle or catheter intended for the subarachnoid space into the subdural space (see Figs. 98-2 and 98-3). If subdural placement is unrecognized, the diagnostic information obtained will be compromised. This problem can be avoided if the operator advances the needle slightly after perceiving the pop of the needle as it pierces the dura, confirms a free flow of spinal fluid, and confirms subarachnoid needle placement by a test dose of water-soluble contrast medium.

Neurologic complications after lumbar myelography are uncommon if proper technique is used. Direct trauma to the spinal cord or nerve roots is usually accompanied

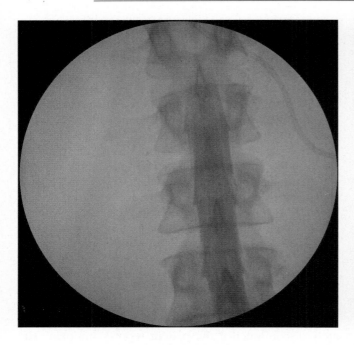

Figure 98-4.
PA view of contrast medium within the thecal sac.

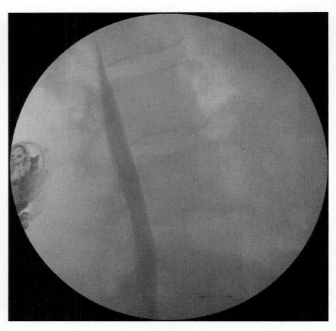

Figure 98-5.
Lateral view of contrast medium within the thecal sac.

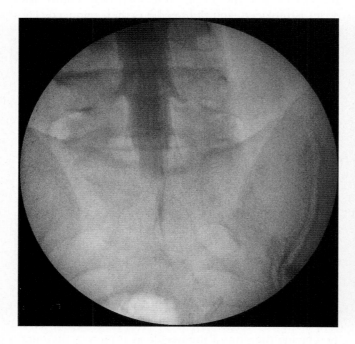

Figure 98-6.
Contrast medium filling the distal thecal sac.

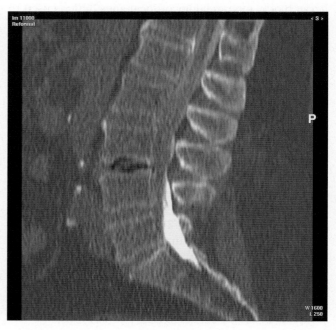

Figure 98-7.
Postmyelography CT demonstrating contrast within the thecal sac.

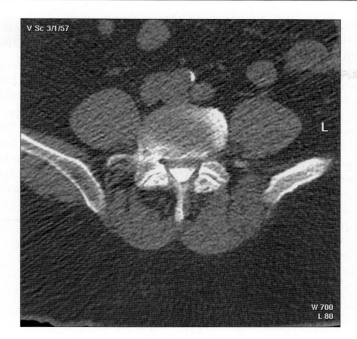

Figure 98-8.

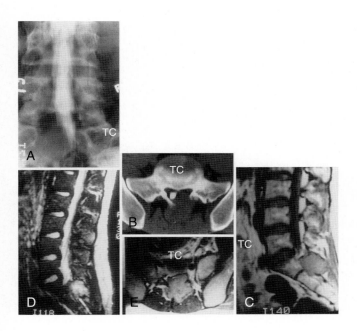

Figure 98-9.
A, Frontal view of the lumbosacral junction showing giant cell tumor causing bone destruction of the left proximal sacrum and mass effect on the thecal sac, pushing it to the left.
B, Axial CT image after myelogram demonstrating a destructive soft tissue mass involving the posterior elements of the sacrum and causing mass effect on the thecal sac.
C, T1-weighted sagittal image of the lumbar spine clearly demonstrates the giant cell tumor involving the posterior aspect of the sacrum. The mass has mixed signal intensity. Evidence of hemorrhage or fluid-fluid levels is not seen.
D, T2-weighted sagittal image of the same giant cell tumor demonstrating mixed signal intensity. Again, evidence of fluid-fluid levels is not seen. **E,** T1-weighted axial image of giant cell tumor of the sacrum demonstrating signal intensity that is mixed but higher than that of muscle. (From Haaga JR, Lanzieri CF: CT and MR imaging of the whole body, 4th ed. St. Louis, Mosby, 2002, p 774.)

by pain. If significant pain occurs during placement of the spinal needle or during injection, the physician should immediately stop and ascertain the cause of the pain to avoid the possibility of additional neural trauma. Delayed neurologic complications due to chemical irritation of the spinal cord and the coverings of the spinal cord and nerves have been reported. Most severe complications have been attributed to contaminants to the contrast medium. Although uncommon, infection in the subarachnoid space remains an ever-present possibility, especially in the immunocompromised AIDS or cancer patient. If epidural abscess occurs, emergent surgical drainage to avoid spinal cord compression and irreversible neurologic deficit is usually required. Meningitis occurring after lumbar myelography may require subarachnoid administration of antibiotics. Early detection and treatment of infection is crucial to avoid potentially life-threatening sequelae.

CLINICAL PEARLS

Lumbar myelography is a safe and effective diagnostic modality if careful attention is paid to technique. Failure to accurately identify the midline is the most common reason for difficulty in performing lumbar myelography and increases the risk for complications. The routine use of sedation or general anesthesia before initiation of lumbar myelography is to be discouraged because it will render the patient unable to provide accurate verbal feedback should needle misplacement occur.

CHAPTER 99

Caudal Epidural Nerve Block: Prone Position

CPT-2009 CODE	
Local Anesthetic/Narcotic	62311
Steroid	62311
Neurolytic	62282

Relative Value Units	
Local Anesthetic	10
Steroid	10
Neurolytic	20

INDICATIONS

Because of the simplicity, safety, and lack of pain associated with the caudal approach to the epidural space, caudal epidural nerve block is rapidly replacing the lumbar approach to the epidural space for a number of pain management applications at many pain centers. In addition to applications for surgical and obstetric anesthesia, caudal epidural nerve block with local anesthetic can be used as a diagnostic tool when performing differential neural blockade on an anatomic basis in the evaluation of pelvic, bladder, perineal, genital, rectal, anal, and lower extremity pain. If destruction of the lower lumbar or sacral nerves is being considered, this technique is useful as a prognostic indicator of the degree of motor and sensory impairment that the patient may experience.

Caudal epidural nerve block with local anesthetic may be used to palliate acute pain emergencies in adults and children, including postoperative pain, pain secondary to pelvic and lower extremity trauma, pain of acute herpes zoster, and cancer-related pain, while waiting for pharmacologic, surgical, or antiblastic methods to become effective. Additionally, this technique is valuable in patients suffering from acute vascular insufficiency of the lower extremities secondary to vasospastic and vaso-occlusive disease, including frostbite and ergotamine toxicity.

The administration of local anesthetic, steroids, or both via the caudal approach to the epidural space is useful in the treatment of a variety of chronic benign pain syndromes, including lumbar radiculopathy, low back syndrome, spinal stenosis, postlaminectomy syndrome, vertebral compression fractures, diabetic polyneuropathy, postherpetic neuralgia, reflex sympathetic dystrophy, phantom limb pain, orchalgia, proctalgia, and pelvic pain syndromes.

The caudal approach to the epidural space is especially useful in patients who have previously undergone low back surgery, which may make the lumbar approach to the epidural space less optimal. Because the caudal approach to the epidural space can be used in the presence of anticoagulation or coagulopathy, local anesthetic, opioids, and steroids can be administered via this route even when other regional anesthetic techniques, including the spinal and lumbar epidural approach, are contraindicated. This is advantageous in patients with vascular insufficiency who are fully anticoagulated and in cancer patients who have developed coagulopathy secondary to radiation or chemotherapy.

The caudal epidural administration of local anesthetic in combination with steroids, opioids, or both is useful in the palliation of cancer-related pelvic, perineal, and rectal pain. This technique has been especially successful in the relief of pain secondary to the bony metastases of prostate cancer and the palliation of chemotherapy-related peripheral neuropathy.

Because of the potential for hematogenous spread via Batson's plexus, local infection and sepsis represent absolute contraindications to the caudal approach to the epidural space. Pilonidal cyst and congenital abnormalities of the dural sac and its contents also represent relative contraindications to the caudal approach to the epidural space.

CLINICALLY RELEVANT ANATOMY

Sacrum

The triangular sacrum consists of the five fused sacral vertebrae, which are dorsally convex (Fig. 99-1). The

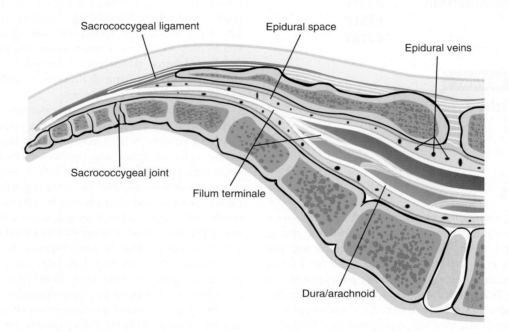

Figure 99-1.

sacrum inserts in a wedgelike manner between the two iliac bones, articulating superiorly with the fifth lumbar vertebra and caudad with the coccyx. On the anterior concave surface, there are four pairs of unsealed anterior sacral foramina that allow passage of the anterior rami of the upper four sacral nerves. The posterior sacral foramina are smaller than their anterior counterparts. Leakage of drugs injected into the sacral canal is effectively prevented by the sacrospinal and multifidus muscles. The vestigial remnants of the inferior articular processes project downward on each side of the sacral hiatus. These bony projections are called the sacral cornua and represent important clinical landmarks when performing caudal epidural nerve block.

Although there are gender- and race-determined differences in the shape of the sacrum, they are of little importance relative to the ultimate ability to successfully perform caudal epidural nerve block on a given patient.

Coccyx

The triangular coccyx is made up of three to five rudimental vertebrae. Its superior surface articulates with the inferior articular surface of the sacrum. The tip of the coccyx is an important clinical landmark when performing caudal epidural nerve block.

Sacral Hiatus

The sacral hiatus is formed by the incomplete midline fusion of the posterior elements of the lower portion of the S4 and the entire S5 vertebrae. This U-shaped space is covered posteriorly by the sacrococcygeal ligament, which also is an important clinical landmark when performing caudal epidural nerve block. Penetration of the sacrococcygeal ligament provides direct access to the epidural space of the sacral canal.

Sacral Canal

A continuation of the lumbar spinal canal, the sacral canal continues inferiorly to terminate at the sacral hiatus. The volume of the sacral canal with all of its contents removed averages about 34 mL in dried bone specimens. It should be emphasized that much smaller volumes of local anesthetic (i.e., 5 to 10 mL) are used in day-to-day pain management practice. The use of large volumes of local anesthetic, especially in the area of pain management, will result in an unacceptable level of local anesthetic-induced side effects, such as incontinence and urinary retention, and should be avoided.

Contents of the Sacral Canal

The sacral canal contains the inferior termination of the dural sac, which ends between S1 and S3 (Fig. 99-2). The five sacral nerve roots and the coccygeal nerve all traverse the canal, as does the terminal filament of the spinal cord, the filum terminale. The anterior and posterior rami of the S1-S4 nerve roots exit from their respective anterior and posterior sacral foramina. The S5 roots and coccygeal nerves leave the sacral canal via the sacral hiatus. These nerves provide sensory and motor innervation to their respective dermatomes and myotomes. They also provide partial innervation to several pelvic organs, including the uterus, fallopian tubes, bladder, and prostate.

The sacral canal also contains the epidural venous plexus, which generally ends at S4 but may continue inferiorly. Most of these vessels are concentrated in the anterior portion of the canal. Both the dural sac and epidural vessels are susceptible to trauma by advancing needles or catheters cephalad into the sacral canal. The remainder of the sacral canal is filled with fat, which is subject to an age-related increase in its density. Some investigators believe this change is responsible for the increased incidence of "spotty" caudal epidural nerve blocks in adults.

TECHNIQUE

The patient is placed in the prone position. The patient's head is placed on a pillow and turned away from the pain management physician. The legs and heels are abducted to prevent tightening of the gluteal muscles, which can make identification of the sacral hiatus more difficult (Fig. 99-3).

Preparation of a wide area of skin with antiseptic solution is then carried out so that all of the landmarks can be palpated aseptically. A fenestrated sterile drape is placed to avoid contamination of the palpating finger. The middle finger of the nondominant hand is placed over the sterile drape into the natal cleft with the fingertip at the tip of the coccyx (Fig. 99-4). This maneuver allows easy confirmation of the sacral midline and is especially important when using the lateral position.

After careful identification of the midline, the area under the proximal interphalangeal joint is located. The middle finger is then moved cephalad to the area that was previously located under the proximal interphalangeal joint. This spot is palpated using a lateral rocking motion to identify the sacral cornua (Fig. 99-5). The sacral hiatus will be found at this level if the pain management physician's glove size is $7\frac{1}{2}$ or 8 (Fig. 99-6). If the pain management physician's glove size is smaller, the location of the sacral hiatus will be just superior to the area located below the operator's proximal inter-

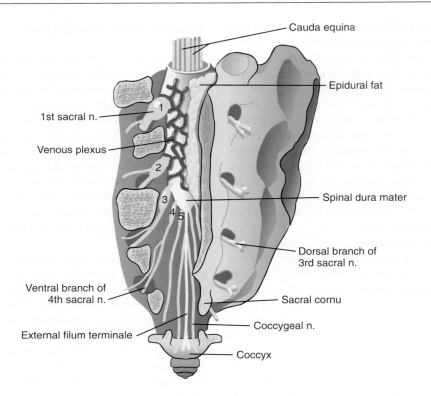

Cauda equina

Epidural fat

1st sacral n.

Venous plexus

Spinal dura mater

Dorsal branch of
3rd sacral n.

Ventral branch of
4th sacral n.

Sacral cornu

External filum terminale

Coccygeal n.

Coccyx

Figure 99-2.

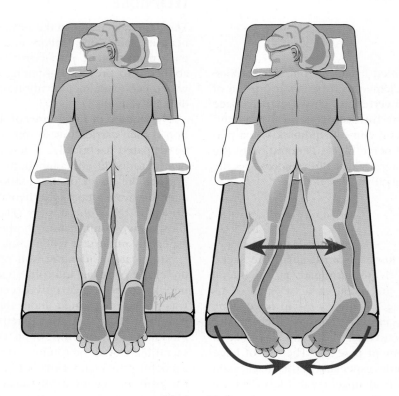

Figure 99-3.

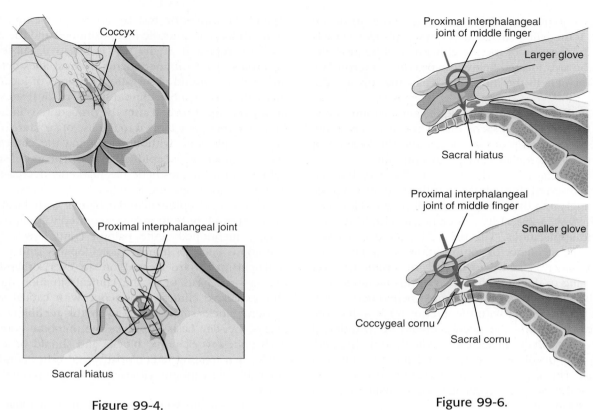

Figure 99-4.

Figure 99-6.

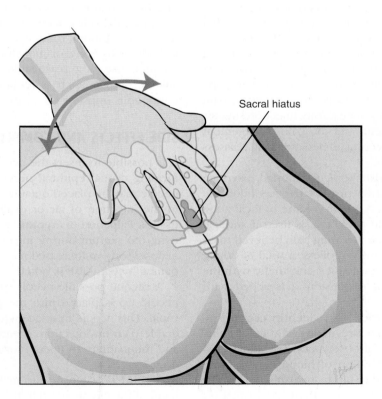

Figure 99-5.

phalangeal joint when the fingertip is at the tip of the coccyx. If the pain management physician's glove size is larger, the location of the sacral hiatus will be just inferior to the area located below the proximal interphalangeal joint when the fingertip is at the tip of the coccyx.

Although there is normally significant anatomic variation of the sacrum and sacral hiatus, the spatial relationship between the tip of the coccyx and the location of the sacral hiatus remains amazingly constant.

After locating the sacral hiatus, a 25-gauge, 1½-inch needle is inserted through the anesthetized area at a 45-degree angle into the sacrococcygeal ligament (Figs. 99-7 through 99-9). A 25-gauge, ⅝-inch needle is indicated for pediatric applications. The use of longer needles will increase the incidence of complications, including intravascular injection and inadvertent dural puncture, yet add nothing to the overall success of this technique.

As the sacrococcygeal ligament is penetrated, a pop will be felt. If contact with the interior bony wall of the sacral canal occurs, the needle should be withdrawn slightly. This will disengage the needle tip from the periosteum. The needle is then advanced about 0.5 cm into the canal. This is to ensure that the entire needle bevel is beyond the sacrococcygeal ligament to avoid injection into the ligament.

An air acceptance test is performed by the injection of 1 mL of air through the needle. There should be no bulging or crepitus of the tissues overlying the sacrum. The force required for injection should not exceed that necessary to overcome the resistance of the needle. If there is initial resistance to injection, the needle should be rotated 180 degrees in case the needle is correctly placed in the canal but the needle bevel is occluded by the internal wall of the sacral canal. Any significant pain or sudden increases in resistance during injection suggest incorrect needle placement, and the pain management physician should stop injecting immediately and reassess the position of the needle.

When the needle is satisfactorily positioned, a syringe containing 5 to 10 mL of 1.0% preservative-free lidocaine is attached to the needle. A larger volume of local anesthetic, on the order of 20 to 30 mL, is used if surgical anesthesia is required. When treating pain believed to be secondary to an inflammatory process, a total of 80 mg of depot-steroid is added to the local anesthetic with the first block, and 40 mg of depot-steroid is added with subsequent blocks.

Gentle aspiration is carried out to identify cerebrospinal fluid or blood. Although rare, inadvertent dural puncture can occur, and careful observation for spinal fluid must be carried out. Aspiration of blood occurs more commonly. This can be due either to damage to veins during insertion of the needle into the caudal canal or, less commonly, to intravenous placement of the needle.

Should the aspiration test be positive for either spinal fluid or blood, the needle is repositioned and the aspiration test repeated. If the test is negative, subsequent injections of 0.5-mL increments of local anesthetic are undertaken. Careful observation for signs of local anesthetic toxicity or subarachnoid spread of local anesthetic during the injection and after the procedure is indicated. Clinical experience has led to the use of smaller volumes of local anesthetic without sacrificing the clinical efficacy of caudal steroid epidural blocks. The use of smaller volumes of local anesthetic has markedly decreased the number of local anesthetic–related side effects.

Daily caudal epidural nerve blocks with local anesthetic, steroid, or both may be required to treat the previously mentioned acute painful conditions. Chronic conditions such as lumbar radiculopathy and diabetic polyneuropathy are treated on an every-other-day to once-a-week basis or as the clinical situation dictates. Our extensive clinical experience with caudal steroid epidural blocks suggests that using this technique on an every-other-day basis improves the outcome compared with once-a-week nerve blocks and should be considered when treating radiculopathy and other conditions amenable to treatment with caudal steroid epidural nerve blocks.

If selective neurolytic block of an individual sacral nerve is desired, incremental 0.1-mL injections of 6.5% phenol in glycerin or alcohol to a total volume of 1 mL may be used after first confirming the level of pain relief and potential side effects with local anesthetic blocks. If the caudal epidural route is chosen for administration of opioids, 4 to 5 mg of morphine sulfate formulated for epidural use is a reasonable initial dose. More lipid-soluble opioids such as fentanyl must be delivered by continuous infusion via a caudal catheter.

SIDE EFFECTS AND COMPLICATIONS

It is possible to insert the needle incorrectly when performing caudal epidural nerve block (Fig. 99-10). The needle may be placed outside the sacral canal, resulting in the injection of air or drugs into the subcutaneous tissues. Palpation of crepitus and bulging of tissues overlying the sacrum during injection indicates this needle malposition. An increased resistance to injection accompanied by pain also is noted.

A second possible needle misplacement is when the needle tip is placed into the periosteum of the sacral canal. This needle misplacement is suggested by considerable pain on injection, a high resistance to injection, and the inability to inject more than a few milliliters of drug.

A third possible needle malposition is partial placement of the needle bevel in the sacrococcygeal ligament. Again, there is significant resistance to injection as well

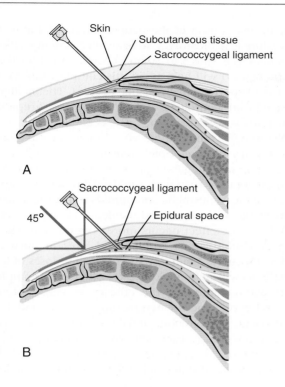

Figure 99-7.

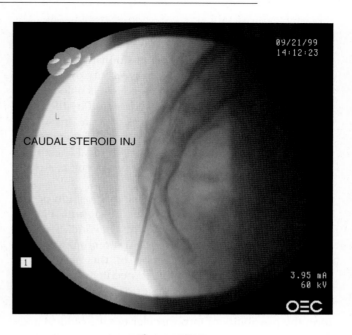

Figure 99-8.
Lateral view of the needle tip within the caudal canal.

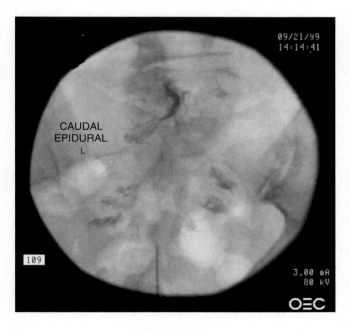

Figure 99-9.
PA view of the needle tip within the caudal canal.

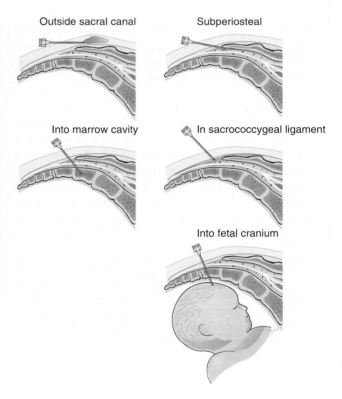

Figure 99-10.

as significant pain as the drugs are injected into the ligament.

A fourth possible needle malposition is to force the point of the needle into the marrow cavity of the sacral vertebra, resulting in very high blood levels of local anesthetic. This needle malposition is detected by the initial easy acceptance of a few milliliters of local anesthetic, followed by a rapid increase in resistance to injection as the noncompliant bony cavity fills with local anesthetic. Significant local anesthetic toxicity can occur as a result of this complication.

The fifth and most serious needle malposition occurs when the needle is inserted through the sacrum or lateral to the coccyx into the pelvic cavity beyond. This can result in the needle entering both the rectum and birth canal, resulting in contamination of the needle. The repositioning of the contaminated needle into the sacral canal will carry with it the danger of infection.

The caudal epidural space is highly vascular; therefore, the possibility of intravascular uptake of local anesthetic is significant with this technique. Careful aspiration and incremental dosing of local anesthetic are important to allow early detection of local anesthetic toxicity.

Careful observation of the patient during and after the procedure is mandatory. Use of smaller volumes of local anesthetic (i.e., the 5 to 10 mL recommended for therapeutic blocks) will help avoid this complication, as will the use of shorter, smaller-gauge needles. The incidence of significant neurologic deficit secondary to epidural hematoma after caudal block is exceedingly rare.

Neurologic complications after caudal nerve block are rare. Usually these complications are associated with a preexisting neurologic lesion or with surgical or obstetric trauma rather than with the caudal block. The application of local anesthetic and opioids to the sacral nerve roots results in an increased incidence of urinary retention. This side effect occurs more commonly in elderly men and multiparous women and after inguinal and perineal surgery. Again, the use of smaller doses of local anesthetic will help avoid these bothersome complications without affecting the efficacy of caudal steroid epidural nerve blocks when treating painful conditions.

Although uncommon, infection remains an ever-present possibility, especially in the immunocompromised AIDS or cancer patient. Early detection of infection is crucial to avoid potentially life-threatening sequelae.

CLINICAL PEARLS

Most recently, pain management specialists have recognized the clinical advantages of the caudal over the lumbar approach to the epidural space when performing steroid epidural nerve blocks. The advantages of the caudal approach include the following:

1. The ability to use smaller and sharper needles relative to the larger and blunter Hustead and Tuohy needles required for the lumbar approach to the epidural space (these smaller, sharper needles produce less procedure-related pain and produce less soft tissue trauma, which further decreases the amount of postprocedure pain the patient will experience compared with lumbar epidural blocks performed with Hustead and Tuohy needles).
2. These small needles (e.g., 25-gauge, $1\frac{1}{2}$-inch needles) are significantly less expensive than the specialized Hustead or Tuohy needles.
3. The caudal approach to the epidural space can be used to deliver drugs to the epidural space in the presence of anticoagulation or coagulopathy, which is not possible via the lumbar route.
4. The efficacy of steroids administered into the epidural space via the caudal route is at least as beneficial as delivering the same drugs via the lumbar route.
5. The technique is less technically demanding than the lumbar approach.
6. The caudal approach to the epidural space is safer for patients who have undergone previous surgery of the lumbar spine.
7. Perhaps most important, there is essentially no risk for inadvertent dural puncture, which occurs with an incidence of 0.5% even when experienced clinicians perform lumbar epidural nerve block. This advantage alone has led many contemporary pain management clinicians to abandon the lumbar epidural route in favor of the caudal approach when treating patients suffering from lumbar radiculopathy, spinal stenosis, and other diseases amenable to treatment with epidural steroids.

CHAPTER 100

Caudal Epidural Nerve Block: Lateral Position

CPT-2009 CODE

Local Anesthetic/Narcotic	62311
Steroid	62311
Neurolytic	62282

Relative Value Units

Local Anesthetic	10
Steroid	10
Neurolytic	20

INDICATIONS

Performing caudal epidural nerve block in the lateral position is one of the most technically demanding regional anesthesia techniques. Despite the difficulty of this approach, the use of the lateral position expands the number of patients in whom caudal epidural block can be performed to include those who cannot assume the prone position because of fractures, pregnancy, and severe pulmonary insufficiency. The lateral position allows the pain management specialist to capitalize on the safety and lack of pain associated with the caudal approach to epidural nerve block. For these reasons, as well as the simplicity of the caudal block when performed with the patient in the prone position, caudal epidural nerve block is rapidly replacing the lumbar approach to the epidural space for a number of pain management applications at many pain centers. In addition to applications for surgical and obstetric anesthesia, caudal epidural nerve block with local anesthetic can be used as a diagnostic tool when performing differential neural blockade on an anatomic basis in the evaluation of pelvic, bladder, perineal, genital, rectal, anal, and lower extremity pain. If destruction of the lower lumbar or sacral nerves is being considered, this technique is useful as a prognostic indicator of the degree of motor and sensory impairment that the patient may experience.

Caudal epidural nerve block with local anesthetic may be used to palliate acute pain emergencies in adults and children, including postoperative pain, pain secondary to pelvic and lower extremity trauma, pain of acute herpes zoster, and cancer-related pain, while waiting for pharmacologic, surgical, or antiblastic methods to become effective. Additionally, this technique is valuable in patients suffering from acute vascular insufficiency of the lower extremities secondary to vasospastic and vaso-occlusive disease, including frostbite and ergotamine toxicity. Caudal nerve block also is recommended to palliate the pain of hydradenitis suppurativa of the groin.

The administration of local anesthetic, steroids, or both via the caudal approach to the epidural space is useful in the treatment of a variety of chronic benign pain syndromes, including lumbar radiculopathy, low back syndrome, spinal stenosis, postlaminectomy syndrome, vertebral compression fractures, diabetic polyneuropathy, postherpetic neuralgia, reflex sympathetic dystrophy, phantom limb pain, orchialgia, proctalgia, and pelvic pain syndromes.

The caudal approach to the epidural space is especially useful in patients who have previously undergone low back surgery, which may make the lumbar approach to the epidural space less optimal. Because the caudal approach to the epidural space can be used in the presence of anticoagulation or coagulopathy, local anesthetic, opioids, and steroids can be administered by this route even when other regional anesthetic techniques, including the spinal and lumbar epidural approach, are contraindicated. This is advantageous in patients with vascular insufficiency who are fully anticoagulated and in cancer patients who have developed coagulopathy secondary to radiation or chemotherapy.

The caudal epidural administration of local anesthetic in combination with steroids, opioids, or both is useful in the palliation of cancer-related pelvic, perineal, and rectal pain. This technique has been especially successful in the relief of pain secondary to the bony metastases of prostate cancer and the palliation of chemotherapy-related peripheral neuropathy. As mentioned earlier, the caudal administration of local anesthetic, opioids, and steroids can be used in the presence of anticoagulation or coagulopathy.

Because of the potential for hematogenous spread via Batson's plexus, local infection and sepsis represent absolute contraindications to the caudal approach to the epidural space. Pilonidal cyst and congenital abnormalities of the dural sac and its contents also represent relative contraindications to the caudal approach to the epidural space.

CLINICALLY RELEVANT ANATOMY

Sacrum

The triangular sacrum consists of the five fused sacral vertebrae that are dorsally convex. The sacrum inserts in a wedgelike manner between the two iliac bones, articulating superiorly with the fifth lumbar vertebra and caudad with the coccyx. On the anterior concave surface, there are four pairs of unsealed anterior sacral foramina that allow passage of the anterior rami of the upper four sacral nerves. It is the unsealed nature of the anterior sacral foramina that allows the escape of drugs injected into the sacral canal.

The convex dorsal surface of the sacrum has an irregular surface secondary to the fusing of the elements of the sacral vertebrae. Dorsally, there is a midline crest called the median sacral crest. The posterior sacral foramina are smaller than their anterior counterparts. Leakage of drugs injected into the sacral canal is effectively prevented by the sacrospinal and multifidus muscles. The vestigial remnants of the inferior articular processes project downward on each side of the sacral hiatus. These bony projections are called the sacral cornua and represent important clinical landmarks when performing caudal epidural nerve block.

Although there are gender- and race-determined differences in the shape of the sacrum, they are of little importance relative to the ultimate ability to successfully perform caudal epidural nerve block on a given patient.

Coccyx

The triangular coccyx is made up of three to five rudimental vertebrae. Its superior surface articulates with the inferior articular surface of the sacrum. Two prominent coccygeal cornua adjoin their sacral counterparts. The ventral surface of the coccyx is angulated anteriorly and superiorly. The tip of the coccyx is an important clinical landmark when performing caudal epidural nerve block.

Sacral Hiatus

The sacral hiatus is formed by the incomplete midline fusion of the posterior elements of the lower portion of the S4 and the entire S5 vertebrae. This U-shaped space is covered posteriorly by the sacrococcygeal ligament, which also is an important clinical landmark when performing caudal epidural nerve block. Penetration of the sacrococcygeal ligament provides direct access to the epidural space of the sacral canal.

Sacral Canal

A continuation of the lumbar spinal canal, the sacral canal continues inferiorly to terminate at the sacral hiatus. The canal communicates with the anterior and posterior sacral foramina. The volume of the sacral canal with all of its contents removed averages about 34 mL in dried bone specimens. It should be emphasized that much smaller volumes of local anesthetic (i.e., 5 to 10 mL) are used in day-to-day pain management practice. The use of large volumes of local anesthetic, especially in the area of pain management, results in an unacceptable level of local anesthetic–induced side effects, such as incontinence and urinary retention, and should be avoided.

Contents of the Sacral Canal

The sacral canal contains the inferior termination of the dural sac, which ends between S1 and S3. The five sacral nerve roots and the coccygeal nerve all traverse the canal, as does the terminal filament of the spinal cord, the filum terminale. The anterior and posterior rami of the S1-S4 nerve roots exit from their respective anterior and posterior sacral foramina. The S5 roots and coccygeal nerves leave the sacral canal via the sacral hiatus. These nerves provide sensory and motor innervation to their respective dermatomes and myotomes. They also provide partial innervation to several pelvic organs, including the uterus, fallopian tubes, bladder, and prostate.

The sacral canal also contains the epidural venous plexus, which generally ends at S4 but may continue inferiorly. Most of these vessels are concentrated in the anterior portion of the canal. Both the dural sac and epidural vessels are susceptible to trauma by advancing needles or catheters cephalad into the sacral canal. The remainder of the sacral canal is filled with fat, which is subject to an age-related increase in its density. Some investigators believe this change is responsible for the increased incidence of "spotty" caudal epidural nerve blocks in adults.

TECHNIQUE

Caudal epidural nerve block is carried out in either the prone or the lateral position. Each position has its own advantages and disadvantages. The prone position is easier for the pain management physician, but its use may be limited because of the patient's inability to rest comfortably on his or her abdomen or because of the presence of ostomy appliances such as colostomy and ileostomy bags. Furthermore, easy access to the airway is limited should problems occur while the patient is prone. The lateral position allows better access to the airway but is technically a more demanding approach.

The patient is placed in the lateral position with the left side down for the right-handed pain management physician. The dependent leg is slightly flexed at the hip and knee for patient comfort. The upper leg is flexed so that it lies over and above the lower leg and in contact with the bed (Fig. 100-1). This modified Sims' position separates the buttocks, making identification of the sacral hiatus easier. Owing to sagging of the buttocks in the lateral position, the gluteal fold is usually inferior to the level of the sacral hiatus and is a misleading landmark for needle placement.

Preparation of a wide area of skin with antiseptic solution is then carried out so that all of the landmarks can be palpated aseptically. A fenestrated sterile drape is placed to avoid contamination of the palpating finger. The middle finger of the nondominant hand is placed over the sterile drape with the fingertip at the tip of the coccyx. In most patients, the natal cleft will be below the level of the sacral hiatus, and the pain management physician must correct for this fact accordingly by carefully identifying the bony landmarks before needle placement. This step is especially important when using the lateral position.

After careful identification of the midline and bony landmarks, the area under the proximal interphalangeal joint is located. The middle finger then is moved cephalad to the area that was previously located under the proximal interphalangeal joint. This spot is palpated using a lateral rocking motion to identify the sacral cornua. The sacral hiatus will be found at this level if the pain management physician's glove size is 7½ or 8. If the pain management physician's glove size is smaller, the location of the sacral hiatus will be just superior to the area located below the operator's proximal interphalangeal joint when the fingertip is at the tip of the coccyx. If the pain management physician's glove size is larger, the location of the sacral hiatus will be just inferior to the area located below the proximal interphalangeal joint when the fingertip is at the tip of the coccyx.

Although there is normally significant anatomic variation of the sacrum and sacral hiatus, the spatial relationship between the tip of the coccyx and the location of the sacral hiatus remains amazingly constant. When the approximate position of the sacral hiatus is located by palpating the tip of the coccyx, identifying the midline and locating the area under the proximal interphalangeal joint as described earlier, inability to identify and enter the sacral hiatus should occur less than 0.5% of the time.

After locating the sacral hiatus, a 25-gauge, 1½-inch needle is inserted through the anesthetized area at a 45-degree angle into the sacrococcygeal ligament. A 25-gauge, ⅝-inch needle is indicated for pediatric applications. The use of longer needles as advocated by some earlier investigators will increase the incidence of complications, including intravascular injection and inadvertent dural puncture. Furthermore, the use of longer needles adds nothing to the overall success of this technique.

As the sacrococcygeal ligament is penetrated, a pop or "giving way" will be felt. If contact with the interior bony wall of the sacral canal occurs, the needle should be withdrawn slightly. This will disengage the needle tip from the periosteum. The needle is then advanced about 0.5 cm into the canal. This is to ensure that the entire needle bevel is beyond the sacrococcygeal ligament to avoid injection into the ligament.

At this point, the needle should be held firmly in place by the bone, ligament, and subcutaneous tissues and should not sag if released by the pain management physician. An air acceptance test is performed by the injection of 1 mL of air through the needle. There should be no bulging or crepitus of the tissues overlying the sacrum. The injection of air, as well as the subsequent injection of drugs, should feel like any other injection into the epidural space. The force required for injection should not exceed that necessary to overcome the resistance of the needle. If there is initial resistance to injection, the needle should be rotated 180 degrees in case the needle is correctly placed in the canal but the needle bevel is occluded by the internal wall of the sacral canal. Any significant pain or sudden increases in resistance during injection suggest incorrect needle placement, and the pain management physician should stop injecting immediately and reassess the position of the needle.

When the needle is satisfactorily positioned, a syringe containing 5 to 10 mL of 1.0% preservative-free lidocaine is attached to the needle. A larger volume of local anesthetic on the order of 20 to 30 mL is used if surgical anesthesia is required. When treating pain thought to be secondary to an inflammatory process, a total of 80 mg of depot-steroid is added to the local anesthetic with the first block, and 40 mg of depot-steroid is added with subsequent blocks.

Gentle aspiration is carried out to identify cerebrospinal fluid or blood. Although rare, inadvertent dural

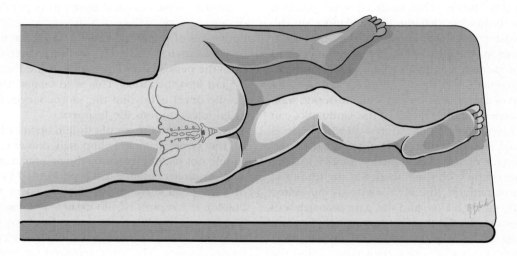

Figure 100-1.

puncture can occur, and careful observation for spinal fluid must be carried out. Aspiration of blood occurs more commonly. This can be due either to damage to veins during insertion of the needle into the caudal canal or, less commonly, to intravenous placement of the needle. Should the aspiration test be positive for either spinal fluid or blood, the needle is repositioned and the aspiration test repeated. If the test is negative, subsequent injections of 0.5-mL increments of local anesthetic are undertaken. Careful observation for signs of local anesthetic toxicity or subarachnoid spread of local anesthetic during the injection and after the procedure is indicated.

The spread of drugs injected into the sacral canal is dependent on the volume and speed of injection, the anatomic variations of the bony canal, and the age and height of the patient. The pregnant patient will require a significantly lower volume to achieve the same level of blockade compared with nongravid patients. Clinical experience has led to the use of smaller volumes of local anesthetic without sacrificing the clinical efficacy of caudal steroid epidural blocks. The use of smaller volumes of local anesthetic has markedly decreased the number of local anesthetic–related side effects.

Daily caudal epidural nerve blocks with local anesthetic, steroid, or both may be required to treat the previously mentioned acute painful conditions. Chronic conditions such as lumbar radiculopathy and diabetic polyneuropathy are treated on an every-other-day to once-a-week basis or as the clinical situation dictates. Our extensive clinical experience with caudal steroid epidural blocks suggests that using this technique on an every-other-day basis improves the outcome compared with once-a-week nerve blocks and should be considered when treating radiculopathy and other conditions amenable to treatment with caudal steroid epidural nerve blocks.

If selective neurolytic block of an individual sacral nerve is desired, incremental 0.1-mL injections of 6.5% phenol in glycerin or alcohol to a total volume of 1 mL may be used after first confirming the level of pain relief and potential side effects with local anesthetic blocks. If the caudal epidural route is chosen for administration of opioids, 4 to 5 mg of morphine sulfate formulated for epidural use is a reasonable initial dose. More lipid-soluble opioids such as fentanyl must be delivered by continuous infusion via a caudal catheter.

SIDE EFFECTS AND COMPLICATIONS

It is possible to insert the needle incorrectly when performing caudal epidural nerve block. The complication of placing the needle outside the sacral canal, resulting in the injection of air or drugs into the subcutaneous tissues, occurs with a greater frequency than when performing caudal block with the patient in the prone position unless careful identification of bony landmarks is carried out before needle placement. Should this complication occur, palpation of crepitus and bulging of tissues overlying the sacrum during injection will be observed. An increased resistance to injection accompanied by pain also is noted.

A second possible needle misplacement is when the needle tip is placed into the periosteum of the sacral canal. This needle misplacement is suggested by considerable pain on injection, a high resistance to injection, and the inability to inject more than a few milliliters of drug. A third possibility of needle malposition is partial placement of the needle bevel in the sacrococcygeal ligament. Again, there is significant resistance to injection as well as significant pain as the drugs are injected into the ligament. A fourth possible needle malposition is to force the point of the needle into the marrow cavity of the sacral vertebra, resulting in high blood levels of local anesthetic. This needle malposition is detected by the initial easy acceptance of a few milliliters of local anesthetic, followed by a rapid increase in resistance to injection as the noncompliant bony cavity fills with local anesthetic. Significant local anesthetic toxicity can occur as a result of this complication. The fifth and most serious needle malposition occurs when the needle is inserted through the sacrum or lateral to the coccyx into the pelvic cavity beyond. This can result in the needle entering both the rectum and birth canal, resulting in contamination of the needle. The repositioning of the contaminated needle into the sacral canal will carry with it the danger of infection. Although in competent hands this complication is exceedingly rare, some investigators believe that the use of caudal analgesia for obstetric applications once the fetal head has entered the pelvis is inadvisable because inadvertent injection of local anesthetic into the fetal head can occur, with resulting fetal demise.

The caudal epidural space is highly vascular; therefore, the possibility of intravascular uptake of local anesthetic is significant with this technique. Careful aspiration and incremental dosing of local anesthetic is important to allow early detection of local anesthetic toxicity. Careful observation of the patient during and after the procedure is mandatory. Use of smaller volumes of local anesthetic (i.e., the 5 to 10 mL recommended for therapeutic blocks) will help avoid this complication.

As mentioned earlier, the epidural venous plexus generally ends at S4 but may descend the entire length of the canal in some patients. Needle trauma to this plexus may result in bleeding, causing postprocedural pain. Subperiosteal injection of drugs also may result in bleeding and is associated with significant pain both during and after injection. Both these complications, as well as the incidence of ecchymosis at the injection site, can be reduced by the use of short, small-gauge needles. The incidence of significant neurologic deficit secondary to epidural hematoma after caudal block is exceedingly rare. Although uncommon, infection remains an ever-present possibility, especially in the immunocompromised AIDS or cancer patient. Early detection of infection is crucial to avoid potentially life-threatening sequelae.

Neurologic complications after caudal nerve block are rare. Usually these complications are associated with a preexisting neurologic lesion or with surgical or obstetric trauma rather than with the caudal block.

The application of local anesthetic and opioids to the sacral nerve roots results in an increased incidence of urinary retention. This side effect of caudal epidural nerve block occurs more commonly in elderly men and multiparous women and after inguinal and perineal surgery.

Overflow incontinence may occur in these patients if they are unable to void or if bladder catheterization is not used. It is advisable that all patients undergoing caudal epidural nerve block void before discharge from the pain center. Again, the use of smaller doses of local anesthetic will help avoid these bothersome complications without affecting the efficacy of caudal steroid epidural nerve blocks when treating painful conditions.

CLINICAL PEARLS

Most recently, pain management specialists have recognized the clinical advantages of the caudal over the lumbar approach to the epidural space when performing steroid epidural nerve blocks.

The advantages of the caudal approach include the following:

1. The ability to use smaller and sharper needles relative to the larger and blunter Hustead and Tuohy needles required for the lumbar approach to the epidural space (these smaller, sharper needles produce less procedure-related pain and produce less soft tissue trauma, which further decreases the amount of postprocedure pain the patient will experience compared with lumbar epidural blocks performed with Hustead and Tuohy needles).
2. These small needles (e.g., 25-gauge, 1½-inch) are significantly less expensive than the specialized Hustead or Tuohy needles.
3. The caudal approach to the epidural space can be used to deliver drugs to the epidural space in the presence of anticoagulation or coagulopathy, which is not possible via the lumbar route.
4. The efficacy of steroids administered into the epidural space via the caudal route is at least as beneficial as delivering the same drugs via the lumbar route.
5. The technique is less technically demanding than the lumbar approach.
6. The caudal approach to the epidural space is safer for patients who have undergone previous surgery of the lumbar spine.
7. Perhaps most important, there is essentially no risk for inadvertent dural puncture, which occurs with an incidence of 0.5% even when experienced clinicians perform lumbar epidural nerve block. This last advantage alone has led many contemporary pain management clinicians to abandon the lumbar epidural route in favor of the caudal approach when treating patients suffering from lumbar radiculopathy, spinal stenosis, and other diseases amenable to treatment with epidural steroids.

Lysis of Epidural Adhesions: Racz Technique

INDICATIONS

Lysis of epidural adhesions has been used to treat a variety of painful conditions. It is postulated that the common denominator in each of these pain syndromes is the compromise of spinal nerve roots as they traverse and exit the epidural space by adhesions and scarring. It is thought that these adhesions and scar tissue not only restrict the free movement of the nerve roots as they emerge from the spinal cord and travel through the intervertebral foramina but also result in dysfunction of epidural venous blood and lymph flow. This dysfunction results in additional nerve root edema, which further compromises the affected nerves. Inflammation may also play a part in the genesis of pain because these nerves are repeatedly traumatized each time the nerve is stretched against the adhesions and scar tissue.

Diagnostic categories thought to be amenable to treatment with lysis of epidural adhesions using the Racz technique include failed back surgery with associated perineural fibrosis, herniated disk, traumatic and nontraumatic vertebral body compression fracture, metastatic carcinoma to the spine and epidural space, multilevel degenerative arthritis, facet joint pain, epidural scarring following infection, and other pain syndromes of the spine that have their basis in epidural scarring and that have failed to respond to more conservative treatments.

CLINICALLY RELEVANT ANATOMY

Sacrum

The triangular sacrum consists of the five fused sacral vertebrae that are dorsally convex. The sacrum inserts in a wedgelike manner between the two iliac bones, articulating superiorly with the fifth lumbar vertebra and caudally with the coccyx. On the anterior concave surface, there are four pairs of unsealed anterior sacral foramina that allow passage of the anterior rami of the upper four sacral nerves. The posterior sacral foramina are smaller than their anterior counterparts. Leakage of drugs injected into the sacral canal is effectively prevented by the sacrospinal and multifidus muscles. The vestigial remnants of the inferior articular processes project downward on each side of the sacral hiatus. These bony projections are called the *sacral cornua* and represent important clinical landmarks when performing epidural lysis of adhesions via the caudal approach. Although there are gender- and race-determined differences in the shape of the sacrum, they are of little importance relative to the ultimate ability to successfully perform caudal epidural nerve block on a given patient.

Coccyx

The triangular coccyx is made up of three to five rudimental vertebrae. Its superior surface articulates with the inferior articular surface of the sacrum. The tip of the coccyx is an important clinical landmark when performing caudal epidural nerve block.

Sacral Hiatus

The sacral hiatus is formed by the incomplete midline fusion of the posterior elements of the lower portion of the S4 and the entire S5 vertebrae. This U-shaped space is covered posteriorly by the sacrococcygeal ligament, which is also an important clinical landmark when performing caudal epidural nerve block. Penetration of the sacrococcygeal ligament provides direct access to the epidural space of the sacral canal and allows the placement of a catheter for lysis of adhesions.

Sacral Canal

A continuation of the lumbar spinal canal, the sacral canal continues inferiorly to terminate at the sacral hiatus. The sacral canal contains the inferior termination of the dural sac, which ends between S1 and S3. The five sacral nerve roots and the coccygeal nerve all traverse the canal, as does the terminal filament of the spinal cord, the filum terminale. The anterior and posterior rami of the S1-S4 nerve roots exit from their respective anterior and posterior sacral foramina. The S5 roots and coccygeal nerves leave the sacral canal via the sacral hiatus. These nerves provide sensory and motor innervation to their respective dermatomes and myotomes. They also provide partial innervation to several pelvic organs, including the uterus, fallopian tubes, bladder, and prostate.

The sacral canal also contains the epidural venous plexus, which generally ends at S4 but may continue inferiorly. Most of these vessels are concentrated in the anterior portion of the canal. Both the dural sac and epidural vessels are susceptible to trauma by advancing needles or catheters cephalad into the sacral canal. The remainder of the sacral canal is filled with fat, which is subject to an age-related increase in its density.

TECHNIQUE

Intravenous access is obtained for administration of intravenous sedation during the injection of solutions via the catheter. Sedation during injection may be necessary because of pain produced by the distraction of the nerve roots as the solution lyses the perineural adhesions. After venous access is obtained, the patient is placed in the prone position with legs moderately abducted and heels inverted to relax the gluteus medius muscles and facilitate identification of the sacral hiatus.

Preparation of a wide area of skin with antiseptic solution is then carried out so that all the landmarks can be palpated aseptically. A fenestrated sterile drape is placed to avoid contamination of the palpating finger. The middle finger of the nondominant hand is placed over the sterile drape into the natal cleft with the fingertip at the tip of the coccyx. This maneuver allows easy confirmation of the sacral midline and is especially important when using the lateral position.

After careful identification of the midline, the area under the proximal interphalangeal joint is located. The middle finger is then moved cephalad to the area that was previously located under the proximal interphalan-

geal joint. This spot is palpated using a lateral rocking motion to identify the sacral cornua. The sacral hiatus is found at this level if the pain management physician's glove size is 7½ or 8. If the pain management physician's glove size is smaller, the location of the sacral hiatus will be just superior to the area located below the operator's proximal interphalangeal joint when the fingertip is at the tip of the coccyx. If the pain management physician's glove size is larger, the location of the sacral hiatus will be just inferior to the area located below the proximal interphalangeal joint when the fingertip is at the tip of the coccyx. Although there is normally significant anatomic variation of the sacrum and sacral hiatus, the spatial relationship between the tip of the coccyx and the location of the sacral hiatus remains amazingly constant.

After locating the sacral hiatus, a point 1 inch lateral and ½ inch below the sacral hiatus is identified, and the skin and subcutaneous tissues down to the sacrococcygeal ligament are infiltrated with local anesthetic. This lateral needle placement facilitates direction of the catheter toward the affected nerve roots. A 16-gauge, 3½-inch styletted needle suitable for catheter placement is inserted through the anesthetized area at a 45-degree angle toward the sacral hiatus. As the sacrococcygeal ligament is penetrated, a pop will be felt. If contact with the interior bony wall of the sacral canal occurs, the needle should be withdrawn slightly. This will disengage the needle tip from the periosteum. The needle is then advanced to about the level of the S2 foramen.

An air acceptance test is performed by the injection of 1 mL of air through the needle. There should be no bulging or crepitus of the tissues overlying the sacrum. The force required for injection should not exceed that necessary to overcome the resistance of the needle. If there is initial resistance to injection, the needle should be rotated slightly in case the needle is correctly placed in the canal but the needle bevel is occluded by the internal wall of the sacral canal. Any significant pain or sudden increase in resistance during injection suggests incorrect needle placement, and the pain management physician should stop injecting immediately and reassess the position of the needle. Needle position should be confirmed by fluoroscopy on both anteroposterior and lateral views (Fig. 101-1).

After negative aspiration for blood and cerebrospinal fluid, 10 mL of a water-soluble contrast medium such as iohexol or metrizamide is slowly injected under fluoroscopy. The pain specialist should check closely for any evidence of contrast medium in the epidural venous plexus, which would suggest intravenous placement of the needle or subdural or subarachnoid placement, which appears as a more concentrated centrally located density. As the epidural space fills with contrast medium,

Text continued on p. 461

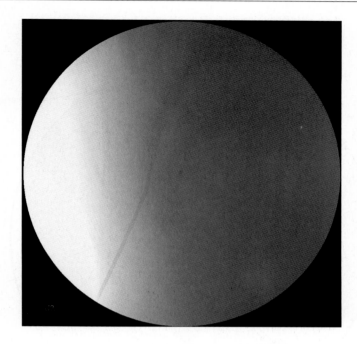

Figure 101-1.
Needle tip within the caudal canal.

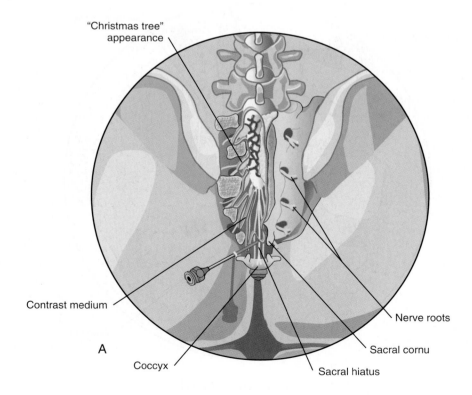

Figure 101-2.
(From Waldman SD: Interventional Pain Management, 2nd ed. Philadelphia, WB Saunders, 2001, p 436.)

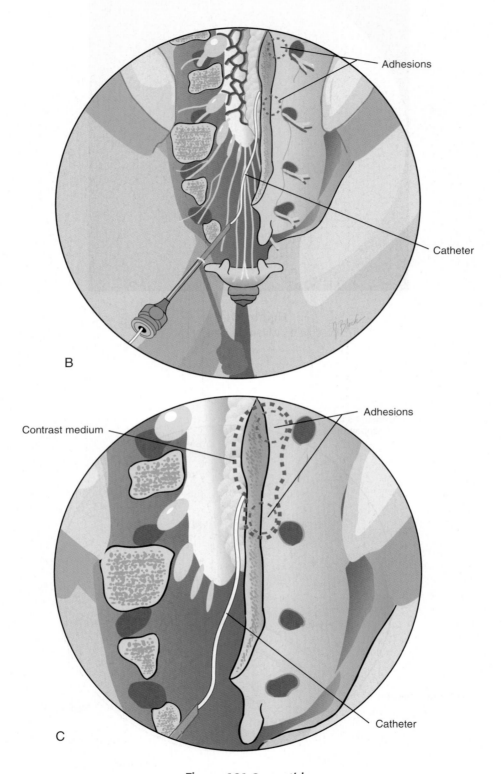

Figure 101-2, cont'd.

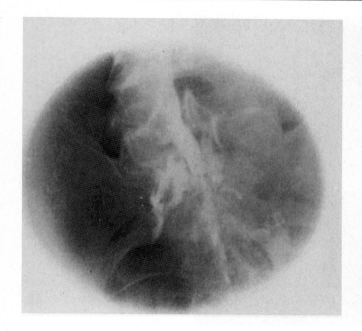

Figure 101-3.
Defects in the Christmas tree appearance. (From Waldman SD: Interventional Pain Management, 2nd ed. Philadelphia, WB Saunders, 2001, p 437.)

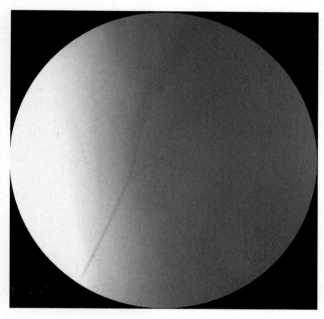

Figure 101-4.
Catheter placed through the needle into the caudal canal.

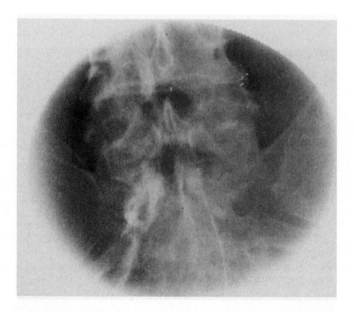

Figure 101-5.
The catheter is placed into the area of epidural adhesions. (From Waldman SD: Interventional Pain Management, 2nd ed. Philadelphia, WB Saunders, 2001, p 437.)

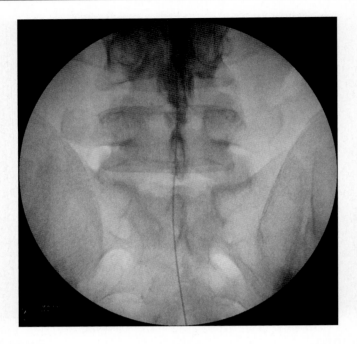

Figure 101-6.
Contrast medium is injected through the catheter.

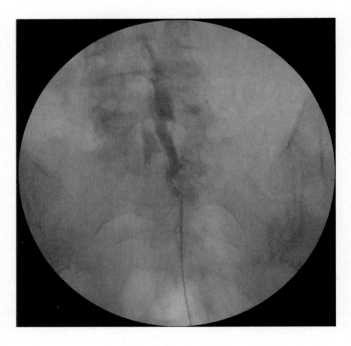

Figure 101-7.
Contrast medium spreading into the epidural space.

a Christmas tree shape will appear as the contrast medium surrounds the perineural structures (Fig. 101-2A). Defects in this classic Christmas tree appearance are indicative of epidural perineural adhesions (Fig. 101-3).

After confirming proper needle placement and ensuring that no blood or cerebrospinal fluid can be aspirated from the needle, 12 to 14 mL of 0.25% preservative-free bupivacaine and 40 mg of triamcinolone acetate are slowly injected through the epidural needle while observing the fluoroscope screen. The local anesthetic will force the contrast medium around the adhesions, further identifying affected nerve roots.

After the area of adhesions is identified on epidurogram, the bevel of the epidural needle is turned toward the ventrolateral aspect of the caudal canal of the affected side. This facilitates passage of the catheter toward the affected nerves and decreases the chance of catheter breakage or shearing. The use of a wire spiral catheter such as the Racz Tun-L-Kath epidural catheter further decreases the incidence of this complication.

The catheter is then passed through the needle into the area of adhesions (Figs. 101-4 and 101-5; see Fig. 101-2B). Multiple attempts may be required to obtain placement of the catheter into the adhesions. The Racz needle allows for the catheter to be withdrawn and repositioned and is preferred over the standard Crawford epidural needle.

After the catheter is placed within the area of adhesions, the catheter is aspirated for blood or cerebrospinal fluid. If the aspiration test is negative, an additional 7 to 10 mL of contrast medium is slowly injected through the catheter. This additional contrast medium should be seen spreading into the area of the adhesion (Figs. 101-6 and 101-7; see Fig. 101-2C). If the contrast material is observed to flow in satisfactory position, an additional 10 mL of 0.25% bupivacaine and 40 mg of triamcinolone are injected through the catheter to further lyse the remaining adhesions. Some investigators also recommend the addition of hyaluronidase to facilitate the spread of solutions injected. About 3% of the population may experience some degree of allergic reaction to this drug, and this fact may limit its use.

Thirty minutes after the second injection of bupivacaine, after negative aspiration, 10 mL of 10% saline is injected in small increments over 20 to 30 minutes. The hyperosmolar properties of the hypertonic saline further shrink the nerve root and help treat the perineural edema caused by the venous obstruction secondary to the adhesions. The injection of 10% saline into the epidural space is quite painful, and intravenous sedation may be required if the saline spreads beyond the area previously anesthetized by the 0.25% bupivacaine. This pain is transient in nature and is generally gone within 10 minutes. After the final injection of 10% saline, the catheter is carefully secured, and a sterile dressing is placed. Intravenous

cephalosporin antibiotics are recommended by Dr. Racz to prevent bacterial colonization of the catheter while it is in place.

This injection procedure of bupivacaine followed by 10% saline is repeated for 3 days. Epidurograms are repeated only if there is a question of catheter migration because the contrast medium can be irritating to the nerve roots and is quite expensive. The catheter is removed after the last injection. The patient is instructed to keep the area clean and dry and to call at the first sign of elevated temperature or infection.

SIDE EFFECTS AND COMPLICATIONS

Complications directly related to epidural lysis of adhesions are generally self-limited, although occasionally, even in the best of hands, severe complications can occur. Self-limited complications include pain at the injection site, transient back pain, ecchymosis and hematoma formation over the sacral hiatus, and unintended subdural or subarachnoid injection of local anesthetic. Severe complications of epidural lysis of adhesions include unintended subdural or subarachnoid injection of hypertonic saline, persistent sensory deficit in the lumbar and sacral dermatomes, paraparesis or paraplegia, persistent bowel or bladder dysfunction, sexual dysfunction, and infection. Although uncommon, unrecognized infection in the epidural space can result in paraplegia and death. Clinically, the signs and symptoms of epidural abscess present as a high temperature, spine pain, and progressive neurologic deficit. If epidural abscess is suspected, blood and urine cultures should be taken, antibiotics started, and emergent magnetic resonance imaging of the spine obtained to allow identification and drainage of any abscess formation before irreversible neurologic deficit.

CLINICAL PEARLS

Lysis of epidural adhesions is a straightforward technique that may provide pain relief in a carefully selected subset of patients. This technique should not be viewed as a starting point or stand-alone treatment in the continuum of pain management modalities but should be carefully integrated into a comprehensive pain management treatment plan. The identification of preexisting neurogenic bowel or bladder dysfunction by the use of urodynamics and careful neurologic examination before performing lysis of epidural adhesions is mandatory to avoid these preexisting problems being erroneously attributed to the procedure. Careful screening for preexisting sexual dysfunction also is indicated before lysis of epidural adhesions, for the same reason.

CHAPTER 102

Sacral Nerve Block: Transsacral Approach

CPT-2009 CODE	
Local Anesthetic/Steroid Single Nerve	64483
Local Anesthetic/Steroid Each	64484
Additional Nerve Neurolytic	64640

Relative Value Units	
Single	10
Multiple	14
Neurolytic	20

INDICATIONS

Sacral nerve block is useful in the evaluation and management of radicular and perineal pain that is believed to be subserved by the sacral nerves. The technique also is useful as an adjunct to provide surgical anesthesia when prior caudal or lumbar epidural block is spotty.

Sacral nerve block via the transsacral approach with local anesthetic can be used as a diagnostic tool when performing differential neural blockade on an anatomic basis in the evaluation of radicular or perineal pain. If destruction of the sacral nerves is being considered, this technique is useful as a prognostic indicator of the degree of motor and sensory impairment that the patient may experience. Sacral nerve block via the transsacral approach with local anesthetic may be used to palliate acute pain emergencies, including postoperative pain relief after transperineal and bladder surgery while waiting for pharmacologic methods to become effective in those patients who would not tolerate the sympathetic block associated with lumbar epidural anesthesia. Sacral nerve block via the transsacral approach with local anesthetic and steroid is occasionally used in the treatment of sacral root or perineal pain when the pain is believed to be secondary to inflammation or when entrapment of the sacral nerve is suspected. Sacral nerve block via the transsacral approach with local anesthetic and steroid also is indicated in the palliation of pain associated with diabetic neuropathy and is useful in the treatment of bladder dysfunction after injury to the cauda equina. Destruction of the sacral nerves via the transsacral approach is occasionally used in the palliation of persistent perineal pain secondary to invasive tumor or bladder dysfunction that is mediated by the sacral nerves and has not responded to more conservative measures (Fig. 102-1).

Because of the potential for hematogenous spread via Batson's plexus, local infection and sepsis represent absolute contraindications to the transsacral approach to sacral nerve block. Pilonidal cyst and congenital abnormalities of the dural sac and its contents also represent relative contraindications to the transsacral approach to sacral nerve block.

CLINICALLY RELEVANT ANATOMY

The convex dorsal surface of the sacrum has an irregular surface secondary to the fusing of the elements of the sacral vertebrae. Dorsally, there is a midline crest called the *median sacral crest*. Eight posterior sacral foramina allow the passage of four pairs of the primary posterior divisions of the sacral nerve roots. The posterior sacral foramina are smaller than their anterior counterparts. Leakage of drugs injected onto the sacral nerves through the posterior neural foramina is effectively prevented by the sacrospinal and multifidus muscles. The fifth sacral nerves exit the sacral canal via the sacral hiatus. The sacral nerves provide sensory innervation to the anorectal region and motor innervation to the external anal sphincter and levator ani muscles. The second through fourth sacral nerves provide the majority of visceral innervation to the bladder and urethra as well as the external genitalia.

TECHNIQUE

Sacral nerve block via the transsacral approach is carried out in either the prone or the lateral position. Each position has its own advantages and disadvantages. The prone position is easier for the pain management physician, but its use may be limited because of the patient's inability to rest comfortably on his or her abdomen or because of the

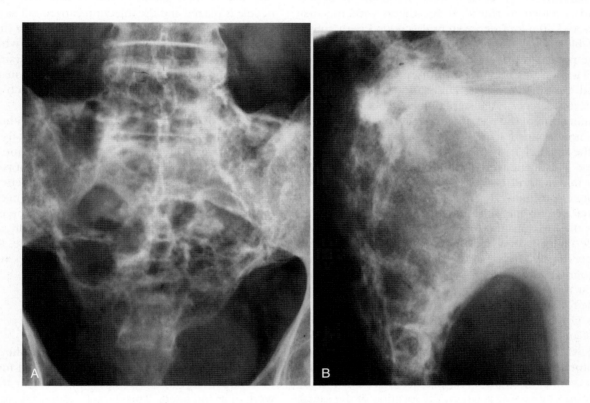

Figure 102-1.
Chordoma. Anteroposterior (**A**) and lateral (**B**) projections of the sacrum showing a large lytic lesion with a trabeculated appearance and well-defined margins. Mineralization of the tumor matrix is suggested. (From Grainger RG, Allison D: Grainger & Allison's Diagnostic Radiology: A Textbook of Medical Imaging, 3rd ed. Edinburgh, Churchill Livingstone, 1997, p 1685.)

presence of ostomy appliances such as colostomy and ileostomy bags. Furthermore, easy access to the airway is limited should problems occur while the patient is prone. The lateral position allows better access to the airway but is technically a more demanding approach. As with the caudal block, identification of the sacral hiatus is crucial to successfully perform sacral nerve block.

Before the procedure is begun, 18 mL of 1.0% preservative-free lidocaine is drawn into a sterile 20-mL syringe. When treating pain believed to be secondary to an inflammatory process, a total of 80 mg of depot-steroid is added to the local anesthetic with the first block, and 40 mg of depot-steroid is added with subsequent blocks.

The patient is placed in the prone position. Preparation of a wide area of skin with antiseptic solution is then carried out so that all the landmarks can be palpated aseptically. A fenestrated sterile drape is placed to avoid contamination of the palpating finger. The middle finger of the nondominant hand is placed over the sterile drape into the natal cleft, with the fingertip at the tip of the coccyx. This maneuver allows easy confirmation of the sacral midline and is especially important when using the lateral position.

After careful identification of the midline, the area under the proximal interphalangeal joint is located. The middle finger is then moved cephalad to the area that was previously located under the proximal interphalangeal joint. This spot is palpated using a lateral rocking motion to identify the sacral cornua. The sacral hiatus will be found at this level if the pain management physician's glove size is $7\frac{1}{2}$ or 8. If the pain management physician's glove size is smaller, the location of the sacral hiatus will be just superior to the area located below the operator's proximal interphalangeal joint when the fingertip is at the tip of the coccyx. If the pain management physician's glove size is larger, the location of the sacral hiatus will be just inferior to the area located below the proximal interphalangeal joint when the fingertip is at the tip of the coccyx.

Although there is normally significant anatomic variation of the sacrum and sacral hiatus, the spatial relationship between the tip of the coccyx and the location of the sacral hiatus remains amazingly constant.

The S5 sacral nerves can be blocked as they exit the sacral foramen. The sacral cornu are identified, and at a point just medial to their inferior border, a 25-gauge, $1\frac{1}{2}$-inch needle is advanced just deep to the cornu, and 2 to 3 mL of solution is injected (Fig. 102-2).

To block the S4 sacral nerves, after locating the sacral hiatus, a point $\frac{1}{2}$ inch superior and $\frac{1}{2}$ inch lateral to the sacral cornu is identified. A 25-gauge, $1\frac{1}{2}$-inch needle is inserted at this point and is advanced slowly perpendicular to the skin into the S4 posterior foramen. If bony contact is made, the needle is withdrawn into the sub-

cutaneous tissues and readvanced in a slightly more superior and lateral trajectory. This maneuver is repeated until the needle is walked off the posterior sacrum into the S4 foramen. The needle is advanced $\frac{1}{2}$ inch into the foramen (see Fig. 102-2). A paresthesia may be elicited, and the patient should be warned of such. Careful aspiration for blood and cerebrospinal fluid is carried out. If the aspiration test is negative, 2 to 3 mL of the solution is injected.

The S3 foramen is then identified about $\frac{1}{2}$ inch superior and $\frac{1}{2}$ inch lateral to the S4 foramen. Again, the needle is placed and the injection carried out as with the technique described for S4 nerve block. This maneuver is repeated for the S2 nerve, the foramen of which is $\frac{1}{2}$ inch superior and $\frac{1}{2}$ inch lateral to the S3 foramen. The maneuver is again repeated in an analogous manner for the S1 nerve, the foramen of which is $\frac{1}{2}$ inch superior and $\frac{1}{2}$ inch lateral to the S2 foramen.

If selective neurolytic block of an individual sacral nerve is desired, incremental 0.1-mL injections of 6.5% phenol in glycerin or alcohol to a total volume of 1 mL may be used after first confirming the level of pain relief and potential side effects with local anesthetic blocks. Because of the potential for spread of drugs injected via the transsacral approach onto other sacral nerves, incremental dosing is crucial to avoid accidentally applying neurolytic solution to the wrong sacral nerve. Radiofrequency lesioning or cryoneurolysis can help avoid this problem.

SIDE EFFECTS AND COMPLICATIONS

Sacral nerve block is a simple and safe procedure as long as there is an understanding of the potential for spread of solutions injected onto nerves for which the drugs were not intended. This fact is especially important when using neurolytic solutions.

This anatomic region is highly vascular; therefore, the possibility of intravascular uptake of local anesthetic is significant with this technique when multiple sacral nerves are blocked. Careful aspiration and incremental dosing of local anesthetic are important to allow early detection of local anesthetic toxicity. Careful observation of the patient during and after the procedure is mandatory.

The epidural venous plexus generally ends at S4 but may descend the entire length of the canal in some patients. Needle trauma to this plexus may result in bleeding, causing postprocedural pain. Subperiosteal injection of drugs also may result in bleeding and is associated with significant pain both during and after injection. Both these complications, as well as the incidence of ecchymosis at the injection site, can be reduced by the use of short, small-gauge needles. The incidence

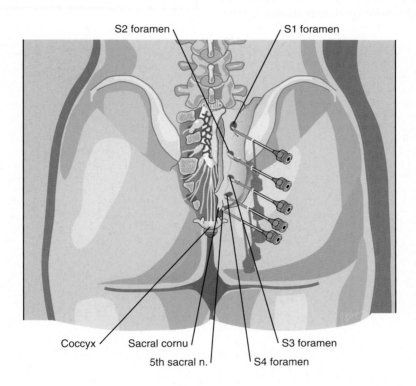

S2 foramen   S1 foramen

Coccyx   Sacral cornu   S3 foramen

5th sacral n.   S4 foramen

Figure 102-2.

of significant neurologic deficit secondary to hematoma after sacral block is exceedingly rare.

Although uncommon, infection remains an ever-present possibility, especially in the immunocompromised AIDS or cancer patient. Early detection of infection is crucial to avoid potentially life-threatening sequelae.

The application of local anesthetic to the sacral nerve roots results in an increased incidence of urinary bladder dysfunction. This side effect of sacral nerve block is seen more commonly in elderly men and multiparous women and after inguinal and perineal surgery. Overflow incontinence or dribbling may occur in this patient population if they are unable to void or bladder catheterization is not used. It is advisable that all patients undergoing sacral nerve block void before discharge from the pain center.

CLINICAL PEARLS

Sacral nerve block is a useful technique in the management of bladder dysfunction in patients who have sustained spinal cord or cauda equina injuries. Combined with pharmacologic modalities, it is possible to use sacral nerve blocks to help decrease bladder spasm and improve detrusor function to allow more complete bladder emptying and decrease the incidence of urinary tract infections. Incremental dosing of neurolytics and performing blockade of individual sacral nerves on sequential visits will help avoid complications.

CHAPTER 103

Hypogastric Plexus Block: Single-Needle Medial Paraspinous Technique

CPT-2009 CODE	
Unilateral	64517
Neurolytic	64681

Relative Value Units	
Unilateral	15
Neurolytic	25

INDICATIONS

Hypogastric plexus block with the single-needle technique is useful in the evaluation and management of sympathetically mediated pain of the pelvic viscera. Included in this category is pain secondary to malignancy, endometriosis, reflex sympathetic dystrophy, causalgia, proctalgia fugax, and radiation enteritis. Hypogastric plexus block also is useful in the palliation of tenesmus secondary to radiation therapy to the rectum. Hypogastric plexus block with local anesthetic can be used as a diagnostic tool when performing differential neural blockade on an anatomic basis in the evaluation of pelvic and rectal pain. If destruction of the hypogastric plexus is being considered, this technique is useful as a prognostic indicator of the degree of pain relief that the patient may experience. Hypogastric plexus block with local anesthetic also is useful in the treatment of acute herpes zoster and postherpetic neuralgia involving the sacral dermatomes. Destruction of the hypogastric plexus is indicated for the palliation of pain syndromes that have temporarily responded to blockade of the hypogastric plexus with local anesthetic and have not been controlled with more conservative measures.

CLINICALLY RELEVANT ANATOMY

In the context of neural blockade, the hypogastric plexus can simply be thought of as a continuation of the lumbar sympathetic chain that can be blocked in a manner analogous to lumbar sympathetic nerve block. The preganglionic fibers of the hypogastric plexus find their origin primarily in the lower thoracic and upper lumbar region of the spinal cord. These preganglionic fibers interface with the lumbar sympathetic chain via the white communicantes. Postganglionic fibers exit the lumbar sympathetic chain and, together with fibers from the parasympathetic sacral ganglion, make up the superior hypogastric plexus. The superior hypogastric plexus lies in front of L4 as a coalescence of fibers. As these fibers descend, at a level of L5, they begin to divide into the hypogastric nerves, following in close proximity the iliac vessels. As the hypogastric nerves continue their lateral and inferior course, they are accessible for neural blockade as they pass in front of the L5-S1 interspace. The hypogastric nerves pass downward from this point, following the concave curve of the sacrum and passing on each side of the rectum to form the inferior hypogastric plexus. These nerves continue their downward course along each side of the bladder to provide innervation to the pelvic viscera and vasculature.

TECHNIQUE
Blind and Fluoroscopic Guidance Technique

The patient is placed in the prone position with a pillow placed under the lower abdomen to gently flex the lumbar spine and maximize the space between the transverse process of L5 and the sacral alae. The L4-L5 interspace is located by identifying the iliac crests and finding the interspace at that level. The skin at this level is prepared with antiseptic solution. A point 6 cm from the midline at this level is identified, and the skin and subcutaneous tissues are anesthetized with 1.0% lidocaine. A 20-gauge, 13-cm needle is then inserted through the previously anesthetized area and directed about 30 degrees caudad and 30 degrees mesiad toward the anterolateral portion of the L5-S1 interspace.

If the transverse process of L5 is encountered, the needle is withdrawn and redirected slightly more caudad. If fluoroscopy is used, the needle should be placed just below the transverse process. If the vertebral body of L5 is encountered, the needle is withdrawn and redirected slightly more lateral until, in a manner analogous to lumbar sympathetic block, the needle is walked off the anterolateral aspect of the vertebral body. If fluoroscopy is used, a 5-mL glass syringe filled with preservative-free saline is then attached to the needle. The needle is then slowly advanced into the prevertebral space while maintaining constant pressure on the plunger of the syringe in a manner analogous to the loss-of-resistance technique used for identification of the epidural space. A pop and loss of resistance will be felt as the needle pierces the anterior fascia of the psoas muscle and enters the prevertebral space (Fig. 103-1). After careful aspiration for blood, cerebrospinal fluid, and urine, 10 mL of 1.0% preservative-free lidocaine is slowly injected in incremental doses while observing the patient closely for signs of local anesthetic toxicity. If fluoroscopy is used, 3 to 4 mL of water-soluble contrast medium is slowly injected after careful aspiration for blood, cerebrospinal fluid, and urine (Fig. 103-2). If there is believed to be an inflammatory component to the pain, the local anesthetic is combined with 80 mg of methylprednisolone and is injected in incremental doses. Subsequent daily nerve blocks are carried out in a similar manner, substituting 40 mg of methylprednisolone for the initial 80-mg dose. The needle is then removed, and an ice pack is placed on the injection site to decrease postblock bleeding and pain. If adequate pain relief is obtained, incremental doses of absolute alcohol or 6.5% aqueous phenol may be injected in a similar manner after it is ascertained that the patient is experiencing no untoward bowel or bladder effects from blockade of the hypogastric plexus.

Computed Tomography–Guided Technique

The patient is placed in the prone position on the computed tomography (CT) gantry with a pillow placed under the lower abdomen to gently flex the lumbar spine and maximize the space between the transverse process of L5 and the sacral alae. A CT scout film of the lumbar spine is taken, and the L4-L5 interspace is identified (Fig. 103-3). The skin overlying the L4-L5 interspace is prepared with antiseptic solution, and sterile drapes are placed. At a point about 6 cm from midline, the skin and subcutaneous tissues are anesthetized with 1% lidocaine using a 25-gauge, 3.8-cm needle. A 20-gauge, 13-cm needle is then inserted through the previously anesthetized area and directed about 30 degrees caudad and 30 degrees mesiad toward the anterolateral portion of the L5-S1 interspace (Fig. 103-4).

If the transverse process of L5 is encountered, the needle is withdrawn and redirected slightly more caudad. If the vertebral body of L5 is encountered, the needle is withdrawn and redirected slightly more lateral and walked off the anterolateral aspect of the vertebral body in a manner analogous to lumbar sympathetic block. A 5-mL glass syringe filled with preservative-free saline is then attached to the needle. The needle is then slowly advanced under CT guidance into the prevertebral space while maintaining constant pressure on the plunger of the syringe (Fig. 103-5). A pop and loss of resistance will be felt as the needle pierces the anterior fascia of the psoas muscle. After careful aspiration, 2 to 3 mL of water-soluble contrast medium is injected through the needle, and a CT scan is taken to confirm current retroperitoneal needle placement (Fig. 103-6). As the contrast is injected under CT guidance, it can be seen to outline the ipsilateral plexus and begin to spread contralaterally (Fig. 103-7). Because of contralateral spread of the contrast medium in the prevertebral space, it is often unnecessary to place a second needle, as is advocated by some pain specialists. A total volume of 10 mL of 1.0% preservative-free lidocaine is then injected in divided doses after careful aspiration for blood, cerebrospinal fluid, and urine. If adequate pain relief is obtained, incremental doses of absolute alcohol or 6.5% aqueous phenol may be injected in a similar manner after it is ascertained that the patient is experiencing no untoward bowel or bladder effects from blockade of the hypogastric plexus.

SIDE EFFECTS AND COMPLICATIONS

The proximity of the hypogastric nerves to the iliac vessels means that the potential for bleeding or inadvertent intravascular injection remains a distinct possibility. The relationship of the cauda equina and exiting nerve roots makes it imperative that this procedure be carried out only by those well versed in the regional anatomy and experienced in performing lumbar sympathetic nerve block. Given the proximity of the pelvic cavity, damage to the pelvic viscera including the ureters during hypogastric plexus block is a distinct possibility. The incidence of this complication is decreased when care is taken to place the needle just beyond the anterolateral margin of the L5-S1 interspace. Needle placement too medial may result in epidural, subdural, or subarachnoid injections or trauma to the intervertebral disk, spinal cord, and exiting nerve roots. Although uncommon, infection remains an ever-present possibility, especially in the immunocompromised cancer patient. Early detection of infection, including diskitis, is crucial to avoid potentially life-threatening sequelae.

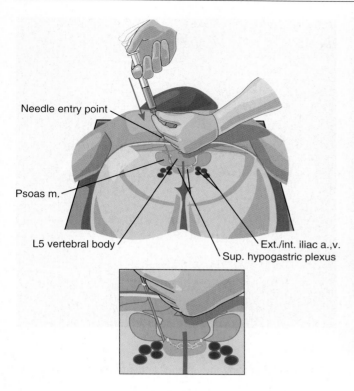

Needle entry point

Psoas m.

L5 vertebral body

Ext./int. iliac a.,v.

Sup. hypogastric plexus

Figure 103-1.

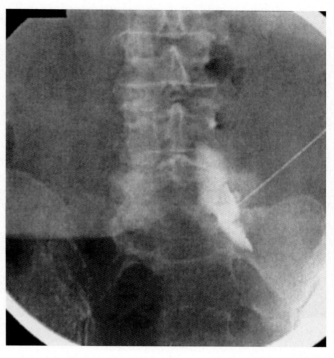

Figure 103-2.
(From Plancarte R, Amescua C, Patt RB: Sympathetic neurolytic blockade. In Patt RB [ed]: Cancer Pain. Philadelphia, JB Lippincott, 1993, pp 377-425.)

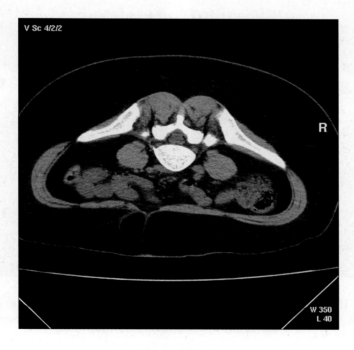

Figure 103-3.
CT scout film for hypogastric plexus.

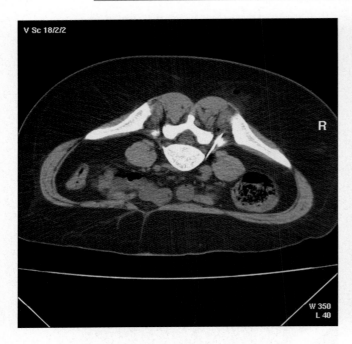

Figure 103-4.
CT of needle directed toward the anterolateral portion of the C5S1 interspace.

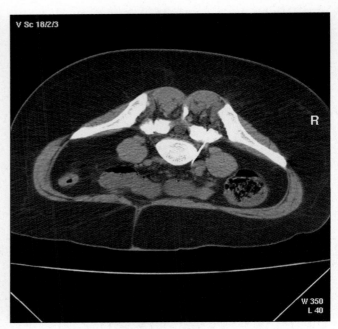

Figure 103-5.
CT of needle piercing the anterior fascia of the psoas muscle.

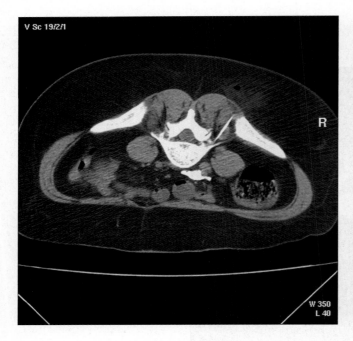

Figure 103-6.
CT of initial contrast medium injection.

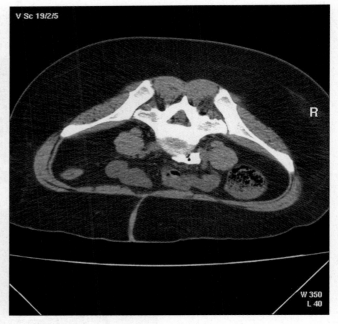

Figure 103-7.
CT of contrast medium beginning to flow to the contralateral sign.

CLINICAL PEARLS

Hypogastric plexus block is a simple technique that can produce dramatic relief for patients suffering from the previously mentioned pain complaints. Neurolytic block with small quantities of absolute alcohol or phenol in glycerin or by cryoneurolysis or radiofrequency lesioning has been shown to provide long-term relief for patients suffering from sympathetically maintained pain that has been relieved with local anesthetic. As with the celiac plexus and lumbar sympathetic nerve blocks, the proximity of the sympathetic nerves to vascular structures mandates repeated careful aspiration and vigilance for signs of unrecognized intravascular injection. CT guidance allows visualization of the major blood vessels and their relationship to the needle, which is a significant advance over blind or fluoroscopically guided techniques. As mentioned earlier, the proximity of the hypogastric plexus to the neuraxis and pelvic viscera makes careful attention to technique mandatory.

CHAPTER 104

Hypogastric Plexus Block: Classic Two-Needle Technique

CPT-2009 CODE	
Unilateral	64517
Neurolytic	64681

Relative Value Units	
Unilateral	15
Neurolytic	25

INDICATIONS

Hypogastric plexus block using the classic two-needle technique is reserved for patients in whom presacral tumor mass or adenopathy prevents contralateral spread of solutions injected through a single needle. This technique is useful in the evaluation and management of sympathetically mediated pain of the pelvic viscera. Included in this category is pain secondary to malignancy, endometriosis, reflex sympathetic dystrophy, causalgia, proctalgia fugax, and radiation enteritis. Hypogastric plexus block also is useful in the palliation of tenesmus secondary to radiation therapy to the rectum. Hypogastric plexus block with local anesthetic can be used as a diagnostic tool when performing differential neural blockade on an anatomic basis in the evaluation of pelvic and rectal pain. If destruction of the hypogastric plexus is being considered, this technique is useful as a prognostic indicator of the degree of pain relief that the patient may experience. Hypogastric plexus block with local anesthetic also is useful in the treatment of acute herpes zoster and postherpetic neuralgia involving the sacral dermatomes. Destruction of the hypogastric plexus is indicated for the palliation of pain syndromes that have temporarily responded to blockade of the hypogastric plexus with local anesthetic and have not been controlled with more conservative measures.

CLINICALLY RELEVANT ANATOMY

In the context of neural blockade, the hypogastric plexus can simply be thought of as a continuation of the lumbar sympathetic chain that can be blocked in a manner analogous to lumbar sympathetic nerve block. The preganglionic fibers of the hypogastric plexus find their origin primarily in the lower thoracic and upper lumbar region of the spinal cord. These preganglionic fibers interface with the lumbar sympathetic chain via the white communicantes. Postganglionic fibers exit the lumbar sympathetic chain and, together with fibers from the parasympathetic sacra ganglion, make up the superior hypogastric plexus. The superior hypogastric plexus lies in front of L4 as a coalescence of fibers. As these fibers descend, at a level of L5, they begin to divide into the hypogastric nerves following in close proximity the iliac vessels. As the hypogastric nerves continue their lateral and inferior course, they are accessible for neural blockade as they pass in front of the L5-S1 interspace. The hypogastric nerves pass downward from this point, following the concave curve of the sacrum and passing on each side of the rectum to form the inferior hypogastric plexus. These nerves continue their downward course along each side of the bladder to provide innervation to the pelvic viscera and vasculature.

TECHNIQUE

Blind and Fluoroscopic Technique

The patient is placed in the prone position with a pillow placed under the lower abdomen to gently flex the lumbar spine and maximize the space between the transverse process of L5 and the sacral alae. The L4-L5 interspace is located by identifying the iliac crests and finding the interspace at that level. The skin at this level is prepared with antiseptic solution. A point 6 cm from the midline at this level is identified, and the skin and subcutaneous tissues are anesthetized with 1.0% lidocaine. A 20-gauge, 13-cm needle is then inserted through the previously anesthetized area and directed about 30 degrees caudad and 30 degrees mesiad toward the antero-lateral portion of the L5-S1 interspace (Fig. 104-1). If the transverse process of L5 is encountered, the needle is withdrawn and redirected slightly more caudad. If the vertebral body of L5 is encountered, the needle is withdrawn and redirected slightly more lateral until, in a manner analogous to lumbar sympathetic block, the needle is walked off the anterolateral aspect of the vertebral body. Fluoroscopy may be useful in helping with accurate needle placement (Figs. 104-2 and 104-3).

A 5-mL glass syringe filled with preservative-free saline is then attached to the needle. The needle is then slowly advanced into the prevertebral space while maintaining constant pressure on the plunger of the syringe in a manner analogous to the loss-of-resistance technique used for identification of the epidural space. A pop and loss of resistance will be felt as the needle pierces the anterior fascia of the psoas muscle and enters the prevertebral space. A contralateral needle is then inserted in a similar manner, using the trajectory and depth of the first needle as a guide (see Figs. 104-1 to 104-3).

After careful aspiration for blood, cerebrospinal fluid, and urine, 5mL of 1.0% preservative-free lidocaine is slowly injected in incremental doses while observing the patient closely for signs of local anesthetic toxicity. If fluoroscopic guidance is being used, after careful aspiration for blood, cerebrospinal fluid, and urine, 5 mL of water-soluble contrast is slowly injected in incremental doses with continuous fluoroscopic guidance to observe the flow of contrast (Figs. 104-4 and 104-5). If there is believed to be an inflammatory component to the pain, the local anesthetic is combined with 80 mg of methylprednisolone and is injected in incremental doses. Subsequent daily nerve blocks are carried out in a similar manner, substituting 40 mg of methylprednisolone for the initial 80-mg dose. Each needle is then removed, and an ice pack is placed on the injection site to decrease postblock bleeding and pain. If adequate pain relief is obtained, incremental doses of absolute alcohol or 6.5% aqueous phenol may be injected in a similar manner after it is ascertained that the patient is experiencing no untoward bowel or bladder effects from blockade of the hypogastric plexus.

Computed Tomography–Guided Technique

The patient is placed in the prone position on the computed tomography (CT) gantry with a pillow placed under the lower abdomen to gently flex the lumbar spine and maximize the space between the transverse process of L5 and the sacral alae. A CT scout film of the lumbar spine is taken, and the L4-L5 interspace is identified. The skin overlying the L4-L5 interspace is prepared with antiseptic solution, and sterile drapes are placed. At a point about 6 cm from midline, the skin and subcutaneous

tissues are anesthetized with 1% lidocaine using a 25-gauge, 3.8-cm needle.

A 20-gauge, 13-cm needle is then inserted through the previously anesthetized area and directed about 30 degrees caudad and 30 degrees mesiad toward the antero-lateral portion of the L5-S1 interspace. If the transverse process of L5 is encountered, the needle is withdrawn and redirected slightly more caudad. If the vertebral body of L5 is encountered, the needle is withdrawn and redirected slightly more lateral and walked off the anterolateral aspect of the vertebral body in a manner analogous to lumbar sympathetic block. A 5-mL glass syringe filled with preservative-free saline is then attached to the needle. The needle is then slowly advanced into the prevertebral space while maintaining constant pressure on the plunger of the syringe. A pop and loss of resistance will be felt as the needle pierces the anterior fascia of the psoas muscle.

After careful aspiration, 2 to 3 mL of water-soluble contrast medium is injected through the needle, and a CT scan is taken to confirm current retroperitoneal needle placement. If no contralateral spread of the contrast medium in the prevertebral space is observed, a contralateral needle is inserted in a similar manner using the trajectory and depth of the first needle as a guide. A total volume of 5 mL of 1.0% preservative-free lidocaine is then injected in divided doses after careful aspiration for blood, cerebrospinal fluid, and urine. If adequate pain relief is obtained, incremental doses of absolute alcohol or 6.5% aqueous phenol may be injected in a similar manner after it is ascertained that the patient is experiencing no untoward bowel or bladder effects from blockade of the hypogastric plexus. Each needle is then removed, and an ice pack is placed on the injection site to decrease postblock bleeding and pain. If adequate pain relief is obtained, incremental doses of absolute alcohol or 6.5% aqueous phenol may be injected in a similar manner after it is ascertained that the patient is experiencing no untoward bowel or bladder effects from blockade of the hypogastric plexus.

SIDE EFFECTS AND COMPLICATIONS

The proximity of the hypogastric nerves to the iliac vessels means that the potential for bleeding or inadvertent intravascular injection remains a distinct possibility. The relationship of the cauda equina and exiting nerve roots makes it imperative that this procedure be carried out only by those well versed in the regional anatomy and experienced in performing lumbar sympathetic nerve block. Given the proximity of the pelvic cavity, damage to the pelvic viscera including the ureters during hypogastric plexus block is a distinct possibility. The incidence of this complication is decreased when care is taken to place the needle just beyond the anterolateral

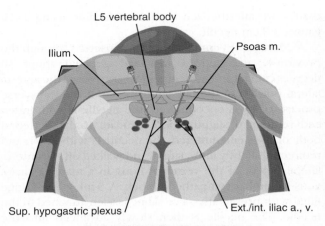

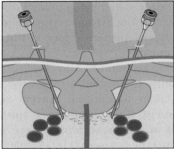

Figure 104-1.

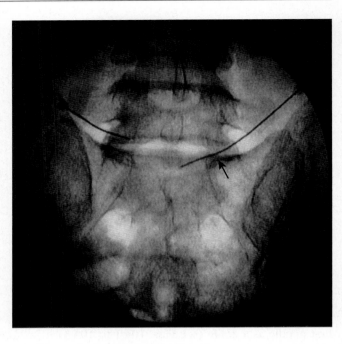

Figure 104-2.

Final needle placement is shown in the anteroposterior view. The left needle is in classic position for superior hypogastric plexus block. Blood was aspirated when the needle tip on the right side was at the point marked with the *arrow*. The right needle was advanced more medially until no blood aspirated. (From Stevens DS, Balatbat GR, Lee FMK: Coaxial imaging technique for superior hypogastric plexus block. Reg Anesth Pain Med 25:643-647, 2000, Fig 3.)

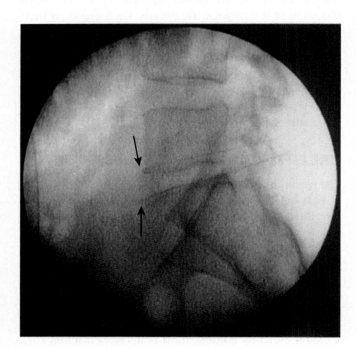

Figure 104-3.

Final needle position is shown in the lateral view. *Arrows* indicate tips of needles. The upper needle is on the left side, and the lower needle is on the right side. Both needles are located just anterior to the most anterior portion of the adjacent vertebra, which is classic position for needle placement for SHP block. (From Stevens DS, Balatbat GR, Lee FMK: Coaxial imaging technique for superior hypogastric plexus block. Reg Anesth Pain Med 25:643-647, 2000, Fig 4.)

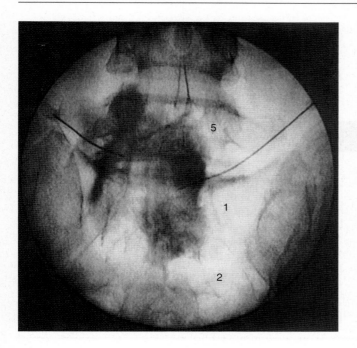

Figure 104-4.
Injection of contrast has been done on each side and is shown in the anteroposterior view. Vertebrae are marked 5 (L5), 1 (S1), and 2 (S2). The left side shows the classic pattern of contrast spread, covering all of L5 and S1 along the lateral portion of each vertebra. The right side shows coverage of the lower portion of L5, all of S1, and part of S2, but the contrast flows more medially than is usually seen. (From Stevens DS, Balatbat GR, Lee FMK: Coaxial imaging technique for superior hypogastric plexus block. Reg Anesth Pain Med 25:643-647, 2000, Fig 5.)

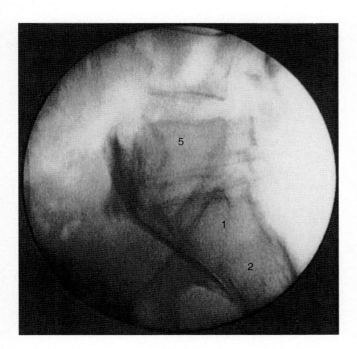

Figure 104-5.
Injection of contrast has been done on each side and is shown in the lateral view. Vertebrae are marked 5 (L5), 1 (S1), and 2 (S2). Contrast is seen to flow along the anterior aspects of L5, S1, and the upper portion of S2. The classic pattern of contrast spread for superior hypogastric plexus block is along the anterior aspect of L5 and S1, in the location of contrast shown in this figure. (From Stevens DS, Balatbat GR, Lee FMK: Coaxial imaging technique for superior hypogastric plexus block. Reg Anesth Pain Med 25:643-647, 2000, Fig 6.)

margin of the L5-S1 interspace. Needle placement too medial may result in epidural, subdural, or subarachnoid injections or trauma to the intervertebral disk, spinal cord, and exiting nerve roots. Although uncommon, infection remains an ever-present possibility, especially in the immunocompromised cancer patient. Early detection of infection, including diskitis, is crucial to avoid potentially life-threatening sequelae.

CLINICAL PEARLS

Hypogastric plexus block is a simple technique that can produce dramatic relief for patients suffering from the previously mentioned pain complaints. Neurolytic block with small quantities of absolute alcohol and phenol in glycerin or by cryoneurolysis or radiofrequency lesioning has been shown to provide long-term relief for patients suffering from sympathetically maintained pain that has been relieved with local anesthetic. As with the celiac plexus and lumbar sympathetic nerve blocks, the proximity of the sympathetic nerves to vascular structures mandates repeated careful aspiration and vigilance for signs of unrecognized intravascular injection. CT guidance allows visualization of the major blood vessels and their relationship to the needle, which is a significant advance over blind or fluoroscopically guided techniques. Furthermore, confirmation of contralateral spread of contrast medium allows the pain specialist to avoid the increased pain and risk of placement of a second needle. As mentioned earlier, the proximity of the hypogastric plexus to the neuraxis and pelvic viscera makes careful attention to technique mandatory.

CHAPTER 105

Hypogastric Plexus Block: Single-Needle Transdiscal Technique

CPT-2009 CODE	
Unilateral	64517
Neurolytic	64681

Relative Value Units	
Unilateral	15
Neurolytic	25

INDICATIONS

Hypogastric plexus block with the single-needle transdiscal technique is useful in the evaluation and management of sympathetically mediated pain of the pelvic viscera. Included in this category is pain secondary to malignancy, endometriosis, reflex sympathetic dystrophy, causalgia, proctalgia fugax, and radiation enteritis. Hypogastric plexus block also is useful in the palliation of tenesmus secondary to radiation therapy to the rectum. Hypogastric plexus block with local anesthetic can be used as a diagnostic tool when performing differential neural blockade on an anatomic basis in the evaluation of pelvic and rectal pain.

If destruction of the hypogastric plexus is being considered, this technique is useful as a prognostic indicator of the degree of pain relief that the patient may experience. Hypogastric plexus block with local anesthetic also is useful in the treatment of acute herpes zoster and postherpetic neuralgia involving the sacral dermatomes. Destruction of the hypogastric plexus is indicated for the palliation of pain syndromes that have temporarily responded to blockade of the hypogastric plexus with local anesthetic and have not been controlled with more conservative measures.

CLINICALLY RELEVANT ANATOMY

In the context of neural blockade, the hypogastric plexus can simply be thought of as a continuation of the lumbar sympathetic chain that can be blocked in a manner analogous to lumbar sympathetic nerve block. The preganglionic fibers of the hypogastric plexus find their origin primarily in the lower thoracic and upper lumbar region of the spinal cord. These preganglionic fibers interface with the lumbar sympathetic chain via the white communicantes.

Postganglionic fibers exit the lumbar sympathetic chain and, together with fibers from the parasympathetic sacral ganglion, make up the superior hypogastric plexus. The superior hypogastric plexus lies in front of L4 as a coalescence of fibers. As these fibers descend, at a level of L5, they begin to divide into the hypogastric nerves, following in close proximity the iliac vessels. As the hypogastric nerves continue their lateral and inferior course, they are accessible for neural blockade as they pass in front of the L5-S1 interspace. The hypogastric nerves pass downward from this point, following the concave curve of the sacrum and passing on each side of the rectum to form the inferior hypogastric plexus. These nerves continue their downward course along each side of the bladder to provide innervation to the pelvic viscera and vasculature.

TECHNIQUE
Fluoroscopic Technique

The patient is placed in the prone position with a pillow placed under the lower abdomen to gently flex the lumbar spine and maximize the space between the transverse process of L5 and the sacral alae. The L5-S1 interspace is located by fluoroscopy. The skin at this level is prepared with antiseptic solution. A point 6 cm from the midline at this level is identified, and the skin and subcutaneous tissues are anesthetized with 1.0% lidocaine. The fluoroscopy tube is then placed in the oblique position and angled 15 to 20 degrees caudad to align the inferior end plates of the adjacent vertebra and more clearly identify the disk space. A 20-gauge, 13-cm needle is then inserted through the previously anesthetized area and directed under fluoroscopic guidance in a slightly cephalad trajectory until it enters the disk (Figs. 105-1 and 105-2). If the transverse process of L5 is encountered, the needle is

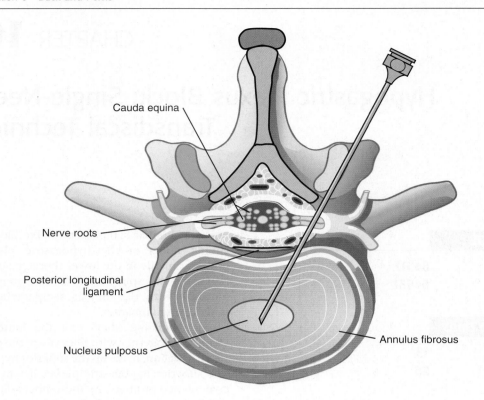

Cauda equina

Nerve roots

Posterior longitudinal ligament

Nucleus pulposus

Annulus fibrosus

Figure 105-1.

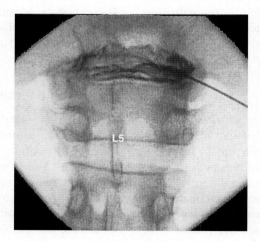

L5

Figure 105-2.
(From Raj PP, Waldman SD, Erdine S, Lou L, Staats PS: Radiographic Imaging for Regional Anesthesia and Pain Management, 1st ed. New York, Churchill Livingstone, 2002, p 235.)

withdrawn and redirected slightly more caudad. After the entry into the disk space has been confirmed on both posterolateral and lateral views, use 1 mL of contrast medium suitable for myelography to further confirm intradiscal placement of the needle tip.

A 5-mL glass syringe filled with preservative-free saline is then attached to the needle. The needle is then slowly advanced through the disk into the prevertebral space while maintaining constant pressure on the plunger of the syringe in a manner analogous to the loss-of-resistance technique used for identification of the epidural space. A pop and loss of resistance will be felt as the needle pierces the anterior annulus of the disk and enters the prevertebral space (Figs. 105-3 and 105-4).

After careful aspiration for blood, cerebrospinal fluid, and urine, 3 mL of water-soluble contrast medium is slowly injected in incremental doses under continuous fluoroscopic guidance to confirm bilateral spread of contrast in the prevertebral space. After proper needle placement is confirmed and aspiration for blood, cerebrospinal fluid, and urine is carried out, 5 to 7 mL of 1% preservative free lidocaine is injected through the needle in small incremental doses while observing the patient closely for signs of local anesthetic toxicity. If there is believed to be an inflammatory component to the pain, the local anesthetic is combined with 80 mg of methylprednisolone and is injected in incremental doses. Subsequent daily nerve blocks are carried out in a similar manner, substituting 40 mg of methylprednisolone for the initial 80-mg dose. The needle is then removed, and an ice pack is placed on the injection site to decrease postblock bleeding and pain. If adequate pain relief is obtained, incremental doses of absolute alcohol or 6.5% aqueous phenol may be injected in a similar manner after it is ascertained that the patient is experiencing no untoward bowel or bladder effects from blockade of the hypogastric plexus.

Computed Tomography–Guided Technique

The patient is placed in the prone position on the computed tomography (CT) gantry with a pillow placed under the lower abdomen to gently flex the lumbar spine and maximize the space between the transverse process of L5 and the sacral alae. A CT scout film of the lumbar spine is taken, and the L5-S1 interspace is located by fluoroscopy. The skin at this level is prepared with antiseptic solution. A point 6 cm from the midline at this level is identified, and the skin and subcutaneous tissues are anesthetized with 1.0% lidocaine. A 20-gauge, 13-cm needle is then inserted through the previously anesthetized area and directed under CT guidance in a slightly cephalad trajectory until it enters the disk. If the transverse process of L5 is encountered, the needle is withdrawn and redirected slightly more caudad. After the

entry into the disk space has been confirmed on CT scan, use 1 mL of contrast medium suitable for myelography to further confirm intradiscal placement of the needle tip (Figs. 105-5 and 105-6).

A 5-mL glass syringe filled with preservative-free saline is then attached to the needle. The needle is then slowly advanced through the disk into the prevertebral space while maintaining constant pressure on the plunger of the syringe in a manner analogous to the loss-of-resistance technique used for identification of the epidural space. A pop and loss of resistance will be felt as the needle pierces the anterior annulus of the disk and enters the prevertebral space. After careful aspiration for blood, cerebrospinal fluid, and urine, 3 mL of water-soluble contrast medium is slowly injected in incremental doses, and a CT scan of the prevertebral area is obtained to confirm bilateral spread of contrast in the prevertebral space. After proper needle placement is confirmed and aspiration for blood, cerebrospinal fluid, and urine is carried out, 5 to 7 mL of 1% preservative-free lidocaine is injected through the needle in small incremental doses while observing the patient closely for signs of local anesthetic toxicity. If there is believed to be an inflammatory component to the pain, the local anesthetic is combined with 80 mg of methylprednisolone and is injected in incremental doses. Subsequent daily nerve blocks are carried out in a similar manner, substituting 40 mg of methylprednisolone for the initial 80-mg dose. The needle is then removed, and an ice pack is placed on the injection site to decrease postblock bleeding and pain.

If adequate pain relief is obtained, incremental doses of absolute alcohol or 6.5% aqueous phenol may be injected in a similar manner after it is ascertained that the patient is experiencing no untoward bowel or bladder effects from blockade of the hypogastric plexus.

SIDE EFFECTS AND COMPLICATIONS

The proximity of the hypogastric nerves to the iliac vessels means that the potential for bleeding or inadvertent intravascular injection remains a distinct possibility. The relationship of the cauda equina and exiting nerve roots makes it imperative that this procedure be carried out only by those well versed in the regional anatomy and experienced in performing lumbar sympathetic nerve block. Given the proximity of the pelvic cavity, damage to the pelvic viscera including the ureters during hypogastric plexus block is a distinct possibility. The incidence of this complication is decreased when care is taken to place the needle just beyond the anterolateral margin of the L5-S1 interspace. Needle placement too medial may result in epidural, subdural, or subarachnoid injections or trauma to the intervertebral disk, spinal

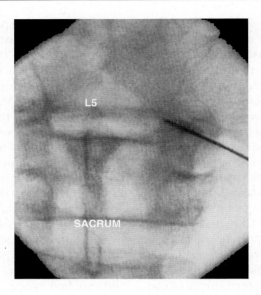

Figure 105-3.
(From Raj PP, Waldman SD, Erdine S, Lou L, Staats PS: Radiographic
Imaging for Regional Anesthesia and Pain Management, 1st ed. New York,
Churchill Livingstone, 2002, p 235.)

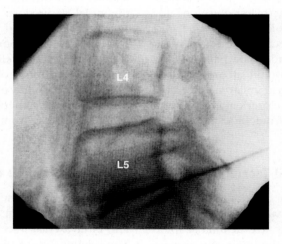

Figure 105-4.
(From Raj PP, Waldman SD, Erdine S, Lou L, Staats PS: Radiographic
Imaging for Regional Anesthesia and Pain Management, 1st ed. New York,
Churchill Livingstone, 2002, p 235.)

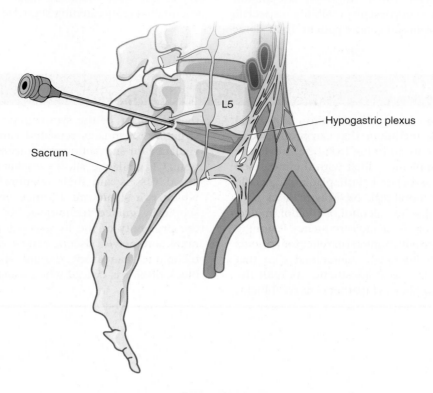

Figure 105-5.

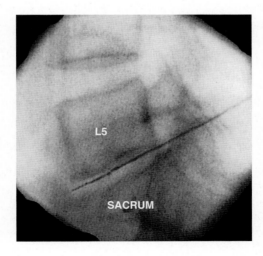

Figure 105-6.
(From Raj PP, Waldman SD, Erdine S, Lou L, Staats PS: Radiographic Imaging for Regional Anesthesia and Pain Management, 1st ed. New York, Churchill Livingstone, 2002, p 235.)

cord, and exiting nerve roots. Although uncommon, infection remains an ever-present possibility, especially in the immunocompromised cancer patient. Early detection of infection, including diskitis, is crucial to avoid potentially life-threatening sequelae.

CLINICAL PEARLS

Hypogastric plexus block using the transdiscal approach is a simple technique that can produce dramatic relief for patients suffering from the previously mentioned pain complaints, albeit with the increased risks for infection associated with placing a needle through the intervertebral disk. Neurolytic block with small quantities of absolute alcohol or phenol in glycerin or by cryoneurolysis or radiofrequency lesioning has been shown to provide long-term relief for patients suffering from sympathetically maintained pain that has been relieved with local anesthetic. As with the celiac plexus and lumbar sympathetic nerve blocks, the proximity of the sympathetic nerves to vascular structures mandates repeated careful aspiration and vigilance for signs of unrecognized intravascular injection. CT guidance allows visualization of the major blood vessels and their relationship to the needle, which is a significant advance over blind or fluoroscopically guided techniques. As mentioned earlier, the proximity of the hypogastric plexus to the neuraxis and pelvic viscera makes careful attention to technique mandatory. Careful observation for postblock diskitis is crucial when using this technique.

CHAPTER 106

Ganglion of Walther (Impar) Block: Prone Technique

CPT-2009 CODE	
Unilateral	64517
Neurolytic	64681

Relative Value Units	
Unilateral	15
Neurolytic	25

INDICATIONS

Ganglion of Walther (also called the *ganglion impar*) block is useful in the evaluation and management of sympathetically mediated pain of the perineum, rectum, and genitalia. This technique has been used primarily in the treatment of pain secondary to malignancy, although theoretical applications for benign pain syndromes, including pain secondary to endometriosis, reflex sympathetic dystrophy, causalgia, proctalgia fugax, and radiation enteritis, can be considered if the pain has failed to respond to more conservative therapies. Ganglion of Walther block with local anesthetic can be used as a diagnostic tool when performing differential neural blockade on an anatomic basis in the evaluation of pelvic and rectal pain. If destruction of the ganglion of Walther is being considered, this technique is useful as a prognostic indicator of the degree of pain relief that the patient may experience. Destruction of the ganglion of Walther is indicated for the palliation of pain syndromes that have temporarily responded to blockade of the ganglion with local anesthetic and have not been controlled with more conservative measures.

CLINICALLY RELEVANT ANATOMY

In the context of neural blockade, the ganglion of Walther can simply be thought of as the terminal coalescence of the sympathetic chain. The ganglion of Walther lies in front of the sacrococcygeal junction and is amenable to blockade at this level. The ganglion receives fibers from the lumbar and sacral portions of the sympathetic and parasympathetic nervous system and provides sympathetic innervation to portions of the pelvic viscera and genitalia.

TECHNIQUE

Blind and Fluoroscopic Technique

The patient is placed in the jackknife position to facilitate access to the inferior margin of the gluteal cleft. The midline is identified, and the skin just below the tip of the coccyx that overlies the anococcygeal ligament is prepared with antiseptic solution. The skin and subcutaneous tissues at this point are anesthetized with 1.0% lidocaine. A 3½-inch spinal needle is then bent at a point 1 inch from its hub to a 30-degree angle to allow placement of the needle tip in proximity to the anterior aspect of the sacrococcygeal junction. Fluoroscopy may aid in placement of the needle if difficulty is encountered. The needle may be bent again at a point 2 inches from the hub to accommodate those patients with an exaggerated coccygeal curve to allow placement of the needle tip to rest against the sacrococcygeal junction.

The bent needle is then placed through the previously anesthetized area and is advanced until the needle tip impinges on the anterior surface of the sacrococcygeal junction (Figs. 106-1 and 106-2). After careful aspiration for blood, cerebrospinal fluid, and urine, 3 mL of 1.0% preservative-free lidocaine is slowly injected in incremental doses. If fluoroscopy is used, 2 mL of water-soluble iodinated contrast is injected to confirm needle position (Figs. 106-3 and 106-4). If there is believed to be an inflammatory component to the pain, the local anesthetic is combined with 80 mg of methylprednisolone and is injected in incremental doses. Subsequent daily nerve blocks are carried out in a similar manner, substituting 40 mg of methylprednisolone for the initial 80-mg dose. The needle is then removed, and an ice pack is placed on the injection site to decrease postblock bleeding and pain.

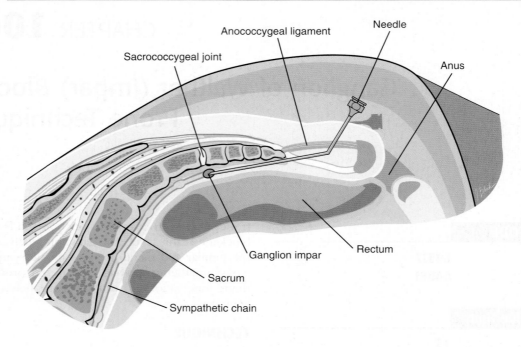

Figure 106-1.

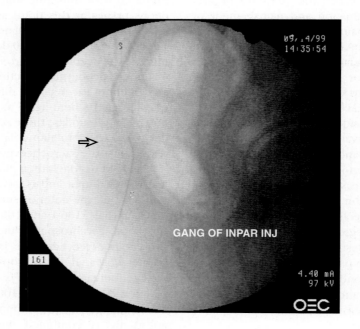

Figure 106-2.
Needle tip against anterior surface of the sacrococcygeal junction.

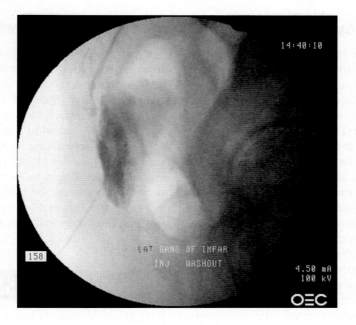

Figure 106-3.
Lateral view of contrast medium anterior to coccyx and sacrum.

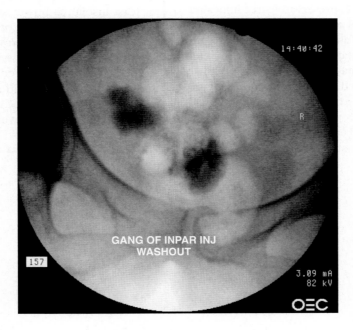

Figure 106-4.
PA view of contrast medium anterior to the coccyx and sacrum.

Computed Tomography–Guided Technique

The patient is placed in the prone position on the computed tomography (CT) gantry with a pillow placed under the pelvis to facilitate access to the inferior gluteal cleft. A CT scout film is taken, and the sacrococcygeal junction and the tip of the coccyx are identified. The midline is also identified, and the skin just below the tip of the coccyx that overlies the anococcygeal ligament is prepared with antiseptic solution. The skin and subcutaneous tissues at this point are anesthetized with 1.0% lidocaine. A 3½-inch spinal needle is then bent at a point 1 inch from its hub to a 30-degree angle to allow placement of the needle tip in proximity to the anterior aspect of the sacrococcygeal junction (see Fig. 106-2). The needle may be bent again at a point 2 inches from the hub to accommodate patients with an exaggerated coccygeal curve to allow the needle tip to rest against the anterior sacrococcygeal junction.

The needle is then placed through the previously anesthetized area and is advanced until the needle tip impinges on the anterior surface of the sacrococcygeal junction. After careful aspiration for blood, cerebrospinal fluid, and urine, 2 to 3 mL of water-soluble contrast medium is injected through the needle, and a CT scan is taken to confirm the spread of contrast medium just anterior to the sacrococcygeal junction (see Figs. 106-3 and 106-4). After correct needle placement is confirmed, a total volume of 3 mL of 1.0% preservative-free lidocaine is injected in divided doses after careful aspiration for blood, cerebrospinal fluid, and urine. If adequate pain relief is obtained, incremental doses of absolute alcohol or 6.5% aqueous phenol may be injected in a similar manner after it is ascertained that the patient is experiencing no untoward bowel or bladder effects from local anesthetic blockade of the ganglion of Walther. The needle is then removed, and an ice pack is placed on the injection site to decrease postblock bleeding and pain.

SIDE EFFECTS AND COMPLICATIONS

The proximity of the ganglion of Walther to the rectum makes perforation and tracking of contaminants back through the needle track during needle removal a distinct possibility. Infection and fistula formation, especially in those patients who are immunocompromised or have received radiation therapy to the perineum, can represent a devastating and potentially life-threatening complication to this block. The relationship of the cauda equina and exiting sacral nerve roots makes it imperative that this procedure be carried out only by those well versed in the regional anatomy and experienced in performing interventional pain management techniques.

CLINICAL PEARLS

Ganglion of Walther block is a straightforward technique that can produce dramatic relief for patients suffering from the previously mentioned pain complaints. Given the localized nature of this neural structure when compared with the superior hypogastric plexus, neurolytic block with small quantities of absolute alcohol or phenol in glycerin or by cryoneurolysis or radiofrequency lesioning may be a reasonable choice over superior hypogastric plexus block, at least insofar as bowel and bladder dysfunction is concerned. Destruction of the ganglion of Walther has been shown to provide long-term relief for patients suffering from sympathetically maintained pain that has been relieved with local anesthetic. CT guidance allows visualization of the regional anatomy and the relationship of the rectum to the needle. This is a significant advance over blind or fluoroscopically guided techniques.

CHAPTER 107

Ganglion of Walther (Impar) Block:
Trans-Coccygeal Technique

CPT-2009 CODE	
Unilateral	64517
Neurolytic	64681

Relative Value Units	
Unilateral	15
Neurolytic	25

INDICATIONS

Ganglion of Walther (also known as the *ganglion impar*) block is useful in the evaluation and management of sympathetically mediated pain of the perineum, rectum, and genitalia. This technique has been used primarily in the treatment of pain secondary to malignancy, although theoretical applications for benign pain syndromes, including pain secondary to endometriosis, reflex sympathetic dystrophy, causalgia, proctalgia fugax, and radiation enteritis, can be considered if the pain has failed to respond to more conservative therapies. Ganglion of Walther block with local anesthetic can be used as a diagnostic tool when performing differential neural blockade on an anatomic basis in the evaluation of pelvic and rectal pain. If destruction of the ganglion of Walther is being considered, this technique is useful as a prognostic indicator of the degree of pain relief that the patient may experience. Destruction of the ganglion of Walther is indicated for the palliation of pain syndromes that have temporarily responded to blockade of the ganglion with local anesthetic and have not been controlled with more conservative measures.

CLINICALLY RELEVANT ANATOMY

In the context of neural blockade, the ganglion of Walther can simply be thought of as the terminal coalescence of the sympathetic chain. The ganglion of Walther lies in front of the sacrococcygeal junction and is amenable to blockade at this level. The ganglion receives fibers from the lumbar and sacral portions of the sympathetic and parasympathetic nervous system and provides sympathetic innervation to portions of the pelvic viscera and genitalia.

TECHNIQUE
Fluoroscopic Technique

The patient is placed in the jackknife position to facilitate access to the inferior margin of the gluteal cleft. The midline is identified, and the skin overlying the coccyx is prepared with antiseptic solution. The skin and subcutaneous tissues at this point are anesthetized with 1.0% lidocaine. Fluoroscopy is used to identify the sacrococcygeal and coccygeal joints. A $3\frac{1}{2}$-inch spinal needle is inserted between the first and second coccygeal bones and slowly advanced until the needle tip rests just beyond the anterior wall of the coccyx in the precoccygeal space (Fig. 107-1). After careful aspiration for blood, cerebrospinal fluid, and urine, 1 mL of water-soluble iodinated contrast medium is slowly injected. After proper needle position and spread of contrast in the precoccygeal space is confirmed on both postero-anterior and lateral fluoroscopic views, 3 mL of 1.0% preservative-free lidocaine is slowly injected in incremental doses (Fig. 107-2). If there is believed to be an inflammatory component to the pain, the local anesthetic is combined with 80 mg of methylprednisolone and is injected in incremental doses. Subsequent daily nerve blocks are carried out in a similar manner, substituting 40 mg of methylprednisolone for the initial 80-mg dose. The needle is then removed, and an ice pack is placed on the injection site to decrease postblock bleeding and pain. If adequate pain relief is obtained, 0.1 mL incremental doses of absolute alcohol or 6.5% aqueous phenol may be injected in a similar manner after it is ascertained that the patient is experiencing no untoward bowel or bladder effects from blockade of the ganglion of Walther.

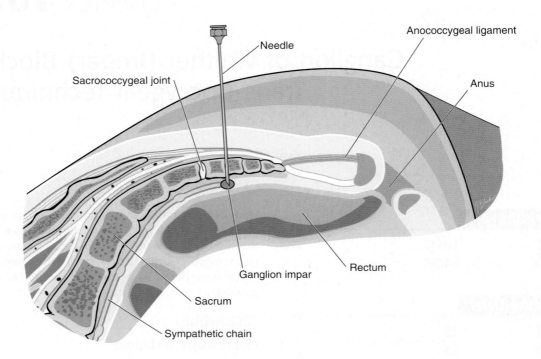

Needle

Anococcygeal ligament

Sacrococcygeal joint

Anus

Ganglion impar

Rectum

Sacrum

Sympathetic chain

Figure 107-1.

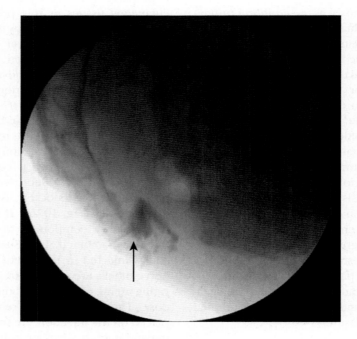

Figure 107-2.
Lateral view of the block of ganglion impar after contrast injection. Note the tip of the needle just anterior to the disk space between the first and second coccyx (*arrow*). (From Hong JH, Jang HS: Block of the ganglion impar using a coccygeal joint approach. Reg Anesth Pain Med 31:583-584, 2006, Fig 2.)

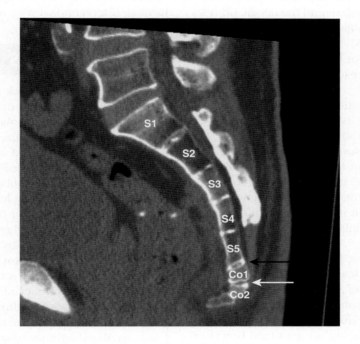

Figure 107-3.
Sagittal view of sacrococcygeal bone by computed tomography. Note the ossification at the sacrococcygeal joint (*black arrow*) and the conserved space between the first and second coccygeal bones (*white arrow*). S, sacrum; Co, coccyx. (From Hong JH, Jang HS: Block of the ganglion impar using a coccygeal joint approach. Reg Anesth Pain Med 31:583-584, 2006, Fig 1.)

Computed Tomography–Guided Technique

The patient is placed in the prone position on the computed tomography (CT) gantry with a pillow placed under the pelvis to facilitate access to the inferior gluteal cleft. A CT scout film is taken, and the sacrococcygeal junction, coccygeal joints, and the tip of the coccyx are identified. The midline is also identified, and the skin overlying the coccyx that overlies the anococcygeal ligament is prepared with antiseptic solution.

The skin and subcutaneous tissues at this point are anesthetized with 1.0% lidocaine. A 3½-inch spinal needle is inserted between the first and second coccygeal bones and slowly advanced until the needle tip rests just beyond the anterior wall of the coccyx in the precoccygeal space (Fig. 107-3).

After careful aspiration for blood, cerebrospinal fluid, and urine, 1 mL of water-soluble iodinated contrast medium is slowly injected.

After proper needle position and spread of contrast in the precoccygeal space is confirmed by repeat CT scan, 3 mL of 1.0% preservative-free lidocaine is slowly injected in incremental doses. If there is believed to be an inflammatory component to the pain, the local anesthetic is combined with 80 mg of methylprednisolone and is injected in incremental doses. Subsequent daily nerve blocks are carried out in a similar manner, substituting 40 mg of methylprednisolone for the initial 80-mg dose.

The needle is then removed, and an ice pack is placed on the injection site to decrease postblock bleeding and pain. If adequate pain relief is obtained, 0.1-mL incremental doses of absolute alcohol or 6.5% aqueous phenol may be injected in a similar manner after it is ascertained that the patient is experiencing no untoward bowel or bladder effects from blockade of the ganglion of Walther.

SIDE EFFECTS AND COMPLICATIONS

The proximity of the ganglion of Walther to the rectum makes perforation and tracking of contaminants back through the needle track during needle removal a distinct possibility. Infection and fistula formation, especially in patients who are immunocompromised or have received radiation therapy to the perineum, can represent a devastating and potentially life-threatening complication to this block. The relationship of the cauda equina and exiting sacral nerve roots makes it imperative that this procedure be carried out only by those well versed in the regional anatomy and experienced in performing interventional pain management techniques.

CLINICAL PEARLS

Ganglion of Walther block is a straightforward technique that can produce dramatic relief for patients suffering from the previously mentioned pain complaints. Given the localized nature of this neural structure when compared with the superior hypogastric plexus, neurolytic block with small quantities of absolute alcohol or phenol in glycerin or by cryoneurolysis or radiofrequency lesioning may be a reasonable choice over superior hypogastric plexus block, at least insofar as bowel and bladder dysfunction is concerned. Destruction of the ganglion of Walther has been shown to provide long-term relief for patients suffering from sympathetically maintained pain that has been relieved with local anesthetic. CT guidance allows visualization of the regional anatomy and the relationship of the rectum to the needle. This is a significant advance over blind or fluoroscopically guided techniques.

CHAPTER 108

Pudendal Nerve Block: Transvaginal Approach

CPT-2009 CODE

Unilateral	64430
Neurolytic	64630

Relative Value Units

Unilateral	12
Neurolytic	20

INDICATIONS

Pudendal nerve block via the transvaginal approach is used primarily in obstetric anesthesia as an adjunct to pain relief during the second stage of labor. It is occasionally used in the evaluation and management of pelvic pain believed to be subserved by the pudendal nerve. The technique also is useful to provide surgical anesthesia for surgery on the labia or scrotum, including lesion removal and laceration repair. Pudendal nerve block with local anesthetic can be used as a diagnostic tool when performing differential neural blockade on an anatomic basis in the evaluation of pelvic pain when peripheral nerve injury or entrapment versus radiculopathy or plexopathy is being evaluated. If destruction of the pudendal nerve is being considered, this technique is useful as a prognostic indicator of the degree of motor and sensory impairment that the patient may experience.

Pudendal nerve block with local anesthetic may be used to palliate acute pain emergencies, including postoperative pain relief, while waiting for pharmacologic methods to become effective. Pudendal nerve block with local anesthetic and steroid also is useful in the treatment of persistent pain after perineal trauma when the pain is believed to be secondary to inflammation or entrapment of the pudendal nerve. Such problems can occur after "straddle injuries" or during forceps deliveries. Pudendal nerve block with local anesthetic and steroid also is useful in the palliation of pain of malignant origin arising from tumors invading the labia or scrotum or the pudendal nerve. The technique also may be useful in palliation of persistent vulvar or vaginal itching that has not responded to topical therapy.

Destruction of the pudendal nerve is occasionally indicated for the palliation of persistent pelvic pain after blunt or open trauma to the pelvis or persistent pain mediated by the pudendal nerve after obstetric deliveries or transvaginal surgery or in the palliation of pain of malignant origin. Pudendal nerve block using a 25-gauge needle may be carried out in the presence of coagulopathy or anticoagulation, albeit with an increased risk for ecchymosis and hematoma formation.

CLINICALLY RELEVANT ANATOMY

The pudendal nerve is made up of fibers from the S2, S3, and S4 nerves. The nerve passes inferiorly between the piriformis and coccygeal muscles. Along with the pudendal vessels, the pudendal nerve leaves the pelvis via the greater sciatic foramen. It then passes around the medial portion of the ischial spine to reenter the pelvis through the lesser sciatic foramen. The pudendal nerve is amenable to blockade at this point via the transvaginal approach. The nerve then divides into three terminal branches:

1. Inferior rectal nerve, which provides innervation to the anal sphincter and perianal region
2. Perineal nerve, which supplies the posterior two thirds of the scrotum or labia majora and muscles of the urogenital triangle
3. Dorsal nerve of the penis or clitoris, which supplies sensory innervation to the dorsum of the penis or clitoris

TECHNIQUE

The patient is placed in the lithotomy position. The index and middle fingers of the pain specialist's nondominant hand are inserted into the vagina to bracket the ischial spine. The needle guide is inserted between the fingers, and its tip is placed against the vaginal mucosa just in front of the ischial spine. A 20-gauge,

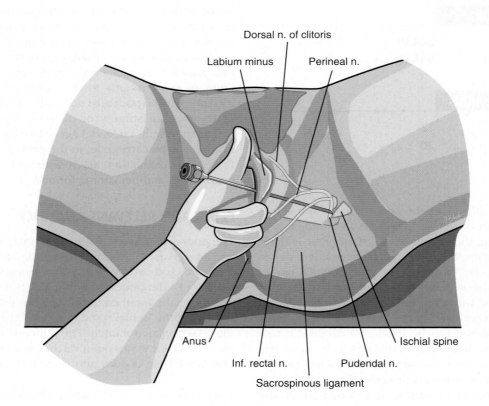

Figure 108-1.

6-inch needle is then placed through the guide and is advanced through the sacrospinous ligament just beyond the ischial spine (Fig. 108-1). A loss of resistance will be felt as the needle passes beyond the ligament. After negative aspiration for blood, 10 mL of 1.0% preservative-free lidocaine is injected. An additional 3 to 4 mL of local anesthetic may be injected as the needle is withdrawn into the vagina to ensure blockade of the inferior rectal nerve.

SIDE EFFECTS AND COMPLICATIONS

The proximity of the pudendal nerve to the pudendal artery and vein makes the potential for intravascular injection a distinct possibility. Despite proximity to the rectum, infection with the transvaginal approach to pudendal nerve block does not appear to be a problem, although, theoretically, infection and fistula formation, especially in those patients who are immunocompromised or have received radiation therapy to the perineum, could represent a devastating and potentially life-threatening complication to this block.

CLINICAL PEARLS

Pudendal nerve block is a simple technique that can produce dramatic relief for patients suffering from the previously mentioned pain complaints. Destruction of the pudendal nerve has been shown to provide long-term relief for patients suffering from pain secondary to invasive tumors of the vulva and scrotum.

CHAPTER 109

Pudendal Nerve Block: Transperineal Approach

CPT-2009 CODE

Unilateral	64430
Neurolytic	64630

Relative Value Units

Unilateral	12
Neurolytic	20

INDICATIONS

Pudendal nerve block via the transperineal approach is used for pudendal nerve block in men and in women when tumor or radiation-induced scarring precludes use of the transvaginal approach. It can by used in the evaluation and management of pelvic pain believed to be subserved by the pudendal nerve. The technique also is useful to provide surgical anesthesia for surgery on the labia or scrotum, including lesion removal and laceration repair.

Pudendal nerve block with local anesthetic can be used as a diagnostic tool when performing differential neural blockade on an anatomic basis in the evaluation of pelvic pain when peripheral nerve injury or entrapment versus radiculopathy or plexopathy is being evaluated. If destruction of the pudendal nerve is being considered, this technique is useful as a prognostic indicator of the degree of motor and sensory impairment that the patient may experience. Pudendal nerve block with local anesthetic may be used to palliate acute pain emergencies, including postoperative pain relief, while waiting for pharmacologic methods to become effective. Pudendal nerve block with local anesthetic and steroid also is useful in the treatment of persistent pain after perineal trauma when the pain is believed to be secondary to inflammation or entrapment of the pudendal nerve. Such problems can occur after "straddle injuries" or during forceps deliveries. Pudendal nerve block with local anesthetic and steroid also is useful in the palliation of pain of malignant origin arising from tumors invading the labia or scrotum or the pudendal nerve. The technique also may be useful in palliation of persistent rectal, vulvar, or vaginal itching that has not responded to topical therapy.

Destruction of the pudendal nerve is occasionally indicated for the palliation of persistent pelvic or rectal pain after blunt or open trauma to the pelvis or persistent pain mediated by the pudendal nerve after obstetric deliveries or transvaginal surgery or in the palliation of pain of malignant origin. Pudendal nerve block using a 25-gauge needle may be carried out in the presence of coagulopathy or anticoagulation, albeit with an increased risk for ecchymosis and hematoma formation.

CLINICALLY RELEVANT ANATOMY

The pudendal nerve is made up of fibers from the S2, S3, and S4 nerves. The nerve passes inferiorly between the piriformis and coccygeal muscles. Along with the pudendal vessels, the pudendal nerve leaves the pelvis via the greater sciatic foramen. It then passes around the medial portion of the ischial spine to reenter the pelvis via the lesser sciatic foramen. The pudendal nerve is amenable to blockade at this point via the transvaginal approach. The nerve then divides into three terminal branches:

1. Inferior rectal nerve, which provides innervation to the anal sphincter and perianal region
2. Perineal nerve, which supplies the posterior two thirds of the scrotum or labia majora and muscles of the urogenital triangle
3. Dorsal nerve of the penis or clitoris, which supplies sensory innervation to the dorsum of the penis or clitoris

TECHNIQUE

The patient is placed in the lithotomy position. The ischial tuberosity is identified by palpation, and an area 1 inch lateral and 1 inch posterior to the tuberosity is then prepared with antiseptic solution. A skin wheal is raised at this point with local anesthetic. The index

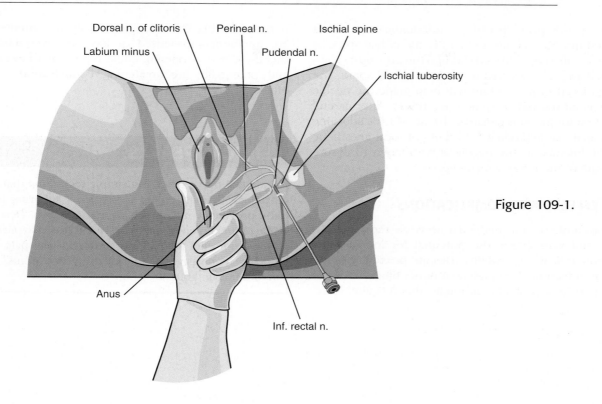

Dorsal n. of clitoris   Perineal n.   Ischial spine

Labium minus   Pudendal n.

Ischial tuberosity

Figure 109-1.

Anus

Inf. rectal n.

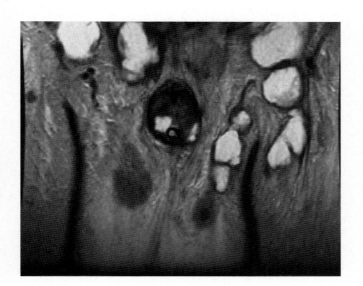

Figure 109-2.
Metastatic disease to the penis. Coronal T2-weighted (4000/108) image of a 58-year-old man with known rectal carcinoma shows abnormal high T2-signal masses within the penis and enlarging inguinal nodes as well as abnormal low signal within both corpora cavernosa. (Courtesy of Dr. Clare Tempany. From Edelman RR, Hesselink JR, Zlatkin MB, Crues JV: Clinical Magnetic Resonance Imaging, 3rd ed. Philadelphia, WB Saunders, 2006, p 3061.)

finger of the pain specialist's nondominant hand is inserted into the rectum to identify the ischial spine. A 6-inch needle is then placed through the previously anesthetized area and directed toward the ischial spine. The finger placed in the rectum will help guide the needle just beyond the ischial spine (Fig. 109-1). After careful aspiration for blood is negative, 10 mL of 1.0% lidocaine is injected. An additional 3 to 4 mL of local anesthetic may be injected as the needle is withdrawn to ensure blockade of the inferior rectal nerve.

SIDE EFFECTS AND COMPLICATIONS

The proximity of the pudendal nerve to the pudendal artery and vein makes the potential for intravascular injection a distinct possibility. Despite proximity to the rectum, infection after pudendal nerve block does not appear to be a problem, although, theoretically, infec-tion and fistula formation, especially in patients who are immunocompromised or have received radiation therapy to the perineum, could represent a devastating and potentially life-threatening complication to this block.

CLINICAL PEARLS

Pudendal nerve block is a simple technique that can produce dramatic relief for patients suffering from the previously mentioned pain complaints. Destruction of the pudendal nerve has been shown to provide long-term relief for patients suffering from pain secondary to invasive tumors of the vulva, penis, and scrotum (Fig. 109-2).

CHAPTER 110

Sacroiliac Joint Injection

CPT-2003 CODE	
Local Anesthetic and Steroid	**27096**

Relative Value Units	
Local Anesthetic	**9**

INDICATIONS

The sacroiliac joint is susceptible to the development of arthritis from a variety of conditions that have in common the ability to damage the joint cartilage. The sacroiliac joint is also susceptible to the development of strain from trauma or misuse. Osteoarthritis of the joint is the most common form of arthritis that results in sacroiliac joint pain; however, rheumatoid arthritis and post-traumatic arthritis are also common causes of sacroiliac pain secondary to arthritis. Less common causes of arthritis-induced sacroiliac pain include the collagen vascular diseases including ankylosing spondylitis, infection, and Lyme disease.

Acute infectious arthritis is usually accompanied by significant systemic symptoms, including fever and malaise, and should be easily recognized by the astute clinician and treated appropriately with culture and antibiotics, rather than injection therapy (Fig. 110-1). The collagen vascular diseases generally manifest as a polyarthropathy rather than a monoarthropathy limited to the sacroiliac joint, although sacroiliac pain secondary to the collagen vascular disease ankylosing spondylitis responds exceedingly well to the intra-articular injection technique described later. Occasionally, the clinician will encounter patients with iatrogenically induced sacroiliac joint dysfunction due to overaggressive bone graft harvesting for spinal fusions.

CLINICALLY RELEVANT ANATOMY

The sacroiliac joint is formed by the articular surfaces of the sacrum and iliac bones (Fig. 110-2). These articular surfaces have corresponding elevations and depressions that give the joints their irregular appearance on radiographs (Fig. 110-3). The strength of the sacroiliac joint comes primarily from the posterior and interosseous ligaments rather than the bony articulations. The sacroiliac joints bear the weight of the trunk and are thus subject to the development of strain and arthritis. As the joint ages, the intra-articular space narrows, making intra-articular injection more challenging. The ligaments and the sacroiliac joint receive their innervation from L3 to S3 nerve roots, with L4 and L5 providing the greatest contribution to the innervation of the joint. This diverse innervation may help explain the ill-defined nature of sacroiliac pain. The sacroiliac joint has a limited range of motion and that motion is induced by changes in the forces placed on the joint by shifts in posture and joint loading.

TECHNIQUE

The goals of this injection technique are explained to the patient. The patient is placed in the supine position, and proper preparation with antiseptic solution of the skin overlying the affected sacroiliac joint space is carried out. A sterile syringe containing 4 mL of 0.25% preservative-free bupivacaine and 40 mg of methylprednisolone is attached to a 24-gauge, 3½-inch needle using strict aseptic technique. With strict aseptic technique, the posterior-superior spine of the ilium is identified. At this point, the needle is carefully advanced through the skin and subcutaneous tissues at a 45-degree angle toward the affected sacroiliac joint (Fig. 110-4). If bone is encountered, the needle is withdrawn into the subcutaneous tissues and redirected superiorly and slightly more lateral. In older patients, fluoroscopic or computed tomographic guidance may simplify intra-articular needle placement (Figs. 110-5 and 110-6). If fluoroscopy is used, a small amount of contrast may be injected into the joint to confirm intra-articular needle placement (Fig. 110-7). After entering the joint space, the contents of the syringe are gently injected. There should be little resistance to injection. If resistance is encountered, the needle is

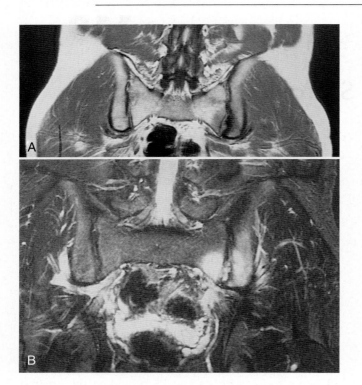

Figure 110-1.
A, Coronal T1-weighted image demonstrates low signal in the left sacral and iliac bones with low signal in a slightly widened irregular joint space. **B,** Fast T2-weighted fat-suppressed image shows abnormal signal in the bones as well as fluid in the joint space. The findings are consistent with sacroiliitis. (From Kaplan P, Helms CA, Dussault R: Musculoskeletal MRI, 1st ed. Philadelphia, WB Saunders, 2001, p 355.)

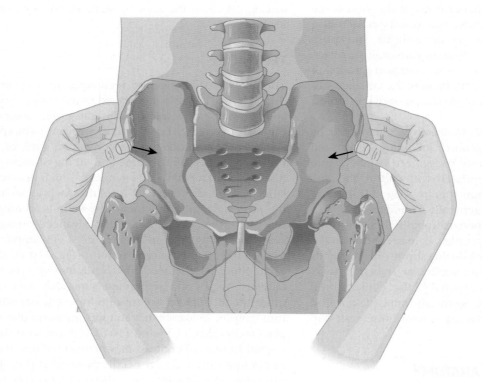

Figure 110-2.

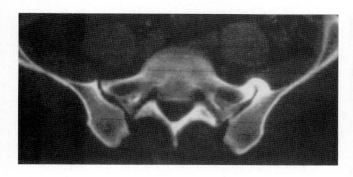

Figure 110-3.
The sacroiliac (SI) joints in a patient with osteoarthritis as viewed with computed tomography. The right SI joint is within normal limits. The left SI joint shows bone sclerosis anteriorly and a large osteophyte bridging the space between the ilium and the sacrum anterior to the true joint. (From Brower AC, Flemming DJ: Arthritis in Black and White, 2nd ed. Philadelphia, WB Saunders, 1997, p 170.)

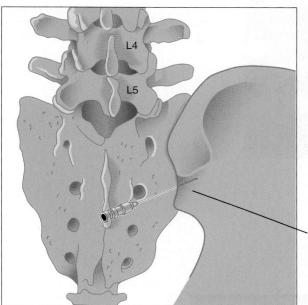

Figure 110-4.

Arthritic and inflamed sacroiliac joint

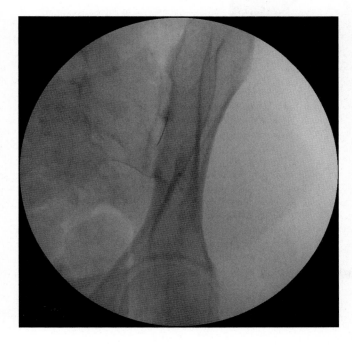

Figure 110-5.
Fluoroscopic view of sacroiliac joint.

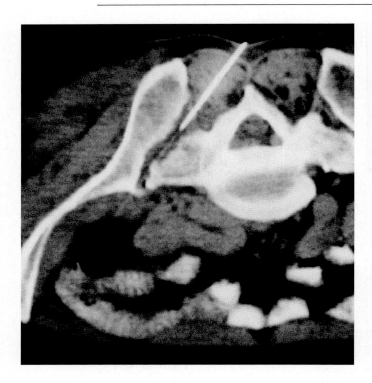

Figure 110-6.
Sacroiliac joint injection in a 73-year-old woman who suffered from local pain without response to analgesics. The needle is placed inside the sacroiliac joint. (From Thanos L, Mylona S, Kalioras V, et al: Percutaneous CT-guided interventional procedures in musculoskeletal system [our experience]. Eur J Radiol 50:273-277, 2004, Fig 3.)

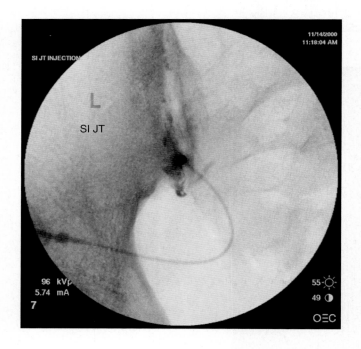

Figure 110-7.
Contrast medium in sacroiliac joint.

probably in a ligament and should be advanced slightly into the joint space until the injection proceeds without significant resistance. The needle is then removed, and a sterile pressure dressing and ice pack are placed at the injection site.

SIDE EFFECTS AND COMPLICATIONS

The major complication of intra-articular injection of the sacroiliac joint is infection. This complication should be exceedingly rare if strict aseptic technique is followed. About 25% of patients complain of a transient increase in pain following intra-articular injection of the sacroiliac joint, and patients should be warned of such. Care must be taken to avoid injection too laterally, or the needle may traumatize the sciatic nerve.

CLINICAL PEARLS

This injection technique is extremely effective in the treatment of the previously mentioned causes of sacroiliac joint pain. Coexistent bursitis and tendinitis may also contribute to sacroiliac pain and may require additional treatment with more localized injection of local anesthetic and depot-steroid. This technique is a safe procedure if careful attention is paid to the clinically relevant anatomy in the areas to be injected. Care must be taken to use sterile technique to avoid infection as well as universal precautions to avoid risk to the operator. The incidence of ecchymosis and hematoma formation can be decreased if pressure is placed on the injection site immediately after injection. The use of physical modalities including local heat as well as gentle range of motion exercises should be introduced several days after the patient undergoes this injection technique for sacroiliac pain. Vigorous exercises should be avoided because they will exacerbate the patient's symptoms. Simple analgesics and nonsteroidal anti-inflammatory agents may be used concurrently with this injection technique.

CHAPTER 111

Sacroiliac Joint: Radiofrequency Lesioning

INDICATIONS

The sacroiliac joint is susceptible to the development of arthritis from a variety of conditions that have in common the ability to damage the joint cartilage. In addition, the sacroiliac joint is susceptible to the development of strain from trauma or misuse. Osteoarthritis of the joint is the most common form of arthritis that results in sacroiliac joint pain. However, rheumatoid arthritis and post-traumatic arthritis also are common causes of sacroiliac pain secondary to arthritis. Less common causes of arthritis-induced sacroiliac pain include the collagen vascular diseases, including ankylosing spondylitis, infection, and Lyme disease.

Acute infectious arthritis is usually accompanied by significant systemic symptoms, including fever and malaise, and should be easily recognized by the astute clinician and treated appropriately with culture and antibiotics, rather than with injection therapy. The collagen vascular diseases generally manifest as a polyarthropathy rather than a monoarthropathy limited to the sacroiliac joint, although sacroiliac pain secondary to the collagen vascular disease ankylosing spondylitis responds exceedingly well to the intra-articular injection technique described later. Occasionally, the clinician encounters patients with iatrogenically induced sacroiliac joint dysfunction due to overaggressive bone graft harvesting for spinal fusions.

Radiofrequency lesioning of the sacroiliac joint is indicated for patients who have received short-term relief of pain following injection of the sacroiliac joint with local anesthetic and have failed treatment with more conservative therapy, including physical therapy, local injec-

tions of steroids, nonsteroidal anti-inflammatory agents, the cyclooxygenase-2 inhibitors, and simple analgesics. It is incumbent on the clinician to rule out treatable causes of sacroiliac joint pain as mentioned.

CLINICALLY RELEVANT ANATOMY

The sacroiliac joint is formed by the articular surfaces of the sacrum and iliac bones (see Fig. 110-1). These articular surfaces have corresponding elevations and depressions that give the joints their irregular appearance on radiographs (see Fig. 110-2). The strength of the sacroiliac joint comes primarily from the posterior and interosseous ligaments rather than the bony articulations. The sacroiliac joints bear the weight of the trunk and are thus subject to the development of strain and arthritis. As the joint ages, the intra-articular space narrows, making intra-articular injection more challenging. The ligaments and the sacroiliac joint receive their innervation from L3 to S3 nerve roots, with L4 and L5 providing the greatest contribution to the innervation of the joint. This diverse innervation may help explain the ill-defined nature of sacroiliac pain. The sacroiliac joint has a limited range of motion, and that motion is induced by changes in the forces placed on the joint by shifts in posture and joint loading.

TECHNIQUE

Although many clinicians denervate the sacroiliac joint by directly placing radiofrequency needles into the joint, many investigators believe that radiofrequency disruption of the posterior innervation of the sacroiliac joint involving lesioning of the L5-S4 lateral branches of the dorsal rami is more efficacious (Fig. 111-1). Each of these can have multiple sub-branches. Because significant variability exists as to both the number and location of these branches, lesioning must be aimed at the potential area in which the nerves may travel in a manner analogous to a field block or attempt a much more specific, albeit tedious, highly specific stereotactic approach as advocated by Yin and Baker. This stereotactic approach

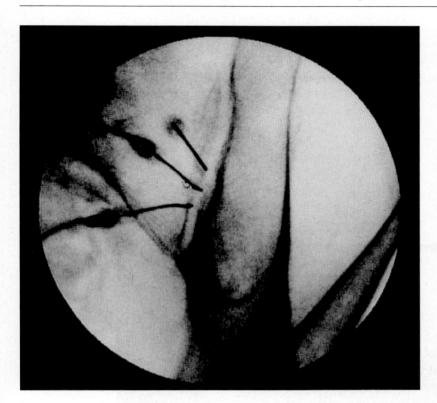

Figure 111-1.
Technique of radiofrequency denervation. Two electrodes are inserted in the joint, and a lesion is made at 90°C for 90 seconds using a bipolar system. A third electrode is placed more cephalad in the joint at a distance less than 1 cm from the next inferior electrode (as viewed fluoroscopically). Sequentially more cephalad lesions are made using this "leapfrog" approach. (From Ferrante FM, King LF, Roche EA, et al: Radiofrequency sacroiliac joint denervation for sacroiliac syndrome. Reg Anesth Pain Med 26:137-142, 2001, Fig 1.)

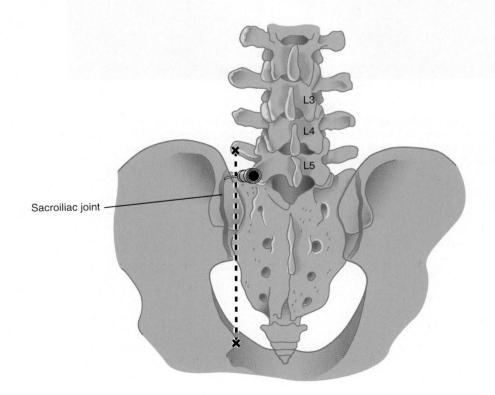

Sacroiliac joint

Figure 111-2.

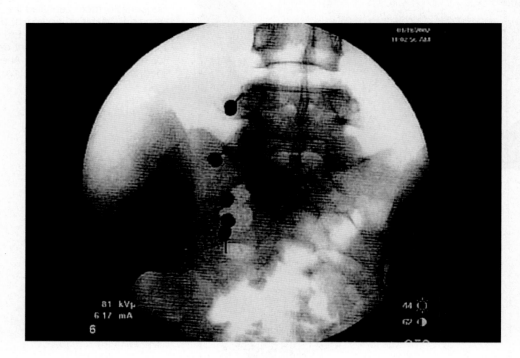

Figure 111-3.
Radiograph demonstrating the location of the needles for nerve blocks performed on the L4 and L5 dorsal rami and S1-3 lateral branches. (From Cohen SP, Abdi S: Lateral branch blocks as a treatment for sacroiliac joint pain: A pilot study. Reg Anesth Pain Med 28:113-119, 2003, Fig 2.)

involves the mapping of the specific branches of the lateral dorsal sacral nerves that may subserve sacroiliac joint pain versus the other lateral dorsal sacral nerves that do not contribute to the patient's sacroiliac joint pain. The more commonly used "field" lesioning approach involves creating a series of lesions along the probable neural pathway subserving the patient's pain.

The goals of this injection technique are explained to the patient. The patient is placed in the prone position with a pillow under the hips, and proper preparation with antiseptic solution of the skin overlying the affected sacroiliac joint space is carried out. Using fluoroscopic guidance, the affected sacroiliac joint is identified. A contralateral oblique view is then obtained, and the image intensifier tube is then adjusted to move the ilium from a position overlying the joint and to allow direct visualization of the joint. A line is drawn on the skin parallel to the joint about one third to one half the distance between the joint and a line connecting the lateral aspects of the posterior S1-S3 foramen. Local anesthetic is then infiltrated in the skin and subcutaneous tissues down to the sacrum along this line parallel to the sacroiliac joint. This line is extended to a point at about the level of the L5 transverse process and a point 1 to 2 cm caudad to the lower edge of the sacrum. A parallel line is now drawn to the inferior edge of the sacrum and sacral ala to indicate the upper and lower needle entry points (Fig. 111-2).

A curved 100-mm radiofrequency needle with a 10-mm active tip is then advanced to the joint starting at the sacral ala. Bone should be contacted within 10 to 12 mm of the sacral ala. Because this is a field lesion, sensory stimulation is not performed, and because no motor nerves are in proximity, no motor stimulation is performed. A radiofrequency lesion is then created by stimulation at 80°C for 90 seconds (Fig. 111-3). The needle is then turned 180 degrees toward the S1 foramen, and a second lesion is then created in a manner analogous to the first lesion. The needle is then advanced inferiorly in 7- to 10-mm increments along the posterior sacrum, and lesions are created using the above parameters.

Under fluoroscopic guidance, a second curved 100-mm radiofrequency needle with a 10-mm active time is placed at the inferior aspect of the affected joint and then advanced superiorly along the course of the joint. An additional 12 lesions are created as the needle is withdrawn in 7- to 10-mm increments along the course

of the joint with the needle alternatively being rotated 180 degrees between each lesion. A total of 24 to 30 lesions should produce an acceptable field block disrupting the lateral branches innervating the sacroiliac joint.

SIDE EFFECTS AND COMPLICATIONS

The major complication of lesioning of the sacroiliac joint is postprocedure pain. Some clinicians recommend the injection of 40 mg of methylprednisolone at the time of radiofrequency lesioning to decrease this side effect. Infection can occur following this technique; this complication should be exceedingly rare if strict aseptic technique is adhered to. Care must be taken to avoid injection too laterally, or the needle may traumatize the sciatic nerve.

CLINICAL PEARLS

This technique is extremely effective in providing long-lasting relief of the previously mentioned causes of sacroiliac joint pain. It should be noted that 4 to 6 weeks may be required to see the full extent of relief from the lesioning procedure. It is a time-consuming procedure, but the results are gratifying if careful attention is paid to technique. Coexistent bursitis and tendinitis also may contribute to sacroiliac pain and may require additional treatment with more localized injection of local anesthetic and depotsteroid. In general, this technique is a safe procedure if careful attention is paid to the clinically relevant anatomy in the areas to be injected. Care must be taken to use sterile technique to avoid infection as well as universal precautions to avoid risk to the operator. The incidence of ecchymosis and hematoma formation can be decreased if pressure is placed on the injection site immediately after injection. The use of physical modalities including local heat and gentle range of motion exercises should be introduced several days after the patient undergoes this injection technique for sacroiliac pain. Vigorous exercises should be avoided because they exacerbate the patient's symptoms. Simple analgesics and nonsteroidal anti-inflammatory agents may be used concurrently with this technique.

Section 7

Lower Extremity

CHAPTER 112

Lumbar Plexus Nerve Block: Winnie 3-in-1 Technique

Local Anesthetic and Steroid	64999
Neurolytic	64640

Relative Value Units

Local Anesthetic and Steroid	12
Neurolytic	20

INDICATIONS

The Winnie 3-in-1 approach to lumbar plexus block has the advantage over the psoas compartment technique in that it is amenable to continuous infusion of local anesthetic by placement of either an 18-gauge intravenous catheter or an over-the-wire central venous catheter into the fascial plane. Lumbar plexus nerve block via the Winnie 3-in-1 technique is used primarily for surgical anesthesia of the lower extremity. It occasionally is used in the area of pain management when treating pain secondary to inflammatory conditions of the lumbar plexus or when tumor has invaded the tissues subserved by the lumbar plexus or the plexus itself.

Lumbar plexus nerve block via the Winnie 3-in-1 technique with local anesthetic occasionally is used diagnostically during differential neural blockade on an anatomic basis in the evaluation of lower extremity and groin pain. If destruction of the lumbar plexus is being considered, this technique is useful as a prognostic indicator of the degree of motor and sensory impairment that the patient may experience.

Lumbar plexus nerve block via the Winnie 3-in-1 technique with local anesthetic may be used to palliate acute pain emergencies, including groin and lower extremity trauma or fracture, acute herpes zoster, and cancer pain, while waiting for pharmacologic, surgical, and antiblastic therapies to become effective. Lumbar plexus nerve block via the Winnie 3-in-1 technique with local anesthetic and steroid also is useful in the treatment of lumbar plexitis secondary to virus or diabetes. For most surgical and pain management applications, epidural or subarachnoid block is a better alternative, although one should expect fewer cardiovascular changes with lumbar plexus block compared with epidural or subarachnoid techniques. Destruction of the lumbar plexus is indicated for the palliation of cancer pain, including invasive tumors of the lumbar plexus and the tissues that the plexus innervates. More selective techniques such as radiofrequency lesioning of specific lumbar paravertebral nerve roots may cause less morbidity than lumbar plexus neurolysis.

CLINICALLY RELEVANT ANATOMY

The lumbar plexus lies within the substance of the psoas muscle. The plexus is made up of the ventral roots of the first four lumbar nerves, and in some patients, a contribution from the 12th thoracic nerve. The nerves lie in front of the transverse processes of their respective vertebrae; as they course inferolaterally, they divide into a number of peripheral nerves. The ilioinguinal and iliohypogastric nerves are branches of the L1 nerves with an occasional contribution of fibers from T12. The genitofemoral nerve is made up of fibers from L1 and L2. The lateral femoral cutaneous nerve is derived from fibers of L2 and L3. The obturator nerve receives fibers from L2-L4, and the femoral nerve is made up of fibers from L2-L4. The pain management specialist should be aware of the considerable interpatient variability in terms of the actual spinal nerves that provide fibers to make up these peripheral branches. This variability means that differential neural blockade on an anatomic basis must be interpreted with caution. Because these nerves pass anteriorly beneath the inguinal ligament, they are accessible to blockade via this technique.

The rationale behind lumbar plexus block using the Winnie 3-in-1 technique is to block the three principal nerves that compose the lumbar plexus as they lie enclosed by the fascial plane between the quadratus lumborum, the iliacus muscle, and the psoas major muscle (Fig. 112-1). Solutions injected in this fascial plane flow cranially to bathe the lateral femoral cutaneous nerve, the

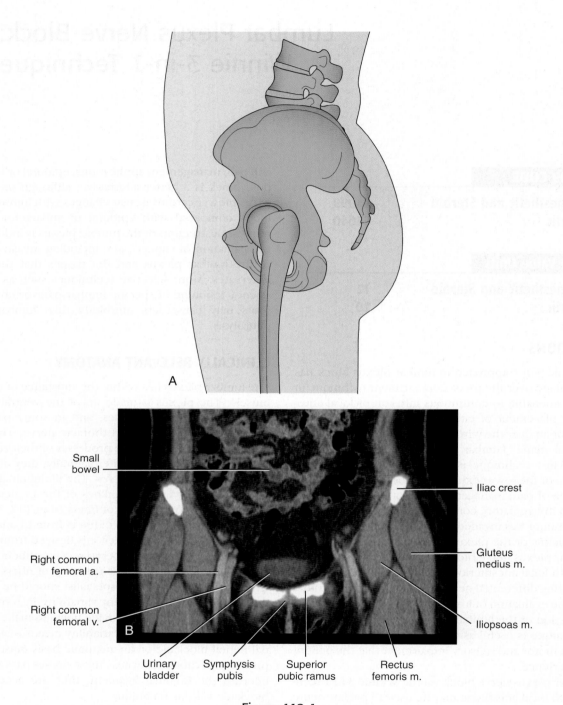

Figure 112-1.

(From El-Khoury GY, Bergman RA, Montgomery WJ: Sectional Anatomy by
MRI and CT, 3rd ed. New York, Churchill Livingstone, 2007, p 558.)

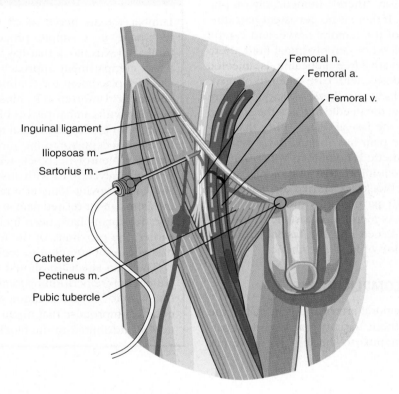

Figure 112-2.

femoral nerve, and the obturator nerve as they pass below the inguinal ligament.

TECHNIQUE

The patient is placed in the supine position. The inguinal ligament and the femoral artery on the side to be blocked are identified. At a point just lateral to the femoral artery and just below the inguinal ligament, the skin is prepared with antiseptic solution. A 22-gauge, 1½-inch needle is advanced slowly in a slightly caudad direction until a paresthesia in the distribution of the femoral nerve is elicited (Fig. 112-2). The patient should be warned of such and instructed to say "there!" immediately on perceiving the paresthesia. If there is no persistent paresthesia in the distribution of the femoral nerve, and careful aspiration reveals no blood or cerebrospinal fluid, 25 to 30 mL of 1.0% preservative-free lidocaine is injected slowly in incremental doses, with care taken to observe the patient for signs of local anesthetic toxicity. Pressure should be applied below the needle to force the solution to flow cranially along the fascial plane rather than distally into the leg. If the pain has an inflammatory component, the local anesthetic is combined with 80 mg of methylprednisolone and is injected in incremental doses. Subsequent daily nerve blocks are carried out in a similar manner, substituting 40 mg of methylprednisolone for the initial 80-mg dose. As mentioned earlier, an intravenous catheter can be placed into the fascial sheath to allow continuous infusion of local anesthetic.

SIDE EFFECTS AND COMPLICATIONS

The proximity to the femoral artery and vein makes the possibility of local anesthetic toxicity real. Persistent paresthesia secondary to trauma to the femoral nerve has rarely been reported after this technique. Although uncommon, infection remains an ever-present possibility, especially in the immunocompromised AIDS or cancer patient. Early detection of infection is crucial to avoid potentially life-threatening sequelae. Postblock groin and back pain, as well as ecchymosis and hematoma of the groin, occur often enough that the patient should be warned of such before beginning lumbar plexus block using the Winnie 3-in-1 technique.

CLINICAL PEARLS

Lumbar plexus nerve block via the Winnie 3-in-1 technique is a simple procedure for performing lumbar plexus block that has the advantage over the psoas compartment approach in that it allows easy catheter placement for continuous infusions of local anesthetic. Unfortunately, most of the things that can be done with lumbar plexus block can be done more easily with epidural or spinal techniques, which may be more acceptable to the surgeon and pain specialist alike. Neurolytic block with small quantities of phenol in glycerin or with absolute alcohol has been shown to provide long-term relief for patients suffering from cancer-related pain in whom more conservative treatments have been ineffectual. As mentioned earlier, the proximity of the femoral artery and vein makes careful attention to technique mandatory.

The pain specialist should carefully examine the patient before performing lumbar plexus block using the Winnie 3-in-1 technique to identify preexisting neural compromise that might subsequently be erroneously attributed to the block.

CHAPTER 113

Lumbar Plexus Nerve Block: Psoas Compartment Technique

CPT-2003 CODE	
Local Anesthetic and Steroid	64999
Neurolytic	64640

Relative Value Units	
Local Anesthetic and Steroid	12
Neurolytic	20

INDICATIONS

Lumbar plexus nerve block via the psoas compartment technique is used primarily for surgical anesthesia of the lower extremity. It is used occasionally in the area of pain management during treatment of pain secondary to inflammatory conditions of the lumbar plexus or when tumor has invaded the tissues subserved by the lumbar plexus or the plexus itself.

Lumbar plexus nerve block via the psoas compartment technique with local anesthetic is used occasionally diagnostically during differential neural blockade on an anatomic basis in the evaluation of lower extremity and groin pain. If destruction of the lumbar plexus is being considered, this technique is useful as a prognostic indicator of the degree of motor and sensory impairment that the patient may experience. Lumbar plexus nerve block via the psoas compartment technique with local anesthetic may be used to palliate acute pain emergencies, including groin and lower extremity trauma or fracture, acute herpes zoster, and cancer pain, while waiting for pharmacologic, surgical, and antiblastic therapies to become effective. This technique used with local anesthetic and steroids also is useful in the treatment of lumbar plexitis secondary to virus or diabetes. For most surgical and pain management applications, epidural or subarachnoid block is a better alternative, although one should expect fewer cardiovascular changes with lumbar plexus block compared with epidural or subarachnoid techniques. Destruction of the lumbar plexus is indicated for the palliation of cancer pain, including invasive

tumors of the lumbar plexus and the tissues that the plexus innervates. More selective techniques such as radiofrequency lesioning of specific lumbar paravertebral nerve roots may cause less morbidity than lumbar plexus neurolysis.

CLINICALLY RELEVANT ANATOMY

The lumbar plexus lies within the substance of the psoas muscle (Fig. 113-1). The plexus is made up of the ventral roots of the first four lumbar nerves and, in some patients, a contribution from the 12th thoracic nerve. The nerves lie in front of the transverse processes of their respective vertebrae; as they course inferolaterally, they divide into a number of peripheral nerves. The ilioinguinal and iliohypogastric nerves are branches of the L1 nerves, with an occasional contribution of fibers from T12. The genitofemoral nerve is made up of fibers from L1 and L2. The lateral femoral cutaneous nerve is derived from fibers of L2 and L3. The obturator nerve receives fibers from L2-L4, and the femoral nerve is made up of fibers from L2-L4. The pain management specialist should be aware of the considerable interpatient variability in terms of the actual spinal nerves that provide fibers to make up these peripheral branches. This variability means that differential neural blockade on an anatomic basis must be interpreted with caution.

The rationale behind lumbar plexus block using the psoas compartment technique is to block the nerves that compose the lumbar plexus because they lie enclosed by the vertebral bodies medially, the quadratus lumborum laterally, and the psoas major muscle ventrally. Solutions injected in this "compartment" flow caudally and cranially to bathe the lumbar nerve roots just as they enter the psoas muscle.

TECHNIQUE

The patient is placed in the lateral or sitting position with the lumbar spine flexed. If the lateral position is chosen, the side to be blocked should be up. The superior iliac crest is identified, and the spinous process is

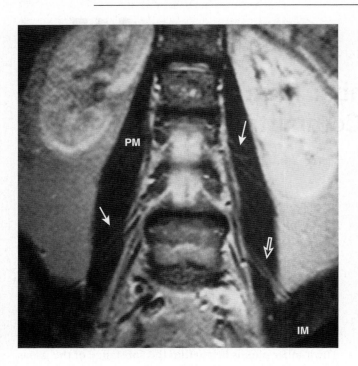

Figure 113-1.
Coronal T2-weighted image of the posterior portion of the psoas major muscle demonstrates lumbar plexus branches outlined by fat signal (*arrows*), traversing the psoas. The femoral nerve (*open arrow*) descends at the junction of the psoas (PM) and iliacus (IM) muscles. (From Stark DD, Bradley WG: Magnetic Resonance Imaging, 3rd ed. St. Louis, Mosby, 1999, p 1908.)

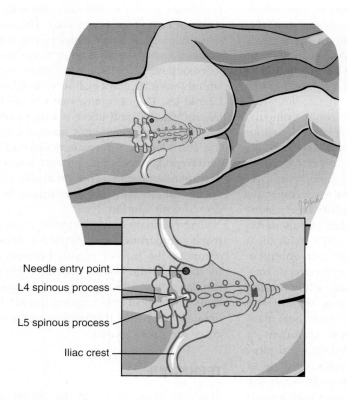

Figure 113-2.

Needle entry point

L4 spinous process

L5 spinous process

Iliac crest

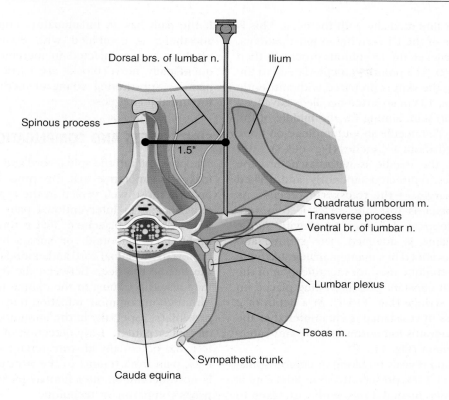

Figure 113-3.

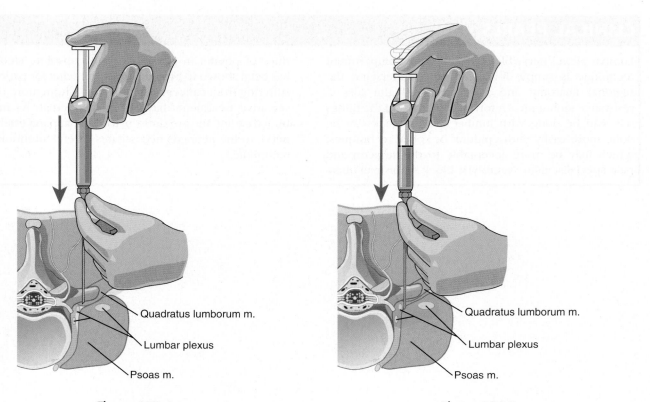

Figure 113-4.

Figure 113-5.

palpated in a direct line medially with the crest. This is the spinous process of the L4 vertebra in most patients. Counting down one level, the L5 spinous process is then identified (Fig. 113-2). At a point 1½ inches lateral to the L5 spinous process, the skin is prepared with antiseptic solution. A 22-gauge, 13-cm styletted needle is advanced perpendicular to the skin, aiming for the middle of the transverse process. The needle should impinge on bone after being advanced about 1½ inches (Fig. 113-3). After bone is contacted, the needle is withdrawn into the subcutaneous tissues, redirected superiorly, and walked off the superior margin of the transverse process. As soon as bony contact is lost, the stylet is removed, and a 5-mL, well-lubricated syringe filled with sterile preservative-free saline is attached. The syringe and needle are slowly advanced in a manner analogous to the loss-of-resistance technique used for identification of the epidural space, with constant pressure being placed on the plunger of the syringe (Fig. 113-4). At a depth of 2 to 2½ inches, a loss of resistance is encountered as the needle exits the quadratus lumborum muscle and enters the psoas compartment (Fig. 113-5).

If careful aspiration reveals no blood or cerebrospinal fluid, 25 to 30 mL of 1.0% preservative-free lidocaine is injected slowly in incremental doses, with care taken to observe the patient for signs of local anesthetic toxicity.

If the pain has an inflammatory component, the local anesthetic is combined with 80 mg of methylprednisolone and is injected in incremental doses. Subsequent daily nerve blocks are carried out in a similar manner, substituting 40 mg of methylprednisolone for the initial 80-mg dose.

SIDE EFFECTS AND COMPLICATIONS

The proximity to the spinal cord and exiting nerve roots makes it imperative that this procedure be performed only by those well versed in the regional anatomy and experienced in interventional pain management techniques. Needle placement that is too medial may result in epidural, subdural, or subarachnoid injections or trauma to the spinal cord and exiting nerve roots. Placing the needle too deep between the transverse processes may result in trauma to the exiting lumbar nerve roots. Although uncommon, infection remains an ever-present possibility, especially in the immunocompromised AIDS or cancer patient. Early detection of infection is crucial to avoid potentially life-threatening sequelae. Postblock back pain from trauma to the paraspinous musculature is not uncommon after lumbar plexus block using the psoas compartment technique.

CLINICAL PEARLS

Lumbar plexus nerve block via the psoas compartment technique is simple for those who understand the regional anatomy and have mastered the loss-of-resistance technique. Unfortunately, most of the things that can be done with lumbar plexus block can be done more easily with epidural or spinal techniques, which may be more acceptable to the surgeon and pain specialist alike. Neurolytic block with small quan-tities of phenol in glycerin or with absolute alcohol has been shown to provide long-term relief for patients suffering from cancer-related pain in whom more conservative treatments have been ineffectual. As mentioned earlier, the proximity of the lumbar paravertebral nerve to the neuraxis necessitates careful attention to technique.

CPT-2009 CODE	
Unilateral	64447
Neurolytic	64640

Relative Value Units	
Unilateral	10
Neurolytic	20

INDICATIONS

Femoral nerve block is useful in the evaluation and management of lower extremity pain thought to be subserved by the femoral nerve. The technique also is useful to provide surgical anesthesia for the lower extremity when combined with lateral femoral cutaneous, sciatic, and obturator nerve block or lumbar plexus block. It is used for this indication primarily in patients who would not tolerate the sympathetic changes induced by spinal or epidural anesthesia and who need lower extremity surgery.

Femoral nerve block with local anesthetic can be used diagnostically during differential neural blockade on an anatomic basis in the evaluation of lower extremity pain. If destruction of the femoral nerve is being considered, this technique is useful as a prognostic indicator of the degree of motor and sensory impairment that the patient may experience. Femoral nerve block with local anesthetic may be used to palliate acute pain emergencies, including femoral neck and shaft fractures, and for postoperative pain relief while waiting for pharmacologic methods to become effective. Femoral nerve block with local anesthetic and steroid is used occasionally in the treatment of persistent lower extremity pain when the pain is thought to be secondary to inflammation or when entrapment of the femoral nerve as it passes under the inguinal ligament is suspected. Femoral nerve block with local anesthetic and steroid also is indicated in the palliation of pain and motor dysfunction associated with diabetic femoral neuropathy. Destruction of the femoral nerve is used occasionally in the palliation of persistent lower extremity pain secondary to invasive tumor that is mediated by the femoral nerve and has not responded to more conservative measures.

CLINICALLY RELEVANT ANATOMY

The femoral nerve innervates the anterior portion of the thigh and medial calf. The femoral nerve is derived from the posterior branches of the L2, L3, and L4 nerve roots. The roots fuse together in the psoas muscle and descend laterally between the psoas and iliacus muscles to enter the iliac fossa. The femoral nerve gives off motor fibers to the iliac muscle and then passes beneath the inguinal ligament to enter the thigh. The femoral nerve is just lateral to the femoral artery as it passes beneath the inguinal ligament and is enclosed with the femoral artery and vein within the femoral sheath. The nerve gives off motor fibers to the sartorius, quadriceps femoris, and pectineus muscles. It also provides sensory fibers to the knee joint as well as the skin overlying the anterior thigh (Fig. 114-1). The nerve is blocked easily as it passes through the femoral triangle.

TECHNIQUE

The patient is placed in the supine position with the leg in neutral position. The femoral artery is identified just below the inguinal ligament by palpation. A point just lateral to the pulsations of the femoral artery and just inferior to the inguinal ligament then is identified and prepared with antiseptic solution (Fig. 114-2). A 25-gauge, $1\frac{1}{2}$-inch needle then is advanced at this point slowly with a cephalad trajectory until a paresthesia in the distribution of the femoral nerve is elicited (Fig. 114-3). The patient should be warned to expect such and should be told to say "there!" immediately on perceiving the paresthesia. Paresthesia usually is elicited at a depth of $\frac{1}{2}$ to $\frac{3}{4}$ inch. If paresthesia is not elicited, the needle is withdrawn and redirected slightly more medially until paresthesia is obtained. Once paresthesia in the distribution of the femoral nerve is elicited, the needle is

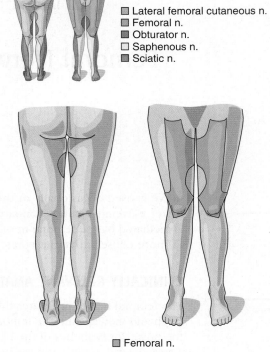

■ Lateral femoral cutaneous n.
■ Femoral n.
■ Obturator n.
□ Saphenous n.
■ Sciatic n.

Figure 114-1.

■ Femoral n.

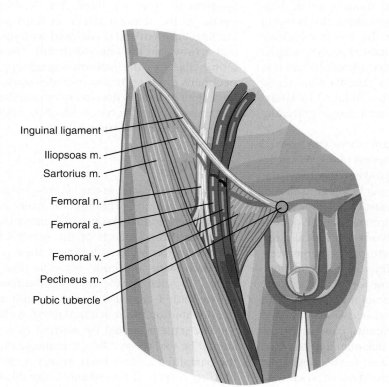

Inguinal ligament
Iliopsoas m.
Sartorius m.
Femoral n.
Femoral a.
Femoral v.
Pectineus m.
Pubic tubercle

Figure 114-2.

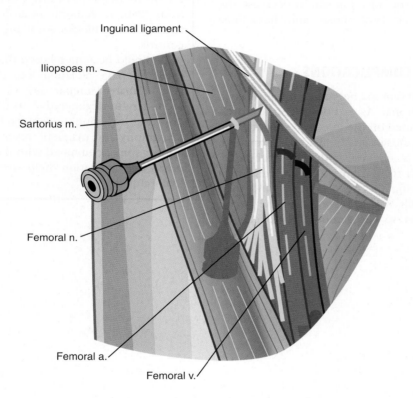

Inguinal ligament

Iliopsoas m.

Sartorius m.

Femoral n.

Femoral a.

Femoral v.

Figure 114-3.

withdrawn 1 mm, and the patient is observed to be sure he or she is not experiencing any persistent paresthesia. If no persistent paresthesia is present and after careful aspiration, 15 to 18 mL of 1.0% preservative-free lidocaine is injected slowly. Care must be taken not to advance the needle into the substance of the nerve during the injection and inject solution intraneurally.

If the pain has an inflammatory component, the local anesthetic is combined with 80 mg of methylprednisolone and is injected in incremental doses. Subsequent daily nerve blocks are performed in a similar manner, substituting 40 mg of methylprednisolone for the initial 80-mg dose. After injection of the solution, pressure is applied to the injection site to decrease the incidence of postblock ecchymosis and hematoma formation.

SIDE EFFECTS AND COMPLICATIONS

The main side effect of femoral nerve block is postblock ecchymosis and hematoma. As mentioned earlier, pressure should be maintained on the injection site after the block to avoid ecchymosis and hematoma formation. Because paresthesia is elicited with this technique, needle-induced trauma to the femoral nerve remains a possibility. By advancing the needle slowly and then withdrawing the needle slightly away from the nerve, needle-induced trauma to the femoral nerve can be avoided.

CLINICAL PEARLS

Femoral nerve block is a simple technique that can produce dramatic relief for patients suffering from the mentioned pain complaints. This technique is especially useful in the emergency department to provide rapid relief for patients suffering from fractures of the femoral neck and shaft. Careful preblock neurologic assessment is important to avoid later attribution of preexisting neurologic deficits to the femoral nerve block. These assessments are especially important in patients who have sustained trauma to the pelvis or lower extremity or who suffer from diabetic femoral neuropathy and in whom femoral nerve blocks are being used for acute pain control.

It should be remembered that the most common cause of pain radiating into the lower extremity is a herniated lumbar disk or nerve impingement secondary to degenerative arthritis of the spine, not disorders involving the femoral nerve per se. Electromyography and magnetic resonance imaging of the lumbar spine, combined with the clinical history and physical examination, help sort out the etiology of femoral pain.

CHAPTER 115

Lateral Femoral Cutaneous Nerve Block

CPT-2009 CODE	
Unilateral	64450
Neurolytic	64640

Relative Value Units	
Unilateral	8
Neurolytic	20

INDICATIONS

Lateral femoral cutaneous nerve block is useful in the evaluation and management of lateral thigh pain thought to be subserved by the lateral femoral cutaneous nerve, including meralgia paresthetica. The technique also is useful to provide surgical anesthesia for skin graft harvest procedures from the lateral thigh and to relieve tourniquet pain.

Lateral femoral cutaneous nerve block with local anesthetic can be used as a diagnostic tool during differential neural blockade on an anatomic basis in the evaluation of lateral pain when peripheral nerve entrapment versus lumbar radiculopathy is being evaluated. If destruction of the lateral femoral cutaneous nerve is being considered, this technique is useful as a prognostic indicator of the degree of motor and sensory impairment that the patient may experience. Lateral femoral cutaneous nerve block with local anesthetic may be used to palliate acute pain emergencies, including postoperative pain relief, while waiting for pharmacologic methods to become effective. Lateral femoral cutaneous nerve block with local anesthetic and steroid also is useful in the treatment of persistent pain after inguinal or bone harvest surgery from the iliac crest when the pain is thought to be secondary to inflammation or entrapment of the lateral femoral cutaneous nerve.

Destruction of the lateral femoral cutaneous nerve occasionally is indicated for the palliation of persistent groin pain after blunt or open trauma to the groin or persistent pain mediated by the lateral femoral cutaneous nerve after groin surgery. A 25-gauge needle may be used for lateral femoral cutaneous nerve block in the presence of coagulopathy or anticoagulation, albeit with an increased risk for ecchymosis and hematoma formation.

CLINICALLY RELEVANT ANATOMY

The lateral femoral cutaneous nerve is formed from the posterior divisions of the L2 and L3 nerves. The nerve leaves the psoas muscle and courses laterally and inferiorly to pass just beneath the ilioinguinal nerve at the level of the anterior-superior iliac spine. The nerve passes under the inguinal ligament and then travels beneath the fascia lata, where it divides into an anterior and a posterior branch. The anterior branch provides limited cutaneous sensory innervation over the anterolateral thigh (Fig. 115-1). The posterior branch provides cutaneous sensory innervation to the lateral thigh from just above the greater trochanter to the knee.

TECHNIQUE

The patient is placed in the supine position with a pillow under the knees if the legs-extended position increases the patient's pain because of traction on the nerve. The anterior-superior iliac spine is identified by palpation. A point 1 inch medial to the anterior-superior iliac spine and just inferior to the inguinal ligament then is identified and prepared with antiseptic solution (Fig. 115-2). A 25-gauge, 1½-inch needle then is advanced slowly perpendicular to the skin until the needle is felt to pop through the fascia. A paresthesia often is elicited. After careful aspiration, 5 to 7 mL of 1.0% preservative-free lidocaine is injected in a fanlike manner as the needle pierces the fascia of the external oblique muscle. Care must be taken not to place the needle too deep and enter the peritoneal cavity and perforate the abdominal viscera.

If the pain has an inflammatory component, the local anesthetic is combined with 80 mg of methylprednisolone and is injected in incremental doses.

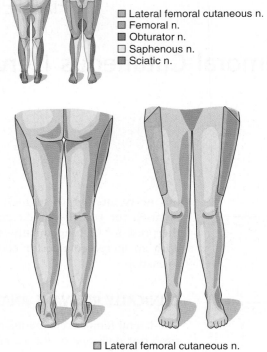

- ☐ Lateral femoral cutaneous n.
- ☐ Femoral n.
- ☐ Obturator n.
- ☐ Saphenous n.
- ☐ Sciatic n.

Figure 115-1.

☐ Lateral femoral cutaneous n.

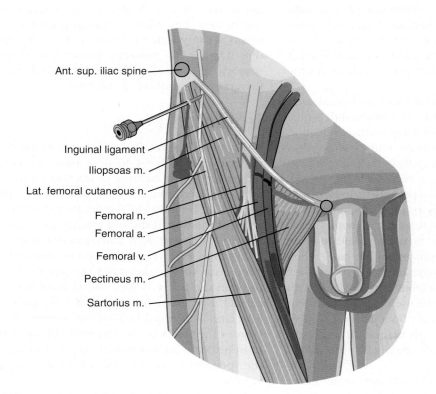

Ant. sup. iliac spine

Inguinal ligament

Iliopsoas m.

Lat. femoral cutaneous n.

Femoral n.

Femoral a.

Femoral v.

Pectineus m.

Sartorius m.

Figure 115-2.

Subsequent daily nerve blocks are carried out in a similar manner, substituting 40 mg of methylprednisolone for the initial 80-mg dose. After injection of the solution, pressure is applied to the injection site to decrease the incidence of postblock ecchymosis and hematoma formation, which can be dramatic, especially in the patient receiving anticoagulants.

SIDE EFFECTS AND COMPLICATIONS

The main side effect of lateral femoral cutaneous nerve block is postblock ecchymosis and hematoma. If the needle is placed too deep and enters the peritoneal cavity, perforation of the colon may result in the formation of intra-abdominal abscess and fistula formation. Early detection of infection is crucial to avoid potentially life-threatening sequelae. If the needle is placed too medial, blockade of the femoral nerve may occur and make ambulation difficult.

CLINICAL PEARLS

Lateral femoral cutaneous nerve block is a simple technique that can produce dramatic relief for patients suffering from the mentioned pain complaints. Neurolytic block with small quantities of phenol in glycerin or by cryoneurolysis or radiofrequency lesioning has been shown to provide long-term relief for patients suffering from chronic pain secondary to trauma to the lateral femoral cutaneous nerve and in whom more conservative treatments have been ineffectual. As mentioned earlier, pressure should be maintained on the injection site after the block to avoid ecchymosis and hematoma formation.

Lateral femoral cutaneous neuralgia often is misdiagnosed as either trochanteric bursitis or lumbar radiculopathy. Also known as meralgia paresthetica, lateral femoral cutaneous neuralgia is characterized as dysesthetic pain and numbness in the lateral thigh. The pain is made worse when sitting or squatting for long periods. This painful condition may also occur second-ary to compression on the nerve by wide belts or tool pouches. Blockade of the lateral femoral cutaneous nerve with local anesthetic should provide prompt relief of symptoms. Electromyography can help confirm the diagnosis. Therapeutic lateral femoral cutaneous nerve blocks with local anesthetic and steroid are extremely beneficial when treating meralgia paresthetica.

If a patient presents with pain suggestive of lateral femoral cutaneous neuralgia and lateral femoral cutaneous nerve blocks are ineffectual, a diagnosis of lesions more proximal in the lumbar plexus or L2-L3 radiculopathy should be considered. Such patients often respond to epidural steroid blocks. Electromyography and magnetic resonance imaging of the lumbar plexus are indicated in this patient population to help rule out other causes of lateral femoral cutaneous pain, including malignancy invading the lumbar plexus or epidural or vertebral metastatic disease at L2-L3.

CHAPTER 116

Obturator Nerve Block

CPT-2003 CODE

Unilateral	64550
Neurolytic	64640

Relative Value Units

Unilateral	8
Neurolytic	20

INDICATIONS

Obturator nerve block is useful in the evaluation and management of hip pain and spasm of the hip adductors thought to be subserved by the obturator nerve. The technique also is useful to provide surgical anesthesia for the lower extremity when combined with lateral femoral cutaneous, femoral, and sciatic nerve block. Obturator nerve block with local anesthetic can be used as a diagnostic tool during differential neural blockade on an anatomic basis in the evaluation of hip pain. If destruction of the obturator nerve is being considered, this technique is useful as a prognostic indicator of the degree of motor and sensory impairment that the patient may experience.

Obturator nerve block with local anesthetic may be used to palliate acute pain emergencies, including postoperative pain relief, while waiting for pharmacologic methods to become effective. Obturator nerve block with local anesthetic also is useful in the management of hip adductor spasm, which may make perineal care or urinary catheterization difficult. Obturator nerve block with local anesthetic and steroid also is useful in the treatment of persistent hip pain when the pain is thought to be secondary to inflammation or entrapment of the obturator nerve. Destruction of the obturator nerve is occasionally indicated for the palliation of persistent hip pain after trauma to the hip that is mediated by the obturator nerve.

CLINICALLY RELEVANT ANATOMY

The obturator nerve provides most of the innervation to the hip joint. It is derived from the posterior divisions of the L2, L3, and L4 nerves. The nerve leaves the medial border psoas muscle and courses inferiorly to pass the pelvis, where it joins the obturator vessels to travel via the obturator canal to enter the thigh. The nerve then divides into an anterior and posterior branch (Fig. 116-1). The anterior branch supplies an articular branch to provide sensory innervation to the hip joint, motor branches to the superficial hip adductors, and a cutaneous branch to the medial aspect of the distal thigh (Fig. 116-2). The posterior branch provides motor innervation to the deep hip adductors and an articular branch to the posterior knee joint.

TECHNIQUE

The patient is placed in the supine position with the legs slightly abducted. The pubic tubercle on the involved side is identified by palpation. A point 1 inch lateral and 1 inch inferior to the pubic tubercle is then identified and prepared with antiseptic solution. A 22-gauge, 3-inch needle is then slowly advanced perpendicular to the skin until the needle is felt to impinge on the superior pubic ramus (Fig. 116-3). The depth of bony contact is noted, and the needle is withdrawn and redirected laterally and slightly inferiorly (Fig. 116-4). The needle is advanced about $\frac{3}{4}$ to 1 inch deeper to place the needle tip in the obturator canal. A paresthesia in the distribution of the obturator nerve may be elicited. After careful aspiration, 10 to 15 mL of 1.0% preservative-free lidocaine is injected. Care must be taken not to place the needle in the obturator artery or vein.

If the pain has an inflammatory component, the local anesthetic is combined with 80 mg of methylprednisolone and is injected in incremental doses. Subsequent daily nerve blocks are carried out in a similar manner, substituting 40 mg of methylprednisolone for the initial 80-mg dose. After injection of the solution, pressure is applied to the injection site to decrease the

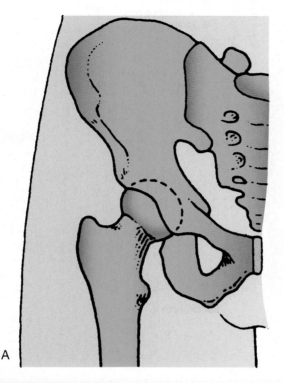

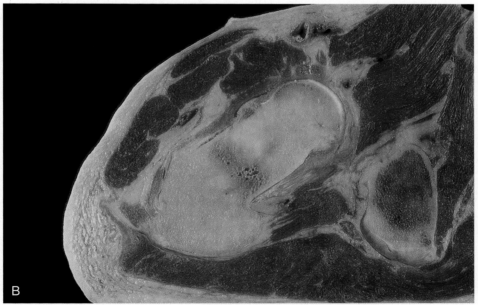

Figure 116-1.
(From Kang HS, Resnick D, Ahn J: MRI of the Extremities: An Anatomic
Atlas, 2nd ed. Philadelphia, WB Saunders 2002, p 251.)

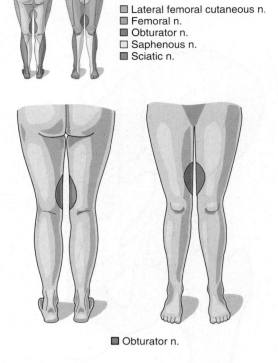

Lateral femoral cutaneous n.
Femoral n.
Obturator n.
Saphenous n.
Sciatic n.

Figure 116-2.

Obturator n.

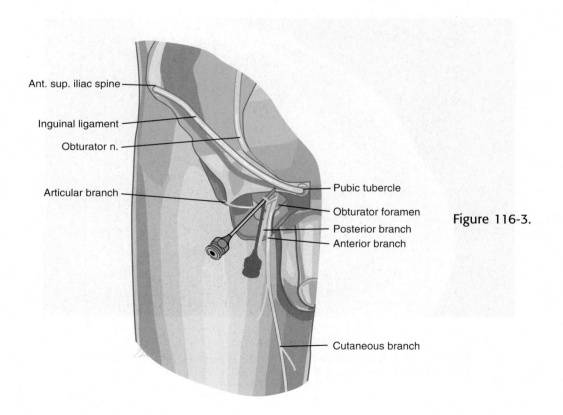

Ant. sup. iliac spine

Inguinal ligament

Obturator n.

Articular branch

Pubic tubercle

Obturator foramen
Posterior branch
Anterior branch

Figure 116-3.

Cutaneous branch

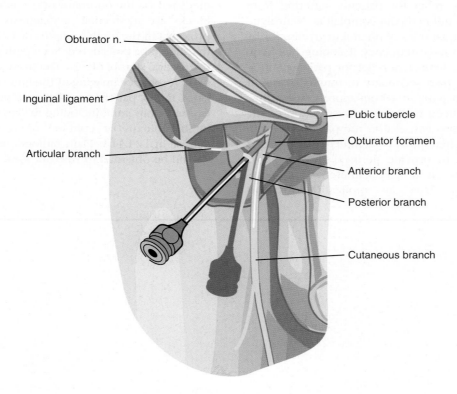

Figure 116-4.

incidence of postblock ecchymosis and hematoma formation.

SIDE EFFECTS AND COMPLICATIONS

The main side effect of obturator nerve block is post-block ecchymosis and hematoma. Because of proximity to the obturator artery and vein, intravascular injection remains an ever-present possibility. As mentioned earlier, pressure should be maintained on the injection site after the block to avoid ecchymosis and hematoma formation.

CLINICAL PEARLS

Obturator nerve block is a simple technique that can produce dramatic relief for patients suffering from the previously mentioned pain complaints. Neurolytic block with small quantities of phenol in glycerin or by cryoneurolysis or radiofrequency lesioning has been shown to provide long-term relief for patients suffering from chronic pain secondary to trauma or tumor involving the hip joint in whom more conservative treatments have been ineffectual. Destruction of the obturator nerve also is useful in the palliation of hip adductor spasm after spinal cord injury or stroke that limits the ability to provide perineal care or allow sexual intercourse or urinary catheterization. Botulinum toxin may have an application for this indication.

If a patient presents with pain that is thought to be mediated via the obturator nerve, and obturator nerve blocks are ineffectual, a diagnosis of lesions more proximal in the lumbar plexus or L2-L3-L4 radiculopathy should be considered. Such patients often respond to epidural steroid blocks. Electromyography and magnetic resonance imaging of the lumbar plexus are indicated in this patient population to help rule out other causes of hip pain, including malignancy invading the lumbar plexus or epidural or vertebral metastatic disease at L2-L3-L4. Plain radiographs of the hip also should be obtained to rule out local pathology.

CHAPTER 117

Sciatic Nerve Block: Anterior Approach

CPT-2009 CODE	
Unilateral	64445
Neurolytic	64640

Relative Value Units	
Unilateral	12
Neurolytic	20

INDICATIONS

Sciatic nerve block via the anterior approach is used for patients who cannot assume the Sims' or lithotomy position because of lower extremity trauma. Sciatic nerve block is useful in the evaluation and management of distal lower extremity pain thought to be subserved by the sciatic nerve. The technique also is useful to provide surgical anesthesia for the distal lower extremity when combined with lateral femoral cutaneous, femoral, and obturator nerve block or lumbar plexus block. It is used for this indication primarily with patients who would not tolerate the sympathetic changes induced by spinal or epidural anesthesia and who need distal extremity amputations or débridement.

Sciatic nerve block with local anesthetic can be used diagnostically during differential neural blockade on an anatomic basis in the evaluation of distal lower extremity pain. If destruction of the sciatic nerve is being considered, this technique is useful as a prognostic indicator of the degree of motor and sensory impairment that the patient may experience. Sciatic nerve block with local anesthetic may be used to palliate acute pain emergencies, including distal lower extremity fractures and postoperative pain relief, while waiting for pharmacologic methods to become effective. Sciatic nerve block with local anesthetic and steroid is occasionally used in the treatment of persistent distal lower extremity pain when the pain is thought to be secondary to inflammation or when entrapment of the sciatic nerve at the level of the lesser trochanter is suspected. Destruction of the sciatic nerve is occasionally indicated for the palliation of persistent distal lower extremity pain secondary to invasive tumor that is mediated by the sciatic nerve and has not responded to more conservative measures.

CLINICALLY RELEVANT ANATOMY

The sciatic nerve innervates the distal lower extremity and foot, with the exception of the medial aspects of the calf and foot, which are subserved by the saphenous nerve. The largest nerve in the body, the sciatic nerve is derived from the L4, L5, and S1-S3 nerve roots (Fig. 117-1). The roots fuse together in front of the anterior surface of the lateral sacrum on the anterior surface of the piriform muscle. The nerve travels inferiorly and leaves the pelvis just below the piriform muscle via the sciatic notch (Fig. 117-2). The sciatic nerve lies anterior to the gluteus maximus muscle and, at this muscle's lower border, lies halfway between the greater trochanter and the ischial tuberosity. The sciatic nerve courses downward past the lesser trochanter to lie posterior and medial to the femur. In the mid-thigh, the nerve gives off branches to the hamstring muscles and the adductor magnus muscle. In most patients, the nerve divides to form the tibial and common peroneal nerves in the upper portion of the popliteal fossa, although these nerves sometimes remain separate through their entire course. The tibial nerve continues downward to provide innervation to the distal lower extremity, whereas the common peroneal nerve travels laterally to innervate a portion of the knee joint and, via its lateral cutaneous branch, to provide sensory innervation to the back and lateral side of the upper calf (Fig. 117-3).

TECHNIQUE

The patient is placed in the supine position with the leg in neutral position. The greater trochanter and the crease of the groin on the involved side are identified by palpation. An imaginary line is then drawn parallel to the crease of the groin that runs from the greater trochanter to the center of the thigh. This center point is then

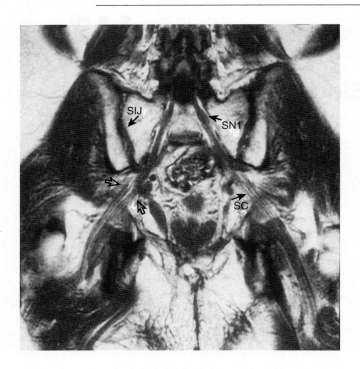

Figure 117-1.
Coronal T1-weighted image. Each S1 nerve (SN1) is joined by the lumbosacral trunk, S2 trunk, and S3 nerve near the inferior aspect of the sacroiliac joints (SIJ), giving rise to the sciatic nerve (SC). The region of the greater sciatic foramen is indicated by the *open arrows*. (From Stark DD, Bradley WG: Magnetic Resonance Imaging, 3rd ed. St. Louis, Mosby, 1999, p 1908.)

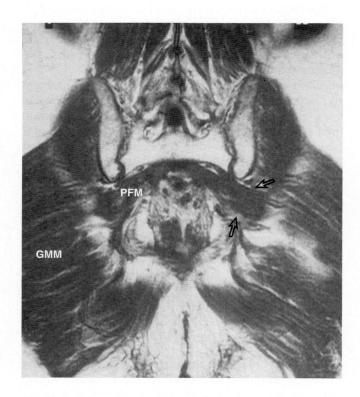

Figure 117-2.
Coronal T1-weighted image, more posterior than the image in Figure 117-1. Each piriformis muscle (PFM) also traverses the greater sciatic foramen (*arrows*). GMM, gluteus maximus muscle. (From Stark DD, Bradley WG: Magnetic Resonance Imaging, 3rd ed. St. Louis, Mosby, 1999, p 1908.)

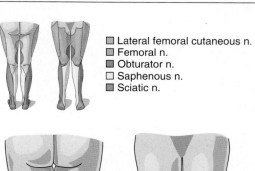

☐ Lateral femoral cutaneous n.
☐ Femoral n.
☐ Obturator n.
☐ Saphenous n.
☐ Sciatic n.

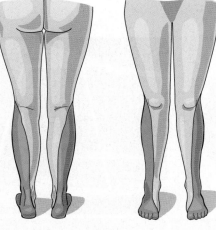

Figure 117-3.

☐ Sciatic n.

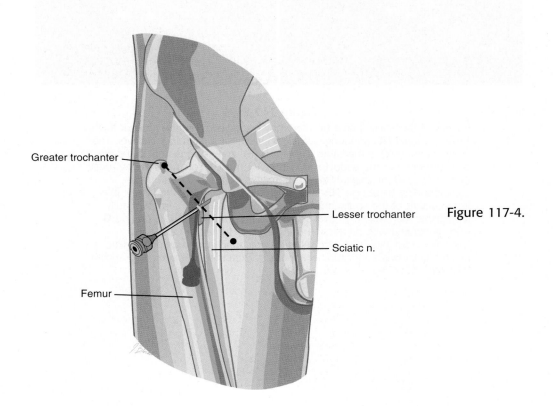

Greater trochanter

Lesser trochanter

Sciatic n.

Figure 117-4.

Femur

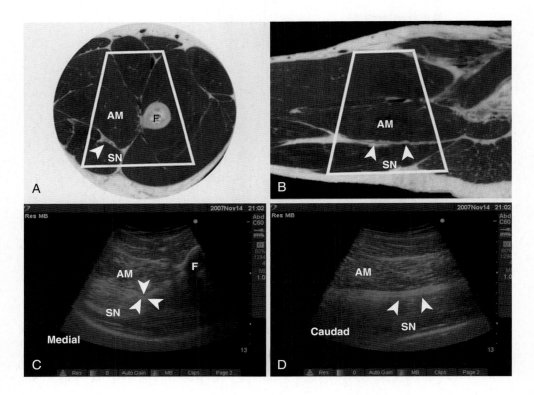

Figure 117-5.

Images of the sciatic nerve (indicated by *arrowheads*) in the anterior thigh. Cross-sectional (**A**) and longitudinal (**B**) views of a thigh in a cadaver. The sciatic nerve (SN) is medial to the femur (F), and its consistent cable-like structure deep to the adductor magus (AM) muscle continues during most of its course in the thigh. Ultrasound images from a live adult using corresponding transverse (**C**) and longitudinal views (**D**). The large cable-like structure of the sciatic nerve in the longitudinal view is more readily identifiable than the small oval shadow in the transverse view. (**A** and **B** were generated with permission using Visible Human Visualization Software. From Tsui BCH, Ozelsel TJP: Ultrasound-guided anterior sciatic nerve block using a longitudinal approach: Expanding the view. Reg Anesth Pain Med 33:275-276, 2008.)

identified and prepared with antiseptic solution. A 25-gauge, 3½-inch needle is then slowly advanced perpendicular to the skin until it impinges on the femur. The needle is then walked slightly superiorly and medially until it walks off the top of the lesser trochanter (Fig. 117-4). A paresthesia in the distribution of the sciatic nerve will be elicited; if a nerve stimulator is used, dorsiflexion and plantar flexion of the foot will be noted. The patient should be warned to expect paresthesia and should be told to say "there!" immediately on perceiving the paresthesia. Paresthesia usually is elicited at a depth 1 inch beyond initial bony contact. Once paresthesia is elicited in the distribution of the sciatic nerve, the needle is withdrawn 1 mm, and the patient is observed to rule out any persistent paresthesia. If no persistent paresthesia is present, and after careful aspiration, 15 to 18 mL of 1.0% preservative-free lidocaine is slowly injected. Care must be taken to not advance the needle into the substance of the nerve during the injection and inject solution intraneurally. Ultrasound guidance may be useful in assisting in needle placement if difficulty is encountered (Fig. 117-5).

If the pain has an inflammatory component, the local anesthetic is combined with 80 mg of methylprednisolone and is injected in incremental doses. Subsequent daily nerve blocks are carried out in a similar manner, substituting 40 mg of methylprednisolone for the initial 80-mg dose. After injection of the solution, pressure is applied to the injection site to decrease the incidence of postblock ecchymosis and hematoma formation.

SIDE EFFECTS AND COMPLICATIONS

The main side effect of sciatic nerve block is postblock ecchymosis and hematoma. As mentioned earlier, pressure should be maintained on the injection site after the block to avoid ecchymosis and hematoma formation. Because this technique elicits paresthesia, needle-induced trauma to the sciatic nerve remains possible. By advancing the needle slowly and withdrawing the needle slightly away from the nerve, one can avoid needle-induced trauma to the sciatic nerve.

CLINICAL PEARLS

Sciatic nerve block via the anterior approach is a simple technique that can produce dramatic relief for patients suffering from the previously mentioned pain complaints. The literature has implied that the sciatic nerve is more prone to needle-induced trauma with resultant persistent paresthesia than are other peripheral nerves. Whether this is true or simply conjecture remains to be seen. In any event, careful preblock neurologic assessment is important to avoid the attribution of preexisting neurologic deficits to the sciatic nerve block. These assessments are especially important in patients who have sustained trauma to the pelvis or lower extremity in whom sciatic nerve blocks are being used for acute pain control.

It should be remembered that the most common causes of sciatica are herniated lumbar disk and degenerative arthritis of the lumbar spine, not disorders involving the sciatic nerve per se. Electromyography and magnetic resonance imaging of the lumbar spine, combined with the clinical history and physical examination, help to sort out the etiology of sciatic pain.

CHAPTER 118

Sciatic Nerve Block: Posterior Approach

CPT-2009 CODE

Unilateral	64445
Neurolytic	64640

Relative Value Units

Unilateral	12
Neurolytic	20

INDICATIONS

Sciatic nerve block via the posterior approach is useful in the evaluation and management of distal lower extremity pain thought to be subserved by the sciatic nerve. The technique also is useful to provide surgical anesthesia for the distal lower extremity when combined with lateral femoral cutaneous, femoral and obturator nerve block, or lumbar plexus block. It is used for this indication primarily for patients who would not tolerate the sympathetic changes induced by spinal or epidural anesthesia and who need distal extremity amputations or débridement.

Sciatic nerve block with local anesthetic can be used diagnostically during differential neural blockade on an anatomic basis in the evaluation of distal lower extremity pain. If destruction of the sciatic nerve is being considered, this technique is useful as a prognostic indicator of the degree of motor and sensory impairment that the patient may experience. Sciatic nerve block with local anesthetic may be used to palliate acute pain emergencies, including distal lower extremity fractures and postoperative pain relief, while waiting for pharmacologic methods to become effective. Sciatic nerve block with local anesthetic and steroid is occasionally used in the treatment of persistent distal lower extremity pain when the pain is thought to be secondary to inflammation or when entrapment of the sciatic nerve by the piriform muscle is suspected (Fig. 118-1). Destruction of the sciatic nerve is occasionally indicated for the palliation of persistent distal lower extremity pain secondary to invasive tumor that is mediated by the sciatic nerve and has not responded to more conservative measures.

CLINICALLY RELEVANT ANATOMY

The sciatic nerve innervates the distal lower extremity and foot with the exception of the medial aspect of the calf and foot, which are subserved by the saphenous nerve. The largest nerve in the body, the sciatic nerve is derived from the L4, L5, and the S1-S3 nerve roots (Fig. 118-2). The roots fuse together in front of the anterior surface of the lateral sacrum on the anterior surface of the piriform muscle. The nerve travels inferiorly and leaves the pelvis just below the piriform muscle via the sciatic notch (Fig. 118-3). The sciatic nerve lies anterior to the gluteus maximus muscle and, at this muscle's lower border, lies halfway between the greater trochanter and the ischial tuberosity. The sciatic nerve courses downward past the lesser trochanter to lie posterior and medial to the femur. In the mid-thigh, the nerve gives off branches to the hamstring muscles and the adductor magnus muscle. In most patients, the nerve divides to form the tibial and common peroneal nerves in the upper portion of the popliteal fossa, although these nerves sometimes remain separate through their entire course. The tibial nerve continues downward to innervate the distal lower extremity, whereas the common peroneal nerve travels laterally to innervate a portion of the knee joint and, via its lateral cutaneous branch, provide sensory innervation to the back and lateral side of the upper calf (see Fig. 118-2).

TECHNIQUE

The patient is placed in the Sims' position with the upper leg flexed. The greater trochanter and the ischial tuberosity on the involved side are identified by palpation. The sciatic nerve lies midway between these two bony landmarks (see Fig. 118-3). This midpoint is then identified and prepared with antiseptic solution. A 25-gauge, 3½-inch needle is then slowly advanced perpendicular to the skin until paresthesia is elicited; if a nerve

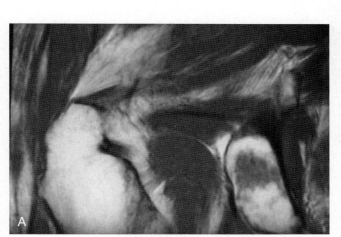

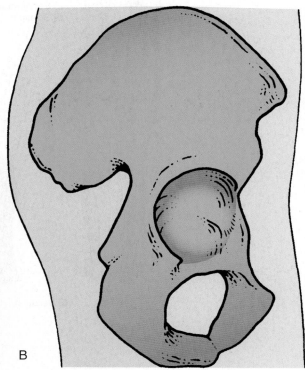

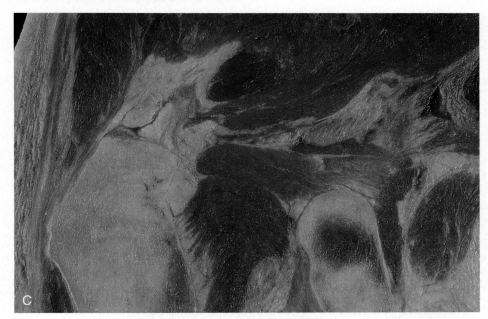

Figure 118-1.
(From Kang HS, Resnick D, Ahn J: MRI of the Extremities: An Anatomic
Atlas, 2nd ed. Philadelphia, WB Saunders, 2002, p 221.)

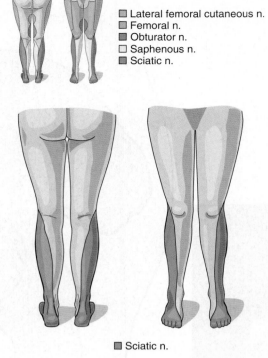

Lateral femoral cutaneous n.
Femoral n.
Obturator n.
Saphenous n.
Sciatic n.

Figure 118-2.

Sciatic n.

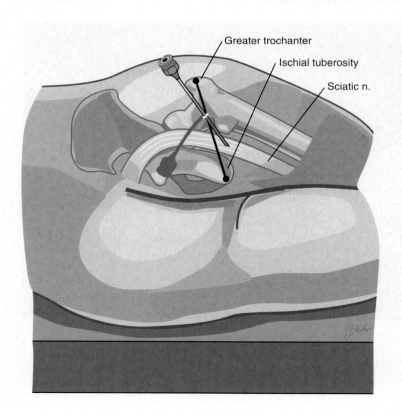

Greater trochanter
Ischial tuberosity
Sciatic n.

Figure 118-3.

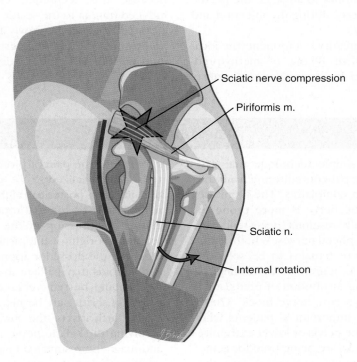

Piriformis Syndrome

Figure 118-4.

stimulator is used, dorsiflexion and plantar flexion of the foot are noted. The patient should be warned to expect a paresthesia and should be told to say "there!" immediately on perceiving the paresthesia. Paresthesia usually is elicited at a depth of $2\frac{1}{2}$ to 3 inches. If the needle is felt to impinge on the bone of the sciatic notch, the needle is withdrawn and redirected laterally and slightly superiorly until paresthesia is elicited. Once paresthesia is elicited in the distribution of the sciatic nerve, the needle is withdrawn 1 mm, and the patient is observed to rule out any persistent paresthesia. If no persistent paresthesia is present, and after careful aspiration, 15 to 18 mL of 1.0% preservative-free lidocaine is slowly injected. Care must be taken not to advance the needle into the substance of the nerve during the injection and inject solution intraneurally.

If the pain has an inflammatory component, the local anesthetic is combined with 80 mg of methylprednisolone and is injected in incremental doses. Subsequent daily nerve blocks are carried out in a similar manner, substituting 40 mg of methylprednisolone for the initial 80-mg dose. After injection of the solution, pressure is applied to the injection site to decrease the incidence of postblock ecchymosis and hematoma formation.

SIDE EFFECTS AND COMPLICATIONS

The main side effect of sciatic nerve block is postblock ecchymosis and hematoma. As mentioned earlier, pressure should be maintained on the injection site after the block to avoid ecchymosis and hematoma formation. Because this technique elicits paresthesia, needle-induced trauma to the sciatic nerve remains possible. By advancing the needle slowly and withdrawing the needle slightly away from the nerve, one can avoid needle-induced trauma to the sciatic nerve.

CLINICAL PEARLS

Sciatic nerve block is a simple technique that can produce dramatic relief for patients suffering from the previously mentioned pain complaints. The literature has implied that the sciatic nerve is more prone to needle-induced trauma with resultant persistent paresthesia than are other peripheral nerves. Whether this is true or simply conjecture remains to be seen. In any event, careful preblock neurologic assessment is important to avoid the later attribution of preexisting neurologic deficits to the sciatic nerve block. These assessments are especially important in patients who have sustained trauma to the pelvis or lower extremity in whom sciatic nerve blocks are being used for acute pain control. In such patients, movement into the Sims' position may be difficult, and the anterior approach to sciatic nerve block may be a better alternative.

Entrapment of the sciatic nerve by the piriform muscle has been described and is called the *piriformis syndrome*. The pain of piriformis syndrome is characteristically localized to the gluteal muscle with radiation into the posterior thigh (Fig. 118-4). The pain is made worse by internal rotation of the femur, which causes compression of the sciatic nerve against the tendinous origin of the piriform muscle. Sciatic nerve block via the posterior approach with local anesthetic and steroids may palliate the painful condition.

It should be remembered that the most common causes of sciatica are herniated lumbar disk and degenerative arthritis of the lumbar spine, not disorders involving the sciatic nerve per se. Electromyography and magnetic resonance imaging of the lumbar spine, combined with the information gleaned from clinical history and physical examination, will help to sort out the etiology of sciatic pain.

CHAPTER 119

Sciatic Nerve Block: Lithotomy Approach

CPT-2009 CODE	
Unilateral	64445
Neurolytic	64640

Relative Value Units	
Unilateral	12
Neurolytic	20

INDICATIONS

Sciatic nerve block via the lithotomy approach is used for patients who cannot assume the Sims' position because of lower extremity trauma. Sciatic nerve block is useful in the evaluation and management of distal lower extremity pain thought to be subserved by the sciatic nerve. The technique also is useful to provide surgical anesthesia for the distal lower extremity when combined with lateral femoral cutaneous, femoral, and obturator nerve block or lumbar plexus block. It is used for this indication primarily with patients who would not tolerate the sympathetic changes induced by spinal or epidural anesthesia and who need distal extremity amputations or débridement.

Sciatic nerve block with local anesthetic can be used diagnostically during differential neural blockade on an anatomic basis in the evaluation of distal lower extremity pain. If destruction of the sciatic nerve is being considered, this technique is useful as a prognostic indicator of the degree of motor and sensory impairment that the patient may experience. Sciatic nerve block with local anesthetic may be used to palliate acute pain emergencies, including distal lower extremity fractures and post-operative pain relief, while waiting for pharmacologic methods to become effective. Sciatic nerve block with local anesthetic and steroid is occasionally used in the treatment of persistent distal lower extremity pain when the pain is thought to be secondary to inflammation or when distal entrapment of the sciatic nerve is suspected. Destruction of the sciatic nerve is occasionally indicated for the palliation of persistent distal lower extremity pain secondary to invasive tumor that is mediated by the sciatic nerve and has not responded to more conservative measures.

CLINICALLY RELEVANT ANATOMY

The sciatic nerve innervates the distal lower extremity and foot with the exception of the medial aspect of the calf and foot, which are subserved by the saphenous nerve. The largest nerve in the body, the sciatic nerve, is derived from the L4, L5, and S1-S3 nerve roots (see Fig. 118-2). The roots fuse together in front of the anterior surface of the lateral sacrum on the anterior surface of the piriform muscle. The nerve travels inferiorly and leaves the pelvis just below the piriform muscle via the sciatic notch (see Fig. 118-3). The sciatic nerve lies anterior to the gluteus maximus muscle and, at this muscle's lower border, lies halfway between the greater trochanter and the ischial tuberosity (Fig. 119-1). The sciatic nerve courses downward past the lesser trochanter to lie posterior and medial to the femur. In the mid-thigh, the nerve gives off branches to the hamstring muscles and the adductor magnus muscle. In most patients, the nerve divides to form the tibial and common peroneal nerves in the upper portion of the popliteal fossa, although these nerves sometimes remain separate through their entire course. The tibial nerve continues downward to innervate the distal lower extremity, whereas the common peroneal nerve travels laterally to innervate a portion of the knee joint and, via its lateral cutaneous branch, provide sensory innervation to the back and lateral side of the upper calf (Fig. 119-2).

TECHNIQUE

The patient is placed in the supine position with the hip maximally flexed. A point just above the gluteal fold and in the middle of the thigh is identified and prepared with antiseptic solution. A 25-gauge, $3\frac{1}{2}$-inch needle is then slowly advanced perpendicular to the skin toward the femur until a paresthesia in the distribution of the sciatic

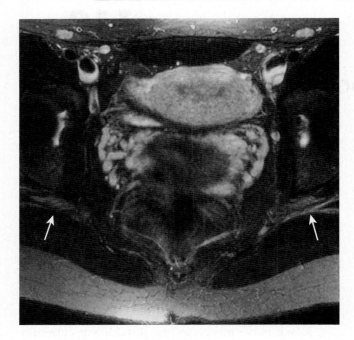

Figure 119-1.
Magnetic resonance neurography of the normal sciatic nerve. Axial, T2-weighted, fast spin-echo image with fat suppression at the level of the femoral head. The striated appearance produced by the nerve fascicles within the sciatic nerves (*arrows*) is shown. (Courtesy of Dr. Kenneth Maravilla, University of Washington School of Medicine.)

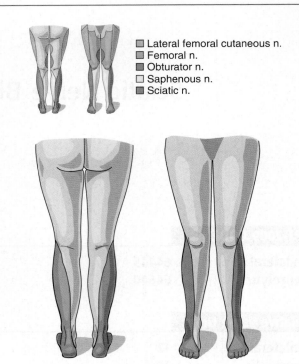

☐ Lateral femoral cutaneous n.
☐ Femoral n.
☐ Obturator n.
☐ Saphenous n.
☐ Sciatic n.

☐ Sciatic n.

Figure 119-2.

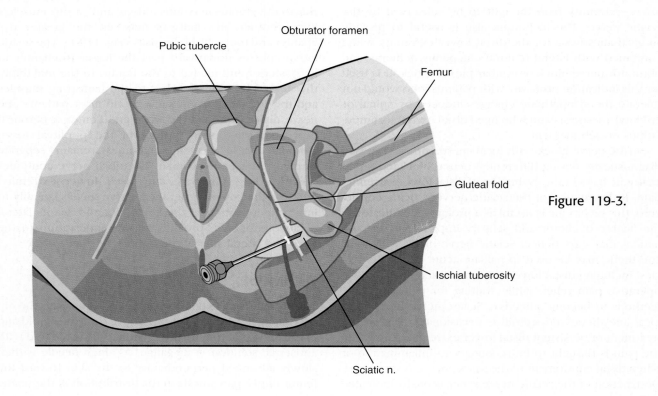

Figure 119-3.

nerve is elicited; if a nerve stimulator is used, dorsiflexion and plantar flexion of the foot will be noted (Fig. 119-3). The patient should be warned to expect a paresthesia and should be told to say "there!" immediately on perceiving the paresthesia. A paresthesia usually is elicited at a depth of about $2\frac{1}{2}$ inches. If a paresthesia is not elicited, the needle is withdrawn and redirected medially until a paresthesia is elicited. Once a paresthesia is elicited in the distribution of the sciatic nerve, the needle is withdrawn 1 mm, and the patient is observed to rule out any persistent paresthesia. If no persistent paresthesia is present, and after careful aspiration, 12 to 15 mL of 1.0% preservative-free lidocaine is slowly injected. Care must be taken not to advance the needle into the substance of the nerve during the injection and inject solution intraneurally.

If the pain has an inflammatory component, the local anesthetic is combined with 80 mg of methylprednisolone and is injected in incremental doses. Subsequent daily nerve blocks are carried out in a similar manner, substituting 40 mg of methylprednisolone for the initial 80-mg dose. After injection of the solution, pressure is applied to the injection site to decrease the incidence of postblock ecchymosis and hematoma formation.

SIDE EFFECTS AND COMPLICATIONS

The main side effect of sciatic nerve block is postblock ecchymosis and hematoma. As mentioned earlier, pressure should be maintained on the injection site after the block to avoid ecchymosis and hematoma formation. Because this technique elicits a paresthesia, needle-induced trauma to the sciatic nerve remains possible. By advancing the needle slowly and withdrawing the needle slightly away from the nerve before injection, one can avoid needle-induced trauma to the sciatic nerve.

CLINICAL PEARLS

Sciatic nerve block via the lithotomy approach is a simple technique that can produce dramatic relief for patients suffering from the previously mentioned pain complaints. The literature has implied that the sciatic nerve is more prone to needle-induced trauma with resultant persistent paresthesia than are other peripheral nerves. Whether this is true or simply conjecture remains to be seen. In any event, careful preblock neurologic assessment is important to avoid later attribution of preexisting neurologic deficits to the sciatic nerve block. These assessments are especially important in patients who have sustained trauma to the pelvis or lower extremity in whom sciatic nerve blocks are being used for acute pain control.

It should be remembered that the most common causes of sciatica are herniated lumbar disk and degenerative arthritis of the lumbar spine, not disorders involving the sciatic nerve per se. Electromyography and magnetic resonance imaging of the lumbar spine, combined with information gleaned from the clinical history and physical examination, will help to sort out the etiology of sciatic pain.

CHAPTER 120

Tibial Nerve Block at the Knee

CPT-2009 CODE	
Unilateral	64450
Neurolytic	64640

Relative Value Units	
Unilateral	10
Neurolytic	20

INDICATIONS

Tibial nerve block at the knee is useful in the evaluation and management of foot and ankle pain thought to be subserved by the tibial nerve. The technique is also useful to provide surgical anesthesia for the distal lower extremity when combined with common peroneal and saphenous nerve block or lumbar plexus block. It is used for this indication primarily in patients who would not tolerate the sympathetic changes induced by spinal or epidural anesthesia and who need distal lower extremity surgery, such as débridement or distal amputation.

Tibial nerve block at the knee with local anesthetic can be used as a diagnostic tool during differential neural blockade on an anatomic basis in the evaluation of lower extremity pain. If destruction of the tibial nerve is being considered, this technique is useful as a prognostic indicator of the degree of motor and sensory impairment that the patient may experience. Tibial nerve block at the knee with local anesthetic may be used to palliate acute pain emergencies, including ankle and foot fractures, and pharmacologic methods to become effective. Tibial nerve block at the knee with local anesthetic and steroid is occasionally used in the treatment of persistent ankle and foot pain when the pain is thought to be secondary to inflammation or when entrapment of the tibial nerve at the popliteal fossa is suspected. Tibial nerve block at the knee with local anesthetic and steroid is also indicated in the palliation of pain and motor dysfunction associated with diabetic neuropathy. Destruction of the tibial nerve block at the knee is occasionally used in the palliation of persistent lower extremity pain secondary to invasive tumor that is mediated by the tibial nerve and has not responded to more conservative measures.

CLINICALLY RELEVANT ANATOMY

The tibial nerve is one of the two major continuations of the sciatic nerve, the other being the common peroneal nerve. The tibial nerve provides sensory innervation to the posterior portion of the calf, the heel, and the medial plantar surface. The tibial nerve splits from the sciatic nerve at the superior margin of the popliteal fossa and descends in a slightly medial course through the popliteal fossa (Figs. 120-1 and 120-2). The tibial nerve block at the knee lies just beneath the popliteal fascia and is readily accessible for neural blockade. The tibial nerve continues its downward course, running between the two heads of the gastrocnemius muscle, passing deep to the soleus muscle. The nerve courses medially between the Achilles tendon and the medial malleolus, where it divides into the medial and lateral plantar nerves, providing sensory innervation to the heel and medial plantar surface (Figs. 120-3 and 120-4). The tibial nerve is occasionally subject to compression at this point and is known as posterior tarsal tunnel syndrome.

TECHNIQUE

The patient is placed in the prone position with the leg slightly flexed. The skin crease of the knee and margins of the semitendinous and biceps femoris muscles in the upper popliteal fossa are palpated. The margins of these muscles can be more easily identified by having the patient flex his or her leg under resistance. An imaginary triangle is envisioned, with the apex being the convergence of these two muscles and the base being the skin crease of the knee (Fig. 120-5). At a point in the center of this imaginary apex, the skin is prepared with antiseptic solution. A 25-gauge, $1\frac{1}{2}$-inch needle is then slowly advanced perpendicular to the skin through this point toward the tibial nerve until a paresthesia is elicited in the distribution of the tibial nerve. The patient should

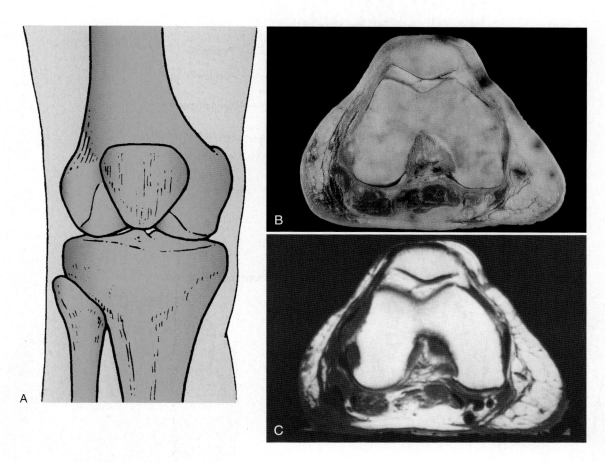

Figure 120-1.
(From Kang HS, Resnick D, Ahn J: MRI of the Extremities: An Anatomic
Atlas, 2nd ed. Philadelphia, WB Saunders 2002, p 212.)

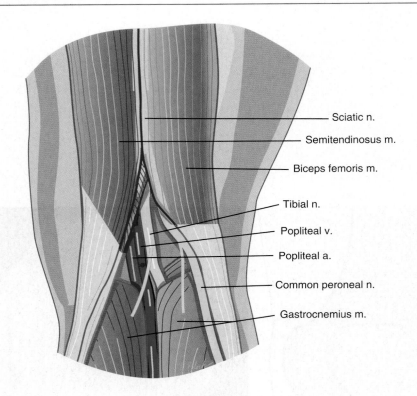

Sciatic n.

Semitendinosus m.

Biceps femoris m.

Tibial n.

Popliteal v.

Popliteal a.

Common peroneal n.

Gastrocnemius m.

Figure 120-2.

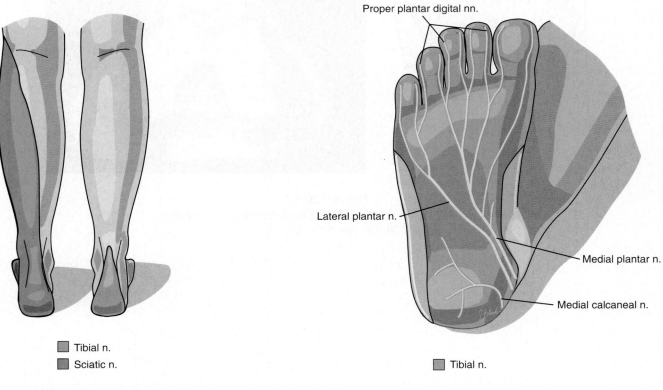

Tibial n.
Sciatic n.

Figure 120-3.

Proper plantar digital nn.

Lateral plantar n.

Medial plantar n.

Medial calcaneal n.

Tibial n.

Figure 120-4.

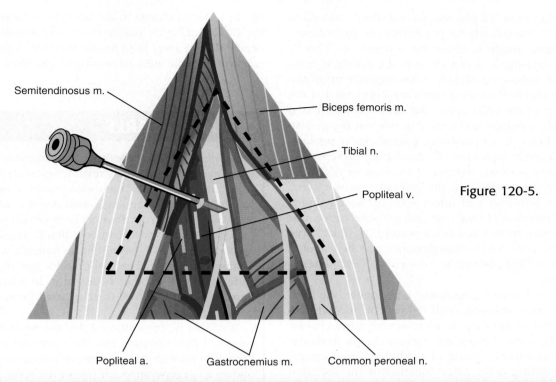

Semitendinosus m.

Biceps femoris m.

Tibial n.

Popliteal v.

Popliteal a.

Gastrocnemius m.

Common peroneal n.

Figure 120-5.

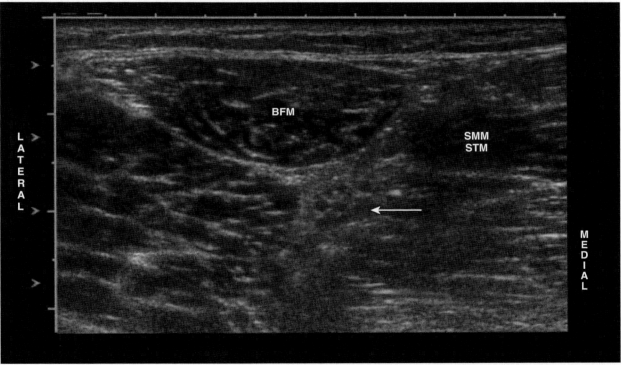

Figure 120-6.

Ultrasound image of the popliteal fossa taken with an Acuson C256, 15-MHz probe. The *arrow* points to the sciatic nerve, with the biceps femoris muscle (BFM) superolateral and the semimembranosus muscle (SMM) and semitendinosus muscle (STM) superomedial. (From Girdharry D, McQuillan P: Popliteal fossa block. Tech Reg Anesth Pain Manage 8:164-166, 2004.)

be warned to expect a paresthesia and should be told to say "there!" immediately on perceiving the paresthesia.

Paresthesia usually is elicited at a depth of ½ to ¾ inch. If a paresthesia is not elicited, the needle is withdrawn and redirected slightly more medially until paresthesia is obtained. Once a paresthesia is elicited in the distribution of the tibial nerve, the needle is withdrawn 1 mm, and the patient is observed to rule out any persistent paresthesia. If no persistent paresthesia is present, and after careful aspiration, 8 mL of 1.0% preservative-free lidocaine is slowly injected. Care must be taken not to advance the needle into the substance of the nerve during the injection and inject solution intraneurally. Given the proximity to the common peroneal nerve, this nerve may also be blocked when performing tibial nerve block at the knee. Ultrasound guidance may be useful in assisting in needle placement if difficulty is encountered (Fig. 120-6).

If the pain has an inflammatory component, the local anesthetic is combined with 80 mg of methylprednisolone and is injected in incremental doses. Subsequent daily nerve blocks are carried out in a similar manner, substituting 40 mg of methylprednisolone for the initial 80-mg dose. After injection of the solution, pressure is applied to the injection site to decrease the incidence of postblock ecchymosis and hematoma formation.

SIDE EFFECTS AND COMPLICATIONS

The main side effect of tibial nerve block at the knee is postblock ecchymosis and hematoma. As mentioned earlier, pressure should be maintained on the injection site after the block to avoid ecchymosis and hematoma formation. Because this technique elicits paresthesia, needle-induced trauma to the tibial nerve remains possible. By advancing the needle slowly and withdrawing the needle slightly away from the nerve before injection, one can avoid needle-induced trauma to the tibial nerve.

CLINICAL PEARLS

Tibial nerve block at the knee is a simple technique that can produce dramatic relief for patients suffering from the previously mentioned pain complaints. Careful preblock neurologic assessment is important to avoid the later attribution of preexisting neurologic deficits to the tibial nerve block. These assessments are especially important in patients who have sustained trauma to the foot or ankle and in patients suffering from diabetic neuropathy in whom tibial nerve block at the knee is being used for acute pain control.

It should be remembered that the most common causes of pain radiating into the lower extremity are herniated lumbar disk and nerve impingement secondary to degenerative arthritis of the spine, not disorders involving the tibial nerve per se. Other pain syndromes that may be confused with tibial nerve entrapment include lesions above the origin of the tibial nerve, such as lesions of the sciatic nerve, and lesions below the division of the tibial nerve, such as posterior tarsal tunnel syndrome. Electromyography and magnetic resonance imaging of the lumbar spine, combined with information gleaned from the clinical history and physical examination, will help to sort out the etiology of distal lower pain.

CHAPTER 121

Tibial Nerve Block at the Ankle

CPT-2009 CODE	
Unilateral	64450
Neurolytic	64640

Relative Value Units	
Unilateral	10
Neurolytic	20

INDICATIONS

Tibial nerve block at the ankle is useful in the evaluation and management of foot and ankle pain thought to be subserved by the tibial nerve. The technique also is useful to provide surgical anesthesia for the ankle and foot when combined with common peroneal and saphenous nerve block or lumbar plexus block. It is used for this indication primarily in patients who would not tolerate the sympathetic changes induced by spinal or epidural anesthesia and who need distal lower extremity surgery, such as débridement or distal amputation.

Tibial nerve block at the ankle with local anesthetic can be used as a diagnostic tool during differential neural blockade on an anatomic basis in the evaluation of lower extremity pain. If destruction of the tibial nerve is being considered, this technique is useful as a prognostic indicator of the degree of motor and sensory impairment. Tibial nerve block at the ankle with local anesthetic may be used to palliate acute pain emergencies, including ankle and foot fractures and postoperative pain relief, when combined with the mentioned blocks, while waiting for pharmacologic methods to become effective. Tibial nerve block at the ankle with local anesthetic and steroid is occasionally used in the treatment of persistent ankle and foot pain when the pain is thought to be secondary to inflammation or when entrapment of the tibial nerve at the posterior tarsal tunnel is suspected. Tibial nerve block at the ankle with local anesthetic and steroid also is indicated in the palliation of pain and motor dysfunction associated with diabetic neuropathy. Destruc-tion of the tibial nerve block at the ankle is occasionally used in the palliation of persistent lower extremity pain secondary to invasive tumor that is mediated by the distal tibial nerve and has not responded to more conservative measures.

CLINICALLY RELEVANT ANATOMY

The tibial nerve is one of the two major continuations of the sciatic nerve, the other being the common peroneal nerve. The tibial nerve provides sensory innervation to the posterior portion of the calf, the heel, and the medial plantar surface. The tibial nerve splits from the sciatic nerve at the superior margin of the popliteal fossa and descends in a slightly medial course through the popliteal fossa. The tibial nerve block at the ankle lies just beneath the popliteal fascia and is readily accessible for neural blockade. The tibial nerve continues its downward course, running between the two heads of the gastrocnemius muscle, passing deep to the soleus muscle. The nerve courses medially between the Achilles tendon and the medial malleolus, where it divides into the medial and lateral plantar nerves, providing sensory innervation to the heel and medial plantar surface (Figs. 121-1 to 121-3). The tibial nerve is subject to compression at this point, which is known as *posterior tarsal tunnel syndrome.*

TECHNIQUE

The patient is placed in the lateral position with the affected leg in the dependent position and slightly flexed. The posterior tibial artery at this level is then palpated. The area between the medial malleolus and the Achilles tendon is identified and prepared with antiseptic solutions. A 25-gauge, $1\frac{1}{2}$-inch needle is inserted at this level and directed anteriorly toward the pulsations of the posterior tibial artery. If the arterial pulsations cannot be identified, the needle is directed toward the posterior-superior border of the medial malleolus. The needle is then advanced slowly toward the tibial nerve, which lies in the posterior groove of the medial malleolus, until a

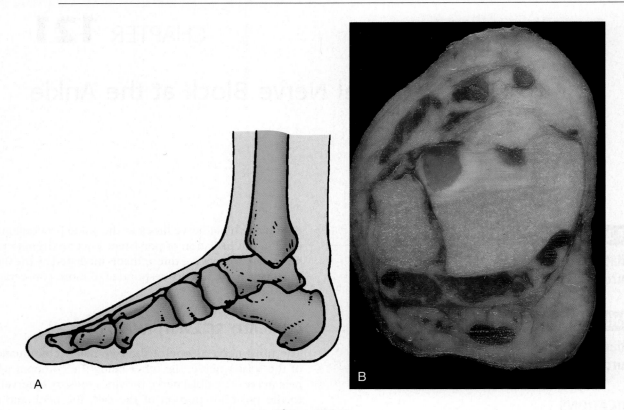

Figure 121-1.
(From Kang HS, Resnick D, Ahn J: MRI of the Extremities: An Anatomic
Atlas, 2nd ed. Philadelphia, WB Saunders, 2002, p 413.)

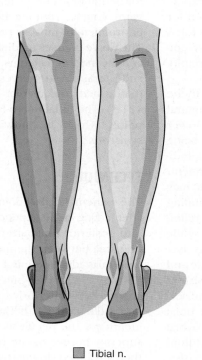

Figure 121-2.

Tibial n.
Sciatic n.

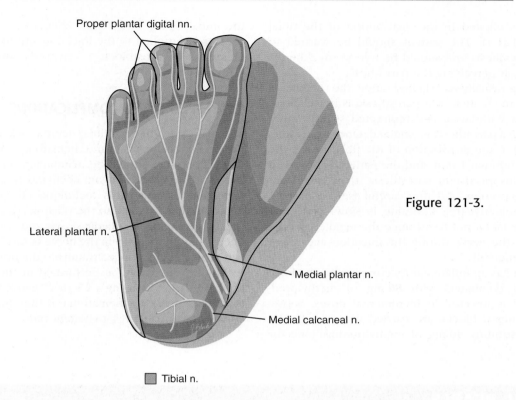

Proper plantar digital nn.

Lateral plantar n.

Medial plantar n.

Medial calcaneal n.

Figure 121-3.

Tibial n.

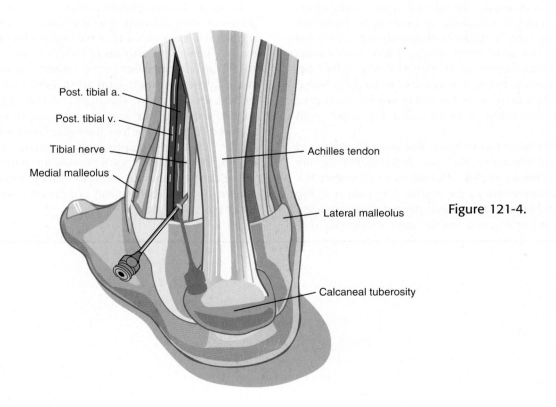

Post. tibial a.

Post. tibial v.

Tibial nerve

Medial malleolus

Achilles tendon

Lateral malleolus

Calcaneal tuberosity

Figure 121-4.

paresthesia is elicited in the distribution of the tibial nerve (Fig. 121-4). The patient should be warned to expect a paresthesia and should be told to say "there!" immediately on perceiving the paresthesia.

Paresthesia usually is elicited after the needle is advanced ½ to ¾ inch. If a paresthesia is not elicited, the needle is withdrawn and redirected slightly more cephalad until a paresthesia is obtained. Once a paresthesia is elicited in the distribution of the tibial nerve, the needle is withdrawn 1 mm, and the patient is observed to rule out any persistent paresthesia. If no persistent paresthesia is present, and after careful aspiration, 6 mL of 1.0% preservative-free lidocaine is slowly injected. Care must be taken not to advance the needle into the substance of the nerve during the injection and inject solution intraneurally.

If the pain has an inflammatory component, the local anesthetic is combined with 80 mg of methylprednisolone and is injected in incremental doses. Subsequent daily nerve blocks are carried out in a similar manner, substituting 40 mg of methylprednisolone for the initial 80-mg dose. After injection of the solution, pressure is applied to the injection site to decrease the incidence of postblock ecchymosis and hematoma formation.

SIDE EFFECTS AND COMPLICATIONS

The main side effect of tibial nerve block at the ankle is postblock ecchymosis and hematoma. As mentioned earlier, pressure should be maintained on the injection site after the block to avoid ecchymosis and hematoma formation. Because this technique elicits paresthesia, needle-induced trauma to the tibial nerve remains possible. By advancing the needle slowly and withdrawing the needle slightly away from the nerve before injection, one can avoid needle-induced trauma to the tibial nerve. This technique can safely be performed in the presence of anticoagulation by using a 25- or 27-gauge needle, albeit at increased risk for hematoma, if the clinical situation dictates a favorable risk-to-benefit ratio.

CLINICAL PEARLS

Tibial nerve block at the ankle is a simple technique that can produce dramatic relief for patients suffering from the previously mentioned pain complaints. Careful preblock neurologic assessment is important to avoid the later attribution of preexisting neurologic deficits to the tibial nerve block. These assessments are especially important in patients who have sustained trauma to the foot or ankle or in patients suffering from diabetic neuropathy and in whom tibial nerve block at the ankle is being used for acute pain control.

Posterior tarsal tunnel syndrome presents as pain in the plantar surface of the foot. It frequently occurs after ankle fractures and dislocations or thrombophlebitis or tenosynovitis in the region. The pain is worse at night and frequently awakens the patient from sleep. The pain is burning and has the same unpleasant dysesthetic quality associated with its analogue, carpal tunnel syndrome.

It should be remembered that the most common causes of pain radiating into the lower extremity are herniated lumbar disk and nerve impingement secondary to degenerative arthritis of the spine, not disorders involving the tibial nerve per se. Other pain syndromes that may be confused with tibial nerve entrapment include lesions above the origin of the tibial nerve, such as lesions of the sciatic nerve, and distal lesions of the tibial nerve, such as posterior tarsal tunnel syndrome. Electromyography and magnetic resonance imaging of the lumbar spine, combined with information gleaned from the clinical history and physical examination, will help to sort out the etiology of distal lower pain.

CHAPTER 122

Saphenous Nerve Block at the Knee

CPT-2009 CODE

Unilateral	64450
Neurolytic	64640

Relative Value Units

Unilateral	10
Neurolytic	20

INDICATIONS

Saphenous nerve block at the knee is useful in the evaluation and management of distal lower extremity pain thought to be subserved by the saphenous nerve. The technique also is useful to provide surgical anesthesia for the distal lower extremity when combined with tibial and common peroneal nerve block or lumbar plexus block. It is used for this indication primarily in patients who would not tolerate the sympathetic changes induced by spinal or epidural anesthesia and who need distal lower extremity surgery, such as débridement or distal amputation.

Saphenous nerve block at the knee with local anesthetic can be used diagnostically during differential neural blockade on an anatomic basis in the evaluation of lower extremity pain. If destruction of the saphenous nerve is being considered, this technique is useful as a prognostic indicator of the degree of motor and sensory impairment that the patient may experience. Saphenous nerve block at the knee with local anesthetic may be used to palliate acute pain emergencies, including distal lower extremity fractures and postoperative pain relief, when combined with the previously mentioned blocks while waiting for pharmacologic methods to become effective. Saphenous nerve block at the knee with local anesthetic and steroid is occasionally used in the treatment of persistent distal lower extremity pain when the pain is thought to be secondary to inflammation or when entrapment of the saphenous nerve as it passes through Hunter's canal is suspected. Saphenous nerve block at the knee with local anesthetic and steroid also is indicated in the palliation of pain and motor dysfunction associated with diabetic neuropathy. Destruction of the saphenous nerve is occasionally used in the palliation of persistent lower extremity pain secondary to invasive tumor that is mediated by the saphenous nerve and has not responded to more conservative measures.

CLINICALLY RELEVANT ANATOMY

The saphenous nerve is the largest sensory branch of the femoral nerve. The saphenous nerve provides sensory innervation to the medial malleolus, the medial calf, and a portion of the medial arch of the foot. The saphenous nerve is derived primarily from the fibers of the L3 and L4 nerve roots. The nerve travels along with the femoral artery through Hunter's canal and moves superficially as it approaches the knee. It passes over the medial condyle of the femur, splitting into terminal sensory branches (Figs. 122-1 and 122-2). The saphenous nerve is subject to trauma or compression anywhere along its course. The nerve is frequently traumatized during vein harvest for coronary artery bypass grafting procedures. The saphenous nerve also is subject to compression as it passes over the medial condyle of the femur.

TECHNIQUE

The patient is placed in the lateral position with the leg slightly flexed. The medial condyle of the femur is palpated. A point just in front of the posterior edge of the medial condyle is then identified and prepared with antiseptic solution. A 25-gauge, $\frac{1}{2}$-inch needle is then slowly advanced through this point toward the medial condyle of the femur until paresthesia is elicited in the distribution of the saphenous nerve (Fig. 122-3). The patient should be warned to expect a paresthesia and should be told to say "there!" immediately on perceiving the paresthesia. Paresthesia usually is elicited at a depth of $\frac{1}{4}$ to $\frac{1}{2}$ inch. If a paresthesia is not elicited, the needle is withdrawn and redirected slightly more anteriorly until

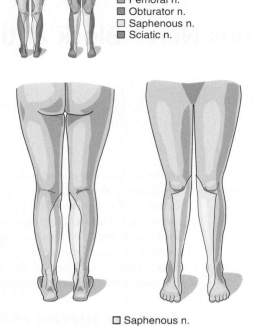

- Lateral femoral cutaneous n.
- Femoral n.
- Obturator n.
- Saphenous n.
- Sciatic n.

Figure 122-1.

- Saphenous n.

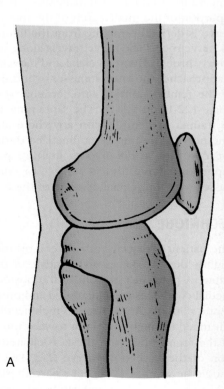
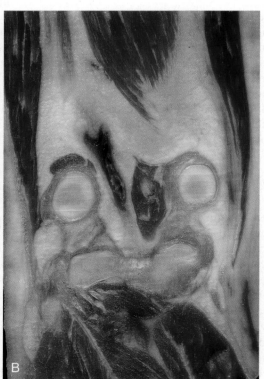

A   B

Figure 122-2.
(From Kang HS, Resnick D, Ahn J: MRI of the Extremities: An Anatomic Atlas, ed 2, Saunders 2002, p 293.)

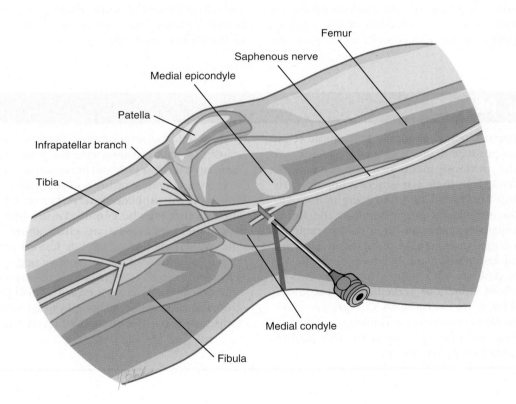

Figure 122-3.

a paresthesia is obtained. Once paresthesia is elicited in the distribution of the saphenous nerve, the needle is withdrawn 1 mm, and the patient is observed to rule out any persistent paresthesia. If no persistent paresthesia is present, and after careful aspiration, 5 mL of 1.0% preservative-free lidocaine is slowly injected. Care must be taken not to advance the needle into the substance of the nerve during the injection and inject solution intraneurally.

If the pain has an inflammatory component, the local anesthetic is combined with 80 mg of methylprednisolone and is injected in incremental doses. Subsequent daily nerve blocks are carried out in a similar manner, substituting 40 mg of methylprednisolone for the initial 80-mg dose. After injection of the solution, pressure is applied to the injection site to decrease the incidence of postblock ecchymosis and hematoma formation.

SIDE EFFECTS AND COMPLICATIONS

The main side effect of saphenous nerve block at the knee is postblock ecchymosis and hematoma because the nerve is close to the greater saphenous artery. As mentioned earlier, pressure should be maintained on the injection site after the block to avoid ecchymosis and hematoma formation. Because this technique elicits a paresthesia, needle-induced trauma to the saphenous nerve remains possible. By advancing the needle slowly and withdrawing the needle slightly away from the nerve before injection, one can avoid needle-induced trauma to the saphenous nerve.

CLINICAL PEARLS

Saphenous nerve block at the knee is a simple technique that can produce dramatic relief for patients suffering from the previously mentioned pain complaints. Careful preblock neurologic assessment is important to avoid the later attribution of preexisting neurologic deficits to the saphenous nerve block at the knee. These assessments are especially important in patients who have sustained trauma to the distal femur, patients who have undergone vascular procedures on the lower extremity, or patients who suffer from diabetic neuropathy in whom saphenous nerve block at the knees is being used for acute pain control. Compressive neuropathy of the saphenous nerve at the knee sometimes occurs in musicians who play the cello. This painful syndrome is called *viol paresthesia*.

It should be remembered that the most common causes of pain radiating into the lower extremity are herniated lumbar disk and nerve impingement secondary to degenerative arthritis of the spine, not disorders involving the saphenous nerve per se. Other pain syndromes that may be confused with saphenous nerve entrapment include lesions either above the origin of the saphenous nerve, such as lesions of the femoral nerve, or lesions of the saphenous nerve at the ankle. Electromyography and magnetic resonance imaging of the lumbar spine, combined with information gleaned from the clinical history and physical examination, will help to sort out the etiology of distal lower pain.

CHAPTER 123

Saphenous Nerve Block at the Ankle

CPT-2009 CODE	
Unilateral	64450
Neurolytic	64640

Relative Value Units	
Unilateral	10
Neurolytic	20

INDICATIONS

Saphenous nerve block at the ankle is useful in the evaluation and management of medial ankle and foot pain thought to be subserved by the distal saphenous nerve. The technique also is useful to provide surgical anesthesia for the ankle and foot when combined with tibial and common peroneal nerve block or lumbar plexus block. It is used for this indication primarily in patients who would not tolerate the sympathetic changes induced by spinal or epidural anesthesia who need distal lower extremity surgery, such as débridement or distal amputation.

Saphenous nerve block at the ankle with local anesthetic can be used as a diagnostic tool when performing differential neural blockade on an anatomic basis in the evaluation of lower extremity pain. If destruction of the distal saphenous nerve is being considered, this technique is useful as a prognostic indicator of the degree of motor and sensory impairment that the patient may experience. Saphenous nerve block at the ankle with local anesthetic may be used to palliate acute pain emergencies, including distal ankle and foot fractures and postoperative pain relief, when combined with the previously mentioned blocks, while waiting for pharmacologic methods to become effective. Saphenous nerve block at the ankle with local anesthetic and steroid occasionally is used in the treatment of persistent distal lower extremity pain when the pain is thought to be secondary to inflammation or when entrapment of the saphenous

nerve at the ankle is suspected. Saphenous nerve block at the ankle with local anesthetic and steroid also is indicated in the palliation of pain and motor dysfunction associated with diabetic neuropathy. Destruction of the distal saphenous nerve occasionally is used in the palliation of persistent lower extremity pain secondary to invasive tumor that is mediated by the saphenous nerve and has not responded to more conservative measures.

CLINICALLY RELEVANT ANATOMY

The saphenous nerve is the largest sensory branch of the femoral nerve. The saphenous nerve provides sensory innervation to the medial malleolus, the medial calf, and a portion of the medial arch of the foot. The saphenous nerve is derived primarily from the fibers of the L3 and L4 nerve roots. The nerve travels along with the femoral artery through Hunter's canal and moves superficially as it approaches the ankle. It passes over the medial condyle of the femur, splitting into terminal sensory branches (Fig. 123-1). The saphenous nerve is subject to trauma or compression anywhere along its course. The nerve frequently is traumatized during vein harvest for coronary artery bypass grafting procedures. The saphenous nerve also is subject to compression as it passes over the medial condyle of the femur. Less commonly, the nerve is damaged or compressed distally as it passes beneath the fascia of the dorsum of the foot.

TECHNIQUE

The patient is placed in the supine position with the leg extended. The extensor hallucis longus tendon is identified by having the patient extend his or her big toe against resistance. A point just medial to the tendon at the skin crease of the ankle is identified and prepared with antiseptic solution (Fig. 123-2). A 25-gauge, $1\frac{1}{2}$-inch needle then is advanced slowly through this point; during injection, the needle is advanced subcutaneously toward the medial malleolus (Fig. 123-3). A total of 7 to 8 mL of 1% preservative-free lidocaine should be injected

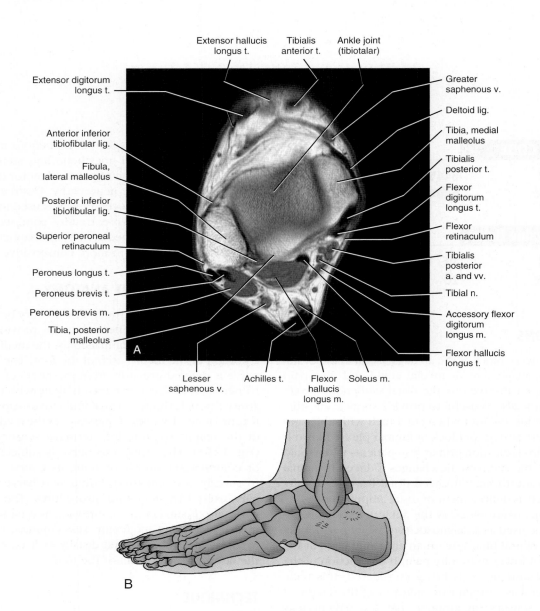

Figure 123-1.
(From El-Khoury GY, Bergman RA, Montgomery WJ: Sectional Anatomy by MRI and CT, 3rd ed. New York, Churchill Livingstone, 2007, p 363.)

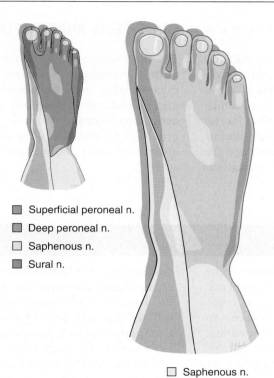

Superficial peroneal n.
Deep peroneal n.
Saphenous n.
Sural n.

Saphenous n.

Figure 123-2.

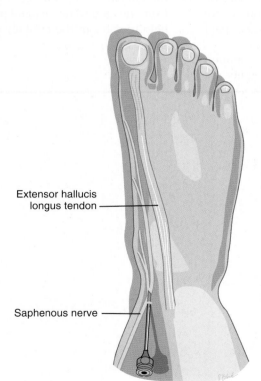

Extensor hallucis longus tendon

Saphenous nerve

Figure 123-3.

to ensure that all the terminal branches of the saphenous nerve are blocked.

If the pain has an inflammatory component, the local anesthetic is combined with 80 mg of methylprednisolone and is injected in incremental doses. Subsequent daily nerve blocks are carried out in a similar manner, substituting 40 mg of methylprednisolone for the initial 80-mg dose. After injection of the solution, pressure is applied to the injection site to decrease the incidence of postblock ecchymosis and hematoma formation.

SIDE EFFECTS AND COMPLICATIONS

The main side effect of saphenous nerve block at the ankle is postblock ecchymosis and hematoma. As mentioned earlier, pressure should be maintained on the injection site after the block to avoid ecchymosis and hematoma formation. Because of the saphenous nerve's proximity to the superficial peroneal nerve, this nerve often is blocked during saphenous nerve block at the ankle.

CLINICAL PEARLS

Saphenous nerve block at the ankle is a simple technique that can produce dramatic relief for patients suffering from the previously mentioned pain complaints. Careful preblock neurologic assessment is important to avoid the later attribution of preexisting neurologic deficits to the saphenous nerve block at the ankle. These assessments are especially important in patients who have sustained trauma to the distal ankle and foot, patients who have undergone vascular procedures on the lower extremity, or patients suffering from diabetic neuropathy in whom saphenous nerve block at the ankles is being used for acute pain control.

It should be remembered that the most common causes of pain radiating into the lower extremity are herniated lumbar disk and nerve impingement secondary to degenerative arthritis of the spine, not disorders involving the saphenous nerve per se. Other pain syndromes that may be confused with saphenous nerve entrapment include lesions above the origin of the saphenous nerve, such as lesions of the femoral nerve, and lesions of the superficial peroneal nerve whose sensory innervation may overlap in some patients. Electromyography and magnetic resonance imaging of the lumbar spine, combined with information gleaned from the clinical history and physical examination, will help to sort out the etiology of distal lower pain.

CHAPTER 124

Common Peroneal Nerve Block at the Knee

CPT-2009 CODE	
Unilateral	64450
Neurolytic	64640

Relative Value Units	
Unilateral	10
Neurolytic	20

INDICATIONS

Common peroneal nerve block is useful in the evaluation and management of distal lower extremity pain thought to be subserved by the common peroneal nerve. The technique also is useful to provide surgical anesthesia for the distal lower extremity when combined with tibial and saphenous nerve block or lumbar plexus block. It is used for this indication primarily in patients who would not tolerate the sympathetic changes induced by spinal or epidural anesthesia and who need distal lower extremity surgery, such as débridement or distal amputation.

Common peroneal nerve block with local anesthetic can be used as a diagnostic tool when performing differential neural blockade on an anatomic basis in the evaluation of lower extremity pain. If destruction of the common peroneal nerve is being considered, this technique is useful as a prognostic indicator of the degree of motor and sensory impairment that the patient may experience. Common peroneal nerve block with local anesthetic may be used to palliate acute pain emergencies, including distal lower extremity fractures and postoperative pain relief, when combined with the previously mentioned blocks while waiting for pharmacologic methods to become effective. Common peroneal nerve block with local anesthetic and steroid occasionally is used in the treatment of persistent distal lower extremity pain when the pain is thought to be secondary to inflammation or when entrapment of the common peroneal nerve as it passes the head of the fibula is suspected. Common peroneal nerve block with local anesthetic and

steroid also is indicated in the palliation of pain and motor dysfunction associated with diabetic neuropathy. Destruction of the common peroneal nerve occasionally is used in the palliation of persistent lower extremity pain secondary to invasive tumor that is mediated by the common peroneal nerve and has not responded to more conservative measures.

CLINICALLY RELEVANT ANATOMY

The common peroneal nerve is one of the two major continuations of the sciatic nerve, the other being the tibial nerve. The common peroneal nerve provides sensory innervation to the inferior portion of the knee joint and the posterior and lateral skin of the upper calf (Fig. 124-1). The common peroneal nerve is derived from the posterior branches of the L4, the L5, and the S1 and S2 nerve roots. The nerve splits from the sciatic nerve at the superior margin of the popliteal fossa and descends laterally behind the head of the fibula (Figs. 124-2 and 124-3).

The common peroneal nerve is subject to compression at this point by such circumstances as improperly applied casts and tourniquets. The nerve also is subject to compression as it continues its lateral course, winding around the fibula through the fibular tunnel, which is made up of the posterior border of the tendinous insertion of the peroneus longus muscle and the fibula. Just distal to the fibular tunnel, the nerve divides into its two terminal branches: the superficial and the deep peroneal nerves. Each of these branches is subject to trauma and may be blocked individually as a diagnostic and therapeutic maneuver.

TECHNIQUE

The patient is placed in the lateral position with the leg slightly flexed. The head of the fibula and the junction of fibular head and neck are palpated. A point just below the fibular head then is identified and prepared with antiseptic solution. A 25-gauge, ½-inch needle then is advanced slowly through this point toward the neck of

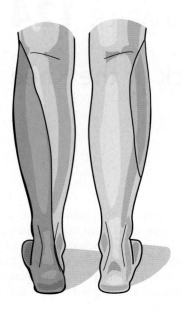
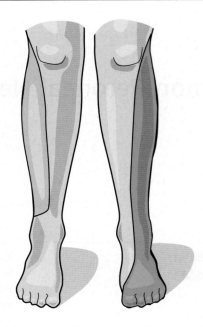

Figure 124-1.

■ Common peroneal n.
■ Sciatic n.

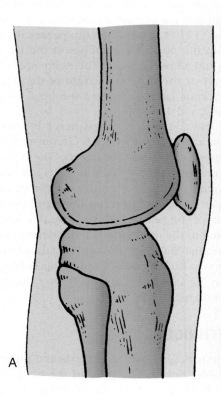
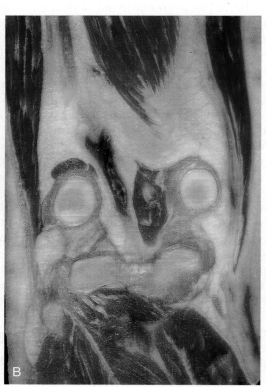

Figure 124-2.
(From Kang HS, Resnick D, Ahn J: MRI of the Extremities: An Anatomic
Atlas, 2nd ed. Philadelphia, WB Saunders, 2002, p 293.)

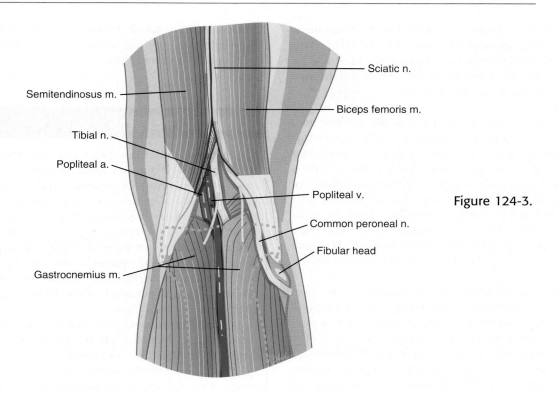

Semitendinosus m.

Tibial n.

Popliteal a.

Gastrocnemius m.

Sciatic n.

Biceps femoris m.

Popliteal v.

Common peroneal n.

Fibular head

Figure 124-3.

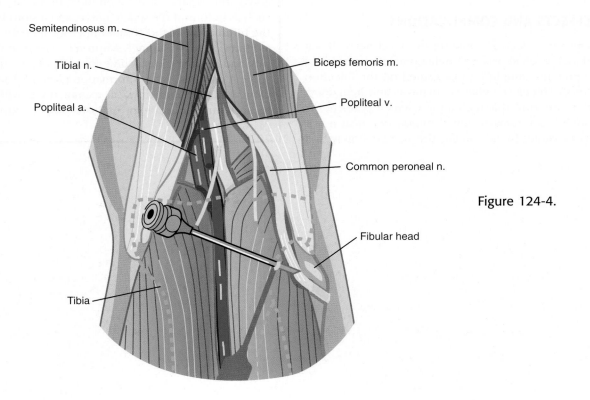

Semitendinosus m.

Tibial n.

Popliteal a.

Tibia

Biceps femoris m.

Popliteal v.

Common peroneal n.

Fibular head

Figure 124-4.

the fibula until a paresthesia is elicited in the distribution of the common peroneal nerve (Fig. 124-4). The patient should be warned to expect a paresthesia and should be told to say "there!" immediately on perceiving the paresthesia. Paresthesia usually is elicited at a depth of $\frac{1}{4}$ to $\frac{1}{2}$ inch.

If a paresthesia is not elicited, the needle is withdrawn and redirected slightly more posteriorly until a paresthesia is obtained. Once a paresthesia is elicited in the distribution of the common peroneal nerve, the needle is withdrawn 1 mm, and the patient is observed to rule out any persistent paresthesia. If no persistent paresthesia is present, and after careful aspiration, 5 mL of 1.0% preservative-free lidocaine is injected slowly. Care must be taken not to advance the needle into the substance of the nerve during the injection and inject solution intraneurally.

If the pain has an inflammatory component, the local anesthetic is combined with 80 mg of methylprednisolone and is injected in incremental doses. Subsequent daily nerve blocks are carried out in a similar manner, substituting 40 mg of methylprednisolone for the initial 80-mg dose. After injection of the solution, pressure is applied to the injection site to decrease the incidence of postblock ecchymosis and hematoma formation.

SIDE EFFECTS AND COMPLICATIONS

The main side effect of common peroneal nerve block is postblock ecchymosis and hematoma. As mentioned earlier, pressure should be maintained on the injection site after the block to avoid ecchymosis and hematoma formation. Because this technique elicits a paresthesia, needle-induced trauma to the common peroneal nerve remains possible. By advancing the needle slowly and withdrawing the needle slightly away from the nerve before injection, one can avoid needle-induced trauma to the common peroneal nerve.

CLINICAL PEARLS

Common peroneal nerve block is a simple technique that can produce dramatic relief for patients suffering from the previously mentioned pain complaints. Careful preblock neurologic assessment is important to avoid the later attribution of preexisting neurologic deficits to the common peroneal nerve block. These assessments are especially important in patients who have sustained trauma to the proximal fibula and in patients suffering from diabetic neuropathy in whom common peroneal nerve blocks are being used for acute pain control.

It should be remembered that the most common causes of pain radiating into the lower extremity are herniated lumbar disk and nerve impingement secondary to degenerative arthritis of the spine, not disorders involving the common peroneal nerve per se. Other pain syndromes that may be confused with common peroneal nerve entrapment include lesions above the origin of the common peroneal nerve, such as lesions of the sciatic nerve, and lesions below the bifurcation of the common peroneal nerve, such as anterior tarsal tunnel syndrome. Electromyography and magnetic resonance imaging of the lumbar spine, combined with information gleaned from the clinical history and physical examination, will help to sort out the etiology of distal lower extremity pain.

CHAPTER 125

Deep Peroneal Nerve Block at the Ankle

CPT-2009 CODE

Unilateral	64450
Neurolytic	64640

Relative Value Units

Unilateral	10
Neurolytic	20

INDICATIONS

Deep peroneal nerve block is useful in the evaluation and management of foot pain thought to be subserved by the deep peroneal nerve. The technique also is useful to provide surgical anesthesia for the foot when combined with tibial and saphenous nerve block or lumbar plexus block. It is used for this indication primarily in patients who would not tolerate the sympathetic changes induced by spinal or epidural anesthesia and who need foot surgery, such as débridement or toe or forefoot amputation.

Deep peroneal nerve block with local anesthetic can be used as a diagnostic tool when performing differential neural blockade on an anatomic basis in the evaluation of distal lower extremity pain. If destruction of the deep peroneal nerve is being considered, this technique is useful as a prognostic indicator of the degree of motor and sensory impairment that the patient may experience. Deep peroneal nerve block with local anesthetic may be used to palliate acute pain emergencies, including foot fractures and postoperative pain relief, when combined with the previously mentioned blocks, while waiting for pharmacologic methods to become effective. Deep peroneal nerve block with local anesthetic and steroid occasionally is used in the treatment of persistent foot pain when the pain is thought to be secondary to inflammation or when entrapment of the deep peroneal nerve as it passes through the anterior tarsal tunnel is suspected. Deep peroneal nerve block with local anesthetic and steroid also is indicated in the palliation of

pain and motor dysfunction associated with diabetic neuropathy. Destruction of the deep peroneal nerve occasionally is used in the palliation of persistent foot pain secondary to invasive tumor that is mediated by the deep peroneal nerve and has not responded to more conservative measures.

CLINICALLY RELEVANT ANATOMY

The common peroneal nerve is one of the two major continuations of the sciatic nerve, the other being the tibial nerve. The common peroneal nerve provides sensory innervation to the inferior portion of the knee joint and the posterior and lateral skin of the upper calf. The common peroneal nerve is derived from the posterior branches of the L4, L5, and S1 and S2 nerve roots. The nerve splits from the sciatic nerve at the superior margin of the popliteal fossa and descends laterally behind the head of the fibula. The common peroneal nerve is subject to compression at this point by such circumstances as improperly applied casts and tourniquets. The nerve also is subject to compression as it continues its lateral course, winding around the fibula through the fibular tunnel, which is made up of the posterior border of the tendinous insertion of the peroneus longus muscle and the fibula itself (Fig. 125-1). Just distal to the fibular tunnel, the nerve divides into its two terminal branches: the superficial and the deep peroneal nerves. Each of these branches is subject to trauma and may be blocked individually as a diagnostic and therapeutic maneuver.

The deep branch continues down the leg in conjunction with the tibial artery and vein to provide sensory innervation to the web space of the first and second toes and adjacent dorsum of the foot (Fig. 125-2). Although this distribution of sensory fibers is small, this area is often the site of Morton's neuroma surgery and thus is important to the regional anesthesiologist. The deep peroneal nerve provides motor innervation to all of the toe extensors and the anterior tibialis muscles. The deep peroneal nerve passes beneath the dense superficial fascia of the ankle, where it is subject to an

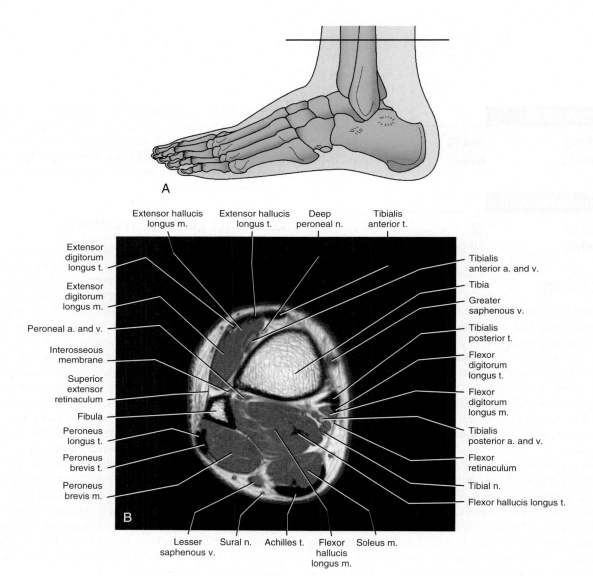

Extensor hallucis
longus m.

Extensor hallucis
longus t.

Deep
peroneal n.

Tibialis
anterior t.

Extensor
digitorum
longus t.

Extensor
digitorum
longus m.

Peroneal a. and v.

Interosseous
membrane

Superior
extensor
retinaculum

Fibula

Peroneus
longus t.

Peroneus
brevis t.

Peroneus
brevis m.

Tibialis
anterior a. and v.

Tibia

Greater
saphenous v.

Tibialis
posterior t.

Flexor
digitorum
longus t.

Flexor
digitorum
longus m.

Tibialis
posterior a. and v.

Flexor
retinaculum

Tibial n.

Flexor hallucis longus t.

Lesser
saphenous v.

Sural n.

Achilles t.

Flexor
hallucis
longus m.

Soleus m.

Figure 125-1.
(From El-Khoury GY, Bergman RA, Montgomery WJ: Sectional Anatomy by
MRI and CT, 3rd ed. New York, Churchill Livingstone, 2007, p 360.)

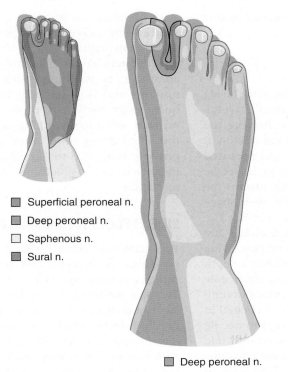

Superficial peroneal n.
Deep peroneal n.
Saphenous n.
Sural n.

Figure 125-2.

Deep peroneal n.

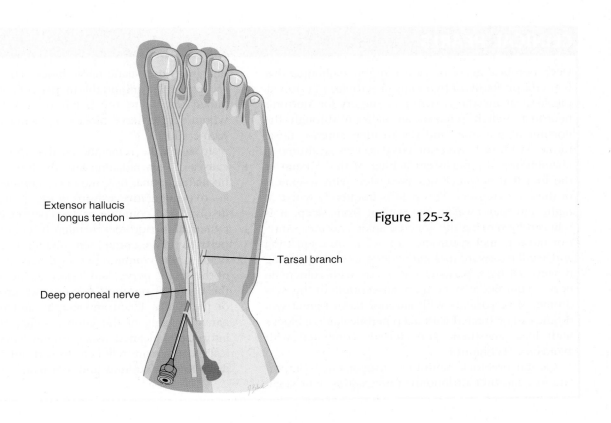

Extensor hallucis longus tendon

Tarsal branch

Deep peroneal nerve

Figure 125-3.

entrapment syndrome known as *anterior tarsal tunnel syndrome*.

TECHNIQUE

The patient is placed in the supine position with the leg extended. The extensor hallucis longus tendon is identified by having the patient extend his or her big toe against resistance. A point just medial to the tendon at the skin crease of the ankle is identified and prepared with antiseptic solution. A 25-gauge, 1½-inch needle then is advanced slowly through this point toward the tibia until a paresthesia is elicited into the web space between the first and second toes (Fig. 125-3). The patient should be warned to expect a paresthesia and should be told to say "there!" immediately on perceiving the paresthesia. Paresthesia usually is elicited at a depth of ¼ to ½ inch. If a paresthesia is not elicited, the needle is withdrawn and redirected slightly more posterior until a paresthesia is obtained. Once paresthesia is elicited in the distribution of the deep peroneal nerve, the needle is withdrawn 1 mm, and the patient is observed to rule out any persistent paresthesia. If no persistent paresthesia is present, and after careful aspiration, 6 to 8 mL of 1.0% preservative-free lidocaine is injected slowly. Care must be taken not to advance the needle into the substance of the nerve during the injection and inject solution intraneurally.

If the pain has an inflammatory component, the local anesthetic is combined with 80 mg of methylprednisolone and is injected in incremental doses. Subsequent daily nerve blocks are carried out in a similar manner, substituting 40 mg of methylprednisolone for the initial 80-mg dose. After injection of the solution, pressure is applied to the injection site to decrease the incidence of postblock ecchymosis and hematoma formation.

SIDE EFFECTS AND COMPLICATIONS

The main side effect of deep peroneal nerve block is postblock ecchymosis and hematoma. As mentioned earlier, pressure should be maintained on the injection site after the block to avoid ecchymosis and hematoma formation. Because this technique elicits a paresthesia, needle-induced trauma to the deep peroneal nerve remains possible. By advancing the needle slowly and withdrawing the needle slightly away from the nerve before injection, one can avoid needle-induced trauma to the deep peroneal nerve.

CLINICAL PEARLS

Deep peroneal nerve block is a simple technique that is useful primarily in two clinical settings: (1) providing surgical anesthesia with foot surgery for Morton's neuroma, which requires an incision through the dorsum of the foot; and (2) treating anterior tarsal tunnel syndrome. Anterior tarsal tunnel syndrome is characterized by persistent aching of the dorsum of the foot that is sometimes associated with weakness of the toe extensors. This pain is frequently worse at night and may awaken the patient from sleep. It is relieved by moving the affected ankle and toes. Anterior tarsal tunnel syndrome can occur after squatting and leaning forward for long periods, as when planting flowers. Diabetic patients and others with vulnerable nerve syndrome may be more susceptible to this syndrome. Most patients with anterior tarsal tunnel syndrome can be treated with deep peroneal nerve blocks with local anesthetic and steroids combined with avoidance techniques.

Careful preblock neurologic assessment is important to avoid later attribution of preexisting neurologic deficits to the sciatic nerve block. These assessments are especially important in patients who have sustained trauma to the pelvis or lower extremity in whom sciatic nerve blocks are being used for acute pain control.

It should be remembered that the most common causes of pain radiating into the lower extremity are herniated lumbar disk and nerve impingement secondary to degenerative arthritis of the spine, not disorders involving the common or deep peroneal nerve per se. Other pain syndromes that may be confused with deep peroneal nerve entrapment include lesions above the origin of the common peroneal nerve, such as lesions of the sciatic nerve, and lesions at the point at which the common peroneal nerve winds around the head of the fibula. Electromyography and magnetic resonance imaging of the lumbar spine, combined with information gleaned from the clinical history and physical examination, will help to sort out the etiology of distal lower extremity and foot pain.

CHAPTER 126

Superficial Peroneal Nerve Block at the Ankle

CPT-2009 CODE

Unilateral	64450
Neurolytic	64640

Relative Value Units

Unilateral	10
Neurolytic	20

INDICATIONS

Superficial peroneal nerve block is useful in the evaluation and management of foot pain thought to be subserved by the superficial peroneal nerve. The technique also is useful to provide surgical anesthesia for the foot when combined with deep peroneal, tibial, and saphenous nerve block or lumbar plexus block. It is used for this indication primarily in patients who would not tolerate the sympathetic changes induced by spinal or epidural anesthesia and who need foot surgery, such as débridement or toe or forefoot amputation.

Superficial peroneal nerve block with local anesthetic can be used as a diagnostic tool when performing differential neural blockade on an anatomic basis in the evaluation of distal lower extremity pain. If destruction of the superficial peroneal nerve is being considered, this technique is useful as a prognostic indicator of the degree of motor and sensory impairment that the patient may experience. Superficial peroneal nerve block with local anesthetic may be used to palliate acute pain emergencies, including foot fractures and postoperative pain relief, when combined with the previously mentioned blocks, while waiting for pharmacologic methods to become effective. Superficial peroneal nerve block with local anesthetic and steroid occasionally is used in the treatment of persistent foot pain when the pain is thought to be secondary to inflammation or when entrapment of the superficial peroneal nerve as it passes underneath the dense fascia of the ankle is suspected. Superficial peroneal nerve block with local anesthetic and steroid also is indicated in the palliation of pain and motor dysfunction associated with diabetic neuropathy. Destruction of the superficial peroneal nerve occasionally is used in the palliation of persistent foot pain secondary to invasive tumor that is mediated by the superficial peroneal nerve and has not responded to more conservative measures.

CLINICALLY RELEVANT ANATOMY

The common peroneal nerve is one of the two major continuations of the sciatic nerve, the other being the tibial nerve. The common peroneal nerve provides sensory innervation to the inferior portion of the knee joint and the posterior and lateral skin of the upper calf. The common peroneal nerve is derived from the posterior branches of the L4, L5, and S1 and S2 nerve roots. The nerve splits from the sciatic nerve at the superior margin of the popliteal fossa and descends laterally behind the head of the fibula. The common peroneal nerve is subject to compression at this point by such circumstances as improperly applied casts and tourniquets. The nerve also is subject to compression as it continues its lateral course, winding around the fibula through the fibular tunnel, which is made up of the posterior border of the tendinous insertion of the peroneus longus muscle and the fibula itself. Just distal to the fibular tunnel, the nerve divides into its two terminal branches, the superficial and the deep peroneal nerves. Each of these branches is subject to trauma and may be blocked individually as a diagnostic and therapeutic maneuver.

The superficial branch continues down the leg in conjunction with the extensor digitorum longus muscle. The nerve divides into terminal branches at a point just above the ankle. The fibers of these terminal branches provide sensory innervation to most of the dorsum of the foot except for the area adjacent to the web space of the first and second toes, which is supplied by the deep peroneal nerve (Fig. 126-1). The superficial

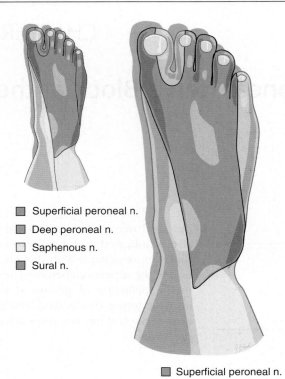

Figure 126-1.

- Superficial peroneal n.
- Deep peroneal n.
- Saphenous n.
- Sural n.

- Superficial peroneal n.

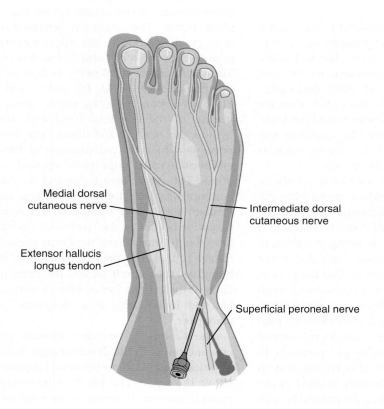

Medial dorsal
cutaneous nerve

Intermediate dorsal
cutaneous nerve

Extensor hallucis
longus tendon

Superficial peroneal nerve

Figure 126-2.

peroneal nerve also provides sensory innervation to the toes, except for the area between the first and second toe, which is supplied by the deep peroneal nerve.

TECHNIQUE

The patient is placed in the supine position with the leg extended. One identifies the extensor hallucis longus tendon by having the patient extend his or her big toe against resistance. A point just medial to the tendon at the skin crease of the ankle is identified and prepared with antiseptic solution. A 25-gauge, 1½-inch needle is then slowly advanced through this point; during injection, the needle is advanced subcutaneously toward the lateral malleolus (Fig. 126-2). A total of 7 to 8 mL of 1.0% preservative-free lidocaine should be injected to ensure that all the terminal branches of the superficial peroneal nerve are blocked.

If the pain has an inflammatory component, the local anesthetic is combined with 80 mg of methylprednisolone and is injected in incremental doses. Subsequent daily nerve blocks are carried out in a similar manner, substituting 40 mg of methylprednisolone for the initial 80-mg dose. After injection of the solution, pressure is applied to the injection site to decrease the incidence of postblock ecchymosis and hematoma formation.

SIDE EFFECTS AND COMPLICATIONS

The main side effect of superficial peroneal nerve block is postblock ecchymosis and hematoma. As mentioned earlier, pressure should be maintained on the injection site after the block to avoid ecchymosis and hematoma formation. Because of proximity to the deep peroneal nerve, this nerve frequently is blocked during superficial peroneal nerve block.

CLINICAL PEARLS

Superficial peroneal nerve block is a simple technique that is useful primarily as an adjunct to surgical anesthesia and to provide pain relief for trauma and postoperative pain involving the dorsum of the foot. The superficial peroneal nerve occasionally is entrapped by the fascia at the ankle. This is less common than entrapment of the deep branch of the peroneal nerve and can usually be sorted out by electromyography and careful neurologic examination.

Careful preblock neurologic assessment is important to avoid the later attribution of preexisting neurologic deficits to the superficial peroneal nerve block. These assessments are especially important in patients who have sustained trauma to the ankle or foot and patients suffering from diabetic neuropathy in whom superficial peroneal nerve blocks are being used for acute pain control.

It should be remembered that the most common causes of pain radiating into the lower extremity are herniated lumbar disk and nerve impingement secondary to degenerative arthritis of the spine, not disorders involving the common or superficial peroneal nerve per se. Other pain syndromes that may be confused with superficial peroneal nerve entrapment include lesions either above the origin of the common peroneal nerve, such as lesions of the sciatic nerve, or lesions at the point at which the common peroneal nerve winds around the head of the fibula. Electromyography and magnetic resonance imaging of the lumbar spine, combined with information gleaned from the clinical history and physical examination, will help to sort out the etiology of distal lower extremity and foot pain.

CHAPTER **127**

Sural Nerve Block at the Ankle

INDICATIONS

Sural nerve block at the ankle is useful in the evaluation and management of foot and ankle pain thought to be subserved by the sural nerve. The technique also is useful to provide surgical anesthesia for the posterior ankle and plantar surface of the foot when combined with common peroneal, posterior tibial, and saphenous nerve block or lumbar plexus block. It is used for this indication primarily in patients who would not tolerate the sympathetic changes induced by spinal or epidural anesthesia and who need distal lower extremity surgery, such as débridement or tendon repair.

Sural nerve block at the ankle with local anesthetic can be used as a diagnostic tool when performing differential neural blockade on an anatomic basis in the evaluation of lower extremity pain. If destruction of the sural nerve is being considered, this technique is useful as a prognostic indicator of the degree of motor and sensory impairment that the patient may experience. Sural nerve block at the ankle with local anesthetic may be used to palliate acute pain emergencies, including heel and foot fractures and postoperative pain relief, when combined with the previously mentioned blocks while waiting for pharmacologic methods to become effective. Sural nerve block at the ankle with local anesthetic and steroid occasionally is used in the treatment of persistent ankle, heel, and foot pain when the pain is thought to be secondary to inflammation or when entrap-

ment of the sural nerve at the ankle is suspected. Sural nerve block at the ankle with local anesthetic and steroid also is indicated in the palliation of pain associated with diabetic neuropathy. Destruction of the sural nerve block at the ankle occasionally is used in the palliation of persistent lower extremity pain secondary to invasive tumor that is mediated by the sural nerve and has not responded to more conservative measures.

CLINICALLY RELEVANT ANATOMY

The sural nerve is a branch of the posterior tibial nerve. The sural nerve passes from the posterior calf around the lateral malleolus to provide sensor innervation of the posterior lateral aspect of the calf and the lateral surface of the foot and fifth toe and the plantar surface of the heel (Figs. 127-1 and 127-2). The sural nerve is subject to compression at the ankle and is known as *boot syndrome* because it is associated with compression of the nerve by boots that are too tight.

TECHNIQUE

The patient is placed in the lateral position with the affected leg in the superior position and slightly flexed. The posterior groove behind the lateral malleolus is identified by palpation. The area between the lateral malleolus and the Achilles tendon is identified and prepared with antiseptic solutions. A 25-gauge, $1\frac{1}{2}$-inch needle is inserted at this level and directed anteriorly toward the lateral malleolus. The needle then is advanced slowly toward the sural nerve, which lies in the posterior groove of the lateral malleolus, until a paresthesia is elicited in the distribution of the sural nerve (Fig. 127-3). The patient should be warned to expect a paresthesia and should be told to say "there!" immediately on perceiving the paresthesia. Paresthesia usually is elicited after the needle is advanced $\frac{1}{2}$ to $\frac{3}{4}$ inch. If a paresthesia is not elicited, the needle is withdrawn and redirected slightly more cephalad until a paresthesia is obtained. Once a paresthesia is elicited in the distribution of the sural

Current Procedural Terminology © 2009 American Medical Association. All Rights Reserved.

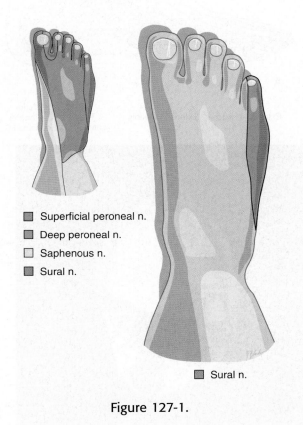

Superficial peroneal n.
Deep peroneal n.
Saphenous n.
Sural n.

Sural n.

Figure 127-1.

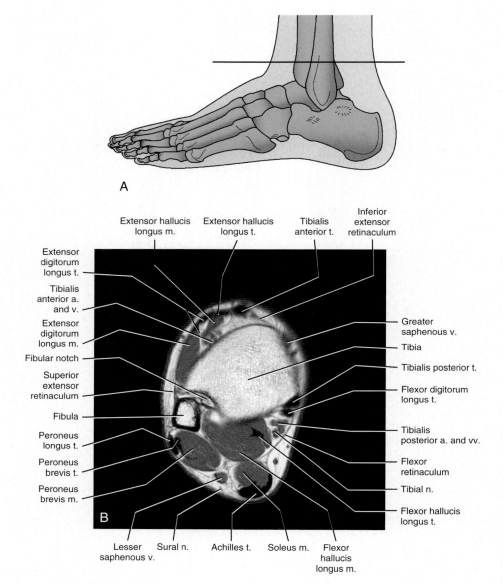

Figure 127-2.
(From El-Khoury GY, Bergman RA, Montgomery WJ: Sectional Anatomy by MRI and CT, 3rd ed. New York, Churchill Livingstone, 2007, p 361.)

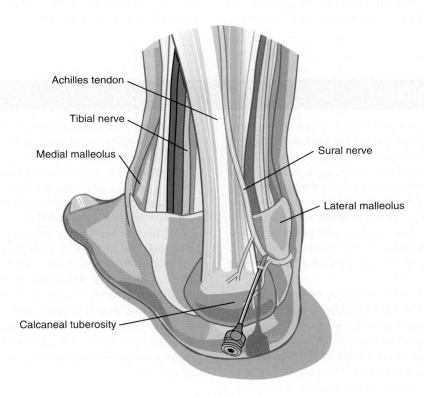

Figure 127-3.

nerve, the needle is withdrawn 1 mm, and the patient is observed to rule out any persistent paresthesia. If no persistent paresthesia is present, and after careful aspiration, 6 mL of 1.0% preservative-free lidocaine is injected slowly. Care must be taken not to advance the needle into the substance of the nerve during the injection and inject solution intraneurally.

If the pain has an inflammatory component, the local anesthetic is combined with 80 mg of methylprednisolone and is injected in incremental doses. Subsequent daily nerve blocks are carried out in a similar manner, substituting 40 mg of methylprednisolone for the initial 80-mg dose. After injection of the solution, pressure is applied to the injection site to decrease the incidence of postblock ecchymosis and hematoma formation.

SIDE EFFECTS AND COMPLICATIONS

The main side effect of sural nerve block at the ankle is postblock ecchymosis and hematoma. As mentioned earlier, pressure should be maintained on the injection site after the block to avoid ecchymosis and hematoma formation. Because this technique elicits a paresthesia, needle-induced trauma to the sural nerve remains possible. By advancing the needle slowly and withdrawing the needle slightly away from the nerve, one can avoid needle-induced trauma to the sural nerve. This technique can be safely performed in the presence of anticoagulation by using a 25- or 27-gauge needle, albeit at increased risk for hematoma, if the clinical situation dictates a favorable risk-to-benefit ratio.

CLINICAL PEARLS

Sural nerve block at the ankle is a simple technique that can produce dramatic relief for patients suffering from the previously mentioned pain complaints. Careful preblock neurologic assessment is important to avoid the later attribution of preexisting neurologic deficits to the sural nerve block. These assessments are especially important in those patients who have sustained trauma to the foot or ankle and patients suffering from diabetic neuropathy in whom sural nerve block at the ankle is being used for acute pain control.

Entrapment of the sural nerve, or boot syndrome, manifests as pain in the heel and lateral aspect of the foot. It occurs after trauma to the sural nerve or from boots with tops that are too tight. It may occur following ankle fractures and dislocations or thrombophlebitis or tenosynovitis in the region. The pain is worse at night and frequently awakens the patient from sleep.

The pain is burning and has the same unpleasant dysesthetic quality associated with its analogue, carpal tunnel syndrome.

It should be remembered that the most common causes of pain radiating into the lower extremity are herniated lumbar disk and nerve impingement secondary to degenerative arthritis of the spine, not disorders involving the sural nerve per se. Other pain syndromes that may be confused with sural nerve entrapment include lesions above the origin of the tibial nerve, such as lesions of the sciatic nerve, and distal lesions of the tibial nerve, such as posterior tarsal tunnel syndrome. Electromyography and magnetic resonance imaging of the lumbar spine, combined with information gleaned from the clinical history and physical examination, will help to sort out the etiology of distal lower pain.

CHAPTER 128

Metatarsal and Digital Nerve Block of the Foot

CPT-2009 CODE	
Unilateral	64450
Bilateral	64450-50
Neurolytic	64650

Relative Value Units	
Unilateral	7
Bilateral	14
Neurolytic	20

INDICATIONS

Metatarsal and digital nerve block is used primarily in two clinical situations: (1) to provide surgical anesthesia in the distribution of the digital nerves for laceration, tendon, and fracture repair, and (2) to provide postoperative pain relief after joint replacement or major surgical procedures on the foot.

CLINICALLY RELEVANT ANATOMY

In a manner analogous to that of the digital nerves of the hand, the digital nerves of the foot travel through the intrametatarsal space to innervate each toe. The plantar digital nerves, which are derived from the posterior tibial nerve, provide sensory innervation to the major portion of the plantar surface. These nerves are subject to entrapment and resultant development of perineural fibrosis and degeneration resulting in the clinical syndrome known as *Morton's neuroma* (Fig. 128-1). The dorsal aspect of the foot is innervated by terminal branches of the deep and superficial peroneal nerves. The overlap in the sensory innervation of these nerves may be considerable.

TECHNIQUE

The patient is placed in a supine position with a pillow placed under the knee to slightly flex the leg. A total of

3 mL per digit of non–epinephrine-containing local anesthetic is drawn up in a 12-mL sterile syringe.

Metatarsal Nerve Block

After preparation of the skin with antiseptic solution, at a point proximal to the metatarsal head, a 25-gauge, 1½-inch needle is inserted just adjacent to the metatarsal bone to be blocked (Fig. 128-2). While slowly injecting, the needle is advanced from the dorsal surface of the foot toward the plantar surface. The plantar digital nerve is situated on the dorsal side of the flexor retinaculum— thus, the needle has to be advanced almost to the plantar surface of the foot in order to produce satisfactory anesthesia. The needle is removed, and pressure is placed on the injection site to avoid hematoma formation.

Digital Nerve Block

After preparation of the skin with antiseptic solution, at a point at the base of the toe, a 25-gauge, 1½-inch needle is inserted just adjacent to the bone of the digit to be blocked (Fig. 128-3). While slowly injecting, the needle is advanced from the dorsal surface of the foot toward the plantar surface. The needle is removed, and pressure is placed on the injection site to avoid hematoma formation.

SIDE EFFECTS AND COMPLICATIONS

Because of the confined nature of the soft tissue surrounding the metatarsals and digits, the potential for mechanical compression of the blood supply after injection of solution must be considered. The pain specialist must avoid rapidly injecting large volumes of solution into these confined spaces, or vascular insufficiency and gangrene may occur. Furthermore, epinephrine-containing solutions must always be avoided to avoid ischemia and possible gangrene.

This technique can be safely performed in the presence of anticoagulation by using a 25- or 27-gauge needle, albeit at increased risk for hematoma, if the clinical situation dictates a favorable risk-to-benefit ratio. These

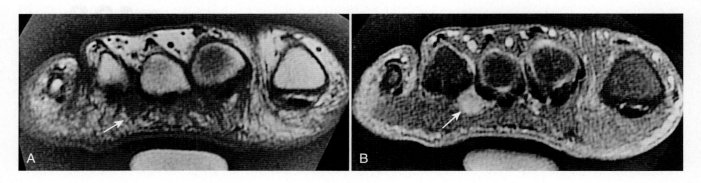

Figure 128-1.
A, T1 short-axis axial image, forefoot. There is a mass (*arrow*) in the third web space beneath the metatarsal heads that is difficult to detect on this sequence. **B,** T1 contrast-enhanced with fat suppression short-axis axial image, forefoot. The mass enhances diffusely (*arrow*) and is an easy diagnosis on this image. (From Kaplan P, Helms CA, Dussault R: Musculoskeletal MRI, 1st ed. Philadelphia, WB Saunders, 2001, p 418.)

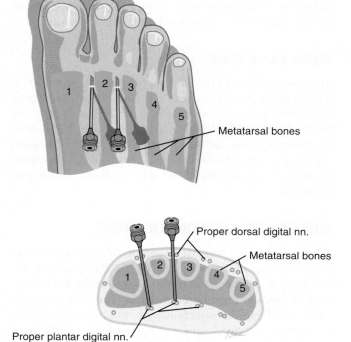

Metatarsal bones

Proper dorsal digital nn.

Metatarsal bones

Proper plantar digital nn.

Figure 128-2.

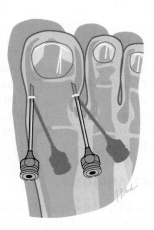

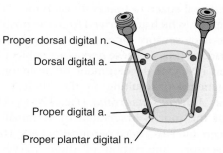

Proper dorsal digital n.

Dorsal digital a.

Proper digital a.

Proper plantar digital n.

Figure 128-3.

complications can be decreased if manual pressure is applied to the area of the block immediately after injection. Application of cold packs for 10-minute periods after the block also decreases the amount of postprocedure pain and bleeding.

CLINICAL PEARLS

Digital nerve block is especially useful in the palliation of postoperative pain after total joint replacement in the foot. For pain secondary to trauma, the pain specialist must ascertain and document the status of the vascular supply before implementing digital nerve block to avoid the erroneous attribution of any subsequent vascular insufficiency to the digital nerve block rather than to preexisting trauma to the vasculature.

Section 8

Advanced Interventional Pain Management Techniques

CHAPTER 129

Cervical Subarachnoid Neurolytic Block

CPT-2009 CODE	
Local Anesthetic/Antispasmodic	62274
Narcotic	62310
Differential Spinal	62318
Continuous Spinal	62318
Neurolytic	62280

Relative Value Units	
Local Anesthetic/Antispasmodic	10
Narcotic	10
Differential Spinal	12
Continuous Spinal	14
Neurolytic	20

INDICATIONS

Cervical subarachnoid neurolytic block is used primarily in patients suffering from pain of malignant origin that is localized to one to three spinal segments and that has failed to respond to other conservative therapy. Because of the potential for serious complications, this technique is rarely used in patients suffering from chronic benign pain, but it may be considered after a careful analysis of the risk-to-benefit ratio in carefully selected patients. Because this technique is most successful when treating pain that is subserved by a limited number of spinal nerves, cervical subarachnoid neurolytic block has its greatest utility in the treatment of pain involving the upper extremity, such as the pain of Pancoast's tumor or metastatic breast malignancy. Given the unique ability of this technique to allow destruction of the sensory component of the spinal root while theoretically sparing the motor component, this technique should probably be considered earlier in the course of a patient's disease than is currently being done. As with neurolytic celiac plexus block, the technique has a highly favorable cost-to-benefit ratio compared with the chronic administration of spinal opioids.

CLINICALLY RELEVANT ANATOMY

The Bell-Magendie law states that the motor fibers exit the ventral aspect of the spinal cord and that the sensory fibers exit the dorsal aspect of the spinal cord. This separation of motor and sensory fibers allows for selective destruction of the sensory fibers without concomitant destruction of the motor fibers at the same level. In the cervical region, the cervical nerve roots exit via the intervertebral foramina above their respective bodies, with C8 exiting above the T1 vertebra (Fig. 129-1). By placing the patient in a position with the dorsal roots uppermost, a hypobaric neurolytic solution such as alcohol can be floated onto the sensory fibers thought to be responsible for subserving the patient's pain while avoiding placing solution on the dependent motor fibers. By placing the patient in a position with the dorsal nerve roots bottommost, a hyperbaric neurolytic solution can be dripped onto the dependent sensory fibers thought to be subserving the patient's pain while at the same time avoiding the solution's floating onto the uppermost motor fibers.

The deep tissues such as bone may receive their innervation from a different spinal level than the skin overlying it. For this reason, if the patient's pain is thought to be primarily due to bony involvement from metastatic disease, it will be necessary to consult a sclerotome chart to determine which spinal nerve root actually provides innervation to the affected area (Fig. 129-2). Failure to consult a sclerotome chart and simply relying on the dermatomal distribution of the pain may result in block of the wrong spinal segment.

In the cervical region, the spinal cord is surrounded by three layers of protective connective tissue: the dura, the arachnoid, and the pia mater. The dura is the outmost layer and is composed of tough fibroelastic fibers that form a mechanical barrier to protect the spinal cord. The next layer is the arachnoid, which is separated from the dura by only a small potential space that is filled with serous fluid. The arachnoid is a barrier to the diffusion of substances and effectively serves to limit the spread of drugs administered into the epidural space from diffusing into the spinal fluid. The innermost layer is the

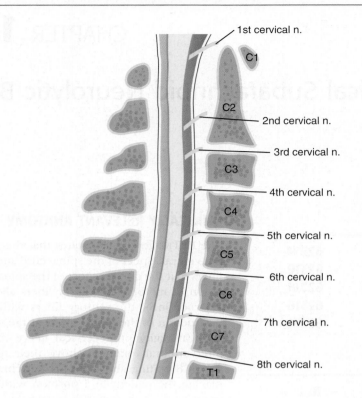

1st cervical n.

C1

C2 — 2nd cervical n.

3rd cervical n.

C3

4th cervical n.

C4

5th cervical n.

C5

6th cervical n.

C6

7th cervical n.

C7

8th cervical n.

T1

Figure 129-1.

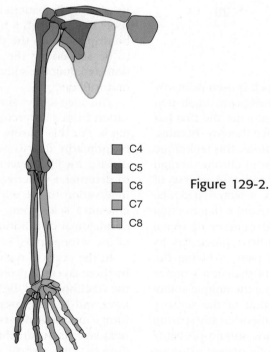

- C4
- C5
- C6
- C7
- C8

Figure 129-2.

pia, a vascular structure that helps provide lateral support to the spinal cord. Drugs administered into the subarachnoid space are placed between the arachnoid and pia, although inadvertent subdural injection is possible. Subdural injection of local anesthetic is characterized by a spotty, incomplete block.

Given the proximity of the spinal cord to needles advanced into the cervical subarachnoid space, the potential for needle trauma to the spinal cord remains an ever-present possibility.

TECHNIQUE

Hypobaric Neurolytic Solution Technique

Cervical subarachnoid neurolytic block is usually carried out in the lateral position, although the sitting position can be used if the patient is unable to lie on the side because of bony metastatic disease or because of respiratory insufficiency that makes lying with the head down difficult. The prone position is occasionally used when bilateral neurolytic block of a cervical segment is desired. Although this position limits the amount of rotation of the spine possible and simplifies midline identification, the inherent dangers of the prone position, including difficulty in monitoring the patient and problems with airway management, militate against the routine use of the prone position for cervical subarachnoid neurolytic block. As with all other regional anesthesia techniques, proper position is crucial to allow successful completion of the block and avoid complications. Regardless of the position chosen, careful attention to patient positioning, including identification of the midline, avoiding rotation of the spine, and ensuring flexion of the cervical spine, is essential to completing cervical subarachnoid neurolytic block successfully.

The patient is placed in the lateral position with the affected side uppermost. The head is placed on a pillow, with the cervical spine flexed and without rotation. The patient is rolled forward toward the abdomen about 45 degrees, with the chest and abdomen bolstered on pillows to allow the patient to remain in this position comfortably for the 30 or 40 minutes required to complete the procedure and allow the block to set up. The spinous process of T1 is identified. The pain specialist then counts upward to identify the cervical segment thought to be subserving the pain. The cervical roots exit the intervertebral foramina above their respective vertebral bodies (Fig. 129-3). If bone or deep structures are thought to be the source of the patient's pain, a sclerotome chart also is consulted to determine the spinal nerve that most likely provides sensory innervation to the affected area (see Fig. 129-2).

The skin overlying the spinal segment thought to subserve the pain, as well as the skin overlying several levels above and below the selected segment, is then prepared

with an antiseptic solution. The spinous process of the selected segment is then identified, and the operator's middle and index fingers are placed on each side of the spinous processes. The position of the interspace is reconfirmed with palpation using a rocking motion in the superior and inferior planes. The midline of this interspace is then identified by palpating the spinous processes above and below the interspace using a lateral rocking motion. Failure to identify the midline accurately is the number one reason for failed cervical subarachnoid neurolytic block.

At a point in the midline of the chosen interspace, local anesthetic is used to infiltrate the skin, subcutaneous tissues, ligamentum nuchae, and interspinous ligament down to the ligamentum flavum. A 22-gauge, $3\frac{1}{2}$-inch spinal needle with the stylet in place is then inserted exactly in the midline through the previously anesthetized area. The stylet is removed, and a well-lubricated, 5-mL glass syringe filled with preservative-free saline is attached to the spinal needle. While maintaining constant pressure on the plunger of the syringe, the nondominant hand advances the needle and syringe as a unit, with care taken to keep the needle fixed against the patient so that any sudden movement by the patient will not allow the needle to advance into the cervical spinal cord. The cervical epidural space is then identified using a loss-of-resistance technique.

After the cervical epidural space has been identified, and if there is no blood or cerebrospinal fluid (CSF) identified in the needle hub, the stylet is replaced, and the needle is carefully advanced through the dura and arachnoid into the subarachnoid space. Care must be taken not to advance the needle in an uncontrolled manner because trauma to the cervical spinal cord with subsequent syrinx formation could occur.

The stylet is removed, and the free flow of CSF is identified. A tuberculin syringe containing 1 mL of absolute alcohol is then attached to the needle. Sequential incremental injections of 0.1 mL of absolute alcohol are then administered (Fig. 129-4). The patient should be forewarned that a strong burning sensation will occur for a few seconds after injection and that he or she will be asked where the burning is felt. The patient's perception of the location of the burning will allow the pain specialist to determine whether the burning is at, above, or below the site of the patient's original pain complaint and allow repositioning of the needle accordingly. This verbal feedback is crucial to the overall success of cervical subarachnoid neurolytic block. For this reason, no local anesthetic should be administered through the spinal needle, and no preblock intravenous sedation should be given in an effort to decrease the amount of procedure-related pain.

If, after injection of alcohol, the burning sensation corresponds to the location of the source of the patient's

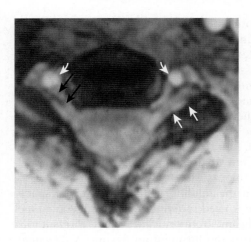

Figure 129-3.
Axial MRI demonstrating the relationship of the subarachnoid space, cervical nerves exiting the neural foramen (*large white arrows*), and vertebral arteries (*curved white arrows*). (From Stark DD, Bradley WG: Magnetic Resonance Imaging, 3rd ed. St. Louis, Mosby, 1999, p 1835.)

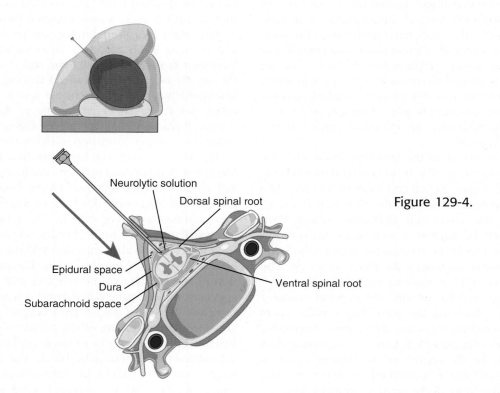

Neurolytic solution

Dorsal spinal root

Epidural space

Dura

Ventral spinal root

Subarachnoid space

Figure 129-4.

pain, up to 0.8 mL of absolute alcohol is injected in 0.1-mL incremental doses, with time given between each dose to ascertain each dose's effects and side effects. If the burning sensation is above or below the site of the patient's pain, the needle is removed and replaced accordingly, and the process is repeated. It is not unusual for several nerves to be blocked in order to provide complete pain relief. This can be done at separate settings in order for the patient to experience the effects of the absolute alcohol on his or her pain and functional ability. After the injection process is completed, the needle is flushed with 0.1 mL of sterile preservative-free saline and the needle is removed. The patient is left in the operative position with the dorsal roots uppermost for an additional 15 minutes. The patient is then returned to the supine position.

Hyperbaric Neurolytic Solution Technique

Phenol (6.5%) in glycerin is the most common neurolytic agent used for hyperbaric cervical subarachnoid neurolytic block. The block is carried out in a manner identical to the hypobaric technique described earlier, except for patient positioning (Fig. 129-5). In order for hyperbaric solutions to block the dorsal sensory fibers without concomitant blockade of the corresponding ventral motor fibers, the patient must be positioned with the affected side down and the patient turned 45 degrees toward his or her back. Pillows or a foam wedge is placed behind the patient's back to allow him or her to rest comfortably in this position for 30 to 40 minutes. As with the hypobaric technique, the pain specialist injects 0.1-mL increments of the neurolytic solution, with time between injections allowed to ascertain the effects and side effects of each increment. The major limitation with the use of hyperbaric solutions is the fact that the patient must lie with the affected side down, making the procedure more painful than using hypobaric solutions, which allow the patient to lie on the nonaffected side.

SIDE EFFECTS AND COMPLICATIONS

Most complications associated with cervical subarachnoid neurolytic block can be greatly decreased if careful attention is paid to the technical details and in particular the positioning of the patient. Motor and sensory deficits after cervical subarachnoid neurolytic block can occur even with the best technique. The patient and patient's family should be forewarned about the potential for complications to ensure a clear understanding of the risk-to-benefit ratio of the proposed procedure. Bowel or bladder dysfunction occurs less frequently after cervical subarachnoid neurolytic block than after thoracic and lumbar subarachnoid neurolytic procedures. Postblock dysesthesias also can occur after seemingly successful neurolytic procedures. Generally, the dysesthesias are thought to represent incomplete destruction of the fibers subserving the pain, and consideration should be given to repeat neurolysis if dysesthesias persist.

Because of the potential for hematogenous spread via Batson's plexus, local infection and sepsis represent absolute contraindications to subarachnoid nerve block. In contradistinction to the caudal approach to the epidural space, anticoagulation and coagulopathy represent absolute contraindications to cervical subarachnoid neurolytic block because of the risk for epidural and subarachnoid hematoma.

Hypotension is a common side effect of cervical subarachnoid neurolytic block and is the result of the profound sympathetic blockade attendant with this procedure. Prophylactic intramuscular or intravenous administration of vasopressors and fluid loading may help avoid this potentially serious side effect of cervical subarachnoid neurolytic block. If it is ascertained that a patient would not tolerate hypotension owing to other serious systemic disease, more peripheral regional anesthetic techniques, such as brachial plexus neurolysis, may be preferable to cervical subarachnoid neurolytic block.

It also is possible to inadvertently place a needle or catheter intended for the subarachnoid space into the subdural space. If subdural placement is unrecognized, the resulting block will be spotty, and the neurolytic solution may spread to nerves that were not intended to be blocked. This problem can be avoided if the operator advances the needle slightly after perceiving the pop of the needle as it pierces the dura.

Neurologic complications due to needle-induced trauma after cervical subarachnoid neurolytic block are uncommon if proper technique is used. Direct trauma to the spinal cord or nerve roots is usually accompanied by pain. If significant pain occurs during placement of the spinal needle, the physician should immediately stop and ascertain the cause of the pain to avoid the possibility of additional neural trauma. Delayed neurologic complications due to chemical irritation of the spinal cords and of coverings of the spinal cord and nerves have been reported. This problem is usually self-limited, although it must be distinguished from meningitis of infectious etiology.

Although uncommon, infection in the subarachnoid space remains an ever-present possibility, especially in the immunocompromised AIDS or cancer patient. If epidural abscess occurs, emergent surgical drainage to avoid spinal cord compression and irreversible neurologic deficit is usually required. Meningitis after cervical subarachnoid neurolytic block may require subarachnoid administration of antibiotics. Early detection and treatment of infection are crucial to avoid potentially life-threatening sequelae.

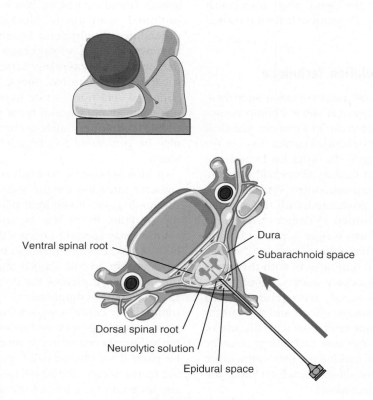

Ventral spinal root

Dura

Subarachnoid space

Dorsal spinal root

Neurolytic solution

Epidural space

Figure 129-5.

CLINICAL PEARLS

Cervical subarachnoid neurolytic block is a straightforward and effective procedure if careful attention is paid to technique. The most common reason for failure to reach the subarachnoid space is failure to identify the midline before needle placement. Given the proximity of the cervical spinal cord and exiting nerve roots to the subarachnoid space, needles placed off the midline can lead to significant neural trauma. The routine use of sedation or general anesthesia before initiation of cervical subarachnoid neurolytic block is to be discouraged because it will render the patient unable to provide accurate verbal feedback should needle misplacement occur.

CHAPTER **130**

Lumbar Subarachnoid Neurolytic Block

INDICATIONS

Lumbar subarachnoid neurolytic block is used primarily in patients suffering from pain of malignant origin that is localized to one to three spinal segments and that has failed to respond to other conservative therapy. Because of the potential for serious complications, this technique is rarely used in patients suffering from chronic benign pain, but it may be considered after a careful analysis of the risk-to-benefit ratio in carefully selected patients. Because this technique is most successful when treating pain that is subserved by a limited number of spinal nerves, lumbar subarachnoid neurolytic block has its greatest utility in the treatment of pain involving lower extremity and lower back pain, such as the pain of tumors invading the lumbar plexus or metastatic prostate or colon malignancy. Given the unique ability of this technique to allow destruction of the sensory component of the spinal root while theoretically sparing the motor component, this technique should probably be considered earlier in the course of a patient's disease than is currently being done. As with neurolytic celiac plexus block, the technique has a highly favorable cost-to-benefit ratio compared with chronic administration of spinal opioids.

CLINICALLY RELEVANT ANATOMY

The Bell-Magendie law states that the motor fibers exit the ventral aspect of the spinal cord and that the sensory fibers exit the dorsal aspect of the spinal cord. This separation of motor and sensory fibers allows for selective destruction of the sensory fibers without concomitant destruction of the motor fibers at the same level. In contradistinction to the cervical region, the lumbar nerve roots leave the spinal cord at levels much higher than they exit the vertebral column (Fig. 130-1). Hence, because the neurolytic solution must be placed on the dorsal root as it leaves the spinal cord, the pain specialist must ascertain the level at which the nerve actually leaves the spinal cord and perform the block at that level rather than at the point at which the spinal nerve root leaves the bony vertebral column.

By placing the patient in a position with the dorsal roots uppermost, a hypobaric neurolytic solution such as alcohol can be floated onto the sensory fibers thought to be responsible for subserving the patient's pain while at the same time avoiding placing solution on the dependent motor fibers. By placing the patient in a position with the dorsal nerve roots being bottommost, a hyperbaric neurolytic solution can be dripped onto the dependent sensory fibers thought to be subserving the patient's pain while avoiding the solution's floating onto the uppermost motor fibers.

The deep tissues such as bone may receive their innervation from a different spinal level than the skin overlying it. For this reason, if the patient's pain is thought to be primarily due to bony involvement from metastatic disease, it will be necessary to consult a sclerotome chart to determine which spinal nerve root actually provides innervation to the affected area (Fig. 130-2). Failure to consult a sclerotome chart and simply relying on the dermatomal distribution of the pain may result in block of the wrong spinal segment.

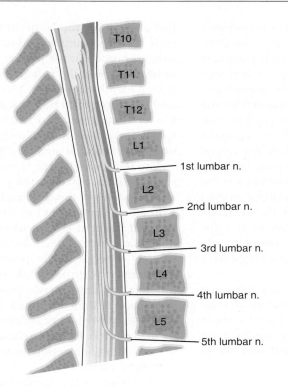

T10
T11
T12
L1
——— 1st lumbar n.
L2
——— 2nd lumbar n.
L3
——— 3rd lumbar n.
L4
——— 4th lumbar n.
L5
——— 5th lumbar n.

Figure 130-1.

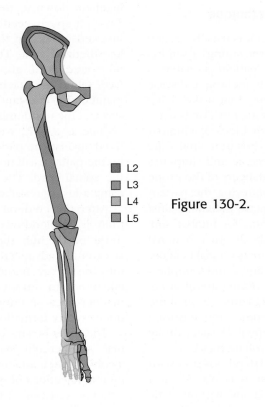

- L2
- L3
- L4
- L5

Figure 130-2.

In the lumbar region, the spinal cord is surrounded by three layers of protective connective tissue: the dura, the arachnoid, and the pia mater. The dura is the outmost layer and is composed of tough fibroelastic fibers that form a mechanical barrier to protect the spinal cord. The next layer is the arachnoid, which is separated from the dura by only a small potential space that is filled with serous fluid. The arachnoid is a barrier to the diffusion of substances and effectively serves to limit the spread of drugs administered into the epidural space from diffusing into the spinal fluid. The innermost layer is the pia, a vascular structure that helps provide lateral support to the spinal cord. Drugs administered into the subarachnoid space are placed between the arachnoid and pia, although inadvertent subdural injection is possible. Subdural injection of local anesthetic is characterized by a spotty, incomplete block.

The spinal cord ends at L2 in most adults, but given the fact that lumbar subarachnoid neurolytic block must be carried out at the level at which the dorsal sensory fibers actually leave the spinal cord, the potential for needle-induced trauma to the spinal cord remains an ever-present possibility.

TECHNIQUE

Hypobaric Neurolytic Solution Technique

Lumbar subarachnoid neurolytic block is usually carried out in the lateral position, although the sitting or semirecumbent position can be used if the patient is unable to lie on his or her side because of bony metastatic disease or because of respiratory insufficiency that makes lying with the head down difficult. The prone position is occasionally used when bilateral neurolytic block of a lumbar segment is desired. Although this position limits the amount of rotation of the spine possible and simplifies midline identification, the inherent dangers of the prone position, including difficulty in monitoring the patient and problems with airway management, militate against the routine use of the prone position for lumbar subarachnoid neurolytic block. As with all other regional anesthesia techniques, proper position is crucial to allow successful completion of the block and avoid complications. Regardless of the position chosen, careful attention to patient positioning, including identification of the midline, avoiding rotation of the spine, and ensuring flexion of the lumbar spine, is essential to successfully complete lumbar subarachnoid neurolytic block.

After the patient is placed in the lateral position with the affected side uppermost, the head is placed on a pillow, with the lumbar spine flexed and without rotation. The patient is rolled forward toward the abdomen about 45 degrees, with the chest and abdomen bolstered on pillows to allow the patient to comfortably remain in this position for the 30 or 40 minutes required to complete the procedure and allow the block to set up. The spinous process at the level at which the nerve thought to be subserving the patient's pain exits the spinal cord is then identified (see Fig. 130-1). If bone or deep structures are thought to be the source of the patient's pain, a sclerotome chart also is consulted to determine the spinal nerve that most likely provides sensory innervation to the affected area (see Fig. 130-2).

The skin overlying the spinal segment thought to subserve the pain, as well as the skin overlying several levels above and below the selected segment, is then prepared with an antiseptic solution. The spinous process of the selected segment is then identified, and the operator's middle and index fingers are placed on each side of the spinous processes. The position of the interspace is reconfirmed with palpation using a rocking motion in the superior and inferior planes. The midline of this interspace is then identified by palpating the spinous processes above and below the interspace using a lateral rocking motion. Failure to accurately identify the midline is the number one reason for failed lumbar subarachnoid neurolytic block.

At a point in the midline of the chosen interspace, local anesthetic is used to infiltrate the skin, subcutaneous tissues, supraspinous ligament, and interspinous ligament down to the ligamentum flavum. A 22-gauge, $3\frac{1}{2}$-inch spinal needle with the stylet in place is then inserted exactly in the midline through the previously anesthetized area. The stylet is removed, and a well-lubricated, 5-mL glass syringe filled with preservative-free saline is attached to the spinal needle. While maintaining constant pressure on the plunger of the syringe, the nondominant hand advances the needle and syringe as a unit, with care taken to keep the needle fixed against the patient so that any sudden movement by the patient will not allow the needle to advance into the spinal cord. The epidural space is then identified using a loss-of-resistance technique.

After the epidural space has been identified, and if there is no blood or cerebrospinal fluid (CSF) identified in the needle hub, the stylet is replaced, and the needle is carefully advanced through the dura and arachnoid into the subarachnoid space (Fig. 130-3). Care must be taken not to advance the needle in an uncontrolled manner because trauma to the spinal cord with subsequent syrinx formation could occur.

The stylet is removed, and a free flow of CSF is identified. A tuberculin syringe containing 1 mL of absolute alcohol is then attached to the needle. Sequential incremental injections of 0.1 mL of absolute alcohol are then administered (Fig. 130-4). The patient should be forewarned that a strong burning sensation will occur for a few seconds after injection and that he or she will be asked where the burning is felt. The patient's perception

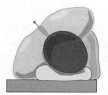

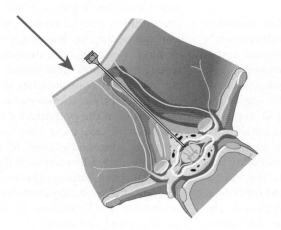

Figure 130-3.

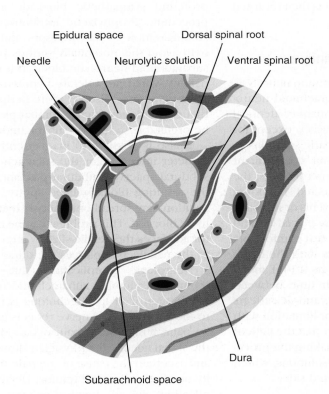

Epidural space

Needle

Neurolytic solution

Dorsal spinal root

Ventral spinal root

Figure 130-4.

Dura

Subarachnoid space

of the location of the burning will allow the pain specialist to determine whether the burning is at, above, or below the site of the patient's original pain complaint and allow repositioning of the needle accordingly. This verbal feedback is crucial to the overall success of lumbar subarachnoid neurolytic block. For this reason, no local anesthetic should be administered through the spinal needle, and no preblock intravenous sedation should be given in an effort to decrease the amount of procedure-related pain.

If, after injection of alcohol, the burning sensation corresponds to the location of the source of the patient's pain, up to 0.8 mL of absolute alcohol is injected in 0.1-mL incremental doses, with time given between each dose to ascertain each dose's effects and side effects. If the burning sensation is above or below the site of the patient's pain, the needle is removed and replaced accordingly, and the process is repeated. It is not unusual for several nerves to be blocked in order to provide complete pain relief. This can be done at separate settings in order for the patient to experience the effects of the absolute alcohol on his or her pain and functional ability. After the injection process is completed, the needle is flushed with 0.1 mL of sterile preservative-free saline and the needle is removed. The patient is left in the operative position with the dorsal roots uppermost for an additional 15 minutes. The patient is then returned to the supine position.

Hyperbaric Neurolytic Solution Technique

Phenol (6.5%) in glycerin is the most common neurolytic agent used for hyperbaric lumbar subarachnoid neurolytic block. The block is carried out in a manner identical to the hypobaric technique described earlier, except for patient positioning. In order for hyperbaric solutions to block the dorsal sensory fibers without concomitant blockade of the corresponding ventral motor fibers, the patient must be positioned with the affected side down and the patient turned 45 degrees toward his or her back (Fig. 130-5). Pillows or a foam wedge is placed behind the patient's back to allow him or her to rest comfortably in this position for 30 to 40 minutes. As with the hypobaric technique, the pain specialist injects 0.1-mL increments of the neurolytic solution, with time between injections allowed to ascertain the effects and side effects of each increment (Fig. 130-6). The major limitation with the use of hyperbaric solutions is the fact that the patient must lie with the affected side down, making the procedure more painful than using hypobaric solutions, which allow the patient to lie on the nonaffected side.

SIDE EFFECTS AND COMPLICATIONS

Most complications associated with lumbar subarachnoid neurolytic block can be greatly decreased if careful attention is paid to the technical details and in particular the positioning of the patient. Motor and sensory deficits after lumbar subarachnoid neurolytic block can occur even with the best technique. The patient and the patient's family should be forewarned about the potential for the complications to ensure a clear understanding of the risk-to-benefit ratio of the proposed procedure. Bowel or bladder dysfunction occurs with greater frequency after lumbar subarachnoid neurolytic block when compared with cervical and upper thoracic subarachnoid neurolytic procedures. Postblock dysesthesias also can occur after seemingly successful neurolytic procedures. Generally, the dysesthesias are thought to represent incomplete destruction of the fibers subserving the pain, and consideration should be given to repeat neurolysis if dysesthesias persist.

Because of the potential for hematogenous spread via Batson's plexus, local infection and sepsis represent absolute contraindications to the subarachnoid nerve block. In contradistinction to the caudal approach to the epidural space, anticoagulation and coagulopathy represent absolute contraindications to lumbar subarachnoid neurolytic block because of the risk for epidural and subarachnoid hematoma.

Hypotension is a common side effect of lumbar subarachnoid neurolytic block and is the result of the profound sympathetic blockade attendant with this procedure. Prophylactic intramuscular or intravenous administration of vasopressors and fluid loading may help avoid this potentially serious side effect of lumbar subarachnoid neurolytic block. If it is ascertained that a patient would not tolerate hypotension owing to other serious systemic disease, more peripheral regional anesthetic techniques, such as lumbar plexus neurolysis, may be preferable to lumbar subarachnoid neurolytic block.

It also is possible to inadvertently place a needle or catheter intended for the subarachnoid space into the subdural space. If subdural placement is unrecognized, the resulting block will be spotty, and the neurolytic solution may spread onto nerves that were not intended to be blocked. This problem can be avoided if the operator advances the needle slightly after perceiving the pop of the needle as it pierces the dura.

Neurologic complications due to needle-induced trauma after lumbar subarachnoid neurolytic block are uncommon if proper technique is used. Direct trauma to the spinal cord or nerve roots is usually accompanied by pain. If significant pain occurs during placement of the spinal needle, the physician should immediately stop and ascertain the cause of the pain to avoid the possibility of additional neural trauma. Delayed neurologic complications due to chemical irritation of the spinal cord and the coverings of the spinal cord and nerves have been reported. This problem is usually self-limited, although it must be distinguished from meningitis of infectious etiology.

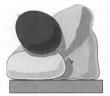

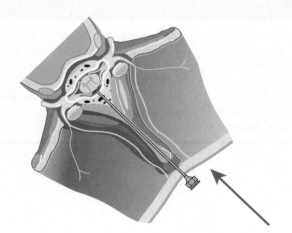

Figure 130-5.

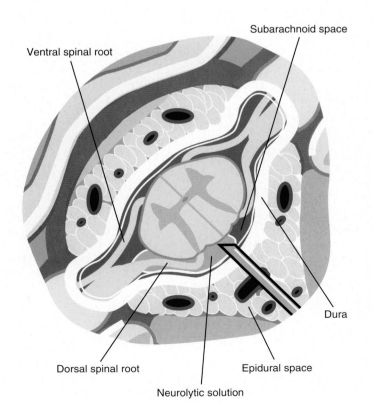

Figure 130-6.

Subarachnoid space

Ventral spinal root

Dura

Dorsal spinal root

Epidural space

Neurolytic solution

Although uncommon, infection in the subarachnoid space remains an ever-present possibility, especially in the immunocompromised AIDS or cancer patient. If epidural abscess occurs, emergent surgical drainage to avoid spinal cord compression and irreversible neurologic deficit is usually required. Meningitis after lumbar subarachnoid neurolytic block may require subarachnoid administration of antibiotics. Early detection and treatment of infection are crucial to avoid potentially life-threatening sequelae.

CLINICAL PEARLS

Lumbar subarachnoid neurolytic block is a straightforward and effective procedure if careful attention is paid to technique. The most common reason for failure to reach the subarachnoid space is failure to identify the midline before needle placement. Given the proximity of the spinal cord and exiting nerve roots to the subarachnoid space, needles placed off the midline can lead to significant neural trauma. The routine use of sedation or general anesthesia before initiation of lumbar subarachnoid neurolytic block is to be discouraged because it will render the patient unable to provide accurate verbal feedback should needle misplacement occur.

Implantation of Subcutaneously Tunneled One-Piece Epidural Catheters

Implantation of Subcutaneously Tunneled Epidural Catheter	**62350**
Implantation of Subcutaneously Tunneled Epidural Catheter With Laminectomy	**62351**
Removal of Previously Implanted Catheter	**62355**

Relative Value Units

Implantation Procedure	**25**
Implantation With Laminectomy	**35**
Removal of Previously Implanted Catheter	**25**

INDICATIONS

Implantation of a subcutaneously tunneled one-piece epidural catheter is indicated for the injection or infusion of drugs into the epidural space in four clinical situations:

1. For the patient who has sustained multiple trauma and in whom it is expected that acute and postoperative pain management will be required for a period longer than a few days
2. For the administration of epidural drugs for the palliation of pain in cancer patients with a life expectancy of weeks to months
3. For catheter placement as the first step in the implantation of totally implantable drug delivery systems including pumps and ports
4. In settings in which easy catheter removal is desired

Given the decreased incidence of infection associated with subcutaneously tunneled epidural catheters compared with simple percutaneously placed catheters, tunneled catheters are being used more frequently in settings in which a simple percutaneous catheter would have been used in the past.

CLINICALLY RELEVANT ANATOMY

The superior boundary of the epidural space is the fusion of the periosteal and spinal layers of dura at the foramen magnum. The epidural space continues inferiorly to the sacrococcygeal membrane. The epidural space is bounded anteriorly by the posterior longitudinal ligament and posteriorly by the vertebral laminae and the ligamentum flavum. The vertebral pedicles and intervertebral foramina form the lateral limits of the epidural space. The cervical epidural space is 3 to 4 mm at the C7-T1 interspace with the cervical spine flexed. The lumbar epidural space is 5 to 6 mm at the L2-L3 interspace with the lumbar spine flexed. The epidural space contains fat, veins, arteries, lymphatics, and connective tissue. Epidural catheters can be placed anywhere along the spine from the cervical to the caudal region.

TECHNIQUE

Catheter placement may be carried out with the patient in the sitting, lateral, or prone position. Selection of position is based on the patient's ability to maintain the chosen position for the 15 to 20 minutes needed to place the catheter subcutaneously. Because most catheters are placed on an outpatient basis, choosing the most comfortable position is important to minimize the need for adjunctive intravenous narcotics or sedation.

After aseptic preparation of the skin to include the site of tunneling and catheter exit site, a 17-gauge Tuohy needle is placed into the epidural space at the level of desired catheter placement. The Silastic one-piece catheter is then advanced through the Tuohy needle into the epidural space (Fig. 131-1A). Silastic catheters have a tendency to drag against the internal needle wall and fold back onto themselves. This can be avoided by wetting both the needle and catheter with saline before attempting to advance the catheter through the needle.

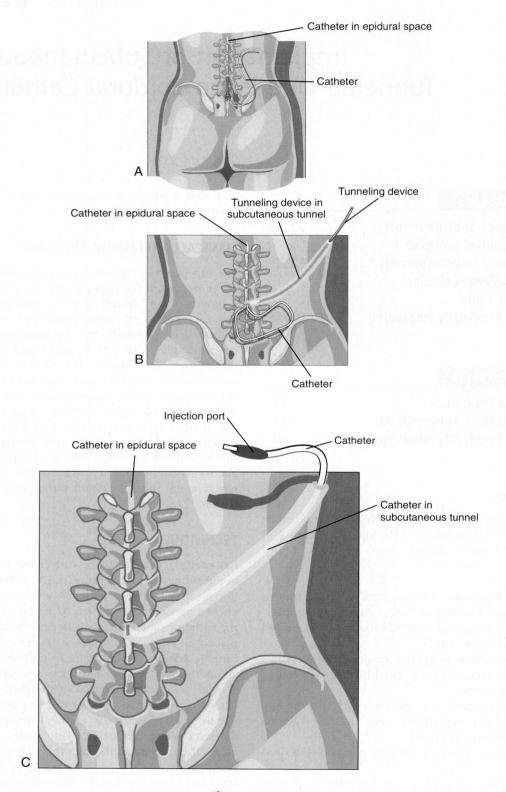

Figure 131-1.

After the catheter enters the epidural space, it is gently advanced an additional 3 to 4 cm. A small incision is made with a No. 15 scalpel extending cranially and caudally about 0.5 cm with the needle still in place to avoid inadvertent damage to the catheter. Care must be taken to completely dissect all tissue away from the needle to allow the catheter to fall freely into the incision as the tunneling tool is advanced. The needle is then carefully withdrawn back along the catheter until the tip is outside the skin. The catheter wire stylet is withdrawn, and the Tuohy needle is removed from the catheter. The injection port is then attached to the distal end of the catheter, and after aspiration, 4 to 5 mL of 1.5% lidocaine is injected into the epidural space via the catheter to provide dense segmental sensory block for the subcutaneous tunneling. This approach avoids the need for painful subcutaneous infiltration at the tunneling site. Injection through the catheter at this point also allows for inspection for any leaks before subcutaneous tunneling.

The malleable tunneling device is then shaped to match the contour of the flank. The skin is now lifted with thumb forceps, and the tunneling device is introduced subcutaneously and guided laterally. When the tip of the tunneling device has reached the exit point laterally, it is turned away from the patient; this forces the tip against the skin. The scalpel is then used to cut down onto the tip. The tunneling device is then advanced through the incision. This approach allows for a straight catheter path and decreases the incidence of catheter failure secondary to subcutaneous catheter kinking. The injection port is removed, and the distal end of the catheter is then threaded onto the stud on the proximal end of the tunneling device (see Fig. 131-1**B**). The tunneling device is then withdrawn through the second incision, bringing the catheter with it through the subcutaneous tunnel (see Fig. 131-1**C**). A subcutaneous reservoir or implantable drug delivery system may then be attached to the distal end of the catheter after making a small subcutaneous pocket, or the catheter may simply be injected via the injection port.

By repeating the tunneling procedure once or twice, the catheter can be advanced to a position anteriorly on the anterior chest or in the mid-subcostal area if the patient is expected to inject his or her own catheter. If nursing staff or family members are expected to inject the catheter, it may be left posteriorly. At this point, the injection port is reinserted into the distal catheter, and a small amount of preservative-free saline is injected to ensure catheter integrity. The wounds at each incision are closed with one or two 4-0 nylon interrupted sutures, and a sterile dressing is applied. Sutures should be removed in about 10 days. The catheter is now ready for injection or attachment to an external continuous infusion pump.

SIDE EFFECTS AND COMPLICATIONS

Because of the potential for hematogenous spread via Batson's plexus, local infection and sepsis represent absolute contraindications to the placement of catheters into the epidural space. Anticoagulation and coagulopathy represent absolute contraindications to placement of epidural catheters because of the risk for epidural hematoma.

Inadvertent dural puncture during identification of the epidural space should occur less than 0.5% of the time. Failure to recognize inadvertent dural puncture can result in immediate total spinal anesthetic with associated loss of consciousness, hypotension, and apnea. If epidural doses of opioids are accidentally placed into the subarachnoid space, significant respiratory and central nervous system depression will result. It is also possible to inadvertently place a needle or catheter intended for the epidural space into the subdural space. If subdural placement is unrecognized and epidural doses of local anesthetic are administered, the signs and symptoms are similar to those of massive subarachnoid injection, although the resulting motor and sensory block may be spotty.

The epidural space is highly vascular. The intravenous placement of the epidural needle or catheter occurs in about 0.5% to 1% of patients undergoing placement of epidural catheters. This complication is increased in patients with distended epidural veins, that is, parturient patients and patients with a large intra-abdominal tumor mass. If the misplacement is unrecognized, injection of local anesthetic directly into an epidural vein results in significant local anesthetic toxicity.

Needle trauma to the epidural veins may result in self-limited bleeding, which may cause postprocedural pain. Uncontrolled bleeding into the epidural space may result in compression of the spinal cord with the rapid development of neurologic deficit. Although the incidence of significant neurologic deficit secondary to epidural hematoma after placement of epidural catheters is exceedingly rare, this devastating complication should be considered whenever there is rapidly developing neurologic deficit after placement of epidural catheters.

Neurologic complications after placement of epidural catheters are uncommon if proper technique is used. Direct trauma to the spinal cord or nerve roots is usually accompanied by pain. If significant pain occurs during placement of the epidural needle or catheter or during injection, the physician should immediately stop and ascertain the cause of the pain to avoid the possibility of additional neural trauma.

Although uncommon, infection in the epidural space remains an ever-present possibility, especially in the immunocompromised AIDS or cancer patient. If epidural abscess occurs, emergent surgical drainage to avoid spinal cord compression and irreversible neurologic deficit is usually required. Early detection and treatment of infection is crucial to avoid potentially life-threatening sequelae. Infections at the tunnel exit site can usually be managed with systemic and topical antibiotics. With close observation of the patient for spread of infection proximally down the tunnel into the epidural space, the catheter does not need to be removed.

CLINICAL PEARLS

Subcutaneous tunneling of epidural one-piece catheters is a safe and effective procedure if careful attention is paid to technique. Failure to accurately identify the midline is the most common reason for difficulty in identifying the epidural space and increases the risk for complications. The routine use of sedation or general anesthesia before identification of the epidural space is to be discouraged because it will render the patient unable to provide accurate verbal feedback should needle misplacement occur.

Many pain centers have begun using tunneled catheters for patients suffering from acute and postoperative pain in whom pain control will be required for longer than 2 or 3 days. Such patients include those who have suffered multiple trauma and those undergoing surgical procedures such as extensive skin grafting or orthopedic procedures over several days. The one-piece catheter is easier to remove than the two-piece catheter with a Dacron cuff and is ideally suited for such patients.

CHAPTER 132

Implantation of Subcutaneously Tunneled Two-Piece Epidural Catheters

Implantation of Subcutaneously Tunneled Epidural Catheter	62350
Implantation of Subcutaneously Tunneled Epidural Catheter With Laminectomy	62351
Removal of Previously Implanted Catheter	62355

Relative Value Units

Implantation Procedure	25
Implantation With Laminectomy	35
Removal of Previously Implanted Catheter	25

INDICATIONS

The use of a two-piece subcutaneously tunneled epidural catheter has both advantages and disadvantages when compared with a one-piece epidural catheter. There are two major advantages of the two-piece catheter: (1) the incidence of infection deep into the tunnel or epidural space is decreased because of the Dacron cuff affixed to the distal catheter segment; and (2) the incidence of accidental catheter displacement or removal is decreased because of the Dacron cuff.

The two major disadvantages of a two-piece catheter are that (1) implantation is more technically demanding, and (2) removal is much more difficult when compared with a one-piece subcutaneously tunneled epidural catheter.

Implantation of a subcutaneously tunneled two-piece epidural catheter is indicated for the injection or infusion of drugs into the epidural space primarily in situations in which the pain management specialist plans to continue the administration of epidural drugs for a period of weeks to months. In clinical situations in which epidural administration of drugs is expected to be used for shorter periods of time, a one-piece catheter is preferred because of the ease of removal.

CLINICALLY RELEVANT ANATOMY

The superior boundary of the epidural space is the fusion of the periosteal and spinal layers of dura at the foramen magnum. The epidural space continues inferiorly to the sacrococcygeal membrane. The epidural space is bounded anteriorly by the posterior longitudinal ligament and posteriorly by the vertebral laminae and the ligamentum flavum. The vertebral pedicles and intervertebral foramina form the lateral limits of the epidural space. The cervical epidural space is 3 to 4 mm at the C7-T1 interspace with the cervical spine flexed. The lumbar epidural space is 5 to 6 mm at the L2-L3 interspace with the lumbar spine flexed. The epidural space contains fat, veins, arteries, lymphatics, and connective tissue. Epidural catheters can be placed anywhere along the spine from the cervical to the caudal region.

TECHNIQUE

Catheter placement may be carried out with the patient in the sitting, lateral, or prone position. Selection of position is based on the patient's ability to maintain the chosen position for the 15 to 20 minutes needed to place the catheter subcutaneously. Because most catheters are placed on an outpatient basis, choosing the most comfortable position is important to minimize the need for adjunctive intravenous narcotics or sedation.

After aseptic preparation of the skin to include the site of tunneling and catheter exit site, a 17-gauge Tuohy needle is placed into the epidural space at the level of desired catheter placement. The proximal portion of a Silastic catheter is then advanced through the Tuohy needle into the epidural space (Fig. 132-1A). Silastic catheters have a tendency to drag against the internal needle wall and fold back onto themselves. This can be avoided by wetting both the needle and catheter with saline before attempting to advance the catheter through the needle.

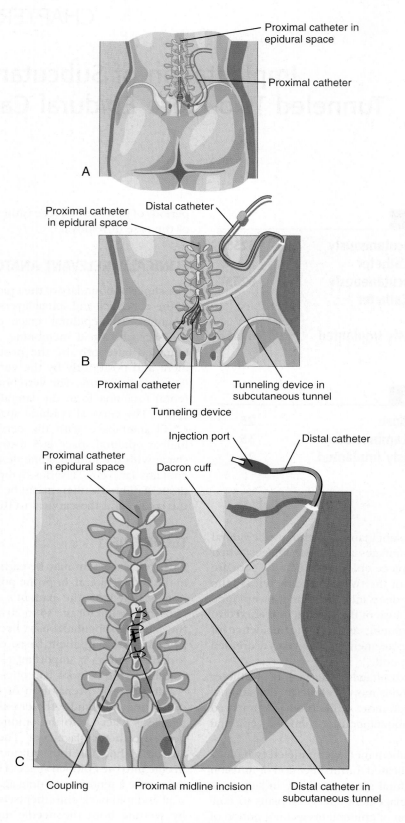

Figure 132-1.

After the catheter enters the epidural space, it is gently advanced an additional 3 to 4 cm. A small incision is made with a No. 15 scalpel extending cranially and caudally about 1 cm with the needle still in place to avoid inadvertent damage to the catheter. Care must be taken to completely dissect all tissue away from the needle to allow the catheter to fall freely into the incision as the tunneling tool is advanced. The needle is then carefully withdrawn back along the catheter until the tip is outside the skin. The catheter wire stylet is withdrawn, and the Tuohy needle is removed from the catheter. The injection port is then attached to the distal end of the catheter, and after aspiration, 4 to 5 mL of 1.5% lidocaine is injected into the epidural space via the catheter to provide dense segmental sensory block for the subcutaneous tunneling. This approach avoids the need for painful subcutaneous infiltration at the tunneling site. Injection through the catheter at this point also allows for inspection for any leaks before subcutaneous tunneling.

The distal portion of the catheter is then implanted by tunneling it from the distal catheter exit site to the proximal midline incision (see Fig. 132-1B). To accomplish this, a small stab wound is made anteriorly past the anterior axillary line. If the patient is planning to self-inject the catheter, the exit site incision is made on the side opposite the patient's dominant hand. The exit site should not be positioned to rest under beltlines or brassieres or where ostomy belts may place pressure on the catheter. After the stab wound is made, a malleable tunneling device is then shaped to match the contour of the flank. The skin is now lifted with thumb forceps, and the tunneling device is introduced subcutaneously and guided toward the midline incision containing the proximal catheter segment. When the tip of the tunneling device has reached the midline incision, the tip of the tunneling device is then advanced out of the incision, with care taken not to damage the proximal catheter segment. This approach allows for a straight catheter path and decreases the incidence of catheter failure secondary to subcutaneous catheter kinking.

The end of the distal catheter segment is then threaded onto the stud on the end of the tunneling device extending out of the exit site incision. The tunneling device is then drawn out through the midline incision, bringing the catheter with it through the subcutaneous tunnel. Care must be taken to facilitate passage of the Dacron cuff past the exit incision into the subcutaneous tunnel created by the tunneling tool. The pain management specialist should expect significant drag on the catheter as the Dacron cuff is drawn through the subcutaneous tunnel. Firm steady tension of the end of the distal catheter segment will be more effective in drawing the Dacron cuff into the subcutaneous tunnel compared with sudden pulling or jerking on the catheter.

After the Dacron cuff has been drawn 2 to 3 inches into the subcutaneous tunnel, any excess portion of the catheter segment extending out of the midline incision is cut off, and the proximal and distal catheter segments are united using the coupling provided with the two-piece catheter (see Fig. 132-1C). Silk sutures are used to secure the catheter to the coupling. The catheter and coupling are then gently placed into the midline incision, and the distal catheter is injected with sterile preservative-free saline to ensure catheter integrity and to ascertain that the catheter is functional. The midline incision is then closed with two or three interrupted sutures, with care taken to ensure that the suture needle does not damage the implanted catheter segments. Sutures can be removed in 10 to 14 days.

SIDE EFFECTS AND COMPLICATIONS

Because of the potential for hematogenous spread via Batson's plexus, local infection and sepsis represent absolute contraindications to the placement of catheters into the epidural space. Anticoagulation and coagulopathy represent absolute contraindications to placement of epidural catheters because of the risk for epidural hematoma.

Inadvertent dural puncture during identification of the epidural space should occur less than 0.5% of the time. Failure to recognize inadvertent dural puncture can result in immediate total spinal anesthetic with associated loss of consciousness, hypotension, and apnea. If epidural doses of opioids are accidentally placed into the subarachnoid space, significant respiratory and central nervous system depression will result. It also is possible to inadvertently place a needle or catheter intended for the epidural space into the subdural space. If subdural placement is unrecognized and epidural doses of local anesthetic are administered, the signs and symptoms are similar to those of massive subarachnoid injection, although the resulting motor and sensory block may be spotty.

The epidural space is highly vascular. The intravenous placement of the epidural needle or catheter occurs in about 0.5% to 1% of patients undergoing placement of epidural catheters. This complication is increased in patients with distended epidural veins, that is, parturient patients and patients with a large intra-abdominal tumor mass. If the misplacement is unrecognized, injection of local anesthetic directly into an epidural vein results in significant local anesthetic toxicity.

Needle trauma to the epidural veins may result in self-limited bleeding, which may cause postprocedural pain. Uncontrolled bleeding into the epidural space may result in compression of the spinal cord with the rapid development of neurologic deficit. Although the incidence of significant neurologic deficit secondary to epidural hematoma after placement of epidural catheters is exceedingly rare, this devastating complication should be considered whenever there is rapidly developing neurologic deficit after placement of epidural catheters.

Neurologic complications after placement of epidural catheters are uncommon if proper technique is used. Direct trauma to the spinal cord or nerve roots is usually accompanied by pain. If significant pain occurs during placement of the epidural needle or catheter or during injection, the physician should immediately stop and ascertain the cause of the pain to avoid the possibility of additional neural trauma.

Although uncommon, infection in the epidural space remains an ever-present possibility, especially in the immunocompromised AIDS or cancer patient. If epidural abscess occurs, emergent surgical drainage to avoid spinal cord compression and irreversible neurologic deficit is usually required. Early detection and treatment of infection is crucial to avoid potentially life-threatening sequelae. Infections at the tunnel exit site can usually be managed with systemic and topical antibiotics. With close observation of the patient for spread of infection proximally down the tunnel into the epidural space, the catheter does not need to be removed.

CLINICAL PEARLS

Subcutaneous tunneling of two-piece epidural catheters is a safe and effective procedure if careful attention is paid to technique. Failure to accurately identify the midline is the most common reason for difficulty in identifying the epidural space and increases the risk for complications. The routine use of sedation or general anesthesia before identification of the epidural space is to be discouraged because it will render the patient unable to provide accurate verbal feedback should needle misplacement occur.

Many pain centers have begun using tunneled catheters for patients suffering from acute and postopera-

tive pain in whom pain control will be required for longer than 2 or 3 days. Such patients include those who have suffered multiple trauma and those undergoing surgical procedures such as extensive skin grafting or orthopedic procedures over several days. The one-piece catheter is easier to remove than the two-piece catheter with a Dacron cuff and is ideally suited for such patients. If it is anticipated that the catheter will need to be left in place for more than a few weeks, a two-piece catheter with a Dacron cuff is a better choice.

CHAPTER 133

Neuradenolysis of the Pituitary: Needle-Through-Needle Technique

CPT-2009 CODE

Destruction of Pituitary—Chemical	61715

Relative Value Units

Neuradenolysis Procedure	40

INDICATIONS

Neuradenolysis of the pituitary is an appropriate treatment modality for patients who suffer from bilateral facial or upper body cancer pain, bilateral diffuse cancer pain, intractable visceral pain, and pain secondary to compression of neural structures in whom all antiblastic methods and other pain-relieving measures have been exhausted. Patients in whom medical hormonal control of pain is lost also may benefit from the procedure. Most investigators observe better results in patients whose pain is secondary to hormone-dependent tumors, although the procedure also is effective in the palliation of pain resulting from non–hormonally responsive malignancies.

Contraindications to neuradenolysis of the pituitary include local infection, sepsis, coagulopathy, significantly increased intracranial pressure, and empty sella syndrome. Relative contraindications to neuradenolysis of the pituitary include poor anesthetic risk, disulfiram therapy, and significant behavioral abnormalities. Obviously, owing to the desperate circumstances surrounding most patients considered for neuradenolysis of the pituitary, the risk-to-benefit ratio is shifted toward performing the procedure on both ethical and humanitarian grounds.

CLINICALLY RELEVANT ANATOMY

The pituitary rests in the bony sella turcica. It is easily reached via the transsphenoidal approach by a needle placed through the nasal mucosa. To reach the pituitary gland, the needle must pass through the nasal mucosa, the sphenoid bone, the sphenoid sinus, and the anterior wall of the sella turcica (Fig. 133-1). The needle must be placed through the nasal mucosa to avoid Kiesselbach's plexus, or vigorous epistaxis will occur. In some patients, there is a midline septum in the sphenoid sinus that may make the passage of a needle difficult. In such patients, the needle is simply advanced along the wall of the septum, with care being taken to ensure that the ultimate entry point of the sella turcica is in the midline. Lateral to the sella turcica are the internal carotid arteries. Just superior and lateral to the carotid arteries are the oculomotor nerves. Behind and lateral to the stalk of the pituitary are the optic nerves and optic chiasm. Above the pituitary is the hypothalamus.

TECHNIQUE
Preoperative Preparations

Screening laboratory tests, consisting of a complete blood count, chemistry profile, electrolyte determination, urinalysis, coagulation profile, chest radiography, and electrocardiogram, are performed as for any other patient undergoing general anesthesia. Anteroposterior and lateral skull films also are obtained to evaluate the size and relative position of the sella turcica and to rule out sphenoid sinus infection, which may be clinically silent. Preoperative treatment of all patients with an intravenous dose of a cephalosporin and aminoglycoside antibiotic 1 hour before induction of anesthesia is indicated to decrease the risk for infection in these immunocompromised patients. Most investigators perform neuradenolysis of the pituitary with the patient under general endotracheal anesthesia, although in view of the lack of pain associated with the procedure, the procedure can be performed using local anesthesia. Opioids are avoided as premedicants as well as intraoperatively to avoid pupillary miosis, which might obscure the pupil-

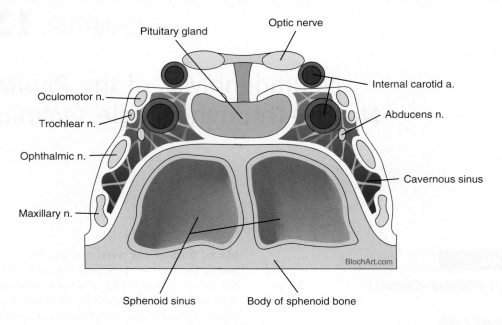

Pituitary gland

Optic nerve

Oculomotor n.

Trochlear n.

Ophthalmic n.

Maxillary n.

Internal carotid a.

Abducens n.

Cavernous sinus

Sphenoid sinus

Body of sphenoid bone

BlochArt.com

Figure 133-1.

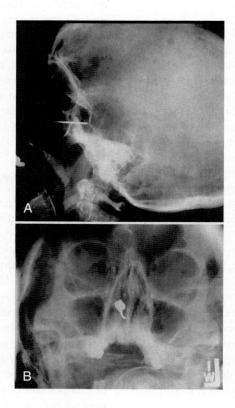

Figure 133-2.
Plain radiographs confirming placement of the 17-gauge, 3½-inch needle in a midline position with the tip resting against the anterior wall of the sella turcica. **A,** Lateral view. **B,** Anteroposterior view. (From Waldman SD: Interventional Pain Management, 2nd ed. Philadelphia, WB Saunders, 2001, p 679.)

lary dilation observed when alcohol inadvertently spills out of the sella turcica onto the oculomotor nerve.

Needle-Through-Needle Technique

With the intubated patient in the supine position on the biplanar fluoroscopy table, the nose is packed with pledgets soaked in 7.5% cocaine solution to provide vasoconstriction and shrinkage of the nasal mucosa. After 10 minutes, the packs are removed, and the anterior nasal mucosa and face are prepared with povidone-iodine solution. Sterile drapes are placed over the nose and face. The anterior medial mucosa and deep tissues are infiltrated with a solution of 1.0% lidocaine and 1:200,000 epinephrine. During infiltration and subsequent needle placement, care must be taken to avoid Kiesselbach's plexus, or vigorous bleeding may ensue. It is imperative that the head be kept in a precise midline position to allow accurate needle placement.

A 17-gauge, $3\frac{1}{2}$-inch spinal needle with the stylet in place is advanced under biplanar fluoroscopic guidance, with care taken to ensure that the needle remains exactly in the midline to avoid trauma to the adjacent structures, including the carotid arteries. The needle is advanced until its tip rests against the anterior wall of the sella turcica (Figs. 133-2 and 133-3). At this point, plain radiographs are taken to confirm needle position. After satisfactory position is verified, the stylet is removed from the 17-gauge needle. A 20-gauge, 13-cm styletted needle is placed through the 17-gauge spinal needle and is carefully advanced through the anterior wall of the sella turcica (Fig. 133-4). This process feels like passing a needle through an eggshell. The 13-cm needle is then further advanced under biplanar fluoroscopic guidance through the substance of the pituitary gland, until the tip rests against the posterior wall of the sella turcica. Needle position is again confirmed with plain radiographs.

The patient's eyes are then exposed, and alcohol in aliquots of 0.2 mL is injected as the 13-cm needle is gradually withdrawn back through the pituitary. Depending on the size of the sella, a total of 4 to 6 mL of alcohol is injected. During the injection process, the pupils are constantly monitored for dilation. Pupillary dilation indicates that the alcohol has spilled outside the sella turcica and has come in contact with an oculomotor nerve. If pupillary dilation is observed, injection of alcohol is discontinued, and the needle is withdrawn to a more anterior position. The injection process is then resumed. In most instances, if the alcohol injection is discontinued at the first sign of pupillary dilation, any resultant visual disturbance is transitory.

After the injection of alcohol is completed, 0.5 mL of cyanomethacrylate resin is injected via the 13-cm needle to seal the hole in the sella turcica and to prevent cere-brospinal fluid (CSF) leakage. Both needles are removed. The nasal mucosa is observed for bleeding or CSF leakage. Nasal packing is not generally required with this modified procedure. The patient is then extubated and taken to the recovery room. It takes about 30 minutes to perform neuradenolysis of the pituitary using the needle-through-needle technique.

Postoperative Care

All patients are continued on antibiotics for 24 hours. Endocrine replacement, consisting of 15 mg of prednisone and 0.15 mg of levothyroxine sodium every morning, is required for every patient.

Accurate monitoring of intake and output is mandatory because transient diabetes insipidus occurs in about 40% of patients undergoing neuradenolysis of the pituitary. In most instances, the diabetes insipidus is self-limited, but vasopressin administration should be considered in patients who are unable to drink as much as they excrete or in whom urinary output exceeds 2.5 L/day. Failure to identify and treat diabetes insipidus is the leading cause of morbidity and mortality in patients undergoing neuradenolysis of the pituitary. All patients are continued on preoperative levels of oral narcotics for 24 hours, and then dosages are tapered. Patients generally resume their normal diet and activities the day of the procedure.

SIDE EFFECTS AND COMPLICATIONS

Complications directly related to neuradenolysis of the pituitary are generally self-limited, although occasionally, even with the best technique, severe complications can occur. Essentially all patients who undergo neuradenolysis of the pituitary complain of a bilateral frontal headache, which resolves spontaneously within 24 to 48 hours. Diabetes insipidus occurs in about 40% of patients who undergo the procedure. Failure to recognize this complication can lead to unnecessary patient deaths. About 35% of patients experience transient temperature increases of up to 1.5°C after neuradenolysis of the pituitary. These temperature aberrations are thought to be due to disturbance of the temperature regulating mechanism of the hypothalamus. About 20% of patients experience an increase in pulmonary secretions and mild orthopnea that clinically resembles congestive heart failure. This problem is self-limited if careful attention is paid to the patient's fluid status. It has been postulated that this phenomenon represents a centrally mediated process.

Although the potential for serious ocular disturbances exists, a review of the literature suggests that transient visual disturbances including diplopia, blurred vision, and loss of visual field occur in less than 10% of patients

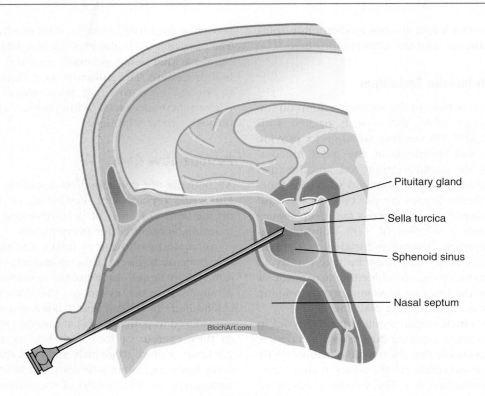

Figure 133-3.

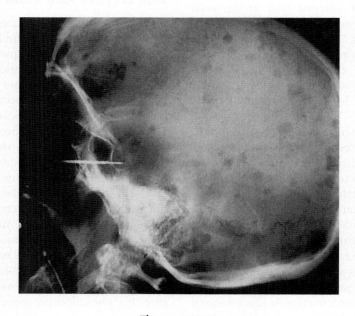

Figure 133-4.

Plain radiograph confirms that the tip of the Hinck needle is resting against the posterior wall of the sella turcica. (From Waldman SD: Interventional Pain Management, 2nd ed. Philadelphia, WB Saunders, 2001, p 680.)

who undergo neuradenolysis of the pituitary gland. Permanent visual disturbances occur much less commonly, with an average incidence of about 5%. CSF leakage, infection, and pituitary hemorrhage occur in less than 1% of patients but represent some of the most devastating complications. If they are not immediately recognized and treated, death can result.

CLINICAL PEARLS

Neuradenolysis of the pituitary gland is a safe, effective method to palliate diffuse pain of malignant origin that is unresponsive to conservative treatment modalities. Its technical simplicity and relative safety make neuradenolysis of the pituitary an ideal procedure for the oncology patient who has undergone a vast array of disease treatments. Although spinal administration of opioids has replaced neuradenolysis of the pituitary as the procedure of choice for many cancer pain syndromes, it is the belief of many cancer pain specialists that neuradenolysis of the pituitary is still currently underused. With use of the needle-through-needle modification described, a more favorable risk-to-benefit ratio is expected. As Bonica has stated, "Neuroadenolysis of the pituitary is one of the most, if not the most, effective ablative procedures for the relief of severe diffuse cancer pain."

The use of phenol, cryoneurolysis, radiofrequency lesions, and electrical stimulation in place of alcohol also has been advocated for neuradenolysis of the pituitary. More experience is needed with each of these modalities to determine whether some of the theoretical advantages and disadvantages of each modification translate into clinically relevant benefits.

CHAPTER **134**

Cervical Diskography

INDICATIONS

Cervical diskography is indicated as a diagnostic maneuver in a carefully selected subset of patients suffering from neck and cervical radicular pain. Patients who may benefit from diskography include the following:

1. Patients with persistent neck or cervical radicular pain in whom traditional diagnostic modalities, such as magnetic resonance imaging (MRI), computed tomography (CT), and electromyography, have failed to delineate a cause of the pain
2. Patients in whom equivocal findings such as bulging cervical disks are identified on traditional diagnostic modalities, to determine whether such abnormalities are in fact responsible for the pain
3. Patients who are to undergo cervical fusion, in which diskography may help identify what levels need to be fused
4. Patients who have previously undergone fusion of the cervical spine, in which diskography may help identify whether levels above and below the fusion are responsible for persistent pain
5. Patients in whom recurrent disk herniation cannot be separated from scar tissue with traditional imaging techniques

In each of these select patient populations, the pain management specialist must correlate the data obtained from the injection, the provocation of pain on injection, the radiographic appearance of the diskogram obtained, and in selected patients, the relief of pain after the disk is injected with local anesthetic. A failure to carefully correlate all this diagnostic information in the context of the patient's clinical presentation will lead the pain management specialist to erroneously interpret the results of diskography and will adversely influence clinical decision making.

CLINICALLY RELEVANT ANATOMY

From a functional anatomic viewpoint, cervical disks must be thought of as distinct from lumbar disks insofar as a source of pain is concerned. Radicular symptoms solely from disk herniation are much less common in the cervical region than in the lumbar region. The reason for this is twofold: (1) In order for the cervical disk to impinge on the cervical nerve roots, it must herniate posteriorly and laterally. The cervical nerve roots are in part protected from impingement from cervical disk herniation by the facet joints, which interpose a bony wall between the disk and the nerve root. (2) The disk is completely enclosed posteriorly by the dense, double-layered posterior longitudinal ligament. This ligament is much more developed than its lumbar counterpart, which is thinner in its lateral aspects and composed of a single layer.

The nuclear material in the cervical disk is placed more anterior than its lumbar counterpart. The anterior portion of the cervical disk space is larger than the posterior portion, making it difficult for the nuclear material to move posteriorly unless great forces are placed on the disk. The tough outer annulus also is thicker in the posterior portion of the disk, making posterior bulging of the cervical disk difficult. It is this annular layer that receives sensory innervation from a variety of sources. Posteriorly, the annulus receives fibers from the sinovertebral nerves, which also provide sensory innervation to the posterior elements including portions of the facet joints. Laterally, fibers from the exiting spinal nerve roots provide sensory innervation, with the anterior portion of the disk receiving fibers from the sympathetic chain. Whether part or all of these fibers play a role in diskogenic pain is a subject of controversy among pain specialists.

The cervical nerve roots leave the spinal cord and travel laterally through the intervertebral foramina. If the posterior cervical disk herniates laterally, it can impinge on the cervical root as it travels through the intervertebral foramen, producing classic radicular symptoms. If the cervical disk herniates posteromedially, it may impinge on the spinal cord, producing myelopathy that may include upper and lower extremity as well as bowel and bladder symptoms. Severe compression of the cervical spinal cord may result in quadriparesis or, rarely, quadriplegia.

TECHNIQUE

The patient is placed in the supine position with the neck in neutral position as if for a stellate ganglion block. The skin of the anterior neck is then prepared with antiseptic solution. CT views are taken through the disks to be imaged, and the relative positions of the carotid artery, esophagus, and trachea are noted. As an alternative, fluoroscopic guidance may be used if CT guidance is unavailable. The right side of the anterior neck is usually chosen for needle entry because the esophagus tracks to the left as it descends the neck. A skin wheal of local anesthetic is placed at the medial border of the sternocleidomastoid muscle at the level to be evaluated. A 22-gauge, 13-cm styletted needle is then advanced toward the superior margin of the vertebral body just below the disk to be evaluated, with care taken to avoid the carotid artery, jugular vein, trachea, and esophagus.

After the needle impinges on bone, the depth of bony contact is noted, and the needle is withdrawn into the subcutaneous tissues and readvanced with a more superior trajectory into the anterior disk annulus (Fig. 134-1). The needle is then advanced in incremental steps into the nucleus (Figs. 134-2 and 134-3). Sequential scanning is indicated to avoid advancing the needle completely through the disk and into the cervical spinal cord. Water-soluble contrast medium suitable for intrathecal use is then slowly injected through the needle into the disk in a volume of 0.2 to 0.6 mL (Fig. 134-4). The resistance to injection should be noted, with an intact disk exhibiting firm resistance at these volumes. Simultaneously, the patient's pain response during injection is noted. The location of the patient's pain and its quality and similarity to the patient's ongoing clinical symptoms are evaluated. A verbal analogue scale may be useful to help the patient quantify the amount of pain experienced compared with the injection of adjacent disks.

The nucleogram of a normal cervical disk appears as a lobulated mass with posterolateral clefts that occur as part of the normal aging process of the disk (Fig. 134-5A). In the damaged disk, the contrast material may flow into tears of the inner annulus, producing a characteristic transverse pattern (see Fig. 134-5B). If the tears in the annulus extend to the outer layer, a radial pattern is produced (Fig. 134-6A). Contrast material also may flow between the layers of annulus, producing a circumferential pattern (see Fig. 134-6B). Complete disruption of the annulus allows the contrast material to flow into the epidural space or into the cartilaginous end plate of the vertebra (Fig. 134-7). Although the greater the damage to the annulus, the greater the likelihood that the disk being evaluated is the source of the patient's pain, the pain management specialist must evaluate all the information obtained during the diskography procedure and place this information into the context of the patient's pain symptoms.

After evaluation of the nucleogram, a decision must be made whether to proceed with diskography of adjacent disks or to inject local anesthetic into the disk currently being imaged. Analgesic diskography is useful in patients whose clinical pain pattern is reproduced or provoked during the injection of contrast medium. If the pain that was provoked during the injection of contrast medium is relieved by a subsequent injection of local anesthetic into the disk, an inference can be drawn that the disk is the likely source of the patient's pain. Remember that if there is disruption of the annulus, the injected local anesthetic may spread into the epidural space and anesthetize somatic and sympathetic nerves that may subserve disks at an adjacent level. If this occurs, erroneous information may be obtained if diskography is then performed on adjacent disks.

After injection procedures are completed, the patient is observed for 30 minutes before discharge. The patient should be warned to expect minor postprocedure discomfort, including some difficulty swallowing. Placing ice packs on the injection site for 20-minute periods will help decrease these untoward effects. The patient should be instructed to call immediately if fever or other systemic symptoms occur that might suggest infection.

SIDE EFFECTS AND COMPLICATIONS

Complications directly related to diskography are generally self-limited, although occasionally, even with the best technique, severe complications can occur. The most common severe complication after diskography is infection of the disk, which is commonly referred to as *diskitis*. Because of the limited blood supply of the disk, such infections can be extremely hard to eradicate. Diskitis usually manifests as an increase in spine pain several days to a week after diskography. Acutely, there will be no change in the patient's neurologic examination as a result of disk infection.

Epidural abscess, which can rarely occur after diskography, generally manifests within 24 to 48 hours.

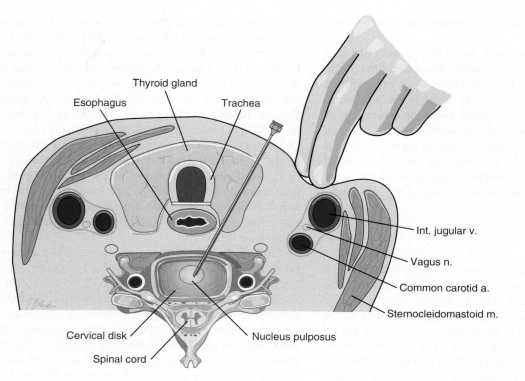

Figure 134-1.

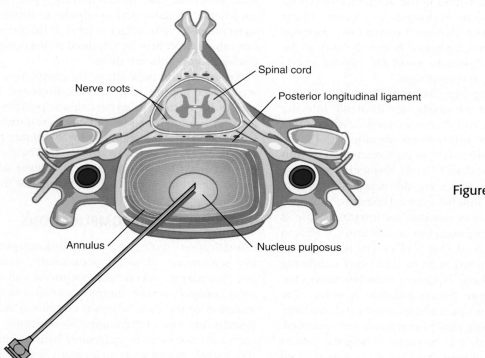

Figure 134-2.

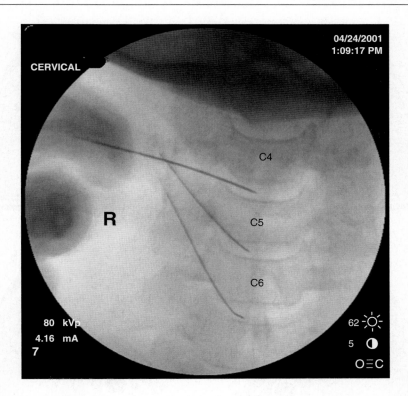

Figure 134-3.
Needles placed in the cervical disks.

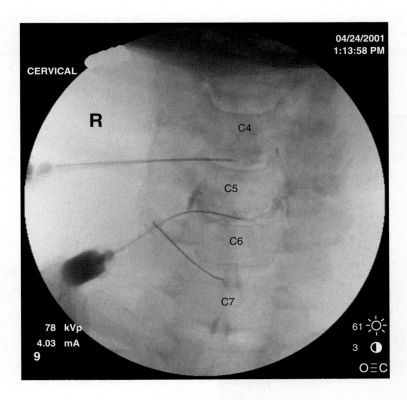

Figure 134-4.
Contrast medium injected into the cervical disks.

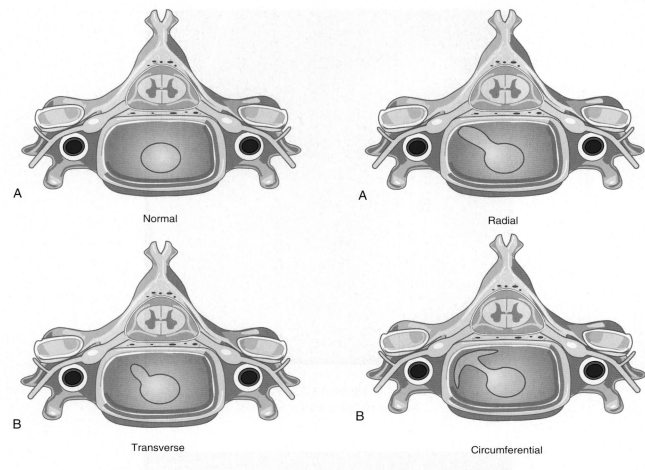

Normal

Radial

Transverse

Circumferential

Figure 134-5.

Figure 134-6.

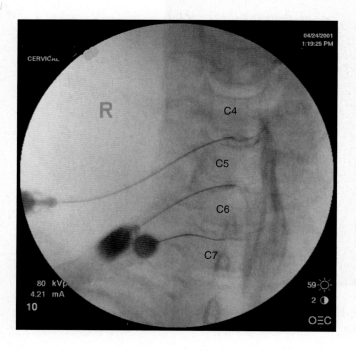

Figure 134-7.
Contrast medium flowing from the cervical disks into the epidural space.

Clinically, the signs and symptoms of epidural abscess are high fever, spine pain, and progressive neurologic deficit. If either diskitis or epidural abscess is suspected, blood and urine cultures should be taken, antibiotics started, and emergent MRI of the spine obtained to allow identification and drainage of any abscess formation to prevent irreversible neurologic deficit.

In addition to infectious complications, pneumothorax may occur after cervical diskography. This complication should rarely occur if CT guidance is used during needle placement. Small apical pneumothorax after cervical diskography can often be treated conservatively, and tube thoracostomy can be avoided.

Direct trauma to the nerve roots and the spinal cord can occur if the needle is allowed to traverse the entire disk or is placed too lateral. These complications should rarely occur if incremental CT scans are taken while advancing the needle. Such needle-induced trauma to the cervical spinal cord can result in syrinx formation with attendant progressive neurologic deficit, including quadriplegia.

CLINICAL PEARLS

Cervical diskography is a straightforward technique that may provide useful clinical information in carefully selected patients. The information obtained from cervical diskography must always be analyzed in the context of the patient's clinical presentation. Failure to do so will lead to a variety of clinical misadventures, including additional spine surgeries that are doomed to failure. The use of CT guidance adds a measure of safety compared with fluoroscopy because it allows the pain specialist to clearly identify anatomic structures and needle position. These advantages more than outweigh the possible added cost when compared with fluoroscopically guided procedures.

CHAPTER 135

Thoracic Diskography

INDICATIONS

Although performed less frequently than cervical and lumbar diskography, thoracic diskography probably provides more clinically useful information than when this diagnostic technique is used at other levels. The reason for this paradox is threefold:

1. Less is known about the thoracic disk in health and disease.
2. Herniated thoracic disks occur less frequently than lumbar and cervical disk herniations.
3. Clinicians are less comfortable attributing pain symptoms to thoracic diskogenic disease.

For these reasons, thoracic diskography can help the pain management specialist determine whether a damaged thoracic disk is in fact the true source of a patient's pain complaints. This information is extremely valuable given the difficulty and risks associated with surgery on the thoracic disks.

Thoracic diskography is indicated as a diagnostic maneuver in a carefully selected subset of patients suffering from thoracic radicular and occasionally myelopathic pain. Patients who may benefit from diskography include the following:

1. Those patients with persistent thoracic radicular or myelopathic pain in whom traditional diagnostic

modalities, such as magnetic resonance imaging (MRI), computed tomography (CT), and electromyography, have failed to delineate a cause of the pain
2. Patients in whom equivocal findings such as bulging thoracic disks are identified on traditional diagnostic modalities, to determine whether such abnormalities are in fact responsible for the pain
3. Patients who are to undergo instrumentation and fusion of the thoracic spine, in which diskography may help identify what levels need to be fused
4. Patients who have previously undergone instrumentation and fusion of the thoracic spine, in which diskography may help identify whether levels above and below the fusion are responsible for persistent pain
5. Patients in whom recurrent disk herniation cannot be separated from scar tissue with traditional imaging techniques

In each of these patient populations, the pain management specialist must correlate the data obtained from the injection, the provocation of pain on injection, the radiographic appearance of the diskogram obtained, and in selected patients, the relief of pain after the disk is injected with local anesthetic. A failure to carefully correlate all this diagnostic information in the context of the patient's clinical presentation will lead the pain management specialist to erroneously interpret the results of diskography and will adversely influence clinical decision making.

CLINICALLY RELEVANT ANATOMY

The gelatinous nucleus pulposus of the thoracic disk is surrounded by a dense, laminated fibroelastic network of fibers known as the *annulus*. The annular fibers are arranged in concentric layers that run obliquely from adjacent vertebrae. It is this annular layer that receives sensory innervation from a variety of sources. Posteriorly, the annulus receives fibers from the sinovertebral nerves, which also provide sensory innervation to the posterior elements including portions of the facet joints. Laterally, fibers from the exiting spinal nerve roots provide sensory innervation, with the anterior portion of the disk receiving fibers from the sympathetic chain. Whether part or all of these fibers play a role in diskogenic pain is a subject of controversy among pain specialists. Each thoracic disk is situated between the cartilaginous end plates of the vertebrae above and below it.

The thoracic nerve roots leave the spinal cord and travel laterally through the intervertebral foramina. If the posterior thoracic disk herniates laterally, it can impinge on the thoracic root as it travels through the intervertebral foramen, producing classic radicular symptoms. If the thoracic disk herniates posteromedially, it may impinge on the spinal cord, producing myelopathy that may include thoracic and lower extremity as well as bowel and bladder symptoms. Severe compression of the thoracic spinal cord may result in paraparesis or, rarely, paraplegia.

TECHNIQUE

The patient is placed in the prone position with a pillow under the lower chest to slightly flex the thoracic spine as if for a thoracic sympathetic block. CT views are taken through the disks to be imaged, and the relative positions of the pleural space, lung, ribs, nerve roots, and spinal cord are noted. As an alternative, fluoroscopy may be used if CT. is unavailable. The spinous process of the vertebra just above the disk to be evaluated is palpated. At a point just below and 1½ inches lateral to the spinous process, the skin is prepared with antiseptic solution, and the skin and subcutaneous tissues are infiltrated with local anesthetic.

A 22-gauge, 13-cm styletted needle is advanced through the skin under CT guidance, with the target being the middle of the disk to be imaged (Fig. 135-1). Given the proximity of the somatic nerve roots, a paresthesia in the distribution of the corresponding thoracic paravertebral nerve may be elicited. If this occurs, the needle should be withdrawn and redirected slightly more cephalad. The needle is readvanced in incremental steps under CT guidance, with care taken to keep the needle trajectory medial to avoid pneumothorax.

The needle is then advanced in incremental steps into the central nucleus (Fig. 135-2). Sequential scanning is indicated to avoid advancing the needle completely through the disk and into the thoracic spinal cord or allowing the needle to track too lateral into the pleural cavity. Water-soluble contrast medium suitable for intrathecal use is then slowly injected through the needle into the disk in a volume of 0.2 to 0.6 mL. The resistance to injection should be noted, with an intact disk exhibiting firm resistance at these volumes. Simultaneously, the patient's pain response during injection is noted. The location of the patient's pain and its quality and similarity to the patient's ongoing clinical symptoms are evaluated.

A verbal analogue scale may be useful to help the patient quantify the amount of pain experienced when compared with the injection of adjacent disks.

The nucleogram of a normal thoracic disk appears as a lobulated mass with occasional posterolateral clefts that occur as part of the normal aging process of the disk (Fig. 135-3A). In the damaged disk, the contrast material may flow into tears of the inner annulus, producing a characteristic transverse pattern (see Fig. 135-3B). If the tears in the annulus extend to the outer layer, a radial pattern is produced (Fig. 135-4A). Contrast material also may flow between the layers of annulus, producing a circumferential pattern (see Fig. 135-4B). Complete disruption of the annulus allows the contrast material to flow into the epidural space or into the cartilaginous end plate of the vertebra. Although the greater the damage to the annulus, the greater the likelihood that the disk being evaluated is the source of the patient's pain, the pain management specialist must evaluate all the information obtained during the diskography procedure and place this information into the context of the patient's pain symptoms.

After evaluation of the nucleogram, a decision must be made whether to proceed with diskography of adjacent disks or to inject local anesthetic into the disk currently being imaged. Analgesic diskography is useful in patients whose clinical pain pattern is reproduced or provoked during the injection of contrast medium. If the pain that was provoked during the injection of contrast medium is relieved by a subsequent injection of local anesthetic into the disk, an inference can be drawn that the disk is the likely source of the patient's pain. It must be remembered that if there is disruption of the annulus, the injected local anesthetic may spread into the epidural space and anesthetize somatic and sympathetic nerves that may subserve disks at an adjacent level. If this occurs, erroneous information may be obtained if diskography is then performed on adjacent disks.

After injection procedures are completed, the patient is observed for 30 minutes before discharge. The patient should be warned to expect minor postprocedure discomfort, including some soreness of the paraspinous musculature. Placing ice packs on the injection site for 20-minute periods will help decrease these untoward effects. The patient should be instructed to call immediately if fever or other systemic symptoms occur that might suggest infection.

SIDE EFFECTS AND COMPLICATIONS

Complications directly related to diskography are generally self-limited, although occasionally, even with the best technique, severe complications can occur. The most common severe complication after diskography is infection of the disk, which is commonly referred to as

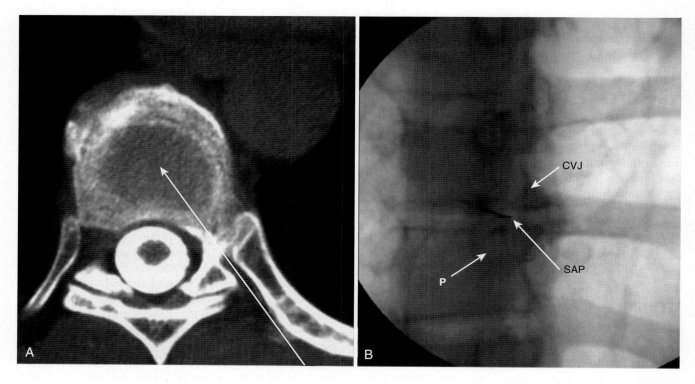

Figure 135-1.
Target point for needle insertion at thoracic spine (oblique view). CVJ, costovertebral joint; P, pedicle; SAP, superior articular process. (From Derby R, Lee SH, Chen Y: Discograms: Cervical, thoracic, and lumbar. Tech Reg Anesth Pain Manage 9:97-105, 2005.)

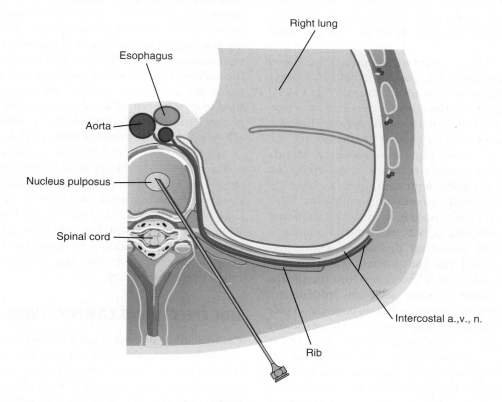

Figure 135-2.

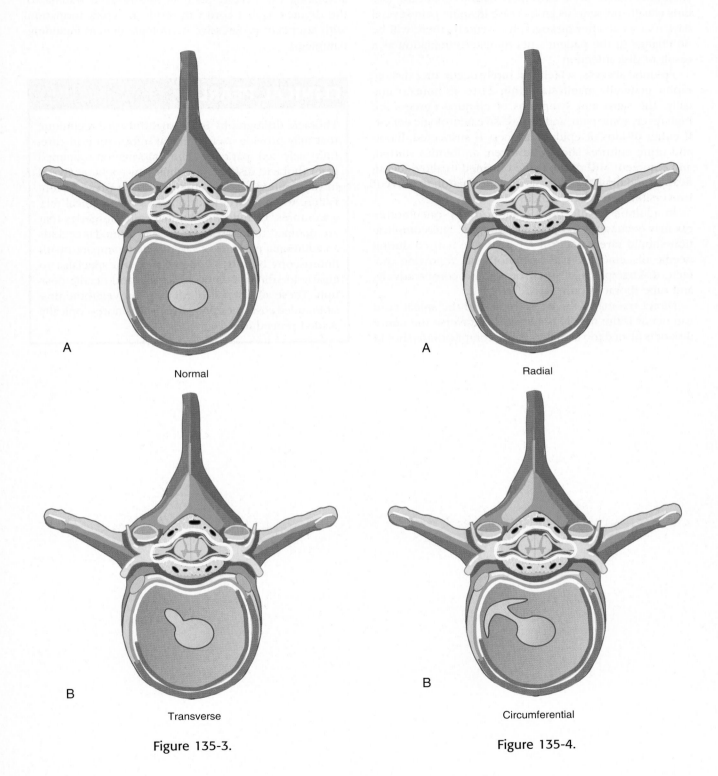

A

Normal

B

Transverse

Figure 135-3.

A

Radial

B

Circumferential

Figure 135-4.

diskitis. Because of the limited blood supply of the disk, such infections can be extremely hard to eradicate. Diskitis usually presents as an increase in spine pain several days to a week after diskography. Acutely, there will be no change in the patient's neurologic examination as a result of disk infection.

Epidural abscess, which can rarely occur after diskography, generally manifests within 24 to 48 hours. Clinically, the signs and symptoms of epidural abscess are high fever, spine pain, and progressive neurologic deficit. If either diskitis or epidural abscess is suspected, blood and urine cultures should be taken, antibiotics started, and emergent MRI of the spine obtained to allow identification and drainage of any abscess formation to prevent irreversible neurologic deficit.

In addition to infectious complications, pneumothorax may occur after thoracic diskography. This complication should rarely occur if CT guidance is used during needle placement. Small pneumothorax following thoracic diskography can often be treated conservatively, and tube thoracostomy can be avoided.

Direct trauma to the nerve roots and the spinal cord can occur if the needle is allowed to traverse the entire disk or is placed too laterally. These complications should rarely occur if incremental CT scans are taken while advancing the needle. Such needle-induced trauma to the thoracic spinal cord can result in syrinx formation with attendant progressive neurologic deficit, including paraplegia.

CLINICAL PEARLS

Thoracic diskography is a straightforward technique that may provide useful clinical information in carefully selected patients. The information obtained from thoracic diskography must always be analyzed in the context of the patient's clinical presentation. Failure to do so will lead to a variety of clinical misadventures, including additional spine surgeries that are doomed to failure. The use of CT guidance adds an additional measure of safety when compared with fluoroscopy because it allows the pain specialist to clearly identify anatomic structures and needle position. These advantages more than outweigh the possible added cost when compared with fluoroscopically guided procedures.

CHAPTER 136

Lumbar Diskography

CPT-2009 CODE

Injection Procedure, Each Level	62290
Radiographic Interpretation of Diskogram	72295

Relative Value Units

Injection Procedure, Each Level	20
Radiographic Interpretation of Diskogram	10

INDICATIONS

Lumbar diskography is indicated as a diagnostic maneuver in a carefully selected subset of patients suffering from back and lumbar radicular pain. Patients who may benefit from diskography include the following:

1. Patients with persistent back or lumbar radicular pain in whom traditional diagnostic modalities, such as magnetic resonance imaging (MRI), computed tomography (CT), and electromyography, have failed to delineate a cause of the pain
2. Patients in whom equivocal findings such as bulging lumbar disks are identified on traditional diagnostic modalities, to determine whether such abnormalities are in fact responsible for the pain
3. Patients who are to undergo lumbar fusion, in which diskography may help identify what levels need to be fused
4. Patients who have previously undergone fusion of the lumbar spine, in which diskography may help identify whether levels above and below the fusion are responsible for persistent pain
5. Patients in whom recurrent disk herniation cannot be separated from scar tissue with traditional imaging techniques

In each of these patient populations, the pain management specialist must correlate the data obtained from the injection, the provocation of pain on injection, the radiographic appearance of the diskogram obtained, and in selected patients, the relief of pain after the disk is injected with local anesthetic. A failure to carefully correlate all this diagnostic information in the context of the patient's clinical presentation will lead the pain management specialist to erroneously interpret the results of diskography and adversely influence clinical decision making.

CLINICALLY RELEVANT ANATOMY

From a functional anatomic viewpoint, lumbar disks must be thought of as distinct from cervical disks insofar as a source of pain is concerned. Radicular symptoms solely from disk herniation are much more common in the lumbar region when compared with the cervical and thoracic regions. The reason for this is twofold: (1) In order for the lumbar disk to impinge on the lumbar nerve roots, it must herniate posteriorly and laterally. The lumbar nerve roots are not protected from impingement from lumbar disk herniation by the bony wall of the facet joints as are the cervical nerve roots. (2) The posterior longitudinal ligament in the lumbar region is only a single layer, which is thinner and less well developed in its lateral aspects. It is this lateral region in which lumbar disk herniation with impingement on exiting nerve roots is most likely to occur.

The nuclear material in the lumbar disk is placed more posterior than its cervical counterpart. The gelatinous nucleus pulposus of the lumbar disk is surrounded by a dense, laminated fibroelastic network of fibers known as the *annulus*. The annular fibers are arranged in concentric layers that run obliquely from adjacent vertebrae. It is this annular layer that receives sensory innervation from a variety of sources. Posteriorly, the annulus receives fibers from the sinovertebral nerves, which also provide sensory innervation to the posterior elements, including portions of the facet joints. Laterally, fibers from the exiting spinal nerve roots provide sensory innervation, with the anterior portion of the disk receiving fibers from the sympathetic chain. Whether part or all of these fibers play a role in diskogenic pain is a subject of controversy among pain specialists.

The lumbar nerve roots leave the spinal cord and travel laterally through the intervertebral foramina. If the posterior lumbar disk herniates laterally, it can impinge on the lumbar root as it travels through the intervertebral foramen, producing classic radicular symptoms. If the lumbar disk herniates posteromedially, it may impinge on the spinal cord, producing myelopathy that may include lower extremity as well as bowel and bladder symptoms. Severe compression of the lumbar spinal cord may result in cauda equina syndrome, paraparesis, or, rarely, paraplegia.

TECHNIQUE

The patient is placed in the prone position with a pillow under the abdomen to slightly flex the lumbar spine as if for a lumbar sympathetic block. CT views are taken through the disks to be imaged, and the relative positions of the lung, ribs, aorta, vena cava, kidneys, nerve roots, and spinal cord are noted (Figs. 136-1 and 136-2). As an alternative, fluoroscopy can be used for needle placement if CT guidance is not available. The spinous process of the vertebra just above the disk to be evaluated is palpated. At a point just below and 1½ inches lateral to the spinous process, the skin is prepared with antiseptic solution, and the skin and subcutaneous tissues are infiltrated with local anesthetic.

A 22-gauge, 13-cm styletted needle is advanced through the skin under CT guidance, with the target being the middle of the disk to be imaged. Given the proximity of the somatic nerve roots, a paresthesia in the distribution of the corresponding lumbar paravertebral nerve may be elicited. If this occurs, the needle should be withdrawn and redirected slightly more cephalad. The needle is again readvanced in incremental steps under CT guidance, with care taken to keep the needle trajectory medial to avoid pneumothorax.

The needle is then advanced in incremental steps into the central nucleus (Fig. 136-3). Sequential scanning is indicated to avoid advancing the needle completely through the disk and into the lower limits of the spinal cord or cauda equina. The pain management specialist also must take care not to allow the needle to track too laterally into the lower pleural or retroperitoneal space. Water-soluble contrast medium suitable for intrathecal use is then slowly injected through the needle into the disk in a volume of 0.2 to 0.6 mL (Figs. 136-4 and 136-5).

The resistance to injection should be noted, with an intact disk exhibiting firm resistance at these volumes. Simultaneously, the patient's pain response during injection is noted. The location of the patient's pain and its quality and similarity to the patient's ongoing clinical symptoms are evaluated. A verbal analogue scale may be useful to help the patient quantify the amount of pain experienced when compared with the injection of adjacent disks.

The nucleogram of a normal lumbar disk appears as a globular mass with occasional posterolateral clefts that occur as part of the normal aging process of the disk (Fig. 136-6A; see Fig. 136-4). In the damaged disk, the contrast material may flow into tears of the inner annulus, producing a characteristic transverse pattern (see Fig. 136-6**B**). If the tears in the annulus extend to the outer layer, a radial pattern is produced (Fig. 136-7**A**). Contrast material also may flow between the layers of annulus, producing a circumferential pattern (see Fig. 136-7**B**). Complete disruption of the annulus allows the contrast material to flow into the epidural space or into the cartilaginous end plate of the vertebra. Although the greater the damage to the annulus, the greater the likelihood that the disk being evaluated is the source of the patient's pain, the pain management specialist must evaluate all the information obtained during the diskography procedure and place this information into the context of the patient's pain symptoms.

After evaluation of the nucleogram, a decision must be made whether to proceed with diskography of adjacent disks or to inject local anesthetic into the disk currently being imaged. Analgesic diskography is useful in patients whose clinical pain pattern is reproduced or provoked during the injection of contrast medium. If the pain that was provoked during the injection of contrast medium is relieved by a subsequent injection of local anesthetic into the disk, an inference can be drawn that the disk is the likely source of the patient's pain. It must be remembered that if there is disruption of the annulus, the injected local anesthetic may spread into the epidural space and anesthetize somatic and sympathetic nerves that may subserve disks at an adjacent level. If this occurs, erroneous information may be obtained if diskography is then performed on adjacent disks.

After injection procedures are completed, the patient is observed for 30 minutes before discharge. The patient should be warned to expect minor postprocedure discomfort, including some soreness of the paraspinous musculature. Placing ice packs on the injection site for 20-minute periods will help decrease these untoward effects. The patient should be instructed to call immediately if fever or other systemic symptoms occur that might suggest infection.

SIDE EFFECTS AND COMPLICATIONS

Complications directly related to diskography are generally self-limited, although occasionally, even with the

Text continued on p. 625

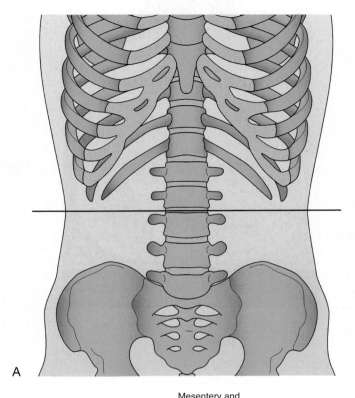

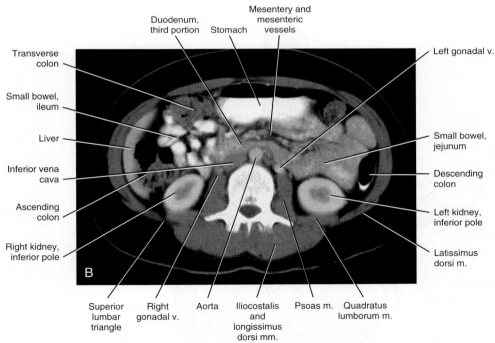

Figure 136-1.
(From El-Khoury GY, Bergman RA, Montgomery WJ: Sectional Anatomy by MRI and CT, 3rd ed. New York, Churchill Livingstone, 2007, p 491.)

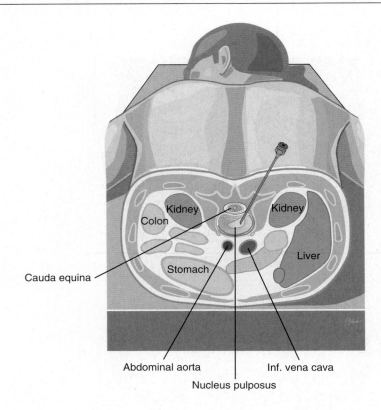

Figure 136-2.

Cauda equina

Abdominal aorta

Nucleus pulposus

Inf. vena cava

Kidney

Colon

Kidney

Stomach

Liver

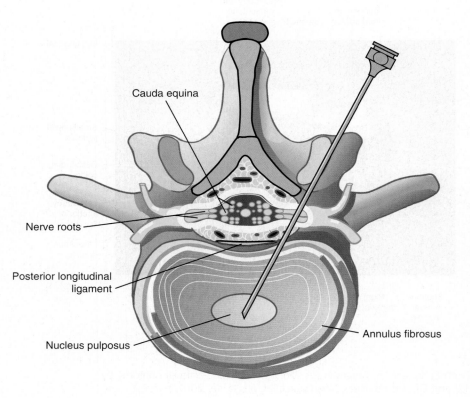

Figure 136-3.

Cauda equina

Nerve roots

Posterior longitudinal ligament

Nucleus pulposus

Annulus fibrosus

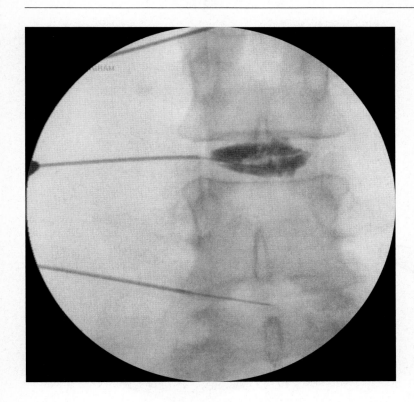

Figure 136-4.
PA view of contrast medium injected into the lumbar disk.

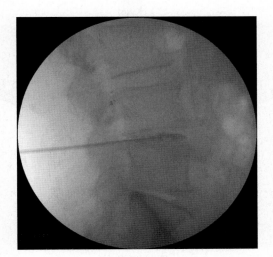

Figure 136-5.
Lateral view of contrast medium injected into the lumbar disk.

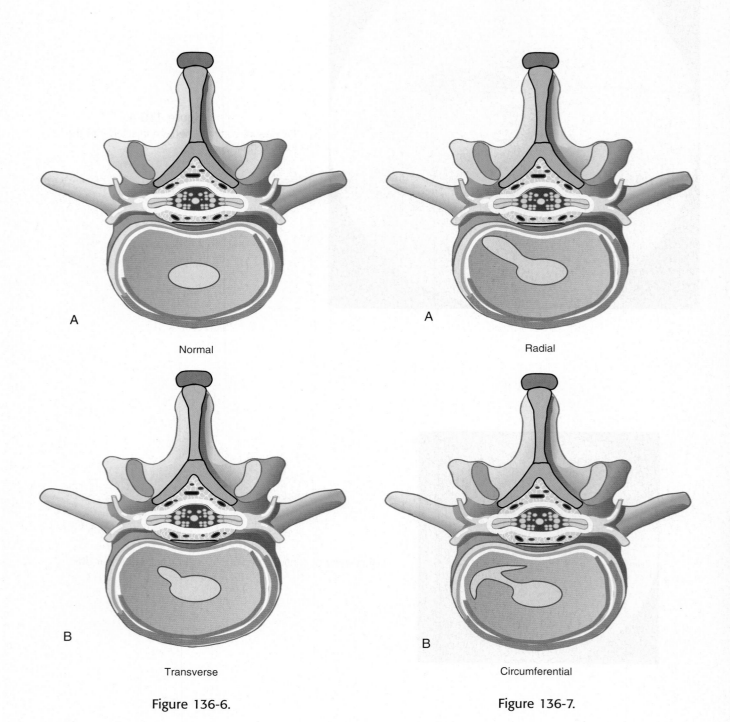

A

Normal

A

Radial

B

Transverse

B

Circumferential

Figure 136-6.

Figure 136-7.

best technique, severe complications can occur. The most common severe complication after diskography is infection of the disk, which is commonly referred to as *diskitis*. Because of the limited blood supply of the disk, such infections can be extremely hard to eradicate. Diskitis usually manifests as an increase in spine pain several days to a week after diskography. Acutely, there will be no change in the patient's neurologic examination as a result of disk infection.

Epidural abscess, which can rarely occur after diskography, generally manifests within 24 to 48 hours. Clinically, the signs and symptoms of epidural abscess are high fever, spine pain, and progressive neurologic deficit. If either diskitis or epidural abscess is suspected, blood and urine cultures should be taken, antibiotics started, and emergent MRI of the spine obtained to allow identification and drainage of any abscess formation to prevent irreversible neurologic deficit.

In addition to infectious complications, pneumothorax may occur after lumbar diskography. This complication should rarely occur if CT guidance is used during needle placement. Small pneumothorax after lumbar diskography can often be treated conservatively, and tube thoracostomy can be avoided. Trauma to retroperitoneal structures, including the kidney, also may occur if CT guidance is not used to avoid and localize these structures.

Direct trauma to the nerve roots and the spinal cord can occur if the needle is allowed to traverse the entire disk or is placed too laterally. These complications should rarely occur if incremental CT scans are taken while advancing the needle. Such needle-induced trauma to the lower lumbar spinal cord and cauda equina can result in deficits, including cauda equina syndrome and paraplegia.

CLINICAL PEARLS

Lumbar diskography is a straightforward technique that may provide useful clinical information in carefully selected patients. The information obtained from lumbar diskography must always be analyzed in the context of the patient's clinical presentation. Failure to do so will lead to a variety of clinical misadventures, including additional spine surgeries that are doomed to failure. The use of CT guidance adds an additional measure of safety when compared with fluoroscopy because it allows the pain specialist to clearly identify anatomic structures and needle position. These advantages more than outweigh the possible added cost when compared with fluoroscopically guided procedures.

CHAPTER **137**

Epiduroscopy

CPT-2009 CODE	
Epiduroscopy	0027T

Relative Value Units	
Epiduroscopy	40

INDICATIONS

Epiduroscopy is a diagnostic and therapeutic technique that is gaining favor in the evaluation and treatment of selected patients with a variety of painful conditions of the lumbar spine and nerve roots. As a diagnostic maneuver, epiduroscopy is useful in the diagnosis of abnormalities of the nerve roots, epidural space, and pathologic conditions following lumbar spine surgery. These abnormalities may manifest themselves clinically as radiculopathy, low back pain, and pseudoclaudication-type symptoms due to perineural fibrosis.

As a therapeutic maneuver, epiduroscopy allows direct visualization of the pathologic process and theoretically allows direct application of steroids onto inflamed nerve roots, direct lysis of adhesions using blunt dissection, cutting or hypertonic saline, and direct placement of electrodes and catheters into areas not readily accessible by percutaneous techniques. As experience is gained with epiduroscopy, this technique also may be used as an adjunct to minimally invasive spine surgery (Fig. 137-1).

CLINICALLY RELEVANT ANATOMY

Although epiduroscopy can theoretically be performed at any level of the spinal column, the caudal approach is technically the most feasible and probably the safest for the treatment of disorders involving the lower lumbar and sacral roots. A clear understanding of the functional anatomy of the sacral canal and its contents is essential to safely perform epiduroscopy.

Sacrum

The triangular sacrum consists of the five fused sacral vertebrae, which are dorsally convex (see Fig. 99-1). The sacrum inserts in a wedgelike manner between the two iliac bones, articulating superiorly with the fifth lumbar vertebra and caudad with the coccyx. On the anterior concave surface, there are four pairs of unsealed anterior sacral foramina that allow passage of the anterior rami of the upper four sacral nerves. The posterior sacral foramina are smaller than their anterior counterparts. Leakage of drugs injected into the sacral canal is effectively prevented by the sacrospinal and multifidus muscles. The vestigial remnants of the inferior articular processes project downward on each side of the sacral hiatus. These bony projections are called the *sacral cornua* and represent important clinical landmarks when performing caudal epidural nerve block.

Although there are gender- and race-determined differences in the shape of the sacrum, they are of little importance relative to the ultimate ability to successfully perform caudal epidural nerve block on a given patient.

Coccyx

The triangular coccyx is made up of three to five rudimental vertebrae. Its superior surface articulates with the inferior articular surface of the sacrum. The tip of the coccyx is an important clinical landmark when performing caudal epidural nerve block.

Sacral Hiatus

The sacral hiatus is formed by the incomplete midline fusion of the posterior elements of the lower portion of the S4 and the entire S5 vertebrae. This U-shaped space is covered posteriorly by the sacrococcygeal ligament, which also is an important clinical landmark when performing caudal epidural nerve block. Penetration of the sacrococcygeal ligament provides direct access to the epidural space of the sacral canal.

Current Procedural Terminology © 2009 American Medical Association. All Rights Reserved.

Sacral Canal

A continuation of the lumbar spinal canal, the sacral canal continues inferiorly to terminate at the sacral hiatus. The volume of the sacral canal with all its contents removed averages about 34 mL in dried bone specimens. It should be emphasized that much smaller volumes of local anesthetic (i.e., 5 to 10 mL) are used in day-to-day pain management practice. The use of large volumes of local anesthetic, especially in the area of pain management, will result in an unacceptable level of local anesthetic–induced side effects, such as incontinence and urinary retention, and should be avoided.

Contents of the Sacral Canal

The sacral canal contains the inferior termination of the dural sac, which ends between S1 and S3 (see Fig. 99-2). The five sacral nerve roots and the coccygeal nerve all traverse the canal, as does the terminal filament of the spinal cord, the filum terminale. The anterior and posterior rami of the S1-S4 nerve roots exit from their respective anterior and posterior sacral foramina. The S5 roots and coccygeal nerves leave the sacral canal via the sacral hiatus. These nerves provide sensory and motor innervation to their respective dermatomes and myotomes. They also provide partial innervation to several pelvic organs, including the uterus, fallopian tubes, bladder, and prostate.

The sacral canal also contains the epidural venous plexus, which generally ends at S4 but may continue inferiorly. Most of these vessels are concentrated in the anterior portion of the canal. Both the dural sac and epidural vessels are susceptible to trauma by advancing needles or catheters cephalad into the sacral canal. The remainder of the sacral canal is filled with fat, which is subject to an age-related increase in its density. Some investigators believe this change is responsible for the increased incidence of "spotty" caudal epidural nerve blocks in adults.

TECHNIQUE

The patient is placed in the prone position with a pillow under the hips for patient comfort. The sacral hiatus is identified as described in detail in Chapter 99. Alternatively, some investigators have begun using a lumbar translaminar approach for placement of the epiduroscope. In more obese patients, fluoroscopy may be a useful adjunct. The skin is then prepared with antiseptic solution, and sterile drapes are placed to allow access to the sacral hiatus. The skin, subcutaneous tissues, and sacrococcygeal ligaments are infiltrated with local anesthetic. A 17-gauge Tuohy needle is then introduced into the sacral canal using a loss-of-resistance technique (Fig.

137-2). A lateral fluoroscopic view may be useful to confirm placement within the sacral canal in larger patients. Then, 10 mL of nonionic contrast medium is injected through the Tuohy needle to provide an epidurogram to aid in identification of epidural scarring, cysts, tumors, or other abnormalities that may be encountered while performing epiduroscopy.

A flexible guidewire is then threaded through the Tuohy needle into the sacral canal and advanced cephalad under fluoroscopic guidance (Fig. 137-3). With the Tuohy needle in place, the entrance site of the needle is enlarged with a No. 11 scalpel to allow easier passage of the dilator and scope sheath. The Tuohy needle is then removed, and the dilator and sheath are introduced over the guidewire into the sacral canal. Using gentle pressure and a twisting movement, the dilator and sheath are passed cephalad over the guidewire. Care must be taken to avoid kinking the guidewire, which will make passage of the dilator and sheath much more difficult if not impossible. The operator should ensure that the guidewire moves freely while advancing the dilator and sheath. If the guidewire becomes kinked due to overzealous advancement of the dilator and sheath, the guidewire will have to be removed and the process started over.

After the dilator and sheath are inserted to the desired depth, the dilator is removed, and the sheath is left in place to allow introduction of the scope. The sidearm of the introducer sheath is then flushed with 1 to 20 mL of preservative-free sterile saline to flush any tissue debris or clot that may obscure visualization of the anatomic structures and to lubricate the introducer lumen. The fiberoptic cable is then placed through the lumen of the steering handle with a sterile saline infusion attached to the second lumen.

The operator should then orient himself or herself by focusing the scope on a sterile instrument such as a towel clamp. The steering handle containing the fiberoptic cable and normal saline infusion are then gently inserted via the introducer sheath (Fig. 137-4). The camera is activated, and the steering handle and fiberoptic cable are gently advanced in a cephalad direction into the epidural space. The saline infusion can be pressurized for brief periods to help distend the epidural space. Care must be taken to avoid prolonged increased pressure in the epidural space because this will compromise perfusion to the neural structures. A volume of 50 to 75 mL of saline is generally sufficient for most epiduroscopies, and excessive infusion of saline should be avoided. Steroid, hyaluronidase, or both can be injected via the second port, or blunt or sharp dissection of adhesions may be carried out under direct vision via the fiberoptic cable. Surgical interventions including the removal of disk fragments using direct visualization of the damaged disk and surrounding structures also has been reported (see Fig. 137-1).

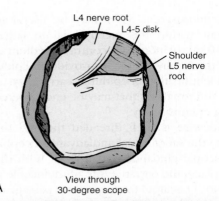

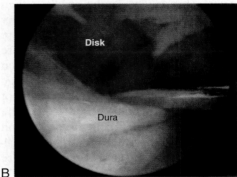

A

View through
30-degree scope

B

Figure 137-1.
A, Line drawing of the view through the arthroscope of the symptomatic nerve root and the disk to be examined. **B,** Digitized image showing the Penfield nerve root retractor being used to retract dura away from the symptomatic disk. (From Antoni DJ, Claro ML, Poehling GG, Hughes SS: Translaminar lumbar epidural endoscopy: Anatomy, technique, and indications. Arthroscopy 12:330-334, 1996.)

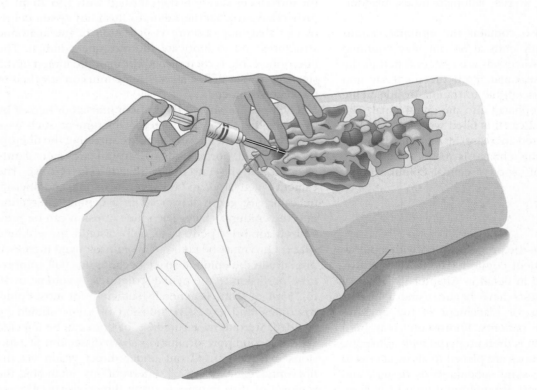

Figure 137-2.

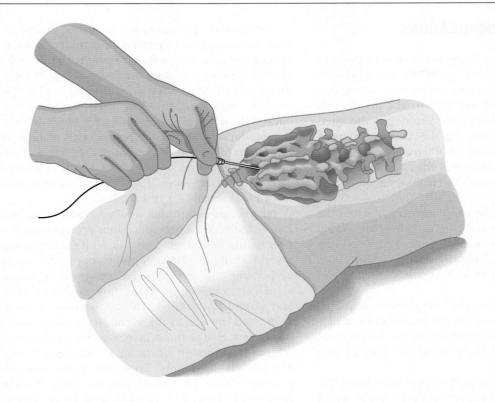

Figure 137-3.

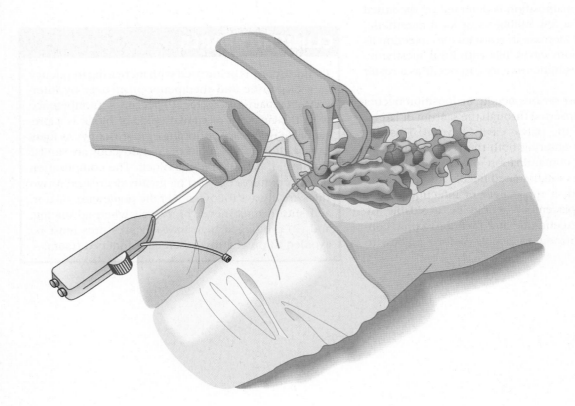

Figure 137-4.

SIDE EFFECTS AND COMPLICATIONS

The side effects of epiduroscopy are similar to those of caudal epidural block. As with caudal block, it is possible to insert the introducer needle incorrectly when performing epiduroscopy (see Fig. 99-10). The needle may be placed outside the sacral canal, resulting in the injection of air, drugs, or both into the subcutaneous tissues. Palpation of crepitus and bulging of tissues overlying the sacrum during injection indicates this needle malposition. An increased resistance to injection, accompanied by pain, also is noted.

A second possible needle misplacement is when the needle tip is placed into the periosteum of the sacral canal. This needle misplacement is suggested by considerable pain on injection, a high resistance to injection, and the inability to inject more than a few milliliters of drug.

A third possibility of needle malposition is partial placement of the needle bevel in the sacrococcygeal ligament. Again, there is significant resistance to injection as well as significant pain as the drugs are injected into the ligament.

A fourth possible needle malposition is to force the point of the needle into the marrow cavity of the sacral vertebra, resulting in high blood levels of local anesthetic. This needle malposition is detected by the initial easy acceptance of a few milliliters of local anesthetic, followed by a rapid increase in resistance to injection as the noncompliant bony cavity fills with local anesthetic. Significant local anesthetic toxicity can occur as a result of this complication.

The fifth and most serious needle malposition occurs when the needle is inserted through the sacrum or lateral to the coccyx into the pelvic cavity beyond. This can result in the needle entering both the rectum and birth canal, resulting in contamination of the needle. The repositioning of the contaminated needle into the sacral canal will carry with it the danger of infection. These pitfalls in needle placement should be avoidable by careful attention to technique and by fluoroscopic confirmation of the introducer needle before guidewire placement.

The caudal epidural space is highly vascular; therefore, the possibility of intravascular uptake of local anesthetics and other drugs is significant with this technique. Careful aspiration and incremental dosing of local anesthetic and all other drugs administered during epiduroscopy is important to allow early detection of local anesthetic or drug toxicity. Careful observation of the patient during and after the procedure is mandatory. The incidence of significant neurologic deficit secondary to epidural hematoma after caudal block is exceedingly rare, but it can occur if forceful advancement of the dilator and sheath is carried out.

Neurologic complications after caudal nerve block are rare. Usually, these complications are associated with a preexisting neurologic lesion or with trauma induced by poor technique during epiduroscopy. As mentioned earlier, the use of prolonged high-pressure saline infusions can compromise blood flow to neural structures and should be avoided. The application of local anesthetic and opioids to the sacral nerve roots during epiduroscopy results in an increased incidence of urinary retention. Although uncommon, infection remains an ever-present possibility, especially in the immunocompromised AIDS or cancer patient. Early detection of infection is crucial to avoid potentially life-threatening sequelae.

CLINICAL PEARLS

Epiduroscopy is being used with increasing frequency as a diagnostic and therapeutic maneuver by interventional pain management specialists. Competence with the nuances of caudal epidural block is a prerequisite to safely performing epiduroscopy. As mentioned, the complications of epiduroscopy are similar to those of caudal epidural block. The complication rate of epiduroscopy can be greatly decreased if two rules are always followed: (1) the guidewire, dilator, and sheath must never be forced when advancing; and (2) prolonged high infusion pressures must be avoided to prevent hydrostatically induced trauma.

CHAPTER 138

Intradiscal Electrothermal Annuloplasty

CPT-2009 CODE

Intradiscal Electrothermal Annuloplasty—First Level	22526
Intradiscal Electrothermal Annuloplasty—Second Level	22527

Relative Value Units

Intradiscal Electrothermal Annuloplasty, Each Level	30

INDICATIONS

Intradiscal electrothermal annuloplasty (IDA) represents another step in the continuum of care for patients suffering from lumbar diskogenic pain. IDA represents a reasonable option in a discrete subset of patients suffering from pain secondary to either an internally disrupted lumbar disk or a disk with limited disk herniation who have failed to respond to conservative therapy including medication management, physical therapy, epidural steroid injections, and bed rest. IDA is not indicated in patients suffering from back or radicular pain secondary to spinal stenosis or significant disk herniation with nerve root compression.

CLINICALLY RELEVANT ANATOMY

The exact mechanisms by which the intervertebral disk serves as a nociceptive generator have yet to be completely elucidated. It is known, however, that the lumbar intervertebral disk does contain nociceptive fibers and is capable of generating pain. These nociceptive fibers are found in greatest numbers in the posterolateral portion of the disk. Pain impulses from these fibers are transmitted to the spinal cord through the dorsal root ganglion. Mechanoreceptors also present in the disk may contribute to afferent impulses via the dorsal root ganglia. Structures surrounding the disk such as the posterior

longitudinal ligament also play an important role in the genesis of back and radicular pain.

Stimulation of the nociceptive fibers within the disk and surrounding structures, such as the posterior longitudinal ligament, may occur from both mechanical and chemical stimulation. Substance P release also has been implicated in the genesis of back and radicular pain secondary to the disrupted lumbar disk, as has the reinnervation of the damaged portion of the disk with small unmyelinated nociceptive fibers. Current thinking suggests that the interplay of all these factors leads to chronic stimulation of the dorsal root ganglia and resultant chronic pain. Plasticity at the spinal cord level also may contribute to the development of chronic pain in response to this continued barrage of afferent nociception from the dorsal root ganglia. Further research is required to clarify how the disrupted lumbar disk causes the clinical constellation of symptoms that pain management specialists currently attribute to diskogenic disease.

TECHNIQUE
Preprocedure Considerations

As with all other interventional pain management modalities, proper patient selection is mandatory to improve patient outcome and to avoid side effects and complications when considering a trial of IDA. As a general rule, patients with chronic back or leg pain being considered for a trial of IDA should have failed to respond to aggressive conservative management of their pain. Medication management with nonsteroidal anti-inflammatory agents, simple analgesics, and skeletal muscle relaxants, combined with bed rest, physical modalities including heat and cold, epidural steroid injections, and a back rehabilitation program, should be undertaken before a trial of IDA. The use of chronic opioid therapy in patients with chronic pain remains controversial and may represent a significant impediment to the overall success of IDA because in most cases, the patient's preexisting back pain increases for a period of time after IDA. For this reason, a careful behavioral assessment of patients who are tolerant to opioids due to chronic use is indicated before a trial of IDA to avoid postprocedure opioid overuse and unwanted drug-seeking behaviors.

Patient Preparation and Positioning

The patient is placed on the fluoroscopic table in either the prone or lateral position, with the choice based on the experience of the pain management specialist and the comfort of the patient. The lateral position has the advantage of easier access to the patient airway should problems occur. The prone position has the advantage of easier and more consistent patient positioning. If the prone position is chosen, putting the patient in a partially oblique position by placing a radiolucent foam wedge under the asymptomatic side may aid in identification of anatomic landmarks. After correct positioning is obtained, the skin is prepared with antiseptic solution, and sterile drapes are placed.

Introducer Needle Placement

The fluoroscope is then used to identify the inferior end plate of the affected spinal level. For the lower spinal interspaces, this requires angling the fluoroscopic beam with a 25- to 35-degree cephalad-to-caudad trajectory. The beam is then rotated to identify the superior articular process and to align it about in the middle of the inferior end plate. The skin overlying a point just lateral to the middle of the superior articular process is marked with a sterile marker to indicate the entry point of the introducer. At this point, the skin and subcutaneous tissues are anesthetized with 1.0% preservative-free lidocaine. A 25-gauge, $3\frac{1}{2}$-inch needle is then placed through the anesthetized area in a trajectory just anterior to the midpoint of the superior articular surface, keeping the needle parallel with the end plates. The patient should be warned to say "there!" should he or she feel any paresthesias indicating the needle has impinged on a nerve root to avoid persistent paresthesia. Then, 1% lidocaine is injected through the needle as it is placed along this trajectory to provide adequate anesthesia for the catheter introducer.

With the 25-gauge needle left in place to provide a radiopaque marker, the 17-gauge, 6-inch introducer needle is advanced just parallel to the 25-gauge needle. Under fluoroscopic guidance, the introducer needle tip should be placed just in front of the superior articular process with the needle bevel facing the posterior wall of the disk. Again, the patient should be warned to say "there!" should any paresthesia be felt. The introducer needle is advanced under fluoroscopic guidance into the annulus of the disk, which will offer significant resistance to needle advancement and exert a "gritty" feel

(Figs. 138-1 and 138-2). There will be a sudden loss of resistance as the introducer needle enters the softer annulus of the disk. The relative placement of the introducer needle to the nuclear cavity is confirmed by obtaining fluoroscopic views in all planes (Figs. 138-3 and 138-4).

Catheter Placement

After satisfactory placement of the introducer needle within the nuclear cavity of the affected disk is confirmed, the bevel of the introducer is placed toward the posterior wall of the disk, and the stylet is removed. The white marker on the tip and handle on the SpineCATH catheter is identified and aligned with the bevel marker on the introducer to aim the curved catheter tip toward the posterior disk. The catheter is then gently advanced through the introducer needle. The first bold marker on the catheter indicates that the catheter tip has reached the bevel of the introducer needle. Under fluoroscopic guidance, the catheter is then gently advanced to place the heating portion of the catheter in proximity to the posterior disk. Ideally, the catheter tip should extend beyond the midline of the posterior disk (Figs. 138-5 and 138-6). The use of small rotational movements while gently advancing the catheter will aid in optimizing needle placement.

Care must be taken that the entire heating portion of the catheter is outside the introducer needle by ensuring that the second bold mark on the catheter is beyond the introducer needle hub. The pain management specialist also should confirm by biplanar fluoroscopy that no portion of the catheter is outside the annulus of the disk before heating. Forceful movements of the catheter are to be discouraged to avoid catheter kinking or breakage. If the catheter becomes kinked, further manipulation of the catheter is to be avoided. If the kinked catheter is in proper position against the posterior disk, the pain management specialist may proceed with the heating sequence. If not, the introducer needle and catheter are withdrawn as a unit under fluoroscopic guidance. The pain management specialist must stop withdrawing the needle and catheter immediately if any significant resistance is felt and ascertain the relative position of both units by fluoroscopy before further attempts at withdrawal.

Heating Sequence

Successful IDA requires the heating of the nociceptive tissues at a high enough temperature for a long enough period of time to produce thermal injury while avoiding thermal injury to surrounding structures and excessive pain to the patient. The following heating protocol is recommended by a number of pain management

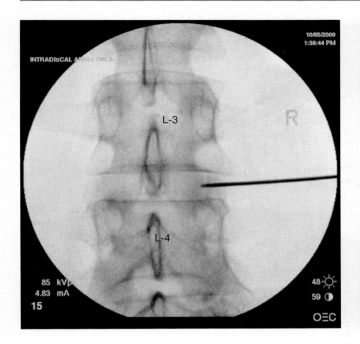

Figure 138-1.
PA view of the introducer needle in the annular of the disk.

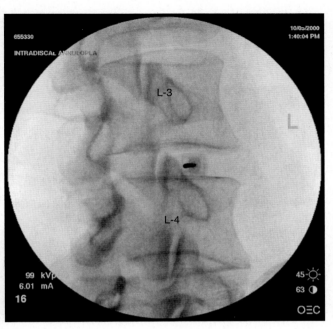

Figure 138-2.
Lateral view of the introducer needle in the annular of the disk.

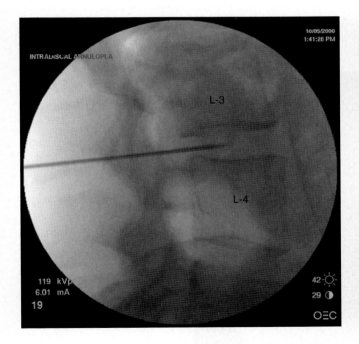

Figure 138-3.
Lateral view of the introducer needle in the nucleus of the disk.

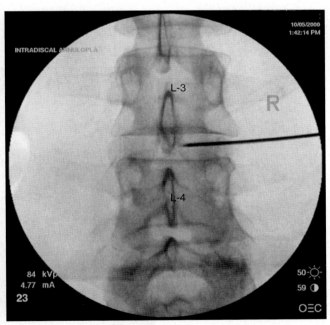

Figure 138-4.
PA view of the introducer needle in the nucleus of the disk.

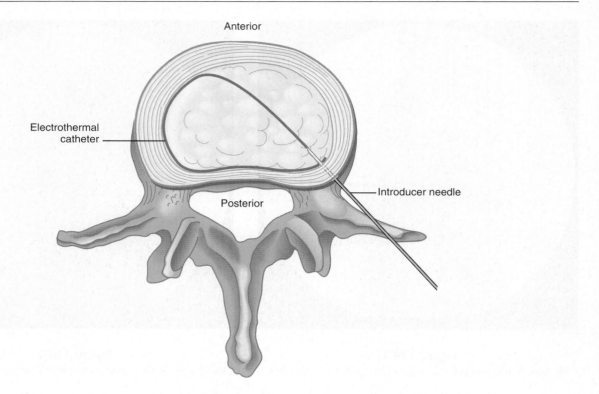

Figure 138-5.

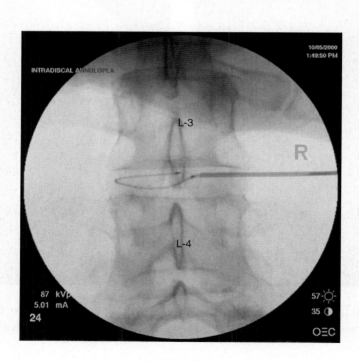

Figure 138-6.
Catheter tip in proper position within the disk.

specialists with experience in IDA, although other heating protocols have been safely and successfully used.

After satisfactory catheter placement, the catheter is heated from 37°C (the patient's body temperature) to a level of 65°C. After the catheter has remained at 65°C for 1 minute and the patient has not complained of excessive pain, the catheter temperature is increased by 1°C each 30 seconds until a catheter temperature of between 80°C and 90°C is reached. The heating sequence will last about 15 minutes, during which time the patient is constantly monitored for the new onset of radicular symptoms or extreme back pain. Clinical experience has shown that if more rapid heating sequences are used, unacceptable levels of patient pain often result. Clinical experience and microscopic analysis of heated disks also have shown that adequate temperature is required to provide long-term pain relief. Heating at levels of less than 76°C often results in a poor outcome in terms of long-term pain relief. After the heating sequence is completed, the introducer needle and catheter are removed as a unit. Some pain management specialists prefer to carefully remove the catheter while leaving the introducer needle in place and then administering intradiscal antibiotics, steroids, or both via the introducer needle before removing it. Sterile dressings over the entry sites are then placed, and the patient is observed until vital signs and neurologic status are stable.

Postprocedure Care

Most patients experience an exacerbation of their preprocedure back or radicular pain following IDA. The patient and family should be warned of this before IDA to reduce the anxiety that "something has gone wrong" with the procedure. This postprocedure flaring of pain generally lasts 3 to 7 days and requires additional analgesics, muscle relaxants, and, above all, reassurance. Occa-

sionally, transcutaneous nerve stimulation and the use of a lumbar support with rigid stays may be beneficial if movement-induced pain and spasm are a problem. As mentioned earlier, patients who have been on chronic opioid therapy may be particularly hard to manage during the early postprocedure period, and the pain management specialist should be prepared to hospitalize such patients to control medication overuse with its attendant problems and risks.

After the immediate postprocedure period, patients may expect to begin to experience pain relief gradually over a period of 4 to 6 weeks. Again, preprocedure communication with the patient and family will help them understand and accept the gradual nature of improvement associated with IDA therapy. After 8 to 12 weeks, all patients who have undergone IDA should begin a careful back rehabilitation program under the direct supervision of a physiatrist or pain management specialist familiar with the rehabilitation of the postoperative spine. Overaggressive therapy often results in an increase in pain and functional disability and should be avoided. Return to work after IDA is based on the patient's rate of recovery, with sedentary workers usually returning to work within 10 to 14 days and those workers performing heavy lifting within 60 to 90 days as recovery allows.

SIDE EFFECTS AND COMPLICATIONS

Acute complications of IDA are related to needle-induced trauma to neural structures and to the vasculature. Poor needle placement also can result in trauma to retroperitoneal structures including the kidney. The incidence of such complications can be greatly reduced if careful attention to the functional anatomy and needle placement is carried out using biplanar fluoroscopic guidance. Thermal injuries due to improper catheter placement also can be avoided with careful attention to technique.

Table 138–1 ■ ADVANTAGES AND DISADVANTAGES OF INTRADISCAL THERMAL DELIVERY SYSTEMS

Delivery System	Advantages	Disadvantages
Laser Fiber Optic *Energy source:* Laser *Delivery method:* Straight or side-firing fiberoptic catheter	Good access to pathology Excellent decompression effect for radiculopathy	Expense Poor temperature control
Radiofrequency Electrode *Energy source:* Radiofrequency *Delivery method:* Straight electrode	Easy intradiscal placement Cost-effective Safe Minimally invasive	Does not heat well discal tissues that have low water content Poor decompressive effect Small treatment area Cannot easily reach posterior disk
Intradiscal Electrothermal Catheter *Energy source:* Electroresistive coil *Delivery method:* Navigable catheter	Easy intradiscal placement Broad target zone Cost-effective Safe Minimally invasive	Poor decompressive effect Cannot reach collapsed disks Poor results for radicular pain

Heating should always be discontinued if the patient experiences new or severe back or radicular pain. Late complications of IDA are related to infection. Diskitis is hard to diagnose clinically but must always be included in the differential diagnosis of persistent or excessive postprocedure pain. Failure to rapidly diagnose infection may result in life-threatening sequelae including epidural abscess and meningitis.

CLINICAL PEARLS

Intradiscal electrothermal annuloplasty is thought to provide amelioration of diskogenic pain by three mechanisms:

1. The thermal destruction of annular nociceptive nerve fibers
2. The thermal injury to collagen fibers of the annulus with subsequent healing
3. The potential reduction in disk volume and intradiscal pressure from thermal destruction of disk tissue

To accomplish these objectives, a heat source capable of controlled heating must be accurately placed in proximity to the source of nociception to produce thermal injury. Several modalities for heat delivery have been developed and include the radiofrequency needle, the fiberoptic laser, and the navigable thermal catheter. Each modality has its advantages and disadvantages as outlined in Table 138-1. The navigable thermal catheter appears to be the most amenable and practical for use by the interventional pain management specialist at this time.

CHAPTER 139

Percutaneous Intradiscal Nucleoplasty

CPT-2003 CODE

Percutaneous Intradiscal Nucleoplasty	0062T (some carriers require the use of 64999)

Relative Value Units

Percutaneous Intradiscal Nucleoplasty, Each Level	35

INDICATIONS

Percutaneous intradiscal nucleoplasty is indicated for a special subset of patients who have low back and radicular pain thought to be caused by contained disk protrusion. This group of patients has failed conservative therapy consisting of a trial of simple analgesics, nonsteroidal anti-inflammatory agents or cyclooxygenase-2 inhibitors, bed rest, and epidural steroids. Some pain management specialists also recommend that a trial of transforaminal epidural steroid nerve blocks should be attempted before percutaneous intradiscal nucleoplasty. To optimize patient selection, the ideal candidate for nucleoplasty should have magnetic resonance imaging (MRI), diskography, and electromyographic changes that correlate with the patient's radicular pain pattern.

CLINICALLY RELEVANT ANATOMY

From a functional anatomic viewpoint, lumbar disks must be thought of as distinct from cervical disks insofar as a source of pain is concerned. Radicular symptoms solely from disk herniation are much more common in the lumbar region than in the cervical and thoracic regions. The reason for this is twofold: (1) In order for the lumbar disk to impinge on the lumbar nerve roots, it must herniate posteriorly and laterally. The lumbar nerve roots are not protected from impingement from lumbar disk herniation by the bony wall of the facet joints, as are the cervical nerve roots. (2) The posterior longitudinal ligament in the lumbar region is only a single layer, which is thinner and less well developed in its lateral aspects. It is in this lateral region that lumbar disk herniation with impingement on exiting nerve roots is most likely to occur.

The nuclear material in the lumbar disk is placed more posterior than its cervical counterpart. The gelatinous nucleus pulposus of the lumbar disk is surrounded by a dense, laminated, fibroelastic network of fibers known as the *annulus*. The annular fibers are arranged in concentric layers that run obliquely from adjacent vertebrae. It is this annular layer that receives sensory innervation from a variety of sources. Posteriorly, the annulus receives fibers from the sinovertebral nerves, which also provide sensory innervation to the posterior elements, including portions of the facet joints. Laterally, fibers from the exiting spinal nerve roots provide sensory innervation, with the anterior portion of the disk receiving fibers from the sympathetic chain. Whether part or all of these fibers play a role in diskogenic pain is a subject of controversy among pain specialists.

The lumbar nerve roots leave the spinal cord and travel laterally through the intervertebral foramina. If the posterior lumbar disk herniates laterally, it can impinge on the lumbar root as it travels through the intervertebral foramen, producing classic radicular symptoms. If the lumbar disk herniates posteromedially, it may impinge on the spinal cord, producing myelopathy that may include lower extremity as well as bowel and bladder symptoms. Severe compression of the lumbar spinal cord may result in cauda equina syndrome, paraparesis, or rarely, paraplegia.

TECHNIQUE

The patient is placed in the lateral or prone position with a pillow under the abdomen to slightly flex the lumbar spine as if for a lumbar sympathetic block. Computed tomography (CT) or fluoroscopic views are taken through the disks to be imaged, and the relative positions of the lung, ribs, aorta, vena cava, kidneys, nerve roots, and spinal cord are noted (see Fig. 120-1). The spinous process of the vertebra just above the disk to be evaluated is palpated. At a point just below and $1\frac{1}{2}$ inches lateral to the spinous process, the skin is prepared with antiseptic solution, and the skin and subcutaneous tissues are infiltrated with local anesthetic. Before inserting the Crawford needle in the patient, the stylet is removed, and the wand is advanced through the needle until the distal end of the reference mark is positioned at the proximal edge of the needle hub. This point is the proximal limit for creating coablation channels.

The wand is then removed and the stylet replaced. The 17-gauge, 6-inch styletted Crawford needle is then advanced through the skin under fluoroscopic or CT guidance, with the target being the middle of the disk to be imaged (Figs. 139-1 and 139-2). Given the proximity of the somatic nerve roots, a paresthesia in the distribution of the corresponding lumbar paravertebral nerve may be elicited. If this occurs, the needle should be withdrawn and redirected slightly more cephalad. The needle is readvanced in incremental steps under CT or fluoroscopic guidance, with care being taken to keep the needle trajectory medial to avoid pneumothorax.

The needle is then advanced in incremental steps until the needle tip rests against or slightly through the annulus of the affected disk (Fig. 139-3). Sequential imaging is indicated to avoid advancing the needle completely through the disk and into the lower limits of the spinal cord or cauda equina. The pain management specialist also must take care not to allow the needle to track too laterally into the lower pleural or retroperitoneal space. The stylet is removed from the Crawford needle, and the coablation wand is then advanced through the Crawford needle into the disk nucleus until the reference mark is all the way to the needle hub. The wand should then be gently advanced under fluoroscopic or CT guidance until the distal end of the tip is felt to impinge on the interior wall of the anterior disk annulus. CT or fluoroscopy is then used to reconfirm that the active portion of the wand tip is in fact outside the needle and not all the way through the disk (Figs. 139-4 to 139-6). After satisfactory position is confirmed, the depth gauge is advanced on the shaft of the wand to the proximal needle hub. This point represents the distal limit for creating coablation channels.

The wand is withdrawn to the proximal reference mark, and it is reconfirmed that the active needle tip is within the disk nucleus with either CT or fluoroscopic imaging. The dot on the wand handle is oriented to the 12-o'clock position and, using the ablation mode, the wand is readvanced to the distal limit as previously marked on the wand handle. CT or fluoroscopic images can be used to confirm wand placement. Ablation is stopped when the wand reaches the distal limit. Using the coagulation mode, the wand is withdrawn to the

proximal reference mark, and coagulation is discontinued. Using the previous technique, additional channels are created at the 4-, 6-, 8-, and 10-o'clock positions (Figs. 139-7 and 139-8). The wand is then withdrawn from the needle, and a postpercutaneous intradiscal nucleoplasty diskogram is performed to demonstrate the coablation channel creation (Fig. 139-9). The needle is then withdrawn from the patient. A sterile dressing is placed over the puncture site.

After the procedure is completed, the patient is observed for 30 minutes before discharge. The patient should be warned to expect minor postprocedure discomfort, including some soreness of the paraspinous musculature. Placing ice packs on the injection site for 20-minute periods will help decrease these untoward effects. The patient should be instructed to call immediately if fever or other systemic symptoms occur that might suggest infection.

SIDE EFFECTS AND COMPLICATIONS

Complications directly related to percutaneous intradiscal nucleoplasty are generally self-limited, although occasionally, even with the best technique, severe complications can occur. The most common severe complication after percutaneous intradiscal nucleoplasty is infection of the disk, which is commonly referred to as *diskitis*. Because of the limited blood supply of the disk, such infections can be extremely hard to eradicate. Diskitis usually presents as an increase in spine pain several days to a week after percutaneous intradiscal nucleoplasty. Acutely, there will be no change in the patient's neurologic examination as a result of disk infection.

Epidural abscess, which can rarely occur after percutaneous intradiscal nucleoplasty, generally presents within 24 to 48 hours. Clinically, the signs and symptoms of epidural abscess are high temperature, spine pain, and progressive neurologic deficit. If either diskitis or epidural abscess is suspected, blood and urine cultures should be taken, antibiotics started, and emergent MRI scan of the spine obtained to allow identification and drainage of any abscess formation to prevent irreversible neurologic deficit.

In addition to infectious complications, pneumothorax may occur after percutaneous intradiscal nucleoplasty. This complication should rarely occur if CT guidance is used during needle placement. Small pneumothorax after percutaneous intradiscal nucleoplasty can often be treated conservatively, and tube thoracostomy can be avoided. Trauma to retroperitoneal structures, including the kidney, also may occur if CT guidance is not used to avoid and localize these structures.

Text continued on p. 643

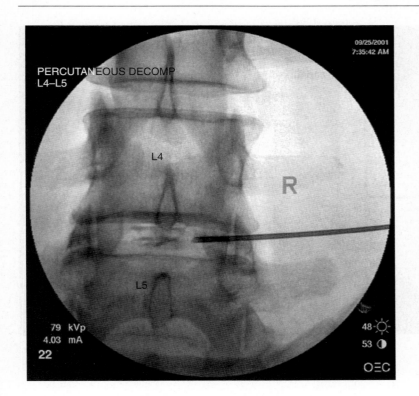

Figure 139-1.
PA view of needle within the nucleus of the disk.

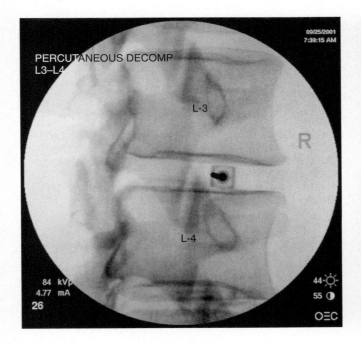

Figure 139-2.
Oblique view of needle within the disk.

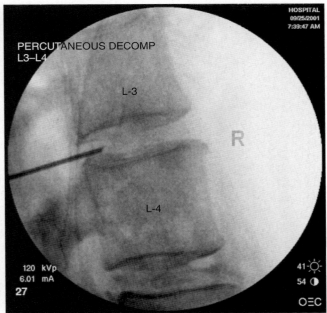

Figure 139-3.
Lateral view of needle within the disk.

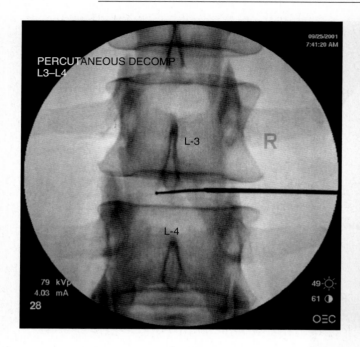

Figure 139-4.
PA view of wand within the disk.

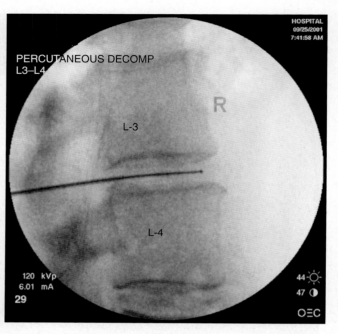

Figure 139-5.
PA view of wand tip within the disk.

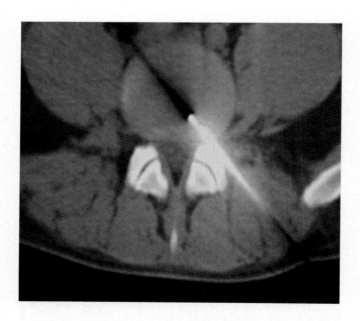

Figure 139-6.
Nucleoplasty: using fluoroscopy, the needle reaches the disk, and then preferably under computed tomography control, the needle is stopped at the presumed nucleus-annulus junction. (From Andreula C, Muto M, Leonardi M: Interventional spinal procedures. Eur J Radiol 50:112-119, 2004.)

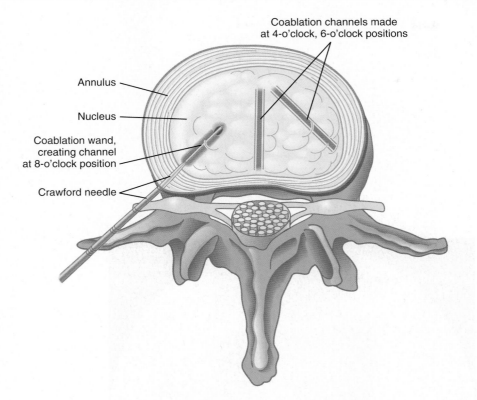

Coablation channels made at 4-o'clock, 6-o'clock positions

Annulus

Nucleus

Coablation wand, creating channel at 8-o'clock position

Crawford needle

Figure 139-7.

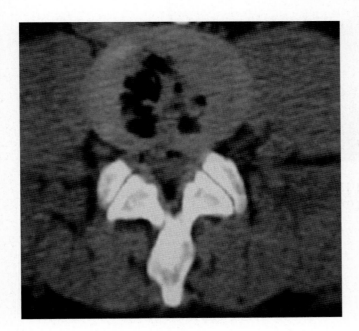

Figure 139-8.

Nucleoplasty: the needle is then retracted about 2 mm (the tip of the needle is now within the posterior margin of the annulus). Using the ablation mode, the wand is advanced into the nucleus to the predetermined depth, and then in coagulation mode, the needle is withdrawn. The coablation technique should be repeated 6 times in 360 degrees, with the result shown in the figure. (From Andreula C, Muto M, Leonardi M: Interventional spinal procedures. Eur J Radiol 50:112-119, 2004.)

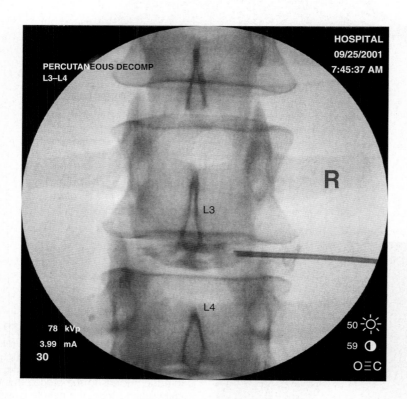

Figure 139-9.
Postablation diskogram showing contrast medium within the disk.

Direct trauma to the nerve roots and the spinal cord can occur if the needle is allowed to traverse the entire disk or is placed too laterally. These complications should rarely occur if incremental fluoroscopic or CT scans are taken while advancing the needle. Such needle-induced trauma to the lower lumbar spinal cord and cauda equina syndrome and paraplegia.

CLINICAL PEARLS

Percutaneous intradiscal nucleoplasty is a straightforward technique that is a reasonable treatment option in carefully selected patients. Proper patient selection is based on correlation with the patient's symptoms and physical examination, MRI, diskogram, and electromyogram results. The use of CT guidance adds a measure of safety when compared with fluoroscopy because it allows the pain specialist to clearly identify anatomic structures and needle position. These advantages more than outweigh the possible added cost compared with fluoroscopically guided procedures.

CHAPTER 140

Percutaneous Diskectomy: Automated Technique

CPT-2009 CODE	
Procedure, Single or Multiple Levels	62287
Radiographic Interpretation of Diskogram	72295

Relative Value Units	
Procedure	35
Radiographic Interpretation of Diskogram	10

INDICATIONS

Percutaneous diskectomy using the automated technique is indicated for a special subset of patients who have low back and radicular pain thought to be caused by contained disk protrusion. This group of patients has failed conservative therapy consisting of a trial of simple analgesics, nonsteroidal anti-inflammatory agents or cyclooxygenase-2 inhibitors, bed rest, and epidural steroids. Some pain management specialists also recommend that a trial of transforaminal epidural steroid nerve blocks should be attempted before percutaneous diskectomy. To optimize patient selection, the ideal candidate for nucleoplasty should have magnetic resonance imaging (MRI), diskography, and electromyographic changes that correlate with the patient's radicular pain pattern.

CLINICALLY RELEVANT ANATOMY

From a functional anatomic viewpoint, lumbar disks must be thought of as distinct from cervical disks insofar as a source of pain is concerned. Radicular symptoms solely from disk herniation are much more common in the lumbar region than in the cervical and thoracic regions. The reason for this is twofold: (1) In order for the lumbar disk to impinge on the lumbar nerve roots, it must herniate posteriorly and laterally. The lumbar nerve roots are not protected from impingement from lumbar disk herniation by the bony wall of the facet joints, as are the cervical nerve roots. (2) The posterior longitudinal ligament in the lumbar region is only a single layer, which is thinner and less well developed in its lateral aspects. It is in this lateral region that lumbar disk herniation with impingement on exiting nerve roots is most likely to occur.

The nuclear material in the lumbar disk is placed more posterior than its cervical counterpart. The gelatinous nucleus pulposus of the lumbar disk is surrounded by a dense, laminated fibroelastic network of fibers known as the *annulus*. The annular fibers are arranged in concentric layers that run obliquely from adjacent vertebrae. It is this annular layer that receives sensory innervation from a variety of sources. Posteriorly, the annulus receives fibers from the sinovertebral nerves, which also provide sensory innervation to the posterior elements, including portions of the facet joints. Laterally, fibers from the exiting spinal nerve roots provide sensory innervation, with the anterior portion of the disk receiving fibers from the sympathetic chain. Whether part or all of these fibers play a role in diskogenic pain is a subject of controversy among pain specialists.

The lumbar nerve roots leave the spinal cord and travel laterally through the intervertebral foramina. If the posterior lumbar disk herniates laterally, it can impinge on the lumbar root as it travels through the intervertebral foramen, producing classic radicular symptoms. If the lumbar disk herniates posteromedially, it may impinge on the spinal cord, producing myelopathy that may include lower extremity as well as bowel and bladder symptoms. Severe compression of the lumbar spinal cord may result in cauda equina syndrome, paraparesis, or rarely, paraplegia.

TECHNIQUE

The patient is placed in the lateral or prone position with a pillow under the abdomen to slightly flex the lumbar spine as if for a lumbar sympathetic block. Computed tomography (CT) or fluoroscopic views are taken through the disks to be imaged, and the relative positions of the lung, ribs, aorta, vena cava, kidneys, nerve roots, and spinal cord are noted (Fig. 140-1). The spinous process of the vertebra just above the disk to be evaluated is palpated. At a point just below and $1\frac{1}{2}$ inches lateral to the spinous process, the skin is prepared with antiseptic solution, and the skin and subcutaneous tissues are infiltrated with local anesthetic. A small stab wound is made at the point of needle entry to facilitate the placement of the introducer cannula.

The stylet is placed into the introducer cannula, and the cannula is then advanced through the skin under fluoroscopic or CT guidance, with the target being the middle of the disk to be decompressed (Figs. 140-2 and 140-3). If fluoroscopic guidance is being used, oblique images may be useful (Fig. 140-4). Given the proximity of the somatic nerve roots, a paresthesia in the distribution of the corresponding lumbar paravertebral nerve may be elicited. If this occurs, the needle should be withdrawn and redirected slightly more cephalad. The needle is readvanced in incremental steps under CT or fluoroscopic guidance. Sequential imaging is always indicated to avoid advancing the needle completely through the disk and into the lower limits of the spinal cord or cauda equina. The pain management specialist also must take care not to allow the needle to track too lateral into the lower pleural or retroperitoneal space.

When the cannula is in satisfactory position in the center of the disk, the stylet is removed, and a small amount of contrast material is injected into the disk to confirm mid-disk needle placement and identify any significant disruption of the annulus (Fig. 140-5). The automated disk decompressor probe is then advanced through the cannula into the center of the disk nucleus until the probe extends beyond the end of the cannula (Fig. 140-6). The activation switch of the device is then turned to the on position for 15-second increments, with the total combined time that the device is activated not to exceed 5 minutes. The device may be gently advanced toward the anterior annulus of the disk being treated under CT or fluoroscopic guidance, with care taken to avoid impinging on the annulus. Disk material will begin to appear in the clear collection chamber after about 1 mL of disk has been removed. After an adequate amount of disk material has been removed, the automated disk decompressor probe is removed from the cannula. A slight rotation of the probe may aid in the easy withdrawal of the probe. The cannula is then removed, and a sterile dressing is placed over the operative site.

After the procedure is completed, the patient is observed for 30 minutes before discharge. The patient should be warned to expect minor postprocedure discomfort, including some soreness of the paraspinous musculature. Placing ice packs placed on the injection site for 20-minute periods will help decrease these untoward effects. The patient should be instructed to call immediately if fever or other systemic symptoms occur that might suggest infection.

SIDE EFFECTS AND COMPLICATIONS

Complications directly related to percutaneous diskectomy using the automated technique are generally self-limited, although occasionally, even with the best technique, severe complications can occur. The most common severe complication after percutaneous diskectomy using the automated technique is infection of the disk, which is commonly referred to as *diskitis*. Because of the limited blood supply of the disk, such infections can be extremely hard to eradicate. Diskitis usually presents as an increase in spine pain several days to a week after percutaneous diskectomy. Acutely, there will be no change in the patient's neurologic examination as a result of disk infection.

Epidural abscess, which can rarely occur after percutaneous diskectomy, generally presents within 24 to 48 hours. Clinically, the signs and symptoms of epidural abscess are high temperature, spine pain, and progressive neurologic deficit. If either diskitis or epidural abscess is suspected, blood and urine cultures should be taken, antibiotics started, and emergent MRI scan of the spine obtained to allow identification and drainage of any abscess formation to prevent irreversible neurologic deficit.

In addition to infectious complications, pneumothorax may occur after percutaneous diskectomy. This complication should rarely occur if CT guidance is used during needle placement. Small pneumothorax after percutaneous diskectomy using the automated technique can often be treated conservatively, and tube thoracostomy can be avoided. Trauma to retroperitoneal structures, including the kidney, also may occur if CT guidance is not used to avoid and localize these structures.

Direct trauma to the nerve roots and the spinal cord can occur if the needle is allowed to traverse the entire disk or is placed too laterally. These complications should rarely occur if incremental fluoroscopic or CT scans are taken while advancing the needle. Such needle-induced trauma to the lower lumbar spinal cord and cauda equina can result in deficits, including cauda equina syndrome and paraplegia.

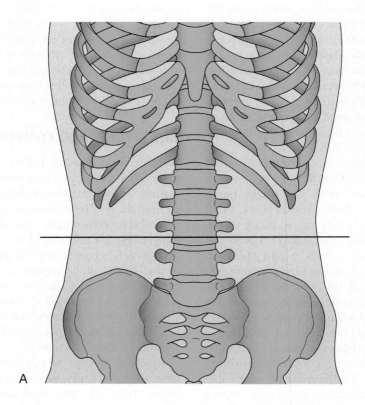

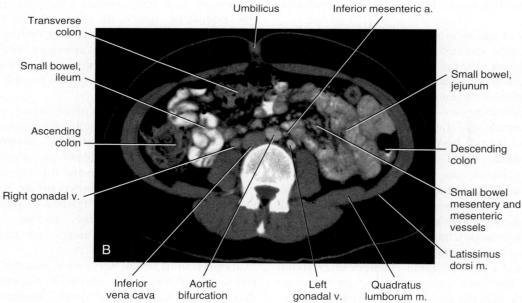

Figure 140-1.
(From El-Khoury GY, Bergman RA, Montgomery WJ: Sectional Anatomy by MRI and CT, 3rd ed. New York, Churchill Livingstone, 2007, p 492.)

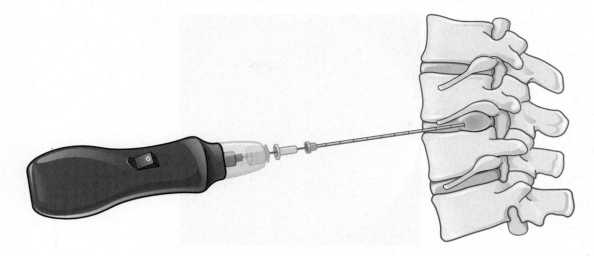

Figure 140-2.

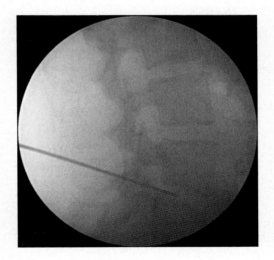

Figure 140-3.
Lateral view of the cannula within the disk.

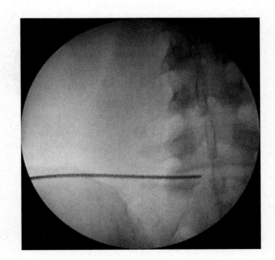

Figure 140-4.
PA view of the cannula within the disk.

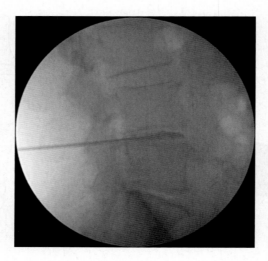

Figure 140-5.
Contrast medium placed via the cannula into the disk.

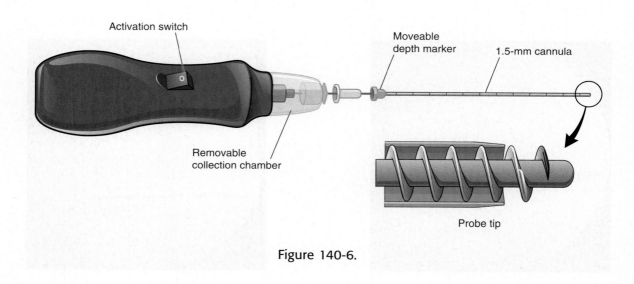

Figure 140-6.

CLINICAL PEARLS

Percutaneous diskectomy using the automated technique is a straightforward procedure that is a reasonable treatment option in carefully selected patients. Proper patient selection is based on correlation with the patient's symptoms and physical examination, MRI, diskogram, and electromyogram results. The use of CT guidance adds a measure of safety compared with fluoroscopy because it allows the pain specialist to clearly identify anatomic structures and needle position. These advantages more than outweigh the possible added cost when compared with fluoroscopically guided procedures.

CHAPTER **141**

Percutaneous Vertebroplasty

INDICATIONS

Percutaneous vertebroplasty is indicated for patients suffering from weakening of the vertebral body due to a number of pathologic processes. Idiopathic osteoporosis is by far the most frequent indication for percutaneous vertebroplasty. Other indications include drug-induced osteoporosis, tumor of the vertebral body, hemangioma, and traumatic vertebral crush fractures. Percutaneous vertebroplasty is indicated for stabilization of a weakened vertebra whether or not pain is present. The best results can be expected when any of the following conditions are met:

1. There is limited compression of the vertebral body.
2. The fracture is less than 12 months old.
3. The lesion is greater than 12 months old and the radionuclide bone scan is still "hot," indicating continued active disease.

Percutaneous vertebroplasty is used most commonly in the mid and lower thoracic and lumbar spine.

CLINICALLY RELEVANT ANATOMY

The vertebral column consists of 24 vertebrae and two fused bones, the sacrum and the coccyx. Its function is to support the body and bear its weight. Its S-shape helps impart strength and adds flexibility. The vertebrae articulate with each other by means of the facet joints, which are true synovial joints, and the intervertebral disks. These disks act as shock absorbers and help distribute any vertical forces placed on the spine horizontally. Although each area of the spine has minor anatomic differences that allow it to better perform its functions, the typical vertebra has many structural features in common (Fig. 141-1). The body, or centrum, of the vertebra bears most of the weight, which is placed in the vertebral column. The lamina is the arch that encloses the posterior portion of the spinal canal.

The spinous process projects posteriorly and serves as an attachment point for the muscles of the back. The vertebral foramina allow passage of the spinal nerve roots from the spinal canal. The articular facet joints allow flexion, extension, and a limited amount of rotation between each spinal segment.

TECHNIQUE

The patient is placed in the prone position on the fluoroscopy table, and the vertebra to be treated is identified with anteroposterior and lateral views. The skin overlying the affected vertebra is marked and then prepared with antiseptic solution and draped in a sterile manner. The skin and subcutaneous tissues are then anesthetized with local anesthetic. A 22-gauge, $3\frac{1}{2}$-inch needle is then directed under fluoroscopic guidance against the pedicle of the affected vertebra, and the deep tissues and periosteum of the pedicle are generously infiltrated with local anesthetic. An 11-gauge trocar is used for the lower thoracic and lumbar vertebrae, and a 13-gauge trocar is used for the smaller mid-thoracic vertebrae. The trocar is advanced through the previously anesthetized area under fluoroscopic guidance in a trajectory that will allow the tip to make contact with the center of the upper outer third of the pedicle of the affected vertebra.

The trocar is embedded into the pedicle using firm pressure and a back-and-forth twisting motion. Care must be taken in severely osteoporotic patients not to

Current Procedural Terminology © 2009 American Medical Association. All Rights Reserved.

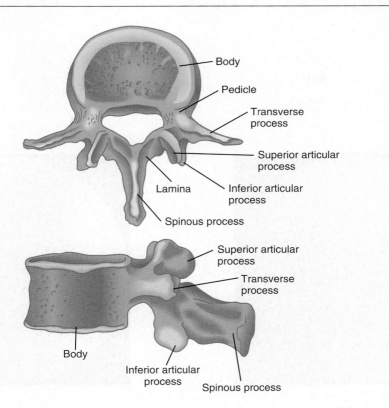

Figure 141-1.

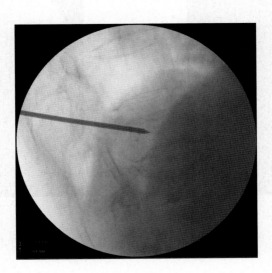

Figure 141-2.
Trocar tip embedded within the pedicle of the fractured vertebra.

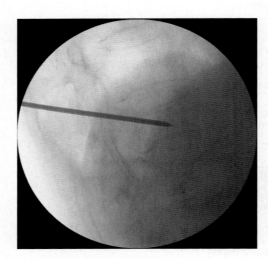

Figure 141-3.
Trocar advanced through the pedicle into the vertebral body.

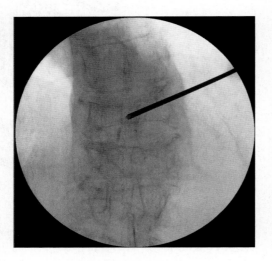

Figure 141-4.
Trocar within the vertebral body.

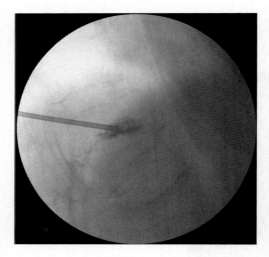

Figure 141-5.
Cement placed via the trocar within the vertebral body.

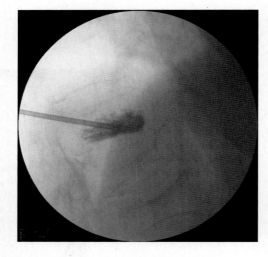

Figure 141-6.
Cement placed via the trocar filling the vertebral body.

fracture the pedicle by overzealous advancement of the trocar. After the tip of the trocar is firmly embedded in the pedicle, the trocar is advanced toward the affected vertebral body under anteroposterior and lateral fluoroscopic guidance (Figs. 141-2 to 141-4). The trocar is advanced until the tip rests in the anterior third of the vertebral body, which bears most of the weight.

A long spinal needle is then used to fill the trocar with sterile saline to avoid injecting air into the epidural veins during the injection of contrast medium. Nonionic iodinated contrast medium is then injected slowly through the trocar under continuous fluoroscopic observation. The contrast should initially fill the vertebral body and will appear as a fine reticular blush pattern before flowing into the epidural and paravertebral veins. If the vertebra is fractured, contrast will be seen to leak out of the defect. Contrast injection also will allow the operator to determine whether the end plates and posterior wall of the vertebral body are intact. If the trocar is seen to be in the lumen of a large vertebral body vein, it should be advanced a few millimeters to avoid injection of the polymethylmethacrylate (PMMA) cement into the vein. Too much contrast injection should be avoided because it can obscure the subsequent injection of the PMMA.

After venograph and vertebral body contrast injection is completed, the trocar is flushed with sterile saline. The PMMA is then mixed according to the manufacturer's directions with the goal of a consistency like that of toothpaste. Most PMMA contains sterile barium sulfate as an opacifying agent. The PMMA is then injected under fluoroscopic observation (Fig. 141-5). If significant venous filling is seen, the operator should wait 1 to 2 minutes to allow the injected PMMA to harden and occlude the veins before resuming injection. If the PMMA extrudes through an incompetent end plate into the intervertebral disk, the same strategy is employed. If the injection becomes difficult, the trocar is withdrawn a few millimeters, and the injection is slowly resumed. This technique is continued until the vertebral body is well filled (Fig. 141-6). It is often necessary to place a second trocar into the vertebral body via the contralateral pedicle to obtain complete filling of the vertebra.

The PMMA will harden in a few minutes. Sitting is allowed after a sedative or anesthetic has worn off, and patients are allowed to stand on the day following the procedure.

SIDE EFFECTS AND COMPLICATIONS

If careful attention is paid to the procedure, complications following percutaneous vertebroplasty are uncommon. The risk for significant intravascular or epidural injection is greatly decreased if fluoroscopic guidance is used during the injection process and if the PMMA is allowed to adequately cure and thicken before injection. Unintentional injection of the PMMA into the spinal canal can result in devastating neurologic complications and should rarely occur if careful attention to technique is used. Severe back pain following percutaneous vertebroplasty can be the result of a new vertebral fracture of a different vertebra or of fracture of the pedicle during the procedure. Encroachment on the intervertebral foramina by PMMA may cause new radicular symptoms that may ultimately require surgical decompression. Infection, although rare, remains a possibility, especially in the immunocompromised patient, such as the patient on chronic steroids or suffering from cancer.

CLINICAL PEARLS

Percutaneous vertebroplasty is a useful addition to the armamentarium of the pain management physician. Rapid use of the technique following acute vertebral compression fracture allows early ambulation, which decreases the morbidity associated with this disease. Kyphoplasty using a balloon to restore vertebral height before injection of PMMA is a reasonable alternative to vertebroplasty and offers some theoretical advantages and some practical disadvantages. Adjuncts to PMMA, including ground coral, also are undergoing clinical trials.

CHAPTER **142**

Percutaneous Kyphoplasty

CPT-2009 CODE

Thoracic—One Level	22523
Lumbar—One Level	22524
Each Additional Thoracic or Lumbar Level	22525

Relative Value Units

Thoracic—One Level	35
Lumbar—One Level	35
Each Additional Level	30

INDICATIONS

Percutaneous kyphoplasty is indicated for patients suffering from weakening of the vertebral body due to a number of pathologic processes. Percutaneous kyphoplasty represents an acceptable alternative to percutaneous vertebroplasty, and both techniques have advantages and disadvantages, with neither vertebroplasty nor kyphoplasty being clearly better. Percutaneous kyphoplasty differs from percutaneous vertebroplasty in that a balloon is used to elevate the vertebral end plates with the aim of restoring vertebral height. Percutaneous kyphoplasty has the added advantage in that the inflated balloon creates a cavity within the vertebral body, theoretically allowing for a more controlled injection of polymethylmethacrylate and decreasing the risk for the extravasation of cement into the vertebral canal or vasculature. Ultimately, the choice of technique generally rests with the experience of the operator.

Idiopathic osteoporosis is by far the most frequent indication for percutaneous kyphoplasty. Other indications include drug-induced osteoporosis, tumor of the vertebral body, hemangioma, and traumatic vertebral crush fractures. Percutaneous kyphoplasty is indicated for stabilization of a weakened vertebra whether or not

pain is present. The best results can be expected when one of the following conditions is met:

1. There is limited compression of the vertebral body.
2. The fracture is less than 12 months old.
3. The lesion is greater than 12 months old and the radionuclide bone scan is still "hot," indicating continued active disease.

Percutaneous kyphoplasty is used most commonly in the mid and lower thoracic and lumbar spine.

CLINICALLY RELEVANT ANATOMY

The vertebral column consists of 24 vertebrae and two fused bones, the sacrum and the coccyx. Its function is to support the body and bear its weight. Its S-shape helps impart strength and adds flexibility. The vertebrae articulate with each other by means of the facet joints, which are true synovial joints, and the intervertebral disks. These disks act as shock absorbers and help distribute any vertical forces placed on the spine horizontally. Although each area of the spine has minor anatomic differences that allow it to better perform its function, the typical vertebra has many structural features in common (Fig. 142-1). The body, or centrum, of the vertebra bears most of the weight, which is placed in the vertebral column. The lamina is the arch that encloses the posterior portion of the spinal canal.

The spinous process projects posteriorly and serves as an attachment point for the muscles of the back. The vertebral foramina allow passage of the spinal nerve roots from the spinal canal. The articular facet joints allow flexion, extension, and a limited amount of rotation between each spinal segment.

TECHNIQUE

The patient is placed in the prone position on the fluoroscopy table, and the vertebra to be treated is identified

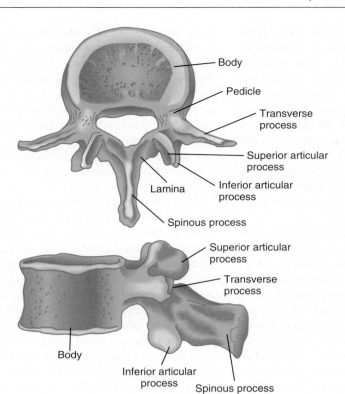

Body

Pedicle

Transverse process

Superior articular process

Inferior articular process

Lamina

Spinous process

Figure 142-1.

Superior articular process

Transverse process

Body

Inferior articular process

Spinous process

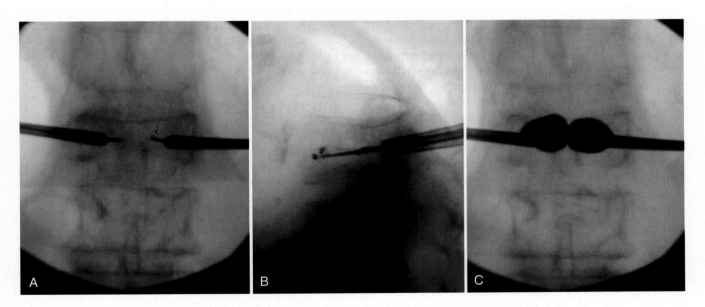

A   B   C

Figure 142-2.
Intraoperative AP (**A**) and lateral (**B**) fluoroscopic images demonstrating balloon placement in the vertebra during a kyphoplasty procedure. **C,** After the balloon is in satisfactory position, it is inflated to create a cavity for the cement. (From Pateder DB, Khanna AJ, Lieberman IH: Vertebroplasty and kyphoplasty for the management of osteoporotic vertebral compression fractures. Orthop Clin North Am 38:409-418, 2007.)

with anteroposterior and lateral views. The skin overlying the affected vertebra is marked and then prepared with antiseptic solution and draped in a sterile manner. The skin and subcutaneous tissues are then anesthetized with local anesthetic. A 22-gauge, $3\frac{1}{2}$-inch needle is then directed under fluoroscopic guidance against the pedicle of the affected vertebra, and the deep tissues and periosteum of the pedicle are generously infiltrated with local anesthetic. An introducer trocar is advanced through the previously anesthetized area under fluoroscopic guidance in a trajectory that will allow the tip to make contact with the center of the upper outer third of the pedicle of the affected vertebra.

The trocar is embedded into the pedicle using firm pressure and a back-and-forth twisting motion. Care must be taken in severely osteoporotic patients not to fracture the pedicle by overzealous advancement of the trocar. After the tip of the trocar is firmly embedded in the pedicle, the trocar is advanced toward the affected vertebral body under anteroposterior and lateral fluoroscopic guidance. The trocar is advanced until the tip rests at a point 3 mm beyond the point at which the pedicle joins the vertebral body. Many clinicians place a second trocar through the contralateral pedicle to allow placement of a second balloon to ensure equal elevation of the end plates and to prevent a single balloon from herniating laterally, and causing a malreduction of the fracture (Fig. 142-2A).

After the trocar or trocars are in satisfactory position, a bone curette is introduced through the trocar to create a cavity within the vertebral body to accommodate the balloon. After the curette is advanced to the anterior one third of the vertebral body under continuous fluoroscopic guidance, it is removed. Nonionic iodinated contrast medium is then injected slowly through the trocar under continuous fluoroscopic observation. The contrast should initially fill the cavity of the vertebral body, and as the vasculature of the bone fills, the contrast will appear as a fine reticular blush pattern before flowing into the epidural and paravertebral veins. If the vertebra is fractured, contrast will be seen to leak out of the defect. Contrast injection also will allow the operator to determine whether the end plates and posterior wall of the vertebral body are intact. If the trocar is seen in the lumen of a large vertebral body vein, it should be advanced or withdrawn a few millimeters to avoid injection of the polymethylmethacrylate (PMMA) cement into the vein. Too much contrast injection should be avoided because it can obscure the subsequent injection of the PMMA.

After venogram and vertebral body contrast injection is satisfactorily completed, an uninflated kyphoplasty balloon is inserted through the trocar into the vertebral body (see Fig. 142-2B). The balloon is then inflated with a mixture of saline and contrast medium under continuous fluoroscopic guidance to ensure that the balloon does not herniate laterally or medially and cause a malreduction of the fracture. Care must be taken not to fracture the end plate of the vertebra as the balloon is being inflated. If a second trocar has been placed, a second uninflated kyphoplasty balloon is inserted through that trocar, and both the first and second balloons are inflated simultaneously to ensure that the fracture is symmetrically reduced (see Fig. 142-2C).

After satisfactory reduction of the vertebral body fracture, the balloon or balloons are deflated and carefully removed from the trocars. The PMMA is then mixed according to the manufacturer's directions. Most PMMA contains sterile barium sulfate as an opacifying agent. The PMMA should cure to the consistency of toothpaste before injection. After the PMMA has cured to the desired consistency, the PMMA is injected under continuous fluoroscopic observation. If significant venous filling is seen, the operator should wait 1 to 2 minutes to allow the injected PMMA to harden and occlude the veins before resuming injection. If the PMMA extrudes through an incompetent end plate into the intervertebral disk, the same strategy is employed. If the injection becomes difficult, the trocar is withdrawn a few millimeters, and the injection is slowly resumed. This technique is continued until the vertebral body is well filled (Fig. 142-3A, B). The PMMA will harden in a few minutes. Postinjection films will confirm final placement of the cement (see Fig. 142-3C, D). Sitting is allowed after the sedative or anesthetic has worn off, and patients are allowed to stand on the day after the procedure.

SIDE EFFECTS AND COMPLICATIONS

If careful attention is paid to the procedure, complications following percutaneous kyphoplasty are uncommon. The risk for significant intravascular or epidural injection is greatly decreased if fluoroscopic guidance is used during the injection process. Unintentional injection of the PMMA into the spinal canal can result in devastating neurologic complications and should rarely occur if careful attention to technique is used. Severe back pain after percutaneous kyphoplasty can be the result of a new vertebral fracture of a different vertebra or from fracture of the pedicle during the procedure. Encroachment on the intervertebral foramina by PMMA may cause new radicular symptoms that may ultimately require surgical decompression. Infection, although rare, remains a possibility, especially in the immunocompromised patient, such as the patient on chronic steroids or suffering from cancer.

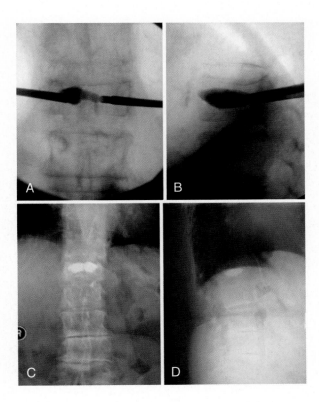

Figure 142-3.
A and **B,** After the balloon is deflated and removed, cement (mixed with barium) is deposited into the cavity under live fluoroscopic guidance in a retrograde fill pattern (from the ventral aspect of the cavity to its dorsal aspect). Final AP (**C**) and lateral (**D**) radiographs are taken to evaluate cement position and overall alignment. (From Pateder DB, Khanna AJ, Lieberman IH: Vertebroplasty and kyphoplasty for the management of osteoporotic vertebral compression fractures. Orthop Clin North Am 38:409-418, 2007.)

CLINICAL PEARLS

Percutaneous kyphoplasty is a useful addition to the armamentarium of the pain management physician. Rapid use of the technique following acute vertebral compression fracture allows early ambulation, which decreases the morbidity associated with this disease. Whether or not use of a balloon to restore vertebral height before injection of PMMA represents an advantage over vertebroplasty remains to be seen.

CHAPTER 143

Cervical Spinal Cord Stimulation: Stage I Trial Stimulation

Percutaneous Implantation of Neurostimulator Electrode	**63650**
Laminectomy for Implantation of Neurostimulator Electrode	**63655**
Removal or Revision of Neurostimulator Electrode	**63660**

Relative Value Units

Percutaneous Implantation of Neurostimulator Electrode	**25**
Laminectomy for Implantation of Neurostimulator Electrode	**30**
Removal or Revision of Neurostimulator Electrode	**20**

INDICATIONS

A trial of spinal cord stimulation in the cervical region is indicated in patients suffering from the following painful conditions that have failed to respond to more conservative therapy:

1. Reflex sympathetic dystrophy of the upper extremities
2. Causalgia of the upper extremities
3. Ischemic pain secondary to peripheral vascular insufficiency
4. Cervical radiculopathies
5. Peripheral neuropathies of the upper extremities
6. Arachnoiditis
7. Postherpetic neuralgia
8. Phantom limb pain
9. Intractable angina

Because spinal cord stimulation is a reversible technique for pain relief, it should be considered before neurodestructive procedures in most patients.

Patients thought to be candidates for a trial of spinal cord stimulation should be psychologically stable and should have exhausted all traditional less invasive treatment modalities. Furthermore, the patient should not exhibit drug misuse, drug overuse, or continued drug-seeking behaviors. The family and patient must demonstrate a clear understanding of the pros and cons of spinal cord stimulation and accept the potential for hardware revisions and electronic reprogramming to obtain optimal pain relief.

CLINICALLY RELEVANT ANATOMY

Spinal cord stimulator electrodes can be placed into the epidural space either percutaneously or via a small laminotomy.

The superior boundary of the cervical epidural space is the fusion of the periosteal and spinal layers of dura at the foramen magnum. The epidural space continues inferiorly to the sacrococcygeal membrane. The cervical epidural space is bounded anteriorly by the posterior longitudinal ligament and posteriorly by the vertebral laminae and the ligamentum flavum. The vertebral pedicles and intervertebral foramina form the lateral limits of the epidural space. The cervical epidural space is 3 to 4 mm at the C7-T1 interspace with the cervical spine flexed. The cervical epidural space contains fat, veins, arteries, lymphatics, and connective tissue. Spinal cord stimulator electrodes can be placed anywhere along the epidural space from the cervical to the caudal region (Fig. 143-1).

TECHNIQUE

Spinal cord stimulator electrode placement may be carried out with the patient in the sitting, lateral, or prone position. Selection of position is based on the patient's ability to maintain the chosen position for the 30 to 45 minutes needed to place the electrode into the epidural space and position it. Because placement of a spinal cord stimulator electrode requires patient feedback, choosing the most comfortable position is

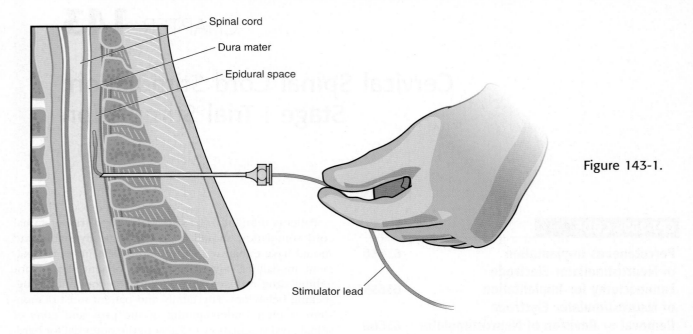

Spinal cord

Dura mater

Epidural space

Stimulator lead

Figure 143-1.

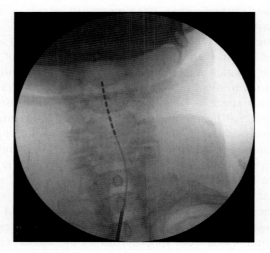

Figure 143-2.
PA view of the electrode in position in the cervical epidural space.

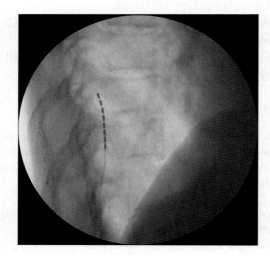

Figure 143-3.
Lateral view of the electrode in the cervical epidural space.

important to minimize the need for adjunctive intravenous narcotics or sedation.

After aseptic preparation of the skin to include the midline and electrode exit site, a Tuohy needle is placed into the epidural space at the level of desired electrode placement. The spinal cord–stimulating electrode is then advanced through the Tuohy needle into the epidural space. Spinal cord stimulator electrodes have a tendency to drag against the internal needle wall, and this may result in damage to the electrode insulation. This can be avoided by wetting both the needle and electrode with saline before attempting to advance the electrode through the needle.

After the electrode enters the epidural space, it is gently advanced under fluoroscopic guidance to a midline position overlying the spinal segments to be stimulated (Figs. 143-2 and 143-3). The needle is then carefully withdrawn back along the electrode and removed. The electrode is now attached to the pulse generator via a sterile screening cable. Trial stimulation is carried out with the patient describing the type and location of stimulation as well as the effect of the stimulation on the patient's ongoing pain. Ideally, the patient should report perception of the stimulation pattern superimposed on the painful area. More than one electrode is occasionally required to adequately relieve the patient's pain.

If an acceptable pattern of stimulation is obtained, the midline incision is then closed with interrupted sutures, and sterile dressings are placed. A 48-hour period of trial stimulation is then carried out with careful quantification of the patient's functional ability and pain relief. If satisfactory results of the period of trial stimulation are obtained, it is reasonable to proceed with stage II permanent implantation of a pulse generator or radiofrequency coupling device.

SIDE EFFECTS AND COMPLICATIONS

Because of the potential for hematogenous spread via the epidural veins, local infection and sepsis represent absolute contraindications to the placement of spinal cord stimulator electrodes into the epidural space. Anticoagulation and coagulopathy represent absolute contraindications to placement of epidural spinal cord stimulator electrodes because of the risk for epidural hematoma.

Inadvertent dural puncture during identification of the epidural space should occur less than 0.5% of the time. Failure to recognize inadvertent dural puncture can result in placement of the stimulating electrode into the subdural or subarachnoid space.

Needle- or electrode-induced trauma to the epidural veins may result in self-limited bleeding, which may cause postprocedural pain. Uncontrolled bleeding into the epidural space may result in compression of the spinal cord with the rapid development of neurologic deficit. Although the incidence of significant neurologic deficit secondary to epidural hematoma after placement of epidural spinal cord stimulator electrodes is exceedingly rare, this devastating complication should be considered whenever there is rapidly developing neurologic deficit after placement of epidural spinal cord stimulator electrodes.

Neurologic complications after placement of epidural spinal cord stimulator electrodes are uncommon if proper technique is used. Direct trauma to the spinal cord or nerve roots is usually accompanied by pain. If significant pain occurs during placement of the epidural needle or electrode placement, the physician should immediately stop and ascertain the cause of the pain to avoid the possibility of additional neural trauma.

Although uncommon, infection in the epidural space remains an ever-present possibility, especially in the immunocompromised AIDS or cancer patient. If epidural abscess occurs, emergent surgical drainage to avoid spinal cord compression and irreversible neurologic deficit is usually required. Early detection and treatment of infection is crucial to avoid potentially life-threatening sequelae.

Although hardware failure occurs with a greatly decreased frequency compared with the early days of spinal cord stimulation, unfortunately, problems still occur. Damage to the insulation of the stimulating electrode during placement can be avoided if the electrode is wetted with sterile saline before advancing it through the epidural needle. The pain management specialist should consult the product package insert before implantation of a spinal cord stimulation system.

CLINICAL PEARLS

A trial of spinal cord stimulation is a reasonable next step for patients with the previously mentioned pain complaints who have failed to respond to more conservative pain-relieving measures, who are psychologically stable, and who have no drug- or medication-related problems. Failure to accurately identify the midline is the most common reason for difficulty in identifying the epidural space and increases the risk for complications. The routine use of sedation or general anesthesia before identification of the epidural space is to be discouraged because it will render the patient unable to provide accurate verbal feedback should needle misplacement occur and make it impossible for the patient to provide the feedback necessary

to optimize electrode placement. As mentioned, occasionally more than one electrode will be required to adequately relieve the patient's pain.

The pain management specialist should recognize that undertaking a trial of spinal cord stimulation requires a high level of ongoing involvement with the patient. Continuity of care is essential if long-term success is to be obtained. This modality should be undertaken only if all members of the pain management care team are committed to a long-term relationship with the patient and will be available to provide support and pulse generator reprogramming for the indefinite future.

CHAPTER 144

Lumbar Spinal Cord Stimulation:
Stage I Trial Stimulation

CPT-2003 CODE	
Percutaneous Implantation	**63650**
of Neurostimulator Electrode	
Laminectomy for Implantation	**63655**
of Neurostimulator Electrode	
Removal or Revision of Neurostimulator	**63660**
Electrode	

Relative Value Units	
Percutaneous Implantation	**25**
of Neurostimulator Electrode	
Laminectomy for Implantation	**30**
of Neurostimulator Electrode	
Removal or Revision of Neurostimulator	**20**
Electrode	

INDICATIONS

A trial of spinal cord stimulation is indicated in patients suffering from the following painful conditions that have failed to respond to more conservative therapy:

1. Reflex sympathetic dystrophy
2. Causalgia
3. Ischemic pain secondary to peripheral vascular insufficiency
4. Radiculopathies
5. Failed back syndrome
6. Arachnoiditis
7. Postherpetic neuralgia
8. Phantom limb pain
9. Intractable angina

Because spinal cord stimulation is a reversible technique for pain relief, it should be considered before neurodestructive procedures in most patients.

Patients thought to be candidates for a trial of spinal cord stimulation should be psychologically stable and should have exhausted all traditional less invasive treatment modalities. Furthermore, the patient should not exhibit drug misuse, drug overuse, or continued drug-seeking behaviors. The family and patient must demonstrate a clear understanding of the pros and cons of spinal cord stimulation and accept the potential for hardware revisions and electronic reprogramming to obtain optimal pain relief.

CLINICALLY RELEVANT ANATOMY

Spinal cord stimulator electrodes can be placed into the epidural space either percutaneously or via a small laminotomy. The superior boundary of the epidural space is the fusion of the periosteal and spinal layers of dura at the foramen magnum. The epidural space continues inferiorly to the sacrococcygeal membrane. The epidural space is bounded anteriorly by the posterior longitudinal ligament and posteriorly by the vertebral laminae and the ligamentum flavum. The vertebral pedicles and intervertebral foramina form the lateral limits of the epidural space. The cervical epidural space is 3 to 4 mm at the C7-T1 interspace with the cervical spine flexed. The lumbar epidural space is 5 to 6 mm at the L2-L3 interspace with the lumbar spine flexed. The epidural space contains fat, veins, arteries, lymphatics, and connective tissue. Spinal cord stimulator electrodes can be placed anywhere along the epidural space from the cervical to the caudal region (Fig. 144-1).

TECHNIQUE

Spinal cord stimulator electrode placement may be carried out with the patient in the sitting, lateral, or prone position. Selection of position is based on the patient's ability to maintain the chosen position for the 30 to 45 minutes needed to place the electrode into the epidural space, position it, and then tunnel the electrode subcutaneously. Because placement of a spinal

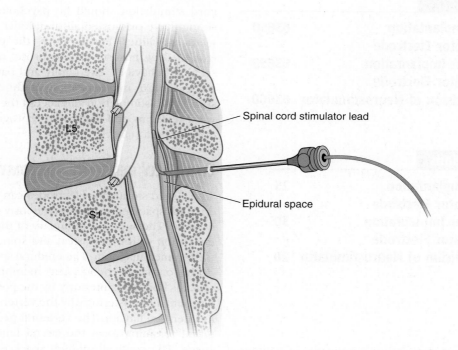

Figure 144-1.

cord stimulator electrode requires patient feedback, choosing the most comfortable position is important to minimize the need for adjunctive intravenous narcotics or sedation.

After aseptic preparation of the skin to include the midline and electrode exit site, a Tuohy needle is placed into the epidural space several levels below the desired level of the spinal segments to be stimulated (Fig. 144-2). The spinal cord–stimulating electrode is then advanced through the Tuohy needle into the epidural space. Spinal cord stimulator electrodes have a tendency to drag against the internal needle wall, and this may result in damage to the electrode insulation. This can be avoided by wetting both the needle and electrode with saline before attempting to advance the electrode through the needle.

After the electrode enters the epidural space, it is gently advanced under fluoroscopic guidance to a midline position overlying the spinal segments to be stimulated (Figs. 144-3 to 144-6). The needle is then carefully withdrawn back along the electrode and removed. The electrode is now attached to the pulse generator via a sterile screening cable. Trial stimulation is carried out with the patient describing the type and location of stimulation as well as the effect of the stimulation on the patient's ongoing pain. Ideally, the patient should report perception of the stimulation pattern superimposed on the painful area. More than one electrode is occasionally required to adequately relieve the patient's pain. After satisfactory electrode position is obtained, the electrode is disconnected from the screening cable. A 48-hour period of trial stimulation is then carried out with careful quantification of the patient's functional ability and pain relief. If satisfactory results of the period of trial stimulation are obtained, it is reasonable to proceed with stage II permanent implantation of a pulse generator or radiofrequency coupling device. If lead migration becomes a problem, a paddle lead can be placed via mini-laminectomy (Fig. 144-7).

SIDE EFFECTS AND COMPLICATIONS

Because of the potential for hematogenous spread via Batson's plexus, local infection and sepsis represent absolute contraindications to the placement of spinal cord stimulator electrodes into the epidural space. Anticoagulation and coagulopathy represent absolute contraindications to placement of epidural spinal cord stimulator electrodes because of the risk for epidural hematoma.

Inadvertent dural puncture during identification of the epidural space should occur less than 0.5% of the time. Failure to recognize inadvertent dural puncture can result in placement of the stimulating electrode into the subdural or subarachnoid space.

Needle- or electrode-induced trauma to the epidural veins may result in self-limited bleeding, which may cause postprocedural pain. Uncontrolled bleeding into the epidural space may result in compression of the spinal cord with the rapid development of neurologic deficit. Although the incidence of significant neurologic deficit secondary to epidural hematoma after placement of epidural spinal cord stimulator electrodes is exceedingly rare, this devastating complication should be considered whenever there is rapidly developing neurologic deficit after placement of epidural spinal cord stimulator electrodes.

Neurologic complications after placement of epidural spinal cord stimulator electrodes are uncommon if proper technique is used. Direct trauma to the spinal cord or nerve roots is usually accompanied by pain. If significant pain occurs during placement of the epidural needle or electrode placement, the physician should immediately stop and ascertain the cause of the pain to avoid the possibility of additional neural trauma.

Although uncommon, infection in the epidural space remains an ever-present possibility, especially in the immunocompromised AIDS or cancer patient. If epidural abscess occurs, emergent surgical drainage to avoid spinal cord compression and irreversible neurologic deficit is usually required. Early detection and treatment of infection is crucial to avoid potentially life-threatening sequelae.

Although hardware failure occurs with a greatly decreased frequency when compared with the early days of spinal cord stimulation, unfortunately, problems still occur.

Damage to the insulation of the stimulating electrode during placement can be avoided if the electrode is wetted with sterile saline before advancing it through the epidural needle. The electrode should never be withdrawn against the tip of the epidural needle, or damage to the insulation or shearing of the electrode can occur. Care must be taken to carefully tighten all set screws when connecting the electrode to the extension set or to the pulse generator so that they do not subsequently loosen and disrupt electrical contact.

Although each spinal cord stimulation system is different, most require that a Silastic cuff be securely placed and sutured over all electrical connections to avoid body fluids from shorting out the connection. The pain management specialist should consult the package insert before implantation of a spinal cord stimulation system.

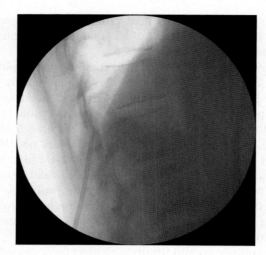

Figure 144-2.
Lateral view of the epidural needle in epidural space.

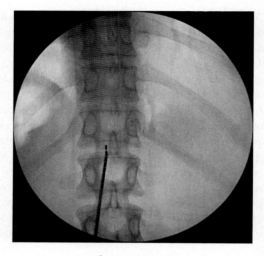

Figure 144-3.
PA view of electrode exiting the epidural space.

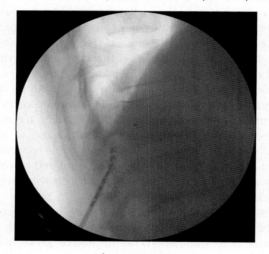

Figure 144-4.
Lateral view of the electrode entering the epidural space.

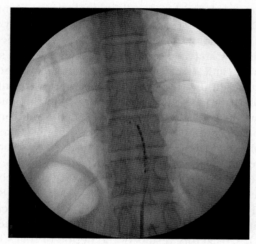

Figure 144-5.
PA view of electrode being advanced into the lower thoracic epidural space.

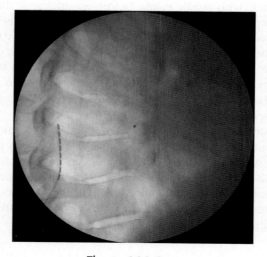

Figure 144-6.
Lateral view of electrode being advanced into the thoracic epidural space.

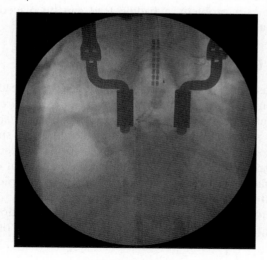

Figure 144-7.
PA view of paddle electrode in the lower thoracic epidural space.

CLINICAL PEARLS

A trial of spinal cord stimulation is a reasonable next step for patients with the previously mentioned pain complaints who have failed to respond to more conservative pain-relieving measures, who are psychologically stable, and who have no drug- or medication-related problems. Failure to accurately identify the midline is the most common reason for difficulty in identifying the epidural space and increases the risk for complications. The routine use of sedation or general anesthesia before identification of the epidural space is to be discouraged because it will render the patient unable to provide accurate verbal feedback should needle misplacement occur and make it impossible for the patient to provide the feedback necessary to optimize electrode placement. As mentioned, occasionally more than one electrode will be required to adequately relieve the patient's pain.

The pain management specialist should recognize that undertaking a trial of spinal cord stimulation requires a high level of ongoing involvement with the patient. Continuity of care is essential if long-term success is to be obtained. This modality should be undertaken only if all members of the pain management care team are committed to a long-term relationship with the patient and will be available to provide support and pulse generator reprogramming for the indefinite future.

CHAPTER 145

Spinal Cord Stimulation: Stage II Pulse Generator Implantation

INDICATIONS

In patients in whom a 48- to 72-hour stage I trial of spinal cord stimulation has been considered successful, it is reasonable to proceed with a stage II permanent implantation of the pulse generator. Before proceeding with permanent implantation of a pulse generator, the pain management specialist should carefully review the results of the trial stimulation period, looking not only at the reported pain relief but also at functional levels, the need for additional pain medication, and other indications of psychological factors that might make permanent implantation inadvisable.

There are two basic types of spinal cord stimulation systems: (1) a totally implantable electrode and pulse generator system with a permanent battery, and (2) a totally implantable electrode with a totally implantable rechargeable pulse generator. Each type of system has advantages and disadvantages, and thus the ultimate choice of system should be based on matching these factors to the needs of the specific patient.

CLINICALLY RELEVANT ANATOMY

Spinal cord stimulator electrodes can be placed into the epidural space either percutaneously or via a small laminotomy. The superior boundary of the epidural space is the fusion of the periosteal and spinal layers of dura at the foramen magnum. The epidural space continues inferiorly to the sacrococcygeal membrane. The epidural space is bounded anteriorly by the posterior longitudinal ligament and posteriorly by the vertebral laminae and the ligamentum flavum. The vertebral pedicles and intervertebral foramina form the lateral limits of the epidural space. The cervical epidural space is 3 to 4 mm at the C7-T1 interspace with the cervical spine flexed. The lumbar epidural space is 5 to 6 mm at the L2-L3 interspace with the lumbar spine flexed. The epidural space contains fat, veins, arteries, lymphatics, and connective tissue. Spinal cord stimulator electrodes can be placed anywhere along the epidural space from the cervical to the caudal region. The pulse generator/receiver antenna pocket should be placed subcutaneously in the anterior subcostal region.

TECHNIQUE

Spinal cord pulse generator placement may be carried out with the patient in the lateral or prone position depending on where the desired site of pulse generator placement is chosen. Because minimal patient cooperation is not required for this technique, intravenous sedation may be given if required for the patient to remain in the selected position for the 30 to 45 minutes needed to implant the pulse generator.

After aseptic preparation of the skin to include the midline incision and pulse generator pocket site, permanent spinal cord stimulator leads are placed as described as in Chapters 143 and 144. Care must be taken to make the midline incision large enough to allow for anchoring of the spinal cord stimulator electrode and to accommodate the tunneling tool. After a satisfactory stimulation pattern is obtained, the area selected for pulse generator implantation is anesthetized with local anesthetic. An incision in the region selected for the pulse

Current Procedural Terminology © 2009 American Medical Association. All Rights Reserved.

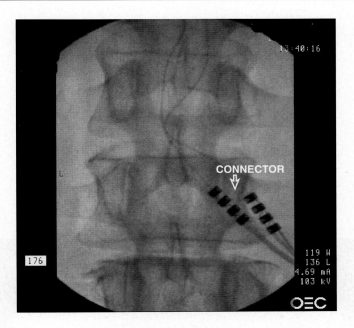

Figure 145-1.
Lead connectors attached to distal end of the electrodes.

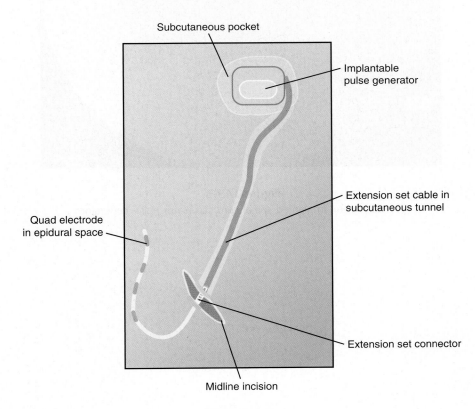

Figure 145-2.

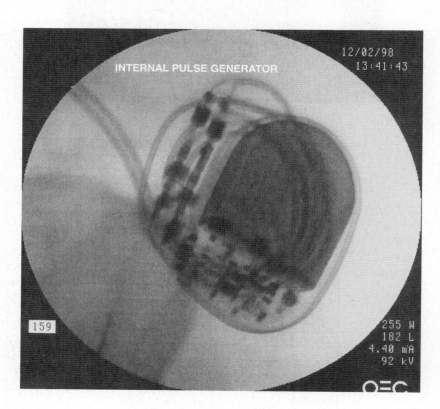

Figure 145-3.
PA view of the implanted spinal cord stimulator pulse generator.

generator is made just large enough to accommodate the pulse generator. A subcutaneous pocket is then created using small, curved, blunt-tipped scissors. The pocket must be commodious enough to accommodate the pulse generator, or the edge of these devices will erode through the skin. However, the pocket must not be made too large, or the devices could turn over on themselves, making subsequent programming or stimulation impossible. After the pocket is created, adequate hemostasis must be obtained, or hematoma formation and infection are a distinct possibility. After adequate hemostasis has been obtained, a malleable tunneling device is then passed from the midline incision to the pulse generator pocket (Fig. 145-1). The spinal cord stimulator electrodes or extension set is passed through the tunneling device back to the pulse generator pocket, and the distal end of the electrode or extension set is attached to the pulse generator (Fig. 145-2). Excess electrode or extension set connector is carefully looped in the pulse generator pocket underneath the pulse generator (Fig. 145-3). The pulse generator is then activated to verify that the system is working. After this is ascertained, the midline and pulse generator pocket incisions are closed with two layers of interrupted sutures, which can be removed in 10 to 14 days.

SIDE EFFECTS AND COMPLICATIONS

Because of the potential for hematogenous spread via Batson's plexus, local infection and sepsis represent absolute contraindications to the placement of spinal cord stimulator systems. Anticoagulation and coagulopathy represent absolute contraindications to placement of epidural spinal cord stimulator electrodes because of the risk for epidural hematoma.

Although uncommon, infection in the epidural space or pulse generator pocket remains an ever-present possibility, especially in the immunocompromised AIDS or cancer patient. If epidural abscess occurs, emergent surgical drainage to avoid spinal cord compression and irreversible neurologic deficit is usually required. Infection in the pulse generator pocket can sometimes be managed without removal of the device by aggressive use of sys-

temic antibiotics, incision and drainage, and careful observation of the patient for spread of the infection along the extension set into the subcutaneous tunnel. Early detection and treatment of infection is crucial to avoid potentially life-threatening sequelae.

Although hardware failure occurs with a greatly decreased frequency compared with the early days of spinal cord stimulation, unfortunately, problems still occur. Damage to the insulation of the stimulating electrode during placement can be avoided if the electrode is wetted with sterile saline before advancing it through the epidural needle. Care must be taken to carefully tighten all set screws when connecting the electrode to the extension set or to the pulse generator so that they do not subsequently loosen and disrupt electrical contact. The pain management specialist should consult the package insert before implantation of a spinal cord stimulation system.

CLINICAL PEARLS

Spinal cord stimulation is a reasonable next step for patients with the previously mentioned pain complaints who have failed to respond to more conservative pain-relieving measures, who are psychologically stable, and who have no drug or medication-related problems. Because of the cost of a spinal cord stimulator system, coupled with the risks associated with this pain treatment modality, a trial of stimulation should be carried out before implantation of a pulse generator or receiver antenna.

The pain management specialist should recognize that undertaking a trial of spinal cord stimulation requires a high level of ongoing involvement with the patient. Continuity of care is essential if long-term success is to be obtained. This modality should be undertaken only if all members of the pain management care team are committed to a long-term relationship with the patient and will be available to provide support and pulse generator reprogramming for the indefinite future.

CHAPTER 146

Occipital Nerve Stimulation

INDICATIONS

Occipital nerve stimulation is indicated for patients suffering from occipital neuralgia who have experienced excellent short-term relief with occipital nerve block with local anesthetic, steroid, or both but in whom the pain returns.

CLINICALLY RELEVANT ANATOMY

The greater occipital nerve arises from fibers of the dorsal primary ramus of the second cervical nerve and to a lesser extent from fibers of the third cervical nerve. The greater occipital nerve pierces the fascia just below the superior nuchal ridge along with the occipital artery. It supplies the medial portion of the posterior scalp as far anterior as the vertex (see Fig. 7-1).

The lesser occipital nerve arises from the ventral primary rami of the second and third cervical nerves. The lesser occipital nerve passes superiorly along the posterior border of the sternocleidomastoid muscle, dividing into cutaneous branches that innervate the lateral portion of the posterior scalp and the cranial surface of the pinna of the ear (see Fig. 7-1).

TECHNIQUE

Percutaneous Lead Placement for Trial Stimulation

Occipital stimulator electrode placement may be carried out with the patient in the sitting, lateral, or prone position. Selection of position is based on the patient's ability to maintain the chosen position for the 30 to 45 minutes needed to place the electrode into the tissues overlying the occipital nerves, and then tunnel the electrode subcutaneously. Because placement of an occipital stimulator electrode requires patient feedback, choosing the most comfortable position is important to minimize the need for adjunctive intravenous narcotics or sedation.

After aseptic preparation of the skin to include the entire occipital and suboccipital region as well as the intended electrode exit site, the level of the first cervical vertebra (atlas) is identified using anteroposterior and lateral fluoroscopy. The skin and subcutaneous tissues at this level are then anesthetized with local anesthetic. A Tuohy needle is placed at the level of the first cervical vertebra and passed subcutaneously toward the midline (Figs. 146-1 and 146-2). The stimulating electrode is then advanced through the Tuohy needle medially to overlie the occipital nerves (Figs. 146-3 and 146-4). Spinal cord stimulator electrodes have a tendency to drag against the internal needle wall, and this may result in damage to the electrode insulation. This can be avoided by wetting both the needle and electrode with saline before attempting to advance the electrode through the needle.

A small incision is then made with a No. 15 scalpel extending cranially and caudally about 0.5 cm with the Tuohy needle still in place to avoid inadvertent damage to the electrode. Care must be taken to completely dissect all tissue away from the needle to allow the electrode to fall freely into the incision as the tunneling tool is advanced. The needle is then carefully withdrawn back along the electrode and removed. The electrode is now attached to the pulse generator via a sterile screening cable. Trial stimulation is carried out with the patient

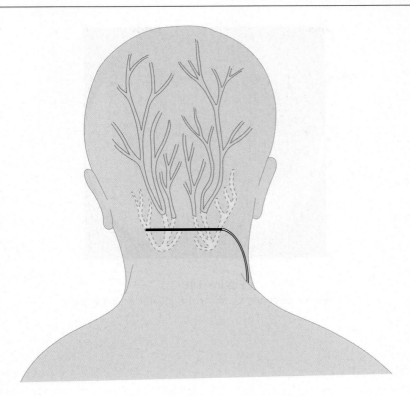

Figure 146-1.

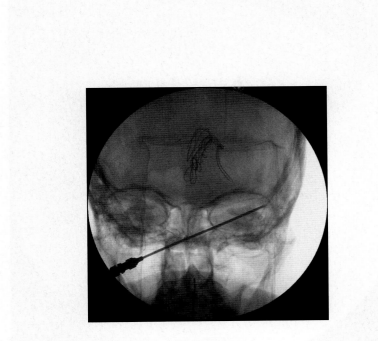

Figure 146-2.
Touhy needle passed subcutaneously with tip overlying the greater occipital nerve.

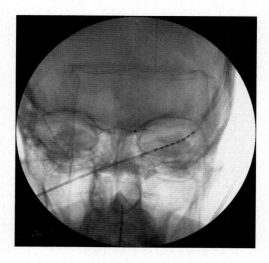

Figure 146-3.
PA view of electrode overlying the greater occipital nerve.

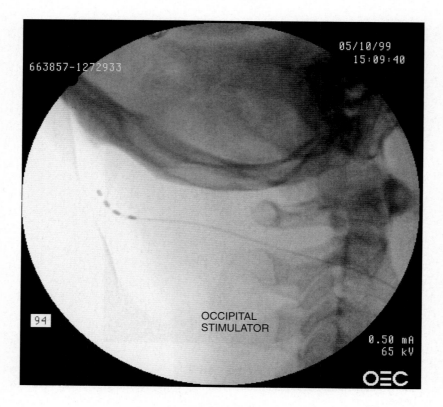

Figure 146-4.
Lateral view of electrode overlying the greater occipital nerve.

describing the type and location of stimulation as well as the effect of the stimulation on the patient's ongoing pain. Ideally, the patient should report perception of the stimulation pattern superimposed on the painful area. More than one electrode is occasionally required to adequately relieve the patient's pain, and bilateral electrodes are required for bilateral pain. After satisfactory electrode position is obtained, the electrode is disconnected from the screening cable, and if a pulse generator is to be implanted, a pocket for the pulse generator in made as described in Chapter 145.

SIDE EFFECTS AND COMPLICATIONS

Local infection and sepsis represent absolute contraindications to the placement of occipital nerve stimulator systems. Anticoagulation and coagulopathy represent absolute contraindications to placement of occipital nerve stimulator electrodes and pulse generator because of the risk for bleeding.

Although uncommon, infection in the stimulator lead tunnel or pulse generator pocket remains an ever-present possibility, especially in the immunocompromised AIDS or cancer patient. If infection occurs, emergent surgical drainage, culture, and initiation of antibiotics are usually required. Infection in the pulse generator pocket can sometimes be managed without removal of the device by aggressive use of systemic antibiotics, incision and drainage, and careful observation of the patient for spread of the infection along the extension set into the subcutaneous tunnel. Early detection and treatment of infection are crucial to avoid potentially life-threatening sequelae.

Although hardware failure occurs with a greatly decreased frequency compared with the early days of spinal cord stimulation, unfortunately, problems still occur. Damage to the insulation of the stimulating electrode during placement can be avoided if the electrode is wetted with sterile saline before advancing it through the Tuohy needle. The electrode should never be withdrawn against the tip of the epidural needle, or damage to the insulation or shearing of the electrode can occur. Care must be taken to carefully tighten all set screws when connecting the electrode to the extension set or to the pulse generator so that they do not subsequently loosen and disrupt electrical contact. The pain management specialist should consult the package insert before implantation of an occipital nerve stimulation system.

CLINICAL PEARLS

Occipital nerve stimulation is a reasonable next step for patients with the previously mentioned pain complaints who have failed to respond to more conservative pain-relieving measures, who are psychologically stable, and who have no drug- or medication-related problems. Because of the cost of a stimulator system, coupled with the risks associated with this pain treatment modality, a trial of stimulation should be carried out before implantation of a pulse generator.

The pain management specialist should recognize that undertaking a trial of occipital nerve stimulation requires a high level of ongoing involvement with the patient. Continuity of care is essential if long-term success is to be obtained. This modality should be undertaken only if all members of the pain management care team are committed to a long-term relationship with the patient and will be available to provide support and pulse generator reprogramming for the indefinite future.

CHAPTER 147

Implantation of Totally Implantable Reservoirs and Injection Ports

CPT-2009 CODE

Implantation of Totally Implantable Reservoir/Port	62360
Removal of Totally Implantable Reservoir/Port	62365

Relative Value Units

Implantation Procedure	35
Removal	25

INDICATIONS

Implantation of a totally implantable reservoir/port is indicated for the injection of drugs into the epidural space in three clinical situations:

1. For the administration of epidural drugs for the palliation of pain in cancer patients with a life expectancy of months to years
2. In patients who have a shorter life expectancy but desire the ability to swim or bathe in a bathtub
3. In patients who will require epidural administration of drugs for a shorter period of time but require hydrotherapy that would necessitate total immersion of the drug delivery system, thus precluding use of a tunneled catheter

Advantages of totally implantable reservoirs/ports include the lower incidence of infection relative to tunneled epidural catheters. Furthermore, once the reservoir/port is implanted, there is a lower incidence of delivery system failure compared with tunneled catheters. Disadvantages of totally implantable reservoirs/ports include the fact that implantation, subsequent injection, and removal are more technically demanding relative to tunneled catheters. Furthermore, the reservoir/port is less amenable to use with an external pump compared with a tunneled catheter.

CLINICALLY RELEVANT ANATOMY

The superior boundary of the epidural space is the fusion of the periosteal and spinal layers of dura at the foramen magnum. The epidural space continues inferiorly to the sacrococcygeal membrane. The epidural space is bounded anteriorly by the posterior longitudinal ligament and posteriorly by the vertebral laminae and the ligamentum flavum. The vertebral pedicles and intervertebral foramina form the lateral limits of the epidural space. The cervical epidural space is 3 to 4 mm at the C7-T1 interspace with the cervical spine flexed. The lumbar epidural space is 5 to 6 mm at the L2-L3 interspace with the lumbar spine flexed. The epidural space contains fat, veins, arteries, lymphatics, and connective tissue. Epidural catheters can be placed anywhere along the spine from the cervical to the caudal region.

TECHNIQUE

Placement of totally implantable reservoirs/ports may be carried out with the patient in the sitting, lateral, or prone position. Selection of position is based on the patient's ability to maintain the chosen position for the 15 to 20 minutes needed to place the catheter subcutaneously. Because most reservoirs/ports are placed on an outpatient basis, choosing the most comfortable position is important to minimize the need for adjunctive intravenous narcotics or sedation.

After aseptic preparation of the skin to include the site of tunneling and reservoir/port implantation site, a 17-gauge Tuohy needle is placed into the epidural space at the level of desired catheter placement. The Silastic one-piece catheter is then advanced through the Tuohy needle into the epidural space (Fig. 147-1A). Silastic catheters have a tendency to drag against the internal needle wall and fold back onto themselves. This can be avoided by wetting both the needle and catheter with saline before attempting to advance the catheter through the needle.

After the catheter enters the epidural space, it is gently advanced an additional 3 to 4 cm. A small incision is made with a No. 15 scalpel extending cranially and

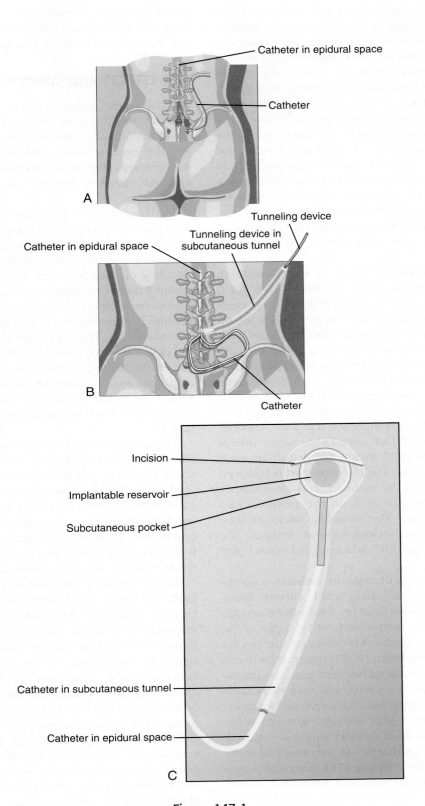

Figure 147-1.

caudally about 0.5 cm with the needle still in place to avoid inadvertent damage to the catheter. Care must be taken to completely dissect all tissue away from the needle to allow the catheter to fall freely into the incision as the tunneling tool is advanced. The needle is then carefully withdrawn back along the catheter until the tip is outside the skin. The catheter wire stylet is withdrawn, and the Tuohy needle is removed from the catheter. The injection port is then attached to the distal end of the catheter, and after aspiration, 4 to 5 mL of 1.5% lidocaine is injected into the epidural space via the catheter to provide dense segmental sensory block for the subcutaneous tunneling. This approach avoids the need for painful subcutaneous infiltration at the tunneling site. Injection through the catheter at this point also allows for inspection for any leaks before subcutaneous tunneling.

The malleable tunneling device is then shaped to match the contour of the flank. The skin is now lifted with thumb forceps, and the tunneling device is introduced subcutaneously and guided laterally. When the tip of the tunneling device has reached the exit point laterally, it is turned away from the patient; this forces the tip against the skin. The scalpel is then used to cut down onto the tip. The tunneling device is then advanced through the incision. This approach allows for a straight catheter path and decreases the incidence of catheter failure secondary to subcutaneous catheter kinking. An incision large enough to accommodate subcutaneous placement of the port is then extended from each side of the tunneling tool. The injection port is removed from the distal end of the catheter, and the catheter is then threaded onto the stud on the proximal end of the tunneling device. The tunneling device is then withdrawn through the second incision, bringing the catheter with it through the subcutaneous tunnel (see Fig. 147-1**B**).

With care taken not to damage the catheter, a subcutaneous pocket is created using small, curved, blunt-tipped scissors. The pocket must be commodious enough to accommodate the reservoir/port, or the edge of the device will erode through the skin. However, the pocket must not be made too large, or the reservoir/port can turn over on itself, making subsequent injection impossible. After the pocket is created, adequate hemostasis must be obtained, or hematoma formation and infection are a distinct possibility. After adequate hemostasis has been obtained, excess distal catheter length is removed, and the reservoir/port is attached to the distal end of the catheter by means of a coupling. The reservoir/port is secured to the catheter by means of interrupted nonabsorbable sutures. The reservoir is then placed into the pocket, with care taken not to twist or kink the catheter (see Fig. 147-1**C**). With the reservoir in place, but before the pocket incision is closed, the reservoir is injected

percutaneously to ensure delivery system integrity. The wound is then closed with interrupted sutures, which may be removed in 10 to 14 days.

SIDE EFFECTS AND COMPLICATIONS

Because of the potential for hematogenous spread via Batson's plexus, local infection and sepsis represent absolute contraindications to the placement of catheters into the epidural space. Anticoagulation and coagulopathy represent absolute contraindications to placement of epidural catheters because of the risk for epidural hematoma.

Inadvertent dural puncture during identification of the epidural space should occur less than 0.5% of the time. Failure to recognize inadvertent dural puncture can result in immediate total spinal anesthetic with associated loss of consciousness, hypotension, and apnea. If epidural doses of opioids are accidentally placed into the subarachnoid space, significant respiratory and central nervous system depression will result. It also is possible to inadvertently place a needle or catheter intended for the epidural space into the subdural space. If subdural placement is unrecognized and epidural doses of local anesthetic are administered, the signs and symptoms are similar to those of massive subarachnoid injection, although the resulting motor and sensory block may be spotty.

The epidural space is highly vascular. The intravenous placement of the epidural needle or catheter occurs in about 0.5% to 1% of patients undergoing placement of epidural catheters. This complication is increased in patients with distended epidural veins, such as parturient patients and patients with a large intra-abdominal tumor mass. If the misplacement is unrecognized, injection of local anesthetic directly into an epidural vein will result in significant local anesthetic toxicity.

Needle trauma to the epidural veins may result in self-limited bleeding, which may cause postprocedural pain. Uncontrolled bleeding into the epidural space may result in compression of the spinal cord with the rapid development of neurologic deficit. Although the incidence of significant neurologic deficit secondary to epidural hematoma after placement of epidural catheters is exceedingly rare, this devastating complication should be considered whenever there is rapidly developing neurologic deficit after placement of epidural catheters.

Neurologic complications after placement of epidural catheters are uncommon if proper technique is used. Direct trauma to the spinal cord or nerve roots is usually accompanied by pain. If significant pain occurs during placement of the epidural needle or catheter or during injection, the physician should immediately stop and ascertain the cause of the pain to avoid the possibility of additional neural trauma.

Although uncommon, infection in the epidural space remains an ever-present possibility, especially in the immunocompromised AIDS or cancer patient. If epidural abscess occurs, emergent surgical drainage to avoid spinal cord compression and irreversible neurologic deficit is usually required. Early detection and treatment of infection is crucial to avoid potentially life-threatening sequelae. Infections of the reservoir/port pocket can usually be managed with systemic and topical antibiotics and, occasionally, incision and drainage. The patient must be observed closely for spread of infection proximally down the subcutaneous tunnel into the epidural space. If this occurs, the entire delivery system should be removed immediately.

CLINICAL PEARLS

Implantation of a totally implantable reservoir/port is a safe and effective procedure if careful attention is paid to technique. Failure to accurately identify the midline is the most common reason for difficulty in identifying the epidural space and increases the risk for complications. The routine use of sedation or general anesthesia before identification of the epidural space is to be discouraged because it will render the patient unable to provide accurate verbal feedback should needle misplacement occur.

The totally implantable reservoir/port has fewer problems associated with it once implanted when compared with tunneled catheters. Difficulty in injection is a major drawback to this type of drug delivery system. Peri-implantation infection will be decreased if care is taken to obtain adequate hemostasis before closing the reservoir/port pocket.

CHAPTER **148**

Implantation of Totally Implantable Infusion Pumps

INDICATIONS

Implantation of a totally implantable infusion pump is indicated for the infusion of drugs into the epidural or more commonly the subarachnoid space in the following clinical situations:

1. For the administration of epidural drugs for the palliation of pain in cancer patients with a life expectancy of months to years
2. In carefully selected patients who suffer from chronic benign pain who have experienced palliation of their pain with trial doses of spinal opioids and who have failed to respond to other more conservative treatments

3. In patients suffering from spasticity who have experienced decreased spasms after trial doses of subarachnoid administration of baclofen

Advantages of totally implantable infusion pumps include the lower incidence of infections relative to tunneled epidural catheters and reservoirs/ports. Furthermore, once the infusion pump is implanted, there is a lower incidence of delivery system failure compared with tunneled catheters. Disadvantages of totally implantable infusion pumps include the fact that implantation, subsequent refill, and pump removal are more technically demanding relative to tunneled catheters and reservoirs/pumps. Additionally, the cost of a totally implantable infusion pump is significantly greater than tunneled catheters or reservoirs/ports, although the lower overall cost of drugs, supplies, and medical bills during the time the pump is used may offset the higher initial cost of the pump.

CLINICALLY RELEVANT ANATOMY

The superior boundary of the epidural space is the fusion of the periosteal and spinal layers of dura at the foramen magnum. The epidural space continues inferiorly to the sacrococcygeal membrane. The epidural space is bounded anteriorly by the posterior longitudinal ligament and posteriorly by the vertebral laminae and the ligamentum flavum. The vertebral pedicles and intervertebral foramina form the lateral limits of the epidural space. The cervical epidural space is 3 to 4 mm at the C7-T1 interspace with the cervical spine flexed. The lumbar epidural space is 5 to 6 mm at the L2-L3 interspace with the lumbar spine flexed. The epidural space contains fat, veins, arteries, lymphatics, and connective tissue. Epidural or subarachnoid catheters can be placed anywhere along the spine from the cervical to the caudal region, although most catheters with a subarachnoid terminus are placed below the level of the spinal cord.

TECHNIQUE

Placement of totally implantable infusion pumps may be carried out with the patient in the sitting, lateral, or prone position. Selection of position is based on the patient's ability to maintain the chosen position for the 25 to 30 minutes needed to place the catheter and pump. Because most infusion pumps are placed on an outpatient basis, choosing the most comfortable position is important to minimize the need for adjunctive intravenous narcotics or sedation. Because each specific type of pump may require additional steps during the implantation process, the pain management specialist should consult the package insert before beginning the implantation procedure.

After aseptic preparation of the skin to include the site of tunneling and infusion pump implantation site, a 17-gauge Tuohy needle is placed into the epidural or subarachnoid space at the level of desired catheter placement. The Silastic one-piece catheter is then advanced through the Tuohy needle into the epidural space (Fig. 148-1**A**). Silastic catheters have a tendency to drag against the internal needle wall and fold back onto themselves. This can be avoided by wetting both the needle and catheter with saline before attempting to advance the catheter through the needle.

After the catheter enters the epidural or subarachnoid space, it is gently advanced an additional 3 to 4 cm. A small incision is made with a No. 15 scalpel extending cranially and caudally about 0.5 cm with the Tuohy needle still in place to avoid inadvertent damage to the catheter. Care must be taken to completely dissect all tissue away from the needle to allow the catheter to fall freely into the incision as the tunneling tool is advanced. If a subarachnoid catheter terminus is planned, a purse-string suture is placed around the needle before removal to help decrease the incidence of hygroma formation as a result of cerebrospinal fluid (CSF) tracking back along the catheter into the pump pocket.

The needle is then carefully withdrawn back along the catheter until the tip is outside the skin. The catheter wire stylet is withdrawn, and the Tuohy needle is removed from the catheter. The injection port is then attached to the distal end of the catheter, and after aspiration, a small amount of preservative-free sterile saline is injected to ensure catheter integrity. If the catheter is placed in the epidural space, 5 to 6 mL of 1.5% lidocaine is injected into the epidural space via the catheter to provide dense segmental sensory block for the subcutaneous tunneling. This approach avoids the need for painful subcutaneous infiltration at the tunneling site. If the catheter is placed into the subarachnoid space, infiltration of a local anesthetic containing epinephrine along the tunneling path is recommended.

The malleable tunneling device is then shaped to match the contour of the flank. The skin is now lifted with thumb forceps, and the tunneling device is introduced subcutaneously and guided laterally. When the tip of the tunneling device has reached the exit point later-

ally in the right upper quadrant of the abdomen, it is turned away from the patient; this forces the tip against the skin. The scalpel is then used to cut down onto the tip. The tunneling device is then advanced through the incision. This approach allows for a straight catheter path and decreases the incidence of catheter failure secondary to subcutaneous catheter kinking. An incision large enough to accommodate subcutaneous placement of the pump is then extended from each side of the tunneling tool. The injection port is removed from the distal end of the catheter, and the catheter is then threaded onto the stud on the proximal end of the tunneling device. The tunneling device is then withdrawn through the second incision, bringing the catheter with it through the subcutaneous tunnel (see Fig. 148-1**B**).

With care taken not to damage the catheter, a subcutaneous pocket is created using small, curved, blunt-tipped scissors. The pocket must be commodious enough to accommodate the infusion pump, or the edge of the pump will erode through the skin. However, the pocket must not be made too large, or the infusion pump can turn over on itself, making subsequent refill impossible. After the pocket is created, adequate hemostasis must be obtained, or hematoma formation and infection are a distinct possibility. After adequate hemostasis has been obtained, excess distal catheter length is removed, and the infusion pump is attached to the distal end of the catheter. The infusion pump is secured to the catheter by means of interrupted nonabsorbable sutures placed over the Silastic boot. The pump is then placed into the pocket, with care taken not to twist or kink the catheter (see Fig. 148-1**C**). The wound is then closed with a double layer of interrupted sutures, which may be removed in 10 to 14 days. Fluoroscopy can be used to assess the position of the pump and catheter if problems arise (Fig. 148-2).

SIDE EFFECTS AND COMPLICATIONS

Because of the potential for hematogenous spread via Batson's plexus, local infection and sepsis represent absolute contraindications to the placement of catheters into the epidural space. Anticoagulation and coagulopathy represent absolute contraindications to placement of epidural catheters because of the risk for epidural hematoma.

Inadvertent dural puncture during identification of the epidural space should occur less than 0.5% of the time. Failure to recognize inadvertent dural puncture can result in immediate total spinal anesthetic with associated loss of consciousness, hypotension, and apnea. If epidural doses of opioids are accidentally placed into the subarachnoid space, significant respiratory and central nervous system depression will result. It also is possible to inadvertently place a needle or catheter intended for

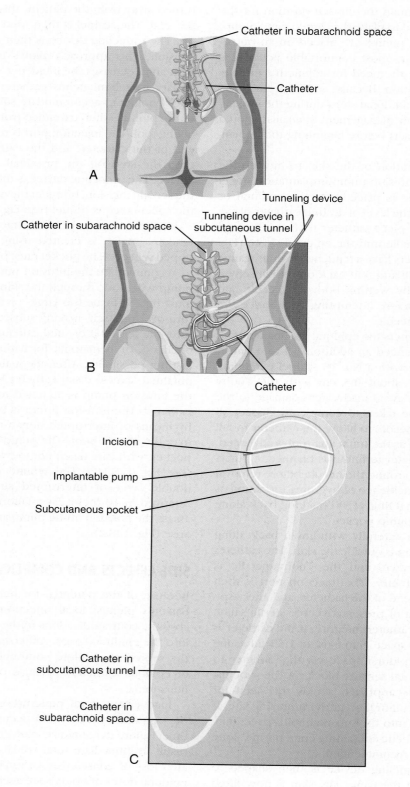

Figure 148-1.

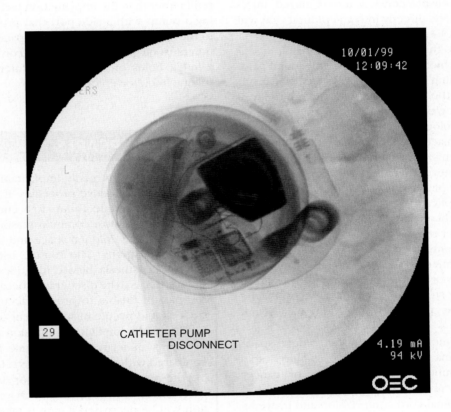

Figure 148-2.
Totally implantable pump with a catheter disconnect.

the epidural space into the subdural space. If subdural placement is unrecognized, and epidural doses of local anesthetic are administered, the signs and symptoms are similar to those of massive subarachnoid injection, although the resulting motor and sensory block may be "spotty."

The epidural space is highly vascular. The intravenous placement of the epidural needle or catheter occurs in about 0.5% to 1% of patients undergoing placement of epidural catheters. This complication is increased in patients with distended epidural veins, such as parturient patients and patients with a large intra-abdominal tumor mass. If the misplacement is unrecognized, injection of local anesthetic directly into an epidural vein will result in significant local anesthetic toxicity.

Needle trauma to the epidural veins may result in self-limited bleeding, which may cause postprocedural pain. Uncontrolled bleeding into the epidural space may result in compression of the spinal cord with the rapid development of neurologic deficit. Although the incidence of significant neurologic deficit secondary to epidural hematoma after placement of epidural catheters is exceedingly rare, this devastating complication should be considered whenever there is rapidly developing neurologic deficit after placement of epidural catheters.

Neurologic complications after placement of epidural or subarachnoid catheters are uncommon if proper technique is used. Direct trauma to the spinal cord or nerve roots is usually accompanied by pain. If significant pain occurs during placement of the epidural or subarachnoid needle or catheter or during injection, the physician should immediately stop and ascertain the cause of the pain to avoid the possibility of additional neural trauma.

Although uncommon, infection in the epidural space or meningitis remains an ever-present possibility, especially in the immunocompromised AIDS or cancer patient. If epidural abscess occurs, emergent surgical drainage to avoid spinal cord compression and irreversible neurologic deficit is usually required. Early detection and treatment of infection is crucial to avoid potentially life-threatening sequelae. Infections of the infusion pump pocket can usually be managed with systemic and topical antibiotics and, occasionally, incision and drainage. The patient must be observed closely for spread of infection proximally down the subcutaneous tunnel into the epidural space. If this occurs, the entire delivery system should be removed immediately.

If a subarachnoid catheter terminus is planned, CSF tracking back along the catheter to the pump pocket with hygroma formation is a possibility. Such hygroma formation makes pump refill more difficult and increases the chance of infection. Hygroma formation can be avoided by placing of a purse-string suture around the needle at the time the catheter is placed and placing a pressure dressing over the pump pocket after the implantation procedure. Although rare, a cutaneous or subarachnoid fistula can occur if CSF leakage continues.

Surprisingly, the major complications that occur with totally implantable infusion pumps are related to pump refill rather than the implantation technique. When refilling a pump with a side port that provides direct access to the subarachnoid or epidural space, scrupulous attention must be given to technique in order to avoid placing a lethal bolus of opioid or baclofen directly into the subarachnoid or epidural space.

CLINICAL PEARLS

Implantation of a totally implantable infusion pump is a safe and effective procedure if careful attention is paid to technique. Failure to accurately identify the midline is the most common reason for difficulty in identifying the epidural space and increases the risk for complications. The routine use of sedation or general anesthesia before identification of the epidural space is to be discouraged because it will render the patient unable to provide accurate verbal feedback should needle misplacement occur.

The totally implantable infusion pump has fewer problems associated with it once implanted when compared with tunneled catheters. Difficulty in refilling the pump and cost are major drawbacks to this type of drug delivery system. Peri-implantation infection will be decreased if care is taken to obtain adequate hemostasis before closing the infusion pump pocket. Failure of the delivery system, although uncommon, can occur. Catheter failure or disconnection from the pump occurs with greater frequency than primary pump failure (see Fig. 148-2). If the pump is equipped with a side port, injection with contrast medium suitable for intrathecal use may help elucidate the problem.

CHAPTER 149

Percutaneous Posterior Facet Joint Spinal Fusion

CPT-2009 CODE	
First Level	22612
Each Additional Level	22614
Structural Bone Allograft	20931

Relative Value Units	
First Level	40
Each Additional Level	35

INDICATIONS

Percutaneous posterior facet joint spinal fusion represents a new option for patients suffering from mechanical low back pain caused by facet joint dysfunction, spine instability following decompressive spine surgeries, and microinstability of spinal segments, and as an adjunct to interbody fusion. By improving spinal segmental stability during flexion, extension, and lateral bending of the spine, percutaneous posterior facet joint spinal fusion can provide significant pain relief in many patients suffering from the above mentioned spinal pathology.

This technique is appropriate as a reasonable next step in those patients suffering from facet joint arthropathy whose pain is relieved with facet joint injections and radiofrequency lesioning of the medial branches of the dysfunctional spinal segments but in whom pain relief is not long lasting. This technique does not preclude additional extension open anterior or posterior spine stabilization techniques should the patient's symptoms recur or progress following percutaneous posterior facet joint spinal fusion.

The fusion device is a specially prepared bone dowel that can be placed percutaneously under fluoroscopic guidance. One of the most commonly used percutaneous posterior facet joint devices is the TruFUSE facet fusion allograft.

CLINICALLY RELEVANT ANATOMY

The lumbar facet joints are formed by the articulations of the superior and inferior articular facets of adjacent vertebrae. The lumbar facet joints are true joints in that they are lined with synovium and possess a true joint capsule. This capsule is richly innervated and supports the notion of the facet joint as a pain generator. The lumbar facet joint is susceptible to arthritic changes and trauma secondary to acceleration-deceleration injuries. Such damage to the joint results in pain secondary to synovial joint inflammation and adhesions.

Each facet joint receives innervation from two spinal levels. Each joint receives fibers from the dorsal ramus at the same level as the vertebra as well as fibers from the dorsal ramus of the vertebra above it (Fig. 149-1). This fact has clinical importance because it helps explain the ill-defined nature of facet-mediated pain and explains why the dorsal nerve from the vertebra above the offending level must often also be blocked in order to provide complete pain relief.

At each level, the dorsal ramus provides a medial branch that exits the intertransverse space, crossing over the top of the transverse process in a groove at the point where the transverse process joins the vertebra. The nerve then travels inferiorly and medially across the posterior surface of the vertebral lamina, where it gives off branches to innervate the facet joint. The medial branch is blocked at the point at which the nerve curves around the top of the transverse process. At the L5 level, it is the actual dorsal ramus of L5 rather than the medial branch that crosses the sacral ala at the junction of the superior articular process. After crossing the sacral ala, the dorsal ramus gives off a medial branch that provides innervation for the lumbosacral facet joint.

TECHNIQUE

To perform percutaneous posterior facet joint spinal fusion, the patient is placed in the prone position on a fluoroscopy table with the lumbar spine flexed to

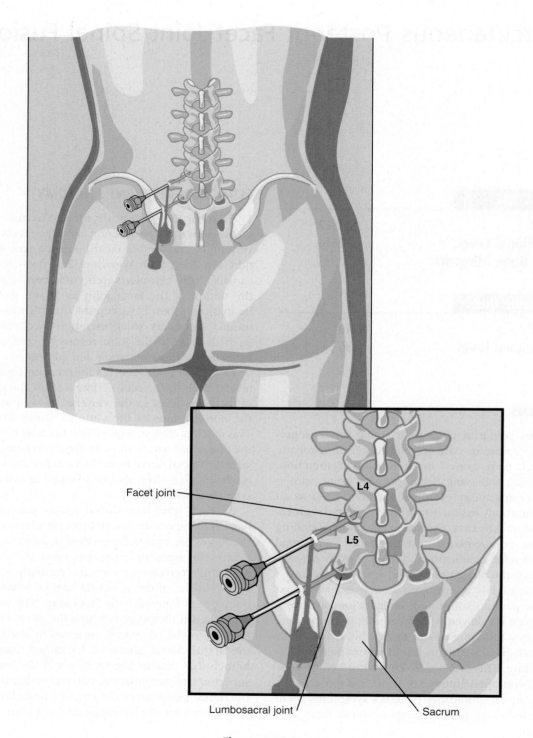

Figure 149-1.

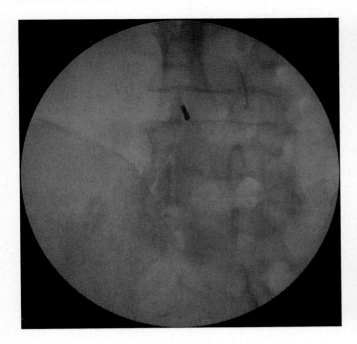

Figure 149-2.

Steinmann pin placed within the facet joint.

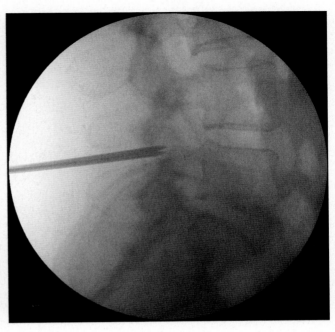

Figure 149-3.

Lateral view of bilateral Steinmann pin placement within the facet joint. Note the similar trajectories for both pins.

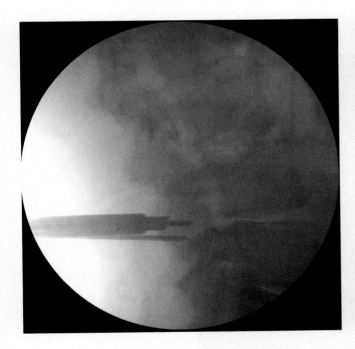

Figure 149-4.

The self-centering spatula is placed over the first Steinmann pin.

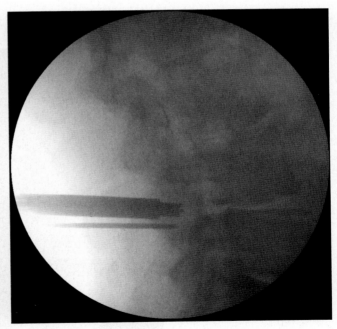

Figure 149-5.

The self-centering spatula is impacted into the facet joint using the previously placed Steinmann pin as a guide.

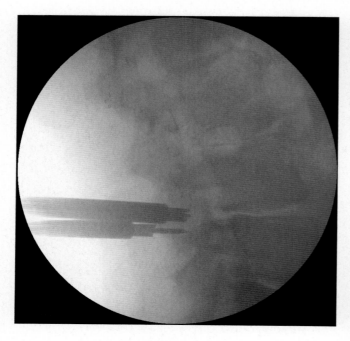

Figure 149-6.
The second self-centering spatula is placed over the contralateral Steinmann pin.

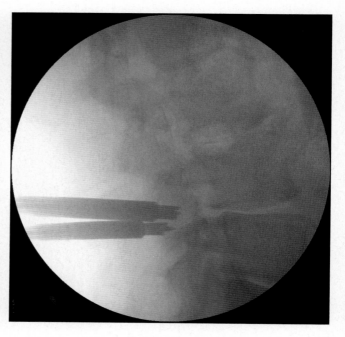

Figure 149-7.
The drill guides are placed over the self-centering spatulas.

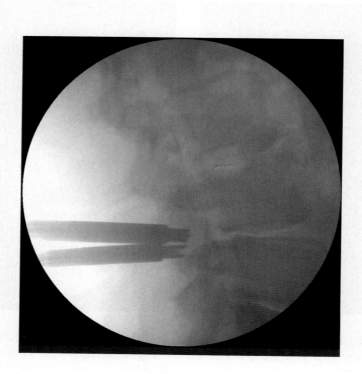

Figure 149-8.
The drill is advanced against the stop on the drill guide.

re-establish facet joint height lost during the degenerative process. This flexion also opens the neuroforamina. Use of a Wilson frame placed on the fluoroscopy table can optimize patient positioning for this procedure.

The facet joints to be fused are first identified on posteroanterior and lateral fluoroscopic views. An oblique view directly through the plane of the facet joint to be fused is then obtained. It is imperative that the exact plane of the facet joint be identified in a manner analogous to the fluoroscopic technique used when performing intra-articular facet injections as the fusion allograft must be placed within this same trajectory to optimize safety and post-procedure pain relief (see Chapter 91).

After the plane of the facet joint is identified, a small stab wound is made through the skin and subcutaneous tissues. A Steinmann pin is placed through the stab wound and directed under fluoroscopic guidance toward the affected facet joint. The pin is advanced into the joint using the bull's-eye approach, with the oblique fluoroscopic beam in the identical trajectory of the facet joint; the pin is advanced in a manner analogous to placing a needle into the facet joint for intra-articular facet joint injection (Fig. 149-2). Posteroanterior and lateral fluoroscopic views also are obtained to confirm both the intra-articular position of the Steinmann pin and the depth to which the pin has been inserted. The Steinmann pin is advanced to approximately the middle of the facet joint to be fused to maximize contact with both the superior and inferior articular surfaces. Because percutaneous posterior facet joint spinal fusion must be performed bilaterally, it is strongly recommended that the second Steinmann pin be placed in the contralateral joint at the same level before proceeding with placement of the first facet fusion device. The trajectory of the second Steinmann pin should be similar to that of the first pin, and any significant variation in trajectory should cause the operator to reconfirm the position of both pins before proceeding with placement of the fusion device (Fig. 149-3).

After satisfactory placement of both Steinmann pins within the facet joints to be fused is confirmed, the self-centering spatula provided with the TruFUSE facet fusion allograft is threaded over the placed Steinmann pins with the beveled edge oriented with the rostral end of the joint (Fig. 149-4). The self-centering spatula is then gently impacted into each facet joint under fluoroscopic guidance using the previously placed Steinmann pins as a guide (Figs. 149-5 and 149-6).

After satisfactory placement of the self-centering spatula within facet joint bilaterally is confirmed with posteroanterior and lateral fluoroscopic views, the drill guide provided with the TruFUSE facet fusion allograft is placed over the spatula with the drill guide handle pointing laterally. The black marks on the drill guide must be aligned with shaft of the spatula to ensure proper intra-articular placement of the drill guide. Teeth

on the superior and inferior aspects of the posterior end of the drill guide will distract the joint to facilitate placement of the fusion device (Fig. 149-7).

The Steinmann pin and spatula are then removed and the drilling is carried out with short 1- to 2-second bursts so that the patient's own compacted subchondral bone (autograft) is not burned, causing osteonecrosis. The bursts continue until the drill has been advanced against the stop on the drill guide, which is a distance of 1 cm (Fig. 149-8). This allows the posterior portion of the facet allograft to be countersunk approximately 2 mm below the posterior surface of the facet joint.

After drilling has been completed, the TruFUSE facet fusion allograft is placed into the graft holder and loaded onto the inserter device. The TruFUSE facet fusion allograft is tapered, and the smaller end is placed toward the anterior portion of the facet joint. The TruFUSE facet fusion allograft is then impacted into the facet joint. The hardware is then removed and the drilling and placement of the TruFUSE facet fusion allograft is carried out on the contralateral joint. The wounds are closed with deep subcutaneous and skin sutures, and small sterile dressings are placed. The patient is then placed in a back brace to limit flexion, extension, and lateral bending for 4 to 6 weeks.

SIDE EFFECTS AND COMPLICATIONS

The proximity to the spinal cord and exiting nerve roots makes it imperative that this procedure only be performed by those well versed in the regional anatomy and experienced in performing interventional pain management techniques. This procedure should not be performed on patients who are anticoagulated, have spondylolysis, or have greater than grade II spondylolisthesis.

CLINICAL PEARLS

Percutaneous posterior facet joint spinal fusion is reasonable for patients who suffer from mechanical low back pain caused by facet joint dysfunction, spine instability following decompressive spine surgeries, and microinstability of spinal segments who have experienced good, albeit transient, pain relief following intra-articular facet injections with local aesthetic and steroid and who have failed to achieve long-lasting relief with radiofrequency facet denervation.

This technique is straightforward when performed by those skilled in placement of needles into the facet joints. Post-procedure bracing will improve long-term outcomes and should be used in all patients undergoing percutaneous posterior facet joint spinal fusion with the TruFUSE allograft.

Index

Note: Page numbers followed by b, f, and t indicate boxes, figures and tables, respectively.

M